T0189031

# Statistical Modeling for Biomedical Researchers

# Statistical Modeling for Biomedical Researchers

## A Simple Introduction to the Analysis of Complex Data

SECOND EDITION

William D. Dupont

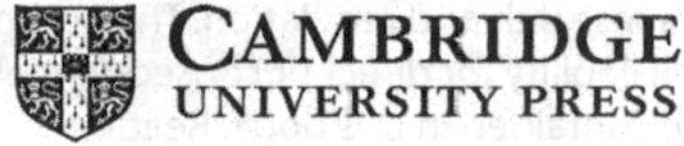

CAMBRIDGE
UNIVERSITY PRESS

**CAMBRIDGE**
**UNIVERSITY PRESS**

University Printing House, Cambridge CB2 8BS, United Kingdom

Cambridge University Press is part of the University of Cambridge.

It furthers the University's mission by disseminating knowledge in the pursuit of education, learning and research at the highest international levels of excellence.

www.cambridge.org
Information on this title: www.cambridge.org/9780521614801



First published 2009
4th printing 2014

*A catalogue record for this publication is available from the British Library*

*Library of Congress Cataloguing in Publication data*
Dupont, William D. (William Dudley), 1946–
Statistical modeling for biomedical researchers : a simple introduction to the analysis of complex data / William D. Dupont. – 2nd ed.
p. ; cm.
Includes bibliographical references and index.
ISBN 978-0-521-84952-4 (hardback) – ISBN 978-0-521-61480-1 (pbk.)
1. Medicine – Research – Statistical methods – Mathematical models. I. Title.
[DNLM: 1. Biometry – methods – Problems and Exercises. 2. Data Interpretation, Statistical – Problems and Exercises. 3. Mathematical Computing – Problems and Exercises. 4. Models, Statistical – Problems and Exercises. WA 18.2 D938s 2008]
R853.M3D865 2008
610.7′27 – dc22 2008026916

ISBN 978-0-521-84952-4 Hardback
ISBN 978-0-521-61480-1 Paperback

# Contents

# Appendices

## A Summary of statistical models discussed in this text 485



## B Summary of Stata commands used in this text 491

# Preface

The purpose of this text is to enable biomedical researchers to use a number of advanced statistical methods that have proven valuable in medical research. The past forty years have seen an explosive growth in the development of biostatistics. As with so many aspects of our world, this growth has been strongly influenced by the development of inexpensive, powerful computers and the sophisticated software that has been written to run them. This has allowed the development of computationally intensive methods that can effectively model complex biomedical data sets. It has also made it easy to explore these data sets, to discover how variables are interrelated, and to select appropriate statistical models for analysis. Indeed, just as the microscope revealed new worlds to the eighteenth century, modern statistical software permits us to see interrelationships in large complex data sets that would have been missed in previous eras. Also, modern statistical software has made it vastly easier for investigators to perform their own statistical analyses. Although very sophisticated mathematics underlies modern statistics, it is not necessary to understand this mathematics to properly analyze your data with modern statistical software. What is necessary is to understand the assumptions required by each method, how to determine whether these assumptions are adequately met for your data, how to select the best model, and how to interpret the results of your analyses. The goal of this text is to allow investigators to effectively use some of the most valuable multivariate methods without requiring a prior understanding of more than high school algebra. Much mathematical detail is avoided by focusing on the use of a specific statistical software package.

This text grew out of my second semester course in biostatistics that I teach in our Master of Public Health program at the Vanderbilt University Medical School. All of the students take introductory courses in biostatistics and epidemiology prior to mine. Although this text is self-contained, I strongly recommend that readers acquire good introductory texts in biostatistics and epidemiology as companions to this one. Many excellent texts are available on these topics. At Vanderbilt we are currently using Katz (2006) for biostatistics and Gordis (2004) for epidemiology. The statistical software used in this text is Stata, version 10 (StataCorp, 2007). It was chosen for the breadth and depth of its statistical methods, for its ease of use, excellent graphics and excellent documentation. There are several other excellent packages available on the market. However, the aim of this text is to teach biostatistics through a specific software package, and length restrictions make it impractical to use more than one package. If you have not yet invested a lot of time learning a different package, Stata is an excellent choice for you to consider. If you are already attached to a different package, you may still find it easier to learn Stata than to master or teach the material covered here from other textbooks. The topics covered in this text are linear regression, logistic regression, Poisson regression, survival analysis, and analysis of variance. Each topic is covered in two chapters: one introduces the topic with simple univariate examples and the other covers more complex multivariate models. The text makes extensive use of a number of real data sets. They all may be downloaded from my web site at `biostat.mc.vanderbilt.edu/dupontwd/wddtext/`. This site also contains complete log files of all analyses discussed in this text.

## Changes in the second edition

I have made extensive modifications and additions to the second edition of this text. These can be summarized as follows.

- Since I wrote the first edition, Stata has undergone major improvements that make it much easier to use and enable more powerful graphics. The examples in this text take advantage of these improvements and comply with Stata's version 10 syntax.
- Stata now has easy-to-use point-and-click commands that may be used as an alternative to Stata's character-based commands. I have provided documentation for both the point-and-click and character-based versions of all commands discussed in this text.
- Appendix A summarizes the types of data discussed in this text and indicates which statistical methods are most appropriate for each type of data.
- Restricted cubic splines are used to analyze non-linear regression models. This is a simple but powerful approach that can be used to extend logistic and proportional hazards regression models as well as linear regression models.
- Density-distribution sunflower plots are used for the exploratory analysis of dense bivariate data.

- The Breslow–Day–Tarone test is used to test the equality of odds ratios across multiple 2 × 2 tables
- Likelihood ratio tests of nested models are used extensively.
- I have added a brief discussion of proportional odds and polytomous logistic regression.
- Predicted survival and log–log plots are used to evaluate the adequacy of the proportional hazards model of survival data.
- Additional exercises have been added to several chapters.

## Acknowledgements

I would like to thank Gordon R. Bernard, Jeffrey Brent, Norman E. Breslow, Graeme Eisenhofer, Cary P. Gross, Frank E. Harrell, Daniel Levy, Steven M. Greenberg, Fritz F. Parl, Paul Sorlie, Wayne A. Ray, and Alastair J. J. Wood for allowing me to use their data to illustrate the methods described in this text. I am grateful to William Gould and the employees of Stata Corporation for publishing their elegant and powerful statistical software and for providing excellent documentation. I would also like to thank the students in our Master of Public Health program who have taken my course. Their energy, intelligence and enthusiasm have greatly enhanced my enjoyment in preparing this material. Their criticisms and suggestions have profoundly influenced this work. I am grateful to David L. Page, my friend and colleague of 31 years, with whom I have learnt much about the art of teaching epidemiology and biostatistics to clinicians. My appreciation goes to Sarah K. Meredith for introducing me to Cambridge University Press; to William Schaffner and Frank E. Harrell, my chairmen during the writing of the first and second editions, respectively, who enabled my spending the time needed to complete this work; to W. Dale Plummer for programing and technical support with Stata and LaTeX; to Nicholas J. Cox for proof-reading this text, for his valuable advice, and for writing the *stripplot* program; to William R. Rising, Patrick G. Arbogast, and Gregory D. Ayers for proof-reading this book and for their valuable suggestions; to Jeffrey S. Pitblado for writing the Stata 8 version of the *sunflower* program and for allowing me to adapt his LaTeX style files for use in this book; to Kristin MacDonald for writing the restricted cubic spline module of the *mkspline* program; to Tebeb Gebretsadik and Knut M. Wittkowski for their helpful suggestions; to Frances Nex for her careful copy editing, to Charlotte Broom, Laura Wood, Richard Marley, and other colleagues at Cambridge University Press, and

Jagdamba Prasad at Aptara Corporation, for producing this beautiful book; and to my mother and sisters for their support during six critical months of this project. Finally, I am especially grateful to my wife, Susan, and sons, Thomas and Peter, for their love and support, and for their cheerful tolerance of the countless hours that I spent on this project.

**Disclaimer:** The opinions expressed in this text are my own and do not necessarily reflect those of the authors acknowledged in this preface, their employers or funding institutions. This includes the National Heart, Lung, and Blood Institute, National Institutes of Health, Department of Health and Human Services, USA.

# 1

# Introduction

This text is primarily concerned with the interrelationships between multiple variables that are collected on study subjects. For example, we may be interested in how age, blood pressure, serum cholesterol, body mass index, and gender affect a patient's risk of coronary heart disease. The methods that we shall discuss involve descriptive and inferential statistics. In descriptive statistics, our goal is to understand and summarize the data that we have actually collected. This can be a major task in a large database with many variables. In inferential statistics, we seek to draw conclusions about patients in the population at large from the information collected on the specific patients in our database. This requires first choosing an appropriate model that can explain the variation in our collected data and then using this model to estimate the accuracy of our results. The purpose of this chapter is to review some elementary statistical concepts that we shall need in subsequent chapters. Although this text is self-contained, I recommend that readers who have not had an introductory course in biostatistics start off by reading one of the many excellent texts on biostatistics that are available (see, for example, Katz, 2006).

## 1.1. Algebraic notation

This text assumes that the reader is familiar with high school algebra. In this section we review notation that may be unfamiliar to some readers.

- We use parentheses to indicate the order of multiplication and addition; brackets are used to indicate the arguments of functions. Thus, $a(b + c)$ equals the product of $a$ and $b + c$, while $a[b + c]$ equals the value of the function $a$ evaluated at $b + c$.
- The function $\log[x]$ denotes the natural logarithm of $x$. You may have seen this function referred to as either $\ln[x]$ or $\log_e[x]$ elsewhere.
- The constant $e = 2.718\ldots$ is the base of the natural logarithm.
- The function $\exp[x] = e^x$ is the constant $e$ raised to the power $x$.

- The function

$$\text{sign}[x] = \begin{cases} 1 : \text{if } x > 0 \\ 0 : \text{if } x = 0 \\ -1 : \text{if } x < 0. \end{cases} \tag{1.1}$$

- The absolute value of $x$ is written $|x|$ and equals

$$|x| = x\ \text{sign}[x] = \begin{cases} x : \text{if } x \geq 0 \\ -x : \text{if } x < 0. \end{cases}$$

- The expression $\int_a^b f[x]dx$ denotes the area under the curve $f[x]$ between $a$ and $b$. That is, it is the region bounded by the function $f[x]$ and the $x$-axis and by vertical lines drawn between $f[x]$ and the $x$-axis at $x = a$ and $x = b$. For example, if $f[x]$ denotes the curve drawn in Figure 1.11 then the area of the shaded region in this figure is $\int_a^b f[x]dx$. With the exception of the occasional use of this notation, no calculus is used in this text.

Suppose that we have measured the weights of three patients. Let $x_1 = 70$, $x_2 = 60$, and $x_3 = 80$ denote the weight of the first, second, and third patient, respectively.

- We use the Greek letter $\Sigma$ to denote summation. For example,

$$\sum_{i=1}^{3} x_i = x_1 + x_2 + x_3 = 70 + 60 + 80 = 210.$$

  When the summation index is unambiguous we will drop the subscript and superscript on the summation sign. Thus, $\sum x_i$ also equals $x_1 + x_2 + x_3$.
- We use the Greek letter $\Pi$ to denote multiplication. For example,

$$\prod_{i=1}^{3} x_i = \prod x_i = x_1\, x_2\, x_3 = 70 \times 60 \times 80 = 336\,000.$$

- We use braces to denote sets of values; $\{i : x_i > 65\}$ is the set of integers for which the inequality to the right of the colon is true. Since $x_i > 65$ for the first and third patient, $\{i : x_i > 65\} = \{1, 3\} =$ the integers one and three. The summation

$$\sum_{\{i:\ x_i > 65\}} x_i = x_1 + x_3 = 70 + 80 = 150.$$

  The product

$$\prod_{\{i:\ x_i > 65\}} x_i = 70 \times 80 = 5600.$$

## 1.2. Descriptive statistics

### 1.2.1. Dot plot

Suppose that we have a sample of $n$ observations of some variable. A **dot plot** is a graph in which each observation is represented by a dot on the $y$-axis. Dot plots are often subdivided by some grouping variable to permit a comparison of the observations between the two groups. For example, Bernard et al. (1997) performed a randomized clinical trial to assess the effect of intravenous ibuprofen on mortality in patients with sepsis. People with sepsis have severe systemic bacterial infections that may be due to a wide number of causes. Sepsis is a life-threatening condition. However, the mortal risk varies considerably from patient to patient. One measure of a patient's mortal risk is the Acute Physiology and Chronic Health Evaluation (APACHE) score (Bernard et al., 1997). This score is a composite measure of the patient's degree of morbidity that was collected just before recruitment into the study. Since this score is highly correlated with survival, it was important that the treatment and control groups be comparable with respect to baseline APACHE score. Figure 1.1 shows a dot plot of the baseline APACHE scores for study subjects subdivided by treatment group. This plot indicates that the treatment and placebo groups are comparable with respect to baseline APACHE score.

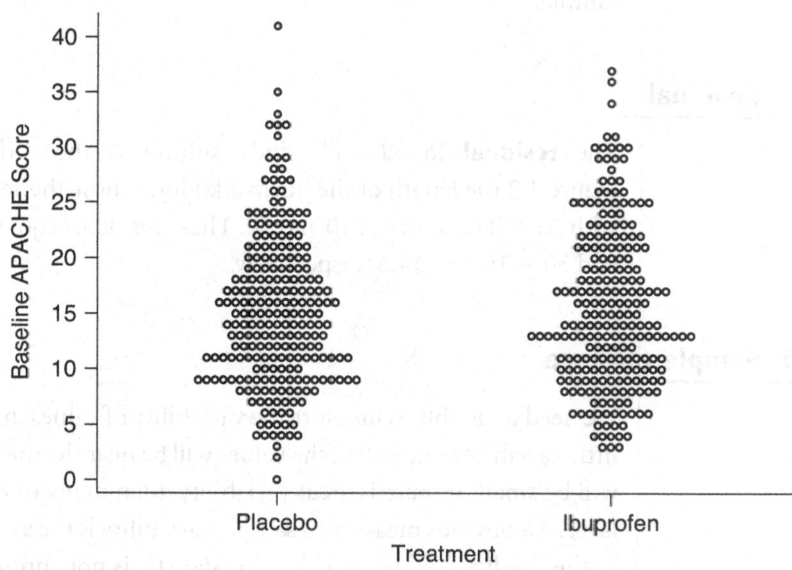


Figure 1.1 Dot plot of baseline APACHE score subdivided by treatment (Bernard et al., 1997).

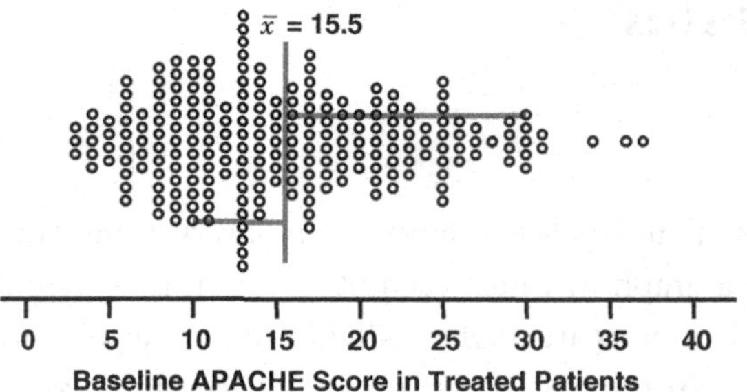


Figure 1.2 Dot plot for treated patients in the Ibuprofen in Sepsis Study. The vertical line marks the sample mean, while the length of the horizontal lines indicates the residuals for patients with APACHE scores of 10 and 30.

### 1.2.2. Sample mean

The **sample mean** $\bar{x}$ for a variable is its average value for all patients in the sample. Let $x_i$ denote the value of a variable for the $i^{\text{th}}$ study subject ($i = 1, 2, \ldots, n$). Then the sample mean is

$$\bar{x} = \sum_{i=1}^{n} x_i/n = (x_1 + x_2 + \cdots + x_n)/n, \tag{1.2}$$

where $n$ is the number of patients in the sample. In Figure 1.2 the vertical line marks the mean baseline APACHE score for treated patients. This mean equals 15.5. The mean is a measure of central tendency of the $x_i$s in the sample.

### 1.2.3. Residual

The **residual** for the $i^{\text{th}}$ study subject is the difference $x_i - \bar{x}$. In Figure 1.2 the length of the horizontal lines show the residuals for patients with APACHE scores of 10 and 30. These residuals equal $10 - 15.5 = -5.5$ and $30 - 15.5 = 14.5$, respectively.

### 1.2.4. Sample variance

We need to be able to measure the variability of values in a sample. If there is little variability, then all of the values will be near the mean and the residuals will be small. If there is great variability, then many of the residuals will be large. An obvious measure of sample variability is the average absolute value of the residuals, $\sum |x_i - \bar{x}|/n$. This statistic is not commonly used because it is difficult to work with mathematically. A more mathematician-friendly measure of variability is the **sample variance**, which is

$$s^2 = \sum (x_i - \bar{x})^2/(n-1). \tag{1.3}$$

You can think of $s^2$ as being the average squared residual. (We divide the sum of the squared residuals by $n-1$ rather than $n$ for mathematical reasons that are not worth explaining at this point.) Note that the greater the variability of the sample, the greater the average squared residual and, hence, the greater the sample variance.

### 1.2.5. Sample standard deviation

The **sample standard deviation** $s$ is the square root of the sample variance. Note that $s$ has the same units as $x_i$. For patients receiving ibuprofen in Figure 1.1 the variance and standard deviation of the APACHE score are 52.7 and 7.26, respectively.

### 1.2.6. Percentile and median

Percentiles are most easily defined by an example; the 75th **percentile** is that value that is greater or equal to 75% of the observations in the sample. The **median** is the 50th percentile, which is another measure of central tendency.

### 1.2.7. Box plot

Dot plots provide all of the information in a sample on a given variable. They are ineffective, however, if the sample is too large and may require more space than is desirable. The mean and standard deviation give a terse description of the central tendency and variability of the sample, but omit details of the data structure that may be important. A useful way of summarizing the data that provides a sense of the data structure is the **box plot** (also called the **box-and-whiskers** plot). Figure 1.3 shows such plots for the APACHE data in each treatment group. In each plot, the sides of the box mark the 25th

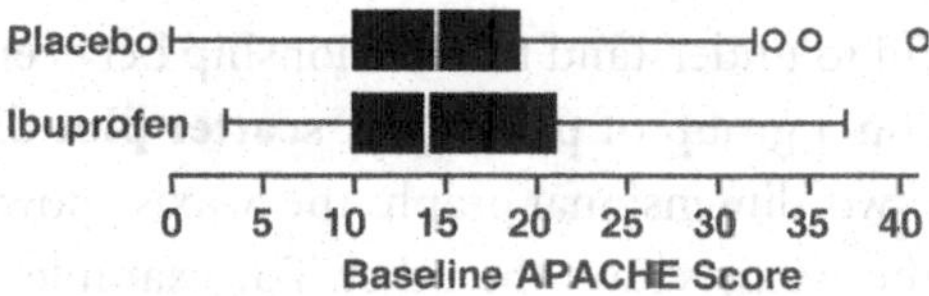


Figure 1.3 Box plots of APACHE scores of patients receiving placebo and ibuprofen in the Ibuprofen in Sepsis Study.

and 75th percentiles, which are also called the **quartiles**. The vertical line in the middle of the box marks the median. The width of the box is called the **interquartile range**. The middle 50% of the observations lie within this range. Whiskers extend on either side of the box. The vertical bars at the end of each whisker mark the most extreme observations that are not more than 1.5 times the interquartile range from their adjacent quartiles. Any values beyond these bars are plotted separately as in the dot plot. They are called **outliers** and merit special consideration because they may have undue influence on some of our analyses. Figure 1.3 captures much of the information in Figure 1.1 in less space.

For both treated and control patients the largest APACHE scores are farther from the median than are the smallest scores. For treated subjects the upper quartile is farther from the median than is the lower quartile. Data sets in which the observations are more stretched out on one side of the median than the other are called **skewed**. They are **skewed to the right** if values above the median are more dispersed than are values below. They are **skewed to the left** when the converse is true. Box plots are particularly valuable when we wish to compare the distributions of a variable in different groups of patients, as in Figure 1.3. Although the median APACHE values are very similar in treated and control patients, the treated patients have a slightly more skewed distribution. (It should be noted that some authors use slightly different definitions for the outer bars of a box plot. The definition given here is that of Cleveland, 1993.)

### 1.2.8. Histogram

This is a graphic method of displaying the distribution of a variable. The range of observations is divided into equal intervals; a bar is drawn above each interval that indicates the proportion of the data in the interval. Figure 1.4 shows a histogram of APACHE scores in control patients. This graph also shows that the data are skewed to the right.

### 1.2.9. Scatter plot

It is often useful to understand the relationship between two variables that are measured on a group of patients. A **scatter plot** displays these values as points in a two-dimensional graph: the $x$-axis shows the values of one variable and the $y$-axis shows the other. For example, Brent et al. (1999) measured baseline plasma glycolate and arterial pH on 18 patients admitted for ethylene glycol poisoning. A scatter plot of plasma glycolate versus arterial pH for these patients is plotted in Figure 1.5. Each circle on this graph shows

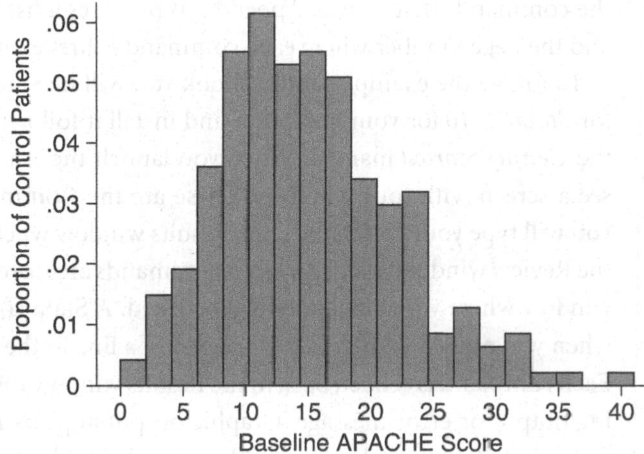


Figure 1.4 Histogram of APACHE scores among control patients in the Ibuprofen in Sepsis Study.

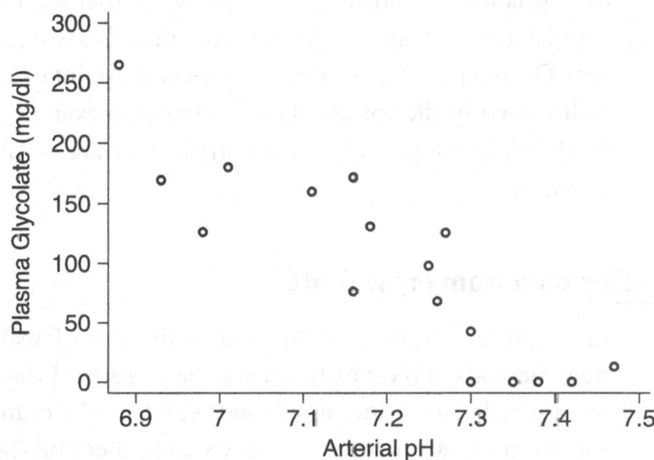


Figure 1.5 Scatter plot of baseline plasma glycolate vs. arterial pH in 18 patients with ethylene glycol poisoning (Brent et al., 1999).

the plasma glycolate and arterial pH for a study subject. Note that patients with high glycolate levels tended to have low pHs, and that glycolate levels tended to decline with increasing pH.

## 1.3. The Stata Statistical Software Package

The worked examples in this text are performed using Stata version 10 (StataCorp, 2007). Excellent documentation is available for this software. At a minimum, I suggest you read their *Getting Started* manual. This text is not intended to replicate the Stata documentation, although it does explain the commands that it uses. Appendix B provides a list of these commands and the page number where each command is first explained.

To follow the examples in this book you will need to purchase a license for *Stata/IC 10* for your computer and install it following the directions in the *Getting Started* manual. When you launch the Stata program you will see a screen with four windows. These are the Command window where you will type your commands, the Results window where output is written, the Review window where previous commands are stored, and the Variables window where variable names will be listed. A Stata command is executed when you press the Enter key at the end of a line in the command window. Each command is echoed back in the Results window followed by the resulting output or error message. Graphic output appears in a separate Graph window. In the examples given in this text, I have adopted the following conventions. All Stata commands and output are written in monospaced fonts. Commands that are entered by the user are written in bold face; variable names, labels and other text chosen by the user are italicized, while command names and options that must be entered as is are printed in an upright font. Output from Stata is written in a smaller point size. Highlighted output is discussed in the comments following each example. Numbers in boxes on the right margin refer to comments that are given at the end of each example.

## 1.3.1. Downloading data from my website

An important feature of this text is the use of real data sets to illustrate methods in biostatistics. These data sets are located at `biostat.mc.vanderbilt.edu/dupontwd/wddtext/`. In the examples, I assume that you are using a Microsoft Windows computer and have downloaded the data into a folder on your C drive called *WDDtext*. I suggest that you create such a folder now. (Of course the location and name of the folder is up to you but if you use a different name you will have to modify the file address in my examples. If you are using Stata on a Macintosh, Linux, or Unix computer you will need to use the appropriate disk and folder naming conventions for these computers.) Next, use your web browser to go to `biostat.mc.vanderbilt.edu/dupontwd/wddtext/` and click on the blue underlined text that says Data Sets. A page of data sets will appear. Click on 1.3.2.Sepsis. A dialog box will ask where you wish to download the sepsis data set. Enter *C:/WDDtext* and click the download button. A Stata data set called *1.3.2.Sepsis.dta* will be copied to your *WDDtext* folder. You are now ready to run the example in the next section.

## 1.3.2. Creating histograms with Stata

The following example shows the contents of the Results window after entering a series of commands in the Command window. Before replicating this example on your computer, you must first download *1.3.2.Sepsis.dta* as described in the preceding section.

```
. * Examine the Stata data set 1.3.2.Sepsis.dta.  Create                 1
. * histograms of baseline APACHE scores in treated and
. * control patients.
. use  C:\WDDtext\1.3.2.Sepsis.dta                                       2
. describe                                                               3

Contains data from c:\WDDtext\1.3.2.Sepsis.dta
  obs:            455
 vars:              2                          16 Apr 2002 15:36
 size:          5,460 (99.5% of memory free)
-------------------------------------------------------------------------------
              storage  display     value
variable name   type   format      label      variable label
-------------------------------------------------------------------------------
treat           float  %9.0g       treatmnt   Treatment
apache          float  %9.0g                  Baseline APACHE Score
-------------------------------------------------------------------------------
Sorted by:
. list  treat apache in 1/3                                              4

     +--------------------+
     |     treat   apache |
     |--------------------|
  1. |   Placebo       27 |
  2. | Ibuprofen       14 |
  3. |   Placebo       33 |
     +--------------------+                                              5

. browse                                                                 6
. histogram apache, by(treat) bin(20) percent                            7
```

**Comments**

1 Command lines that start with an asterisk (*) are treated as comments and are ignored by Stata.

2 The *use* command specifies the name of a Stata data set that is to be used in subsequent Stata commands. This data set is loaded into memory where it may be analyzed or modified. Data sets may also be opened by clicking on the folder icon on the Stata toolbar. In Section 4.21 we will illustrate how to create a new data set using Stata.

3 The *describe* command provides some basic information about the current data set. The *1.3.2.Sepsis* data set contains 455 observations. There are two variables called *treat* and *apache*. The labels assigned to these variables are *Treatment* and *Baseline APACHE Score*.

4 The *list* command gives the values of the specified variables; *in 1/3* restricts this listing to the first three observations in the file.

5 At this point the Review, Variables, Results, and Command windows should look like those in Figure 1.6. (The size of these windows has been changed to fit in this figure.) Note that if you click on any command in the Review window it will appear in the Command window where you can edit and re-execute it. This is particularly useful for fixing command errors. When entering variables in a command you may either type them directly or click on the desired variable from the Variables window. The latter method avoids spelling mistakes.

6 Typing *browse* opens the Stata Data Browser window (there is a button on the toolbar that does this as well). This command permits you to review but not modify the current data set. Figure 1.7 shows this window, which presents the data in a spreadsheet format with one row per patient and one column per variable. (Stata also has an *edit* command that allows you to both view and change the current data. I recommend that you use the *browse* command when you only wish to view your data in order to avoid accidental changes.)

I will refer to rows and columns of the Stata Data Browser as *observations* and *variables*, respectively. An observation consists of all of the variable values in a single row, which will usually consist of all variable values collected on a single patient. A row of variable values is also called a *record*.

7 This command produces Figure 1.8. This figure appears in its own Graph window. The *by(treat)* option causes separate histograms for each treatment to be drawn side by side in the same graph; *bin(20)* groups the data into 20 bins with a separate bar for each bin in each panel. The *percent* option causes the *y*-axis to be the percentage of patients on each

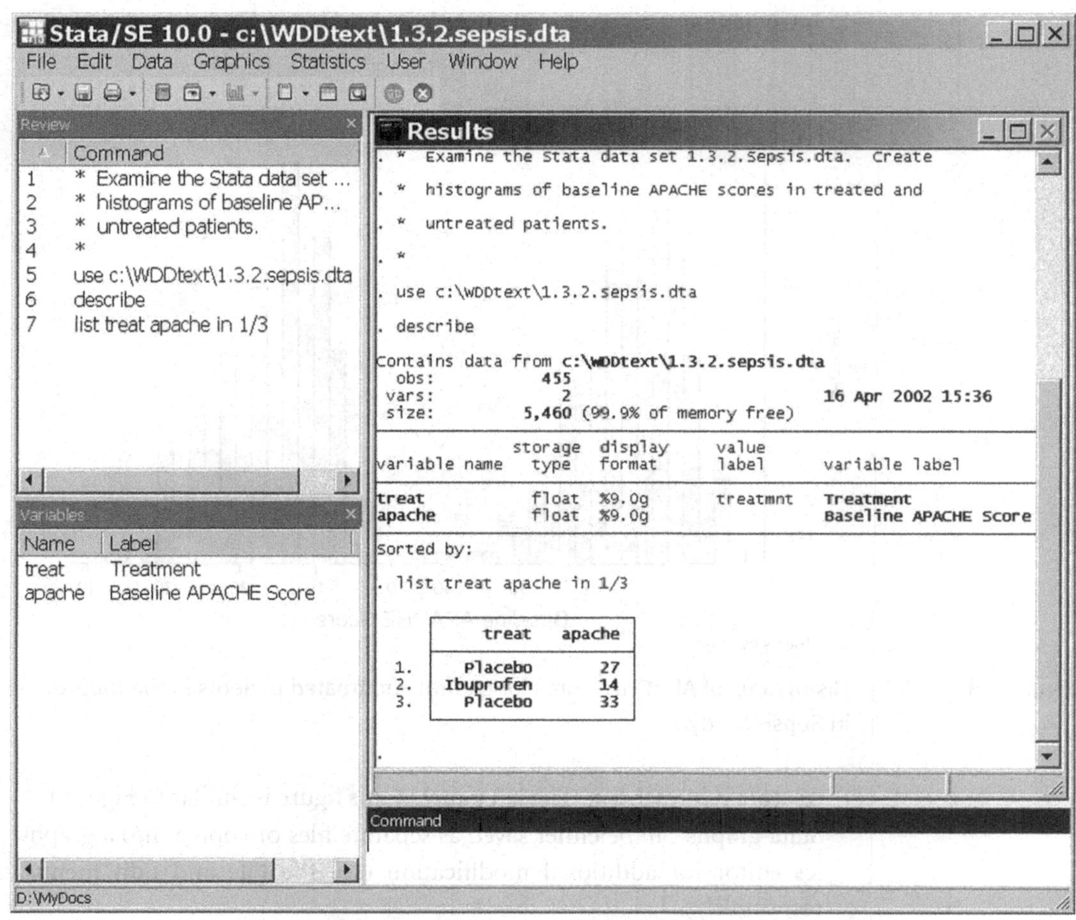


Figure 1.6 The Stata Review, Variables, Results, and Command windows are shown immediately after the *list* command from the example on page 9. The shapes and sizes of these windows have been altered to fit in this figure.

Data Browser

Preserve | Restore | Sort | << | >> | Hide | Delete...

treat[1] = 0

| | treat | apache |
|---|---|---|
| 1 | Placebo | 27 |
| 2 | Ibuprofen | 14 |
| 3 | Placebo | 33 |
| 4 | Ibuprofen | 3 |
| 5 | Placebo | 5 |
| 6 | Ibuprofen | 13 |
| 7 | Ibuprofen | 34 |
| 8 | Placebo | 11 |

Figure 1.7 The Stata Data Browser shows the individual values of the data set, with one row per patient and one column per variable.

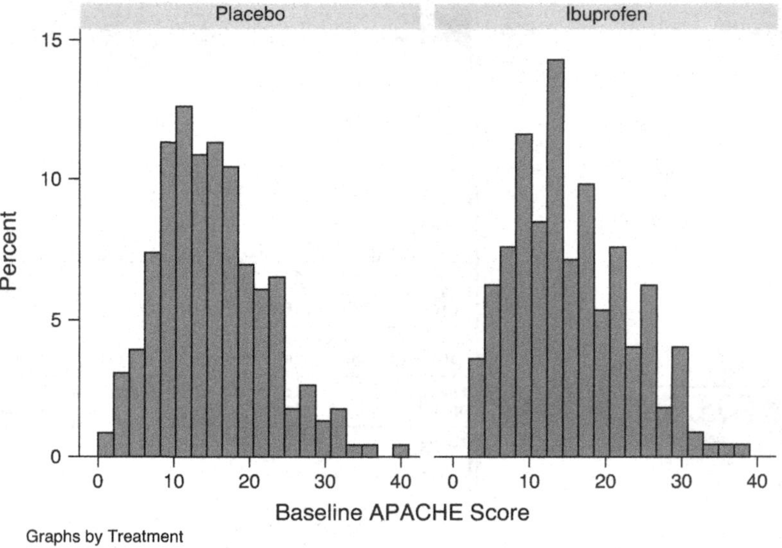


Figure 1.8 Histograms of APACHE scores for control and treated patients in the Ibuprofen in Sepsis Study.

treatment in each bin. The left panel of this figure is similar to Figure 1.4. Stata graphs can be either saved as separate files or copied into a graphics editor for additional modification (see the File and Edit menus, respectively).

### 1.3.3. Stata command syntax

Stata commands are either written in the Command window or issued as point-and-click commands (see Section 1.3.8). Written commands must comply with Stata's grammatical rules. For the most part, Stata will provide error messages when you type something wrong (see Section 1.3.4). There are, however, a few instances where you may be confused by Stata's response to your input.

**Punctuation** The first thing to check if Stata gives a confusing error message is your punctuation. Stata commands are modified by **qualifiers** and **options**. Qualifiers precede options; there must be a comma between the last qualifier and the first option. For example, in the command

**histogram *apache*, by(*treat*) bin(20)**

the variable *apache* is a qualifier while *by(treat)* and *bin(20)* are options. Without the comma, Stata will not recognize *by(treat)* or *bin(20)* as valid options to the *histogram* command. In general, qualifiers apply to most commands while options are more specific to the individual command. A qualifier that precedes the command is called a **command prefix**. Most command prefixes must be separated from the subsequent command by a colon. See the Stata manuals or the Appendix for further details.

**Capitalization** Stata variables and commands are case-sensitive. That is, Stata considers *age* and *Age* to be two distinct variables. In general, I recommend that you use lower case variable names. Sometimes Stata will create variables for you that contain upper case letters. You must use the correct capitalization when referring to these variables.

**Abbreviations** Some commands and options may be abbreviated. The minimum acceptable abbreviation is underlined in the Stata manuals and help files.

### 1.3.4. Obtaining interactive help from Stata

Stata has an extensive interactive help facility that is fully described in the *Getting Started* and *User's Guide* manuals (StataCorp, 2007). I have found the following features to be particularly useful.

- If you type *help command* in the Stata Command window, Stata will open a Viewer window that gives instructions on syntax for the specified command. For example, *help histogram* gives instructions on how to create histograms with Stata. In the upper right-hand corner of the Viewer window are links to the dialog boxes that generate the point-and-click versions of these commands. An excellent way of generating the command you want is to click on these links. Filling out these dialog boxes will also generate the equivalent character-based command in your Review window. These can then be restored to your Command window for further modifications (see Comment 5 on page 10).
- Typing *search word* will provide a table of contents from the Stata database that relates to the word you have specified. You may then click on any command in this table to receive instructions on its use. For example, *search plot* will give a table of contents of all commands that provide plots, one of which is the *dotplot* command.
- Typing *findit word* searches the Internet for Stata programs that are related to *word*. There is a large collection of Stata programs that have been donated by the Stata community but which are not official Stata programs. We will illustrate how to download one of these programs in Section 10.7.

- When you make an error specifying a Stata command, Stata will provide a terse error message followed by the code *r(#)*, where # is some error number. If you then type *search r(#)* you will get a more detailed description of your error. For example, the command *dotplt apache* generates the error message *unrecognized command: dotplt* followed by the error code *r(199)*. Typing *search r(199)* generates a message suggesting that the most likely reason why Stata did not recognize this command was because of a typographical error (*i.e. dotplt* was misspelt).

### 1.3.5. Stata log files

You can keep a permanent record of your commands and Stata's responses in a log file. You can copy commands from a log file back into the Command window to replicate old analyses. In Section 1.3.9 we illustrate the creation of a log file. You will find log files from each example in this text at `biostat.mc.vanderbilt.edu/dupontwd/wddtext/`. It is hard to overemphasize the value of keeping log files of any important analysis that you do. If you hope to present or publish your work it is vital to be able to determine exactly how you did your analysis when you return to it at some future date. Often, the existence of a log file makes the difference between reproducible and irreproducible analyses.

### 1.3.6. Stata graphics and schemes

A real strength of Stata is its graphics capabilities. Reasonable versions of most graphs can be generated with simple commands or by using the pull-down menus. A wide range of options can be added to these commands that allow publication quality graphs that are customized to the user's needs or preferences. Many of these options are illustrated in the Stata examples of this text. Stata also allows users wide control over the default options for their graphs. This is done by defining a Stata scheme. In this text, I have elected to use default graph settings that are slightly different from the standard Stata defaults; my figures were generated using schemes that are available on my web page. For the most part, these schemes control the default size of the text's figures and generate monochromatic graphs that are suitable for a text. There are, however, two minor features of my schemes that differ from the standard Stata schemes and which may cause some confusion. First, the numeric labels of the *y*-axis of my graphs are oriented horizontally as in Figure 1.8. Stata's standard schemes orient these labels parallel to the *y*-axis. Second, in scatter plots I prefer to use open circles to denote observations. Stata's standard schemes use solid circles for these plots. In Comment 13 on page 61 I describe the Stata options that enable these features when a standard Stata scheme is in use. In other examples these options have been omitted. See `biostat.mc.vanderbilt.edu/dupontwd/wddtext/` for further information on the schemes that I have used in this text and Stata's documentation for details on how to customize your own schemes.

Stata has its own graphics editor that can sometimes be helpful for creating graphs that are hard to produce using only character-based commands. I find this editor particularly helpful for annotating graphs. There are also times when it is easier to use an external graphics editor than to figure out how to generate a graph entirely within Stata. Stata graphs can be readily copied into your graphics editor by right-clicking on the Graph window. Right-clicking on this window also provides access to the Stata Graph Editor. I recommend that you experiment with this and other editors to find out what is best for your needs.

### 1.3.7. Stata *do* files

Stata provides users with considerable flexibility in how to run analyses. In this text, I emphasize using the Command window interactively or using Stata's point-and-click commands. However, many users prefer to do analyses via *do* files. These are text files composed of a series of Stata commands that can be executed in Stata as if they were a single command. They make it very easy to rerun previous analyses. Stata typically runs so fast that the time needed to rerun an analysis from scratch is trivial and a complete analysis can be built by incrementally adding commands to your *do* file. Also, if you insert a *log* command into your original *do* file then subsequent modifications will be automatically recorded in your log file.

An introduction to creating and executing these files is given in the *Getting Started with Stata* manual. I recommend that you take a look at this feature after you become comfortable with executing commands interactively. *Do* files for all of the examples given in this text are posted on my web site at `biostat.mc.vanderbilt.edu/dupontwd/wddtext/`.

### 1.3.8. Stata pulldown menus

Stata also allows most commands to be executed using its pulldown menus. This approach has the great advantage of not requiring the user to learn Stata command syntax. When you issue a point-and-click command in this way, Stata generates the corresponding character command and places it in the Review window. This command can then be recalled to the Command window where it can be edited and re-executed or copied and pasted into a *do* file.

In the Stata example comments throughout this text I have given the equivalent point-and-click command for the character-based command being discussed. To do this, we need a compact notation for these commands. This notation is illustrated by the following example.

Suppose that we have loaded the *1.3.2.Sepsis* data set into memory as illustrated in Section 1.3.2. We now wish to generate the histogram shown in Figure 1.8 using point-and-click commands. The notation that we will use to describe how this is done is as follows:

Graphics ▶ Histogram ⌡Main⌊ ┌ Data — Variable: *apache* ┘ ┌ Bins — [✓] *20* Number of bins ┘ ┌ Y axis — ⦿ Percent ┘ ⌡By⌊ ┌ [✓] Draw subgraphs for unique values of variables — Variables: *treat* ┘ [Submit].

A detailed explanation of both the preceding notation and how to execute this command is given below. Its first component is

Graphics ▶ Histogram.

This means: click on *Graphics* at the top of the *Stata/IC 10* window (see Figure 1.6) to display the Graphics menu. Next, click on *Histogram* from this menu. The dialog box given in the top panel of Figure 1.9 will be displayed.

The next command component is

⌡Main⌊ ┌ Data — Variable: *apache* ┘ ┌ Bins — [✓] *20* Number of bins ┘ ┌ Y axis — ⦿ Percent ┘

Stata dialog boxes often have several tabs at the top of the box. The default tab, which is displayed in Figure 1.9, is called *Main*. Clicking on different tabs displays different aspects of the dialog box. When I illustrate a point-and-click command I will always indicate the tab of the dialog box that I am referring to by a schematic tab symbol as shown above.

We next select the variable *apache* from the *Variable* pulldown list as shown in the bottom panel of Figure 1.9. Fields in Stata dialog boxes have text indicating the function of the field (e.g. *Variable:*) and values that the user inserts into these fields (e.g. *apache*). In my command descriptions, text that Stata uses to identify the field is written in a sans-serif font. Values

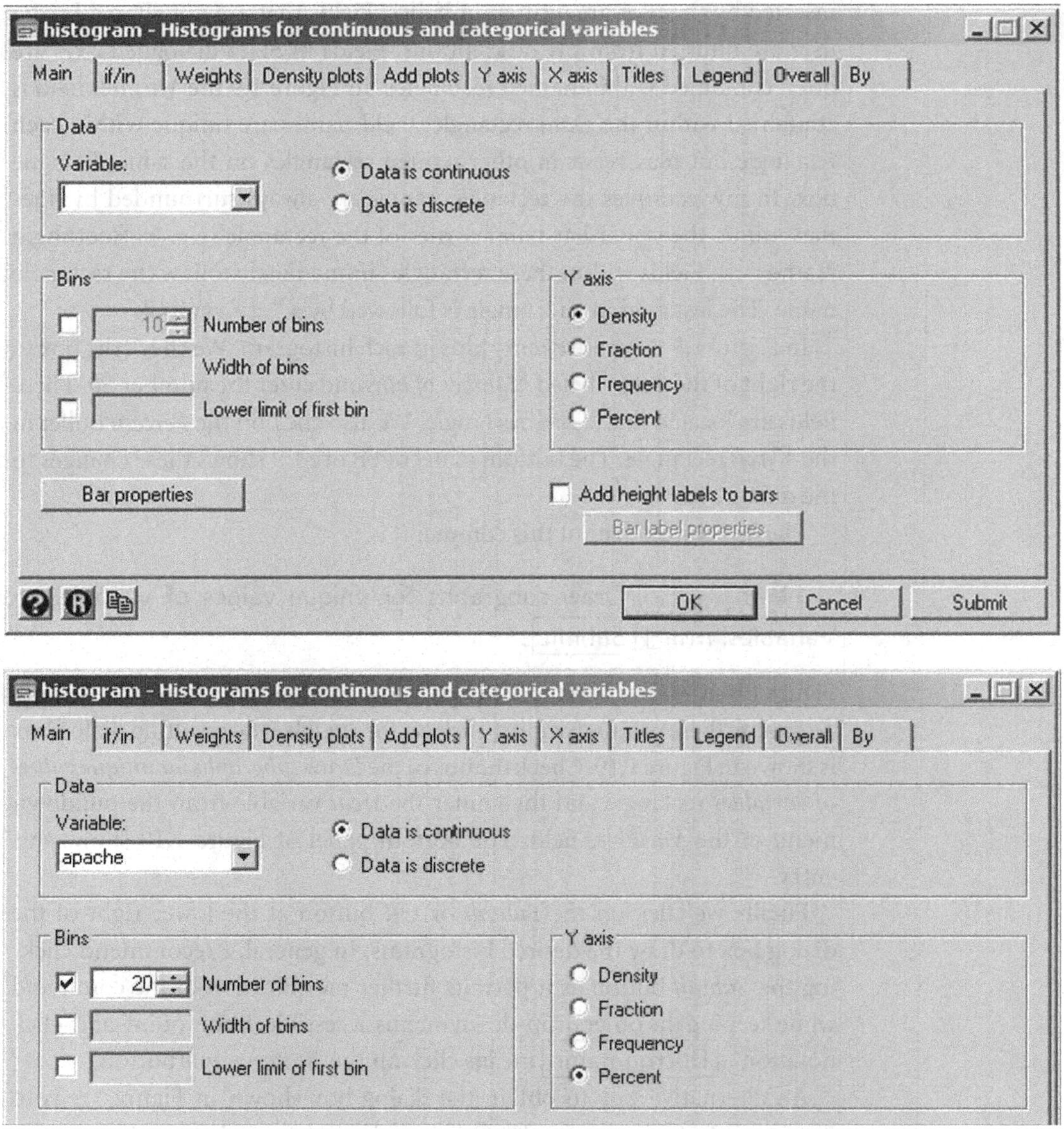

Figure 1.9 The top panel shows the *Main* tab of the histogram dialog box. It is displayed by clicking on the *Graphics* pulldown menu and then clicking on *Histogram*. The first step in creating Figure 1.8 is to enter *apache* in the *Variable* field and then specify 20 bins for the histogram. These entries are shown in the bottom panel of this figure. To draw histograms for each treatment in the same graph we next click on the *By* tab (see Figure 1.10).

inserted by the user are written in italics. Fields that are not altered by the user are omitted from my descriptions. Fields in Stata dialogue boxes are often contained within named rectangles. In Figure 1.9 the *Variable* field is contained within the *Data* rectangle. Field names are unique within each rectangle but may recur in other named rectangles on the same dialogue box. In my examples the rectangle names are always surrounded by lines that mimic the upper left-hand corner of the rectangle (e.g. ┌ Rectangle Name — ). Fields within these rectangles immediately follow the rectangle name. The last field in a rectangle is followed by a " ┘ " symbol.

In Figure 1.8 there are twenty bins in each histogram. We check the box to the right of the field labeled *Number of bins* and enter the number *20.* These fields are located in the *Bins* rectangle. We also click on the *Percent* bullet in the *Y axis* rectangle. The bottom panel of Figure 1.9 shows these changes to the dialog box.

The last component of this command is

┘By└ ┌ [✓] Draw subgraphs for unique values of variables — Variables: *treat* ┘ [Submit].

Figure 1.8 shows histograms of Apache score subdivided by treatment group. To specify these groups we must click on the *By* tab. The resulting dialog box is shown in Figure 1.10. Check the box of the *Draw subgraphs for unique values of variables* rectangle and then enter the *treat* variable from the pulldown menu of the *Variables* field. The bottom panel of Figure 1.10 shows this entry.

Finally we click on the *Submit* or *OK* button at the lower right of the dialog box to draw the desired histograms. In general, I recommend clicking the *Submit* button as it permits further modification of the command while keeping the other drop-down menus accessible. In my point-and-click notation, [Button name] means click on the *Button name* button.

An alternative way to obtain the dialog box shown in Figure 1.9 is to execute *help histogram* in the Command window and then click on the *histogram* link in the upper right-hand corner of the Viewer window. A third way to obtain this dialog box is to give the command

**db *histogram***

All Stata dialog boxes have a question mark in the lower left-hand corner (see Figure 1.9). Clicking on this question mark opens the help window for the associated command.

Two additional examples of my point-and-click notation for Stata commands are as follows. The *describe* command illustrated in Section 1.3.2 is

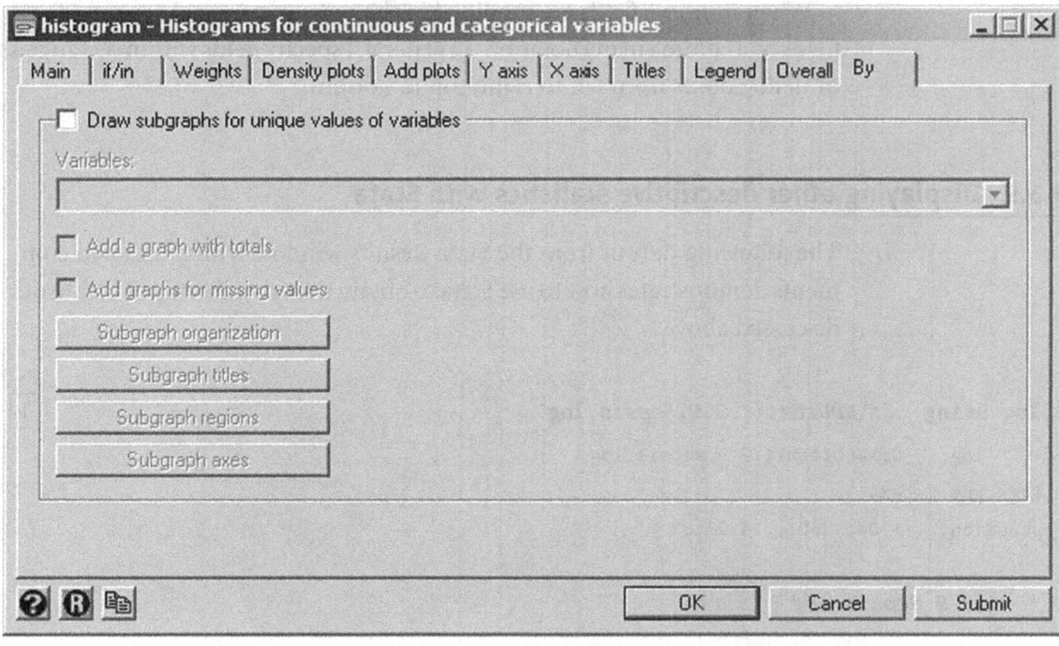


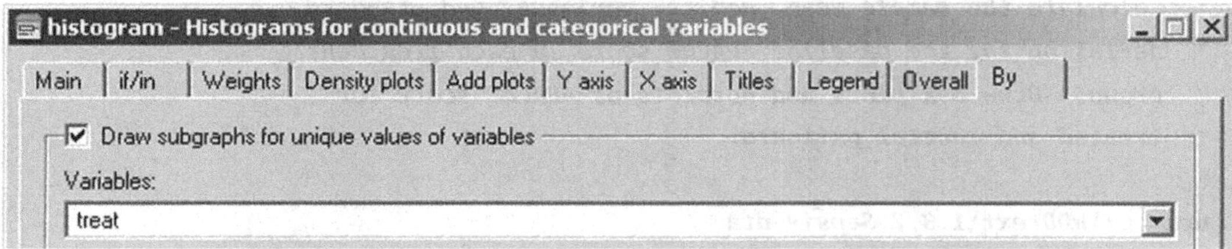


Figure 1.10 The top panel shows the *By* tab of the histogram dialog box (see Figure 1.9). To obtain separate histograms for each treatment on the same graph we check the box labeled "Draw subgraphs ..." and enter *treat* in the *Variables:* field as shown in the bottom panel. To create this graph click the *Submit* button.

implemented as Data ▶ Describe data ▶ Describe data in memory ⌜ [Submit]. Note that the dialog box displayed by the preceding command does not have any tabs. The modified fields of such boxes in my descriptions are preceded by a ⌜ symbol. In this particular example, no fields are modified and hence nothing is written between this symbol and the *Submit* command. The *list* command in Section 1.3.2 is implemented as Data ▶ Describe data ▶ List data ⌋ Main ⌊ Variables: (leave empty for all variables) *treat apache* ⌋ by/if/in ⌊ ⌐ Restrict observations — [✓] Use a range of observations, From *1* to *3* ⌋ [Submit].

When multiple fields are modified in the same rectangle, I separate these fields by a comma in my notation. In general, I specify fields within rectangles or dialog boxes from left to right, top to bottom.

## 1.3.9. Displaying other descriptive statistics with Stata

The following output from the Stata Results window with annotated comments demonstrates how to use Stata to obtain the other descriptive statistics discussed above.

```
. log using  C:\WDDtext\1.3.9.Sepsis.log                                   1

       log:   C:\WDDtext\1.3.9.sepsis.log
  log type:  text
 opened on:   1 Dec 2007, 14:28:33

. *  1.3.9.Sepsis.log
. *
. *  Calculate the sample mean, median, variance, and standard
. *  deviation for the baseline APACHE score in each treatment
. *  group.  Draw box plots and dotplots of APACHE score for
. *  treated and control patients.
. *
. use  C:\WDDtext\1.3.2.Sepsis.dta

. by  treat, sort: summarize  apache, detail                               2

------------------------------------------------------------------------------
-> treat = Placebo

                      Baseline APACHE Score
-------------------------------------------------------------
      Percentiles      Smallest
 1%            3              0
 5%            5              2
10%            7              3       Obs                 230
25%           10              4       Sum of Wgt.         230

50%         14.5                      Mean           15.18696
                        Largest       Std. Dev.      6.922831
75%           19             32
90%           24             33       Variance       47.92559
```

```
95%        28          35       Skewness      .6143051
99%        33          41       Kurtosis      3.383043
-------------------------------------------------------------

-> treat = Ibuprofen

                    Baseline APACHE Score
-------------------------------------------------------------
      Percentiles      Smallest
 1%         3             3
 5%         5             3
10%         7             3       Obs                224
25%        10             4       Sum of Wgt.        224

50%        14                     Mean          15.47768
                        Largest   Std. Dev.     7.261882
75%        21            31
90%        25            34       Variance      52.73493
95%        29            36       Skewness      .5233335
99%        34            37       Kurtosis      2.664936
```

**. graph hbox *apache*, over(*treat*)** 3

**. dotplot *apache*, over(*treat*) center** 4

**. log close** 5

**Comments**

1 The *log using* command creates a log file of the subsequent Stata session. This file, called *1.3.9.Sepsis.log*, will be written in the *WDDtext* folder. Stata creates a simple text log file when the *.log* file name extension is used. There is also a button on the Stata toolbar that permits you to open, close, and suspend log files.

2 The *summarize* command provides some simple statistics on the *apache* variable calculated across the entire data set. With the *detail* option these include means, medians, and other statistics. The command prefix *by treat:* subdivides the data set into as many subgroups as there are distinct values of *treat*, and then calculates the summary statistics for each subgroup. This prefix requires that the data be sorted by the *by* variable *treat*. If the data is not sorted in this way, the prefix *by treat, sort:* can be used to create the desired tables.

In this example, the two values of *treat* are *Placebo* and *Ibuprofen*. For patients on ibuprofen, the mean APACHE score is 15.48 with variance 52.73

and standard deviation 7.26; their interquartile range is from 10 to 21. The equivalent point-and-click command is Statistics ▶ Summaries, tables & tests ▶ Summary and descriptive statistics ▶ Summary statistics ⌡Main⌊ Variables: (leave empty for all variables) *apache* ⌐ Options — ⊙ Display additional statistics ⌋ ⌡by/if/in⌊ ⌐ ☑ Repeat command by groups — Variables that define groups: *treat* ⌋ Submit.

Note that in the preceding command that there is a check box field in the *Repeat command by groups* rectangle name.

3 The *graph hbox* command draws horizontal box plots for the *apache* variable that are similar to those in Figure 1.3. The *over(treat)* option tells Stata that we want a box plot for each treatment drawn in a single graph. The *graph box* command produces box plots that are oriented vertically. The point-and-click command is Graphics ▶ Box plot ⌡Main⌊ ⌐ Orientation — ⊙ Horizontal ⌋ Variables: *apache* ⌡Categories⌊ ⌐ ☑ Over 1 — Grouping variable: *treat* ⌋ Submit.

4 This *dotplot* command generates the graph shown in Figure 1.1. A separate dot plot of the APACHE variable is displayed for each value of the *treat* variable; *center* draws the dots centered over each treatment value. The point-and-click command is Graphics ▶ Distributional graphs ▶ Distribution dot plot ⌡Main⌊ ⌐ Variables to plot — ⊙ Plot single variable, Variable: *apache* ⌋ ⌡Options⌊ ⌐ ☑ Show columnar dot plots — Variable: *treat* ⌋ ☑ Center the dot for each column ⌋ Submit.

5 This command closes the log file *C:\WDDtext\1.3.2.Sepsis.dta.* You can also do this by clicking the *Log* button and choosing *Close log file.*

## 1.4. Inferential statistics

In medical research we are interested in drawing valid conclusions about all patients who meet certain criteria. For example, we would like to know if treating septic patients with ibuprofen improves their chances of survival. The **target population** consists of all patients, both past and future, to whom we would like our conclusions to apply. We select a sample of these subjects and observe their outcome or attributes. We then seek to infer conclusions about the target population from the observations in our sample.

The typical response of subjects in our sample may differ from that of the target population due to chance variation in subject response or to bias in the way that the sample was selected. For example, if tall people are more likely to be selected than short people, it will be difficult to draw valid conclusions about the average height of the target population from the heights of people in the sample. An **unbiased sample** is one in which each member of the target population is equally likely to be included in the sample. Suppose that we select an unbiased sample of patients from the target population and measure some attribute of each patient. We say that this attribute is a **random variable** drawn from the target population. The observations in a sample are mutually **independent** if the probability that an individual is selected is unaffected by the selection of any other individual in the sample. In this text we will assume that we observe unbiased samples of independent observations and will focus on assessing the extent to which our results may be inaccurate due to chance. Of course, choosing an unbiased sample is much easier said than done. Indeed, implementing an unbiased study design is usually much harder than assessing the effects of chance in a properly selected sample. There are, however, many excellent epidemiology texts that cover this topic. I strongly recommend that you peruse such a text if you are unfamiliar with this subject (see, for example, Katz, 2006 or Hennekens and Buring, 1987).

### 1.4.1. Probability density function

Suppose that we could measure the value of a continuous variable on each member of a target population (for example, their height). The distribution of this variable throughout the population is characterized by its probability density function. Figure 1.11 gives an example of such a function. The $x$-axis of this figure gives the range of values that the variable may take in

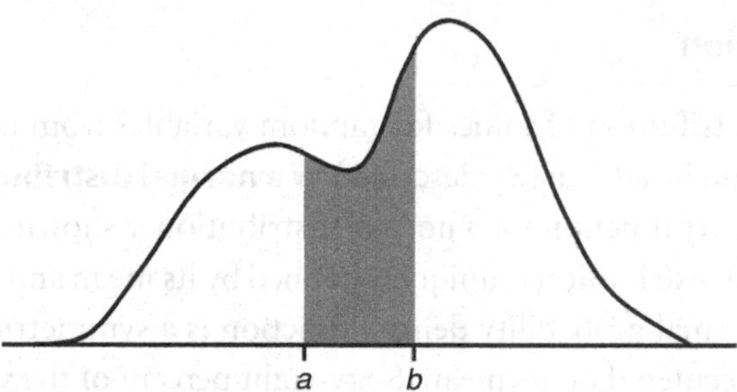


Figure 1.11 Probability density function for a random variable in a hypothetical population. The probability that a member of the population has a value of the variable in the interval $(a, b)$ equals the area of the shaded region.

the population. The **probability density function** is the uniquely defined curve that has the following property. For any interval $(a,b)$ on the $x$-axis, the probability that a member of the population has a value of the variable in the interval $(a, b)$ equals the area under the curve over this interval. In Figure 1.11 this is the area of the shaded region. It follows that the total area under the curve must equal one since each member of the population must have some value of the variable.

### 1.4.2. Mean, variance, and standard deviation

The **mean** of a random variable is its average value in the target population. Its **variance** is the average squared difference between the variable and its mean. Its **standard deviation** is the square root of its variance. The key distinction between these terms and the analogous sample mean, sample variance, and sample standard deviation is that the former are unknown attributes of a target population, while the latter can be calculated from a known sample. We denote the mean, variance, and standard deviation of a variable by $\mu$, $\sigma^2$, and $\sigma$, respectively. In general, unknown attributes of a target population are called **parameters** and are denoted by Greek letters. Functions of the values in a sample, such as $\bar{x}$, $s^2$, and $s$, are called **statistics** and are denoted by Roman letters or Greek letters covered by a caret. (For example, $\hat{\beta}$ might denote a statistic that estimates a parameter $\beta$.) We will often refer to $\bar{x}$, $s^2$, and $s$ as the mean, variance, and standard deviation of the sample when it is obvious from the context that we are talking about a statistic from an observed sample rather than a population parameter.

### 1.4.3. Normal distribution

The distribution of values for random variables from many target populations can be adequately described by a **normal distribution**. The probability density function for a normal distribution is shown in Figure 1.12. Each normal distribution is uniquely defined by its mean and standard deviation. The normal probability density function is a symmetric bell-shaped curve that is centered on its mean. Sixty-eight percent of the values of a normally distributed variable lie within one standard deviation of its mean; 95% of these values lie within 1.96 standard deviations of its mean.

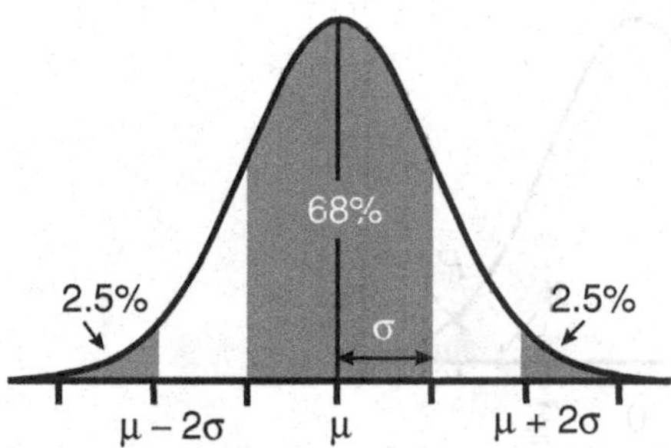


Figure 1.12 Probability density function for a normal distribution with mean $\mu$ and standard deviation $\sigma$. Sixty-eight percent of observations from such a distribution will lie within one standard deviation of the mean. Only 5% of observations will lie more than two standard deviations from the mean.

## 1.4.4. Expected value

Suppose that we conduct a series of identical experiments, each of which consists of observing an unbiased sample of independent observations from a target population and calculating a statistic. The **expected value** of the statistic is its average value from a very large number of these experiments. If the target population has a normal distribution with mean $\mu$ and standard deviation $\sigma$, then the expected value of $\bar{x}$ is $\mu$ and the expected value of $s^2$ is $\sigma^2$. We express these relationships algebraically as $E[\bar{x}] = \mu$ and $E[s^2] = \sigma^2$. A statistic is an **unbiased estimate** of a parameter if its expected value equals the parameter. For example, $\bar{x}$ is an unbiased estimate of $\mu$ since $E[\bar{x}] = \mu$. (The reason why the denominator of Equation (1.3) is $n - 1$ rather than $n$ is to make $s^2$ an unbiased estimate of $\sigma^2$.)

## 1.4.5. Standard error

As the sample size $n$ increases, the variation in $\bar{x}$ from experiment to experiment decreases. This is because the effects of large and small values in each sample tend to cancel each other out. The standard deviation of $\bar{x}$ in this hypothetical population of repeated experiments is called the **standard error**, and equals $\sigma/\sqrt{n}$. If the target population has a normal distribution, so will $\bar{x}$. Moreover, the distribution of $\bar{x}$ converges to normality as $n$ gets large even if the target population has a non-normal distribution. Hence, unless the target population has a badly skewed distribution, we can usually treat $\bar{x}$ as having a normal distribution with mean $\mu$ and standard deviation $\sigma/\sqrt{n}$.

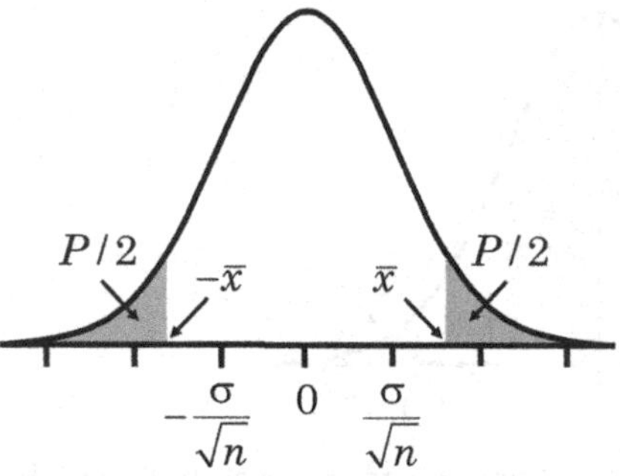


Figure 1.13 The *P*-value associated with the null hypothesis that $\mu = 0$ is given by the area of the shaded region. This is the probability that the sample mean will be greater than $|\bar{x}|$ or less than $-|\bar{x}|$ when the null hypothesis is true.

## 1.4.6. Null hypothesis, alternative hypothesis, and *P*-value

The **null hypothesis** is one that we usually hope to disprove and which permits us to completely specify the distribution of a relevant test statistic. The null hypothesis is contrasted with the **alternative hypothesis** that includes all possible distributions except the null. Suppose that we observe an unbiased sample of size $n$ and mean $\bar{x}$ from a target population with mean $\mu$ and standard deviation $\sigma$. For now, let us make the rather unrealistic assumption that $\sigma$ is known. We might consider the null hypothesis that $\mu = 0$ versus the alternative hypothesis that $\mu \neq 0$. If the null hypothesis is true, then the distribution of $\bar{x}$ will be as in Figure 1.13 and $\bar{x}$ should be near zero. The farther $\bar{x}$ is from zero the less credible the null hypothesis. The ***P* value** is the probability of obtaining a sample mean that is at least as unlikely under the null hypothesis as the observed value $\bar{x}$. That is, it is the probability of obtaining a sample mean greater than $|\bar{x}|$ or less than $-|\bar{x}|$. This probability equals the area of the shaded region in Figure 1.13. When the *P* value is small, then either the null hypothesis is false or we have observed an unlikely event. By convention, if $P < 0.05$ we claim that our result provides statistically significant evidence against the null hypothesis in favor of the alternative hypothesis; $\bar{x}$ is then said to provide evidence against the null hypothesis at the 5% level of significance. The *P* value indicated in Figure 1.13 is called a **two-sided** or **two-tailed** *P* value because the **critical region** of values deemed less credible than $\bar{x}$ includes values less than $-|\bar{x}|$ as well as those greater than $|\bar{x}|$. Recall that the standard error of $\bar{x}$ is $\sigma/\sqrt{n}$. The absolute value of $\bar{x}$ must exceed 1.96 standard errors to have $P < 0.05$. In Figure 1.13, $\bar{x}$ lies between 1 and 2 standard errors. Hence, in this example $\bar{x}$ is not significantly different from zero. If we were testing some other null hypothesis, say $\mu = \mu_0$, then the distribution of $\bar{x}$ would be centered over $\mu_0$ and we would reject this null hypothesis if $|\bar{x} - \mu_0| > 1.96\,\sigma/\sqrt{n}$.

### 1.4.7. 95% confidence interval

In the preceding example, we were unable to reject at the 5% level of significance all null hypotheses $\mu = \mu_0$ such that $|\bar{x} - \mu_0| < 1.96\,\sigma/\sqrt{n}$. A **95% confidence interval** for a parameter contains of all possible values of the parameter that cannot be rejected at the 5% significance level given the observed sample. In this example, this interval is

$$\bar{x} - 1.96\,\sigma/\sqrt{n} \le \mu \le \bar{x} + 1.96\,\sigma/\sqrt{n}. \qquad (1.4)$$

In this and most other examples involving normal distributions, the probability that $\bar{x} - 1.96\,\sigma/\sqrt{n} \le \mu \le \bar{x} + 1.96\,\sigma/\sqrt{n}$ equals 0.95. In other words, the true parameter will lie within the confidence interval in 95% of similar experiments. This interval, $\bar{x} \pm 1.96\,\sigma/\sqrt{n}$, provides a measure of the accuracy with which we can estimate $\mu$ from our sample. Note that this accuracy increases as $\sqrt{n}$ increases and decreases with increasing $\sigma$.

Many textbooks define the 95% confidence interval to be an interval that includes the parameter with 95% certainty. These two definitions, however, are not always equivalent, particularly in epidemiological statistics involving discrete distributions. This has led most modern epidemiologists to prefer the definition given here. It can be shown that the probability that a 95% confidence interval, as defined here, includes its parameter is at least 95%. Rothman and Greenland (1998) discuss this issue in greater detail.

### 1.4.8. Statistical power

If we reject the null hypothesis when it is true we make a **Type I error**. The probability of making a Type I error is denoted by $\alpha$, and is the **significance level** of the test. For example, if we reject the null hypothesis when $P < 0.05$, then $\alpha = 0.05$ is the probability of making a Type I error. If we do not reject the null hypothesis when the alternative hypothesis is true we make a **Type II error**. The probability of making a Type II error is denoted by $\beta$. The **power** of the test is the probability of correctly accepting the alternative hypothesis when it is true. This probability equals $1 - \beta$. It is only possible to derive the power for alternative hypotheses that completely specify the distribution of the test statistic. However, we can plot **power curves** that show the power of the test as a function of the different values of the parameter under the alternative hypothesis. Figure 1.14 shows the power curves for the example

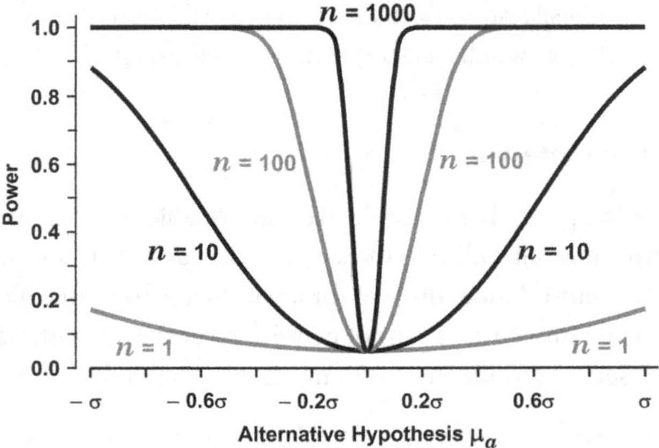


Figure 1.14 Power curves for samples of size 1, 10, 100, and 1000. The null hypothesis is $\mu_0 = 0$. The alternative hypothesis is expressed in terms of $\sigma$, which in this example is assumed to be known.

introduced in Section 1.4.6. Separate curves are drawn for sample sizes of $n = 1$, 10, 100, and 1000 as a function of the mean $\mu_a$ under different alternative hypotheses. The power is always near $\alpha$ for values of $\mu_a$ that are very close to the null ($\mu_0 = 0$). This is because the probability of accepting an alternative hypothesis that is virtually identical to the null equals the probability of falsely rejecting the null hypothesis, which equals $\alpha$. The greater the distance between the alternative and null hypotheses the greater the power, and the rate at which the power rises increases with increasing sample size. Regardless of the sample size, the power eventually approaches 1 (certainty) as the magnitude of $\mu_a$ gets sufficiently large. Note that larger $n$ results in greater ability to correctly reject the null hypothesis in favor of any specific true alternative hypothesis. For example, the power associated with $\mu_a = 0.2\,\sigma$ is 0.055, 0.097, 0.516, and 1.00 when $n = 1$, 10, 100, and 1000, respectively.

Power calculations are particularly useful when designing a study to ensure that the sample size is large enough to detect alternative hypotheses that are clinically important. There are several good software packages available for calculating statistical power. One of these is the *PS* program (Dupont and Plummer, 1990, 1998). This is a self-documented interactive program that produces power and sample size graphs and calculations for most of the commonly used study designs. It is freely available and can be downloaded from the web at `biostatistics.mc.vanderbilt.edu/PowerSampleSize`. Stata also has the *sampsi* command that can be used for power and sample size calculations for a large variety of study designs.

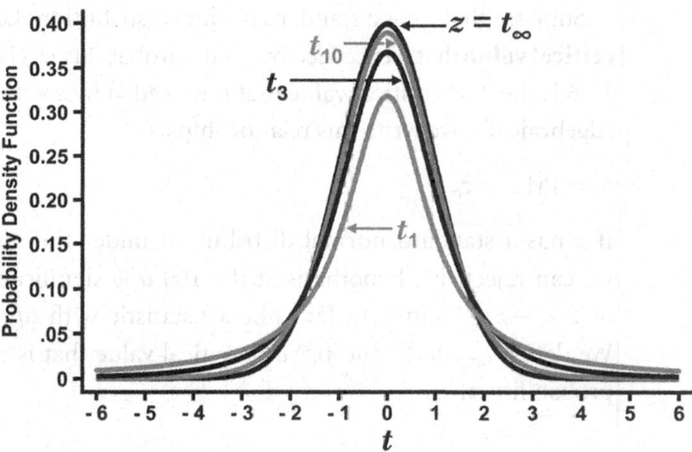


Figure 1.15 Probability density functions for $t$ distributions with one, three, and ten degrees of freedom. These distributions converge to the standard normal distribution as the number of degrees of freedom gets large.

### 1.4.9. The $z$ and Student's $t$ distributions

There are several distributions of special statistics for which we will need to calculate confidence intervals and $P$ values. Two of these are the $z$ and $t$ distributions. The $z$ or **standardized normal distribution** is the normal distribution with mean $\mu = 0$ and standard deviation $\sigma = 1$. If each observation $x_i$ in a sample has a normal distribution with mean $\mu$ and standard deviation $\sigma$, then $(x_i - \mu)/\sigma$ will have a standardized normal distribution. In addition, if the $n$ observations in the sample are independent, then $(\bar{x} - \mu)/(\sigma/\sqrt{n})$ also has a standard normal distribution.

The examples given in the last three sections are rather artificial in that it is unusual to know the true standard deviation of the target population. However, we can estimate $\sigma$ by the sample standard deviation $s$. Moreover, $(\bar{x} - \mu)/(s/\sqrt{n})$ has a completely specified distribution. This is a **Student's $t$ distribution**, which is one of a family of bell-shaped distributions that are symmetric about zero. Each such distribution is indexed by an integer called its **degrees of freedom.** The statistic $t_{n-1} = (\bar{x} - \mu)/(s/\sqrt{n})$ has a $t$ distribution with $n-1$ degrees of freedom. Figure 1.15 shows the probability density functions for $t$ distributions with one, three, and ten degrees of freedom. As the degrees of freedom increase the probability density function converges towards the standard normal distribution, which is also shown in this figure. The standard deviation of a $t$ statistic is greater than that of the standard normal distribution due to imprecision in $s$ as an estimate of $\sigma$. As the sample size increases $s$ becomes a more and more precise estimate of $\sigma$ and $t_{n-1}$ converges to $z$.

Suppose that $z$ has a standard normal distribution. Let $z_\alpha$ be the **100 $\alpha$% critical value** that is exceeded by $z$ with probability $\alpha$. (For example, $z_{0.025} = 1.96$ is the 2.5% critical value that is exceeded by $z$ with probability 0.025.) Algebraically, we write this relationship as

$$\alpha = \Pr[z > z_\alpha]. \tag{1.5}$$

If $z$ has a standard normal distribution under the null hypothesis, then we can reject this hypothesis at the 100 $\alpha$% significance level if $z > z_{\alpha/2}$ or $z < -z_{\alpha/2}$. Similarly, let $t_{df}$ be a $t$ statistic with $df$ degrees of freedom. We define $t_{df,\alpha}$ to be the 100 $\alpha$% critical value that is exceeded by $t_{df}$ with probability $\alpha$.

### 1.4.10. Paired *t* test

Suppose that normally distributed responses $x_{i1}$ and $x_{i2}$ are measured before and after treatment on the $i^{\text{th}}$ member of an independent sample of $n$ patients. We wish to test the null hypothesis that the treatment has no effect on the mean patient response. Let $d_i = x_{i1} - x_{i2}$ be the change in response for the $i^{\text{th}}$ patient. Then under the null hypothesis, $d_i$ has a normal distribution with mean 0 and some unknown standard deviation $\sigma_d$. Let $\bar{d}$ and $s_d$ be the sample mean and standard deviation of the differences $d_i$. Then $s_d/\sqrt{n}$ estimates the standard error of $\bar{d}$. Under the null hypothesis

$$\bar{d}/(s_d/\sqrt{n}) \tag{1.6}$$

has a $t$ distribution with $n-1$ degrees of freedom. The $P$-value associated with this statistic is

$$P = \Pr[t_{n-1} < -|\bar{d}/(s_d/\sqrt{n})| \text{ or } t_{n-1} > |\bar{d}/(s_d/\sqrt{n})|], \tag{1.7}$$

where $t_{n-1}$ has a $t$ distribution with $n-1$ degrees of freedom.

The 95% confidence interval for the true change in response associated with treatment is

$$\bar{d} \pm t_{n-1,0.025}(s_d/\sqrt{n}). \tag{1.8}$$

*Example*

In the Ibuprofen in Sepsis Study, the body temperature of all study subjects was recorded at baseline and after two hours of therapy. All patients received standard care for sepsis. In addition, patients who were randomized to the intervention group received intravenous ibuprofen. There were $n = 208$ patients in the intervention group who had their temperatures recorded at both of these times. The average drop in temperature for these patients is

$\bar{d} = 0.8845$ °F. The sample standard deviation of these differences is $s_d = 1.2425$ °F. The estimated standard error of $\bar{d}$ is $s_d/\sqrt{n} = 1.2425/\sqrt{208} = 0.086\,15$ °F, and the $t$ statistic equals 0.8845/0.086 15 = 10.27 with 207 degrees of freedom. The two-sided $P$-value associated with this test is <0.000 05. This provides overwhelming evidence that the drop in temperature in the first two hours of treatment was not due to chance. The 95% confidence interval for the true mean drop in temperature among septic patients treated with ibuprofen is $\bar{d} \pm t_{n-1,0.025}(s_d/\sqrt{n}) = 0.8845 \pm 1.971 \times 0.086\,15 = (0.71, 1.05)$. Note that the critical value $t_{207,0.025} = 1.971$ is close to $z_{0.025} = 1.960$. This is due to the fact that a $t$ distribution with 207 degrees of freedom is almost identical to the standard normal distribution.

## 1.4.11. Performing paired *t* tests with Stata

The following Stata log file shows the derivation of the statistics from the example in the preceding section.

```
. * 1.4.11.Sepsis.log                                                1
. *
. *  Perform paired t test of temperature change by 2 hours
. *  in septic patients receiving ibuprofen.
. *
. use c:\WDDtext\1.4.11.Sepsis.dta
. codebook treat                                                     2

------------------------------------------------------------------------
treat                                                          Treatment
------------------------------------------------------------------------

                 type:  numeric (float)
                label:  treatmnt

                range:  [0,1]                        units:  1
        unique values:  2                        missing .:  0/455

           tabulation:  Freq.   Numeric  Label
                          231         0  Placebo
                          224         1  Ibuprofen

. keep if treat==1                                                   3
(231 observations deleted)

. codebook temp0 temp1                                               4
```

```
--------------------------------------------------------------------------------
temp0                                              Baseline Temperature (deg. F)
--------------------------------------------------------------------------------

                  type:  numeric (float)

                 range:  [91.58,107]                   units:  .01
         unique values:  96                        missing .:  0/224

                  mean:   100.362
             std. dev:    2.13871

           percentiles:        10%       25%       50%       75%       90%
                              97.7     99.25    100.58    101.48    102.74

--------------------------------------------------------------------------------
temp1                                                Temperature after 2 hours
--------------------------------------------------------------------------------

                  type:  numeric (float)

                 range:  [92.6,106.7]                  units:  .01
         unique values:  78                        missing .:  16/224

                  mean:   99.5211
             std. dev:    1.85405

           percentiles:      10%      25%      50%      75%      90%
                            97.3     98.6     99.5    100.5    101.4
```

**. ttest *temp0* = *temp1*** 5

```
Paired t test
------------------------------------------------------------------------------
Variable |     Obs        Mean    Std. Err.   Std. Dev.   [95% Conf. Interval]
---------+--------------------------------------------------------------------
   temp0 |     208    100.4056    .1493624    2.154135    100.1111       100.7
   temp1 |     208    99.52106    .1285554    1.854052    99.26761     99.7745
---------+--------------------------------------------------------------------
    diff |     208    .8845193    .0861504    1.242479    .7146746    1.054364
------------------------------------------------------------------------------

     mean(diff) = mean(temp0 - temp1)                             t =  10.2672
 Ho: mean(diff) = 0                              degrees of freedom =      207

 Ha: mean(diff) < 0           Ha: mean(diff) != 0           Ha: mean(diff) > 0
 Pr(T < t) = 1.0000         Pr(|T| > |t|) = 0.0000          Pr(T > t) = 0.0000
```

**. log close**

**Comments**

1 In this and subsequent examples I have not shown the *log using* command that opens the log file.

2 This *codebook* command provides information on the variable *treat.* It indicates that *treat* is a numeric variable that takes the values zero and one. The value labels *Placebo* and *Ibuprofen* are assigned to these numeric values. (See Section 4.21 for an explanation of how to assign value labels to numeric variables.) Stata uses these labels whenever possible. However, when we wish to specify a value of *treat* in a Stata command we must use its numeric value.

The *codebook* point-and-click command is Data ▶ Describe data ▶ Describe data contents (codebook) ⌋ Main ⌊ Variable: (leave empty for all) *treat* Submit .

3 The *keep* command is used to designate either observations or variables that are to be kept in the data set. When used with the qualifier *if logicaLexpression* this command keeps all observations (rows of variable values in the data set) for which *logicaLexpression* is true; *treat* == *1* is a logical expression that is true if *treat* equals 1. Hence, this command keeps all observations for which *treat* equals 1. In other words, it keeps the observations on all patients receiving ibuprofen. Stata indicates that 231 observations have been deleted, which are the records of the 231 placebo patients.

Logical expressions can be constructed in Stata using "and" (&), "or" (|) or "not" (!) operators. For example, *treat* != 0 & (*apache* >= 30 | *temp0* < 96) is true for all patients for whom *treat* is not equal to 0 and either *apache* $\geq$ 30 or *temp0* < 96; otherwise it is false. The expression !(*fruit* == "apple") is true whenever (*fruit* == "apple") is false. That is, it is true when *fruit* takes any value other than "apple".

The point-and-click *keep* command is Data ▶ Variable utilities ▶ Keep or drop observations ⌋ Main ⌊ ⌈ Observations to keep — If: (expression) *treat* == *1* ⌋ Submit .

4 The patient's body temperature at baseline and after two hours of therapy are recorded in the *temp0* and *temp1* variables, respectively. This *codebook* command indicates that while all ibuprofen patients have a recorded baseline temperature, there are 16 patients for whom the 2 hour temperature is missing. Hence there are $n = 224 - 16 = 208$ patients in the ibuprofen group who had their temperatures recorded at both times.

5 The *ttest* command performs independent and paired *t* tests. The qualifier *temp0* = *temp1* specifies that a paired test of these two variables is

to be performed. In the notation of Section 1.4.10 $x_{i1}$ and $x_{i2}$ denote *temp0* and *temp1*, respectively. The mean change in temperature is $\bar{d} = 0.8845$ °F, $s_d = 1.242$ °F, $n = 224 - 16 = 208$, $s_d/\sqrt{n} = 0.086\,15$, and the $t$ statistic equals 10.27 with 207 degrees of freedom. The two-sided $P$-value associated with this test is $<0.000\,05$ (see last row of output). The 95% confidence interval for the true drop in temperature is (0.715, 1.054).

The point-and-click version of this *ttest* command is Statistics ▶ Summaries, tables, & tests ▶ Classical tests of hypotheses ▶ Mean comparison test, paired data [Main] First variable: *temp0*, Second variable: *temp1* [Submit].

### 1.4.12. Independent $t$ test using a pooled standard error estimate

Suppose that we have two independent samples of size $n_0$ and $n_1$ from normal populations with means $\mu_0$ and $\mu_1$ and standard deviations both equal to $\sigma$. Let $\bar{x}_0$, $\bar{x}_1$, $s_0$, and $s_1$ be the means and standard deviations from these two samples. Then a pooled estimate of $\sigma$ from both samples is

$$s_p = \sqrt{((n_0 - 1)s_0^2 + (n_1 - 1)s_1^2)/(n_0 + n_1 - 2)}, \tag{1.9}$$

and the estimated standard error of $(\bar{x}_0 - \bar{x}_1)$ is

$$s_p\sqrt{\frac{1}{n_0} + \frac{1}{n_1}}. \tag{1.10}$$

Under the null hypothesis that $\mu_0 = \mu_1$,

$$t_{n_0+n_1-2} = (\bar{x}_0 - \bar{x}_1) \Bigg/ \left(s_p\sqrt{\frac{1}{n_0} + \frac{1}{n_1}}\right) \tag{1.11}$$

has a $t$ distribution with $n_0 + n_1 - 2$ degrees of freedom. A 95% confidence interval for $\mu_0 - \mu_1$ is therefore

$$(\bar{x}_0 - \bar{x}_1) \pm t_{n_0+n_1-2,0.025}\left(s_p\sqrt{\frac{1}{n_0} + \frac{1}{n_1}}\right). \tag{1.12}$$

*Example*

In the previous two sections we showed that the observed drop in temperature in septic patients treated with ibuprofen could not be explained by chance fluctuations. Of course, this does not prove that ibuprofen caused the temperature drop since there are many other factors associated with treatment in an intensive care unit (ICU) that could cause this change. To show a causal relationship between ibuprofen treatment and temperature we need to compare temperature change in treated and untreated patients. In the Ibuprofen in Sepsis Study there were $n_0 = 212$ patients in the control group and $n_1 = 208$ patients in the ibuprofen group who had temperature readings at baseline and after two hours. The average drop in temperature in these two groups was $\bar{x}_0 = 0.3120$ and $\bar{x}_1 = 0.8845$ °F with standard deviations $s_0 = 1.0705$ °F and $s_1 = 1.2425$ °F, respectively. (Note that temperatures fall in both groups, although the average reduction is greater in the ibuprofen group than in the control group.) The pooled estimate of the standard deviation is

$$s_p = \sqrt{\frac{(212-1)\times 1.0705^2 + (208-1)\times 1.2425^2}{212+208-2}} = 1.1589\ °\text{F}.$$

The estimated standard error of

$\bar{x}_0 - \bar{x}_1$ is $1.1589 \times \sqrt{(1/212) + (1/208)} = 0.1131$ °F,

and

$t = (0.3120 - 0.8845)/0.1131 = -5.062$

has a $t$ distribution with $212 + 208 - 2 = 418$ degrees of freedom. The two-sided $P$-value associated with the null hypothesis of equal temperature drops in the two patient groups is $P < 0.000\,05$. This result, together with the fact that these data come from a double-blinded randomized clinical trial, provides convincing evidence of the antipyretic effects of ibuprofen in septic patients. A 95% confidence interval for the true difference in temperature reduction associated with the placebo and treatment groups is $(0.3120 - 0.8845) \pm 1.9657 \times 0.1131 = -0.5725 \pm 0.2223 = (-0.79, -0.35)$, where $t_{418,0.025} = 1.9657$ is the 2.5% critical value for a $t$ statistic with 418 degrees of freedom. In other words, the likely average true reduction in temperature due to ibuprofen, and above and beyond that due to other therapy on the ICU, is between 0.35 and 0.79 °F.

### 1.4.13. Independent $t$ test using separate standard error estimates

Sometimes we wish to compare groups that have markedly different standard error estimates. In this case it makes sense to abandon the assumption that both groups share a common standard deviation $\sigma$. Let

$$t_v = (\bar{x}_0 - \bar{x}_1) \bigg/ \left( \sqrt{\frac{s_0^2}{n_0} + \frac{s_1^2}{n_1}} \right). \tag{1.13}$$

Then $t_v$ will have an approximately $t$ distribution with

$$v = \frac{\left(s_0^2/n_0 + s_1^2/n_1\right)^2}{s_0^4/\left(n_0^2\,(n_0 - 1)\right) + s_1^4/\left(n_1^2\,(n_1 - 1)\right)} \tag{1.14}$$

degrees of freedom (Satterthwaite, 1946). The analogous 95% confidence interval associated with this test is

$$(\bar{x}_0 - \bar{x}_1) \pm t_{v,0.025} \left( \sqrt{\frac{s_0^2}{n_0} + \frac{s_1^2}{n_1}} \right). \tag{1.15}$$

This test is less powerful than the test with the pooled standard error estimate and should only be used when the assumption of identical standard errors in the two groups appears unreasonable.

## 1.4.14. Independent *t* tests using Stata

The following log file and comments illustrate how to perform independent *t* tests with Stata.

```
. *  1.4.14.Sepsis.log
. *
. *  Perform an independent t test comparing change in temperature
. *  from baseline after two hours in the ibuprofen group compared
. *  with that in the control group.
. *
. use C:\WDDtext\1.4.11.Sepsis.dta

. generate tempdif = temp0 - temp1                                  1

(35 missing values generated)

. *
. * Assume equal standard deviations in the two groups
. *
. ttest tempdif, by(treat)                                          2
Two-sample t test with equal variances
```

| Group | Obs | Mean | Std. Err. | Std. Dev. | [95% Conf. | Interval] |
|---|---|---|---|---|---|---|
| Placebo | 212 | .3119811 | .0735218 | 1.070494 | .1670496 | .4569125 |
| Ibuprofe | 208 | .8845193 | .0861504 | 1.242479 | .7146746 | 1.054364 |
| combined | 420 | .5955238 | .0581846 | 1.192429 | .4811538 | .7098938 |
| diff | | -.5725383 | .1130981 | | -.7948502 | -.3502263 |

```
    diff = mean(Placebo) - mean(Ibuprofe)                          t =  -5.0623
Ho: diff = 0                                     degrees of freedom =      418

    Ha: diff < 0               Ha: diff != 0               Ha: diff > 0
 Pr(T < t) = 0.0000      Pr(|T| > |t|) = 0.0000         Pr(T > t) = 1.0000

. *
. * Assume unequal standard deviations in the two groups
. *
. ttest tempdif, by(treat) unequal
```
3

Two-sample t test with unequal variances

| Group | Obs | Mean | Std. Err. | Std. Dev. | [95% Conf. | Interval] |
|---|---|---|---|---|---|---|
| Placebo | 212 | .3119811 | .0735218 | 1.070494 | .1670496 | .4569125 |
| Ibuprofe | 208 | .8845193 | .0861504 | 1.242479 | .7146746 | 1.054364 |
| combined | 420 | .5955238 | .0581846 | 1.192429 | .4811538 | .7098938 |
| diff | | -.5725383 | .1132579 | | -.7951823 | -.3498942 |

```
    diff = mean(Placebo) - mean(Ibuprofe)                          t =  -5.0552
Ho: diff = 0                      Satterthwaite's degrees of freedom =  406.688

    Ha: diff < 0               Ha: diff != 0               Ha: diff > 0
 Pr(T < t) = 0.0000      Pr(|T| > |t|) = 0.0000         Pr(T > t) = 1.0000
.log close
```

**Comments**

1 The *generate* command calculates the values of new variables from old ones. In this example *tempdif* is set equal to the difference between the

patient's baseline temperature (*temp0*) and his or her temperature two hours later (*temp1*). When either *temp0* or *temp1* is missing so is *tempdif*. There are 35 observations where this occurs. The point-and-click version of this command is Data ▶ Create or change variables ▶ Create new variable [Main] New variable name *tempdif*, Contents of new variable (expression) *temp0 - temp1* [Submit].

Note that Stata distinguishes between *apple* = 1, which assigns the value 1 to *apple*, and *apple* == 1, which is a logical expression that is true if *apple* equals 1 and false otherwise.

2 This form of the *ttest* command performs an independent *t* test comparing *tempdif* in the two groups of patients defined by the values of *treat*. The highlighted values in this output correspond to those in the example in Section 1.4.12. The point-and-click command is Statistics ▶ Summaries, tables & tests ▶ Classical tests of hypotheses ▶ Two-group mean-comparison test [Main] Variable name: *tempdif*, Group variable name: *treat* [Submit].

3 The *unequal* option causes Satterthwaite's *t* test for groups with unequal standard deviations to be performed. In this example, the standard deviations in the two groups are similar and the sample sizes are large. Hence, it is not surprising that this test gives very similar results to the test that assumes equal standard deviations. Note that the approximate degrees of freedom are reduced by about 11 and the absolute value of the *t* statistic drops from 5.062 to 5.055. Hence, in this example, the loss in power due to not assuming equal standard deviations is trivial. Stata's *robvar* command may be used to test the hypothesis that the standard deviations of the response variable in the two groups are equal (see Section 10.1 and page 445).

The point-and-click command is identical to that given above except that the Unequal variances box is checked.

### 1.4.15. The chi-squared distribution

Another important standard distribution that we will use is the **chi-squared** distribution. Let $z_1, z_2, \ldots, z_n$ denote $n$ mutually independent variables that have standard normal distributions. Then $\chi_n^2 = \sum z_i^2$ has a chi-squared distribution with $n$ degrees of freedom. The probability density functions for chi-squared distributions with one through six degrees of freedom are plotted in Figure 1.16. We will use this distribution for testing certain null hypotheses involving one or more parameters. A chi-squared statistic always takes a positive value. Low values of this statistic are consistent with

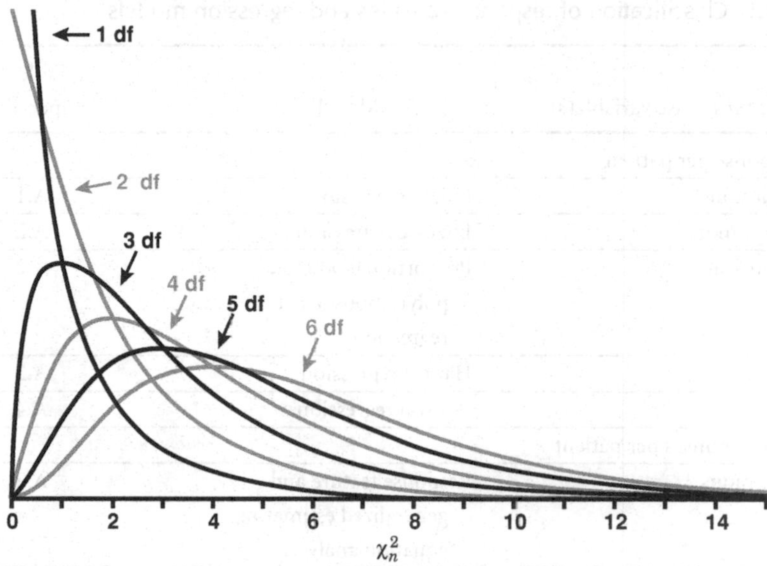


Figure 1.16 Probability density functions for the chi-squared distributions with one through six degrees of freedom (df). High values of a chi-squared statistic provide evidence against the null hypothesis of interest. The expected value of a chi-squared statistic equals its degrees of freedom.

the null hypothesis while high values provide evidence that it is false. The expected value of a chi-squared statistic under the null hypothesis equals its degrees of freedom. The *P*-value associated with an observed value of $\chi_n^2$ is the probability that a chi-squared distribution with *n* degrees of freedom will exceed this value. Note that with the *t* distribution we reject the null hypothesis if *t* is either very large or very small. With the chi-squared distribution we only reject the null hypothesis when $\chi_n^2$ is large.

## 1.5. Overview of methods discussed in this text

Throughout this text we will seek to explain or predict the value of one variable in terms of others. We will refer to this first variable as the **response** or **dependent** variable and the others as **independent** variables or **covariates**. For example, if we wished to predict how change from baseline temperature differed with treatment in Section 1.4.12 then the response variable would be the change from baseline temperature and the independent variable would be the treatment. The first step in any analysis is to select the most appropriate class of models for our data. We do this by first identifying the type of response variable that we will use in our analysis (see Table 1.1).

**Table 1.1.** Classification of response variables and regression models

| Nature of response variable(s) | Model | Table in Appendix A | Chapters |
|---|---|---|---|
| One response per patient | | | |
| Continuous | Linear regression | A.1 | 2, 3, 10 |
| Dichotomous | Logistic regression | A.2 | 4, 5 |
| Categorical | Proportional odds and polytomous logistic regression | A.2 | 5 |
| Survival | Hazard regression | A.3 | 6, 7 |
| Rates | Poisson regression | A.4 | 8, 9 |
| Multiple responses per patient | | | |
| Continuous | Response feature and generalized estimating equation analysis | A.5 | 11 |
| Dichotomous | Response feature and generalized estimating equation analysis | A.5 | 11 |

## 1.5.1. Models with one response per patient

In these models the response variable is only measured once for each patient, and the responses of different patients are independent. They are often called **fixed-effects models** because the parameters being estimated from the target population are fixed and the only variation is due to chance variability of the sampled subjects. The types of fixed effects response variables discussed in this text are outlined below. More detailed guidance on selecting the most appropriate model for your data is summarized in the tables of Appendix A. These tables also give the pages in the text where these methods are explained.

- **Continuous** Models of continuous response variables usually entail linear regression and are discussed in Chapters 2, 3, and 10 (see also Table A.1 in Appendix A).
- **Dichotomous** In these models we are concerned whether patients can be classified as belonging to one of two groups: those who will live or die, do or do not have a disease, etcetera. These data are usually analyzed by logistic regression and are discussed in Chapters 4 and 5 (see also Table A.2).
- **Categorical** In these models the response variable takes one of several distinct values. They are usually analyzed by polytomous or proportional

odds logistic regression. They are briefly introduced in Section 5.36 (see also Table A.2).

- **Survival Data** In survival data the response variables for each patient consist of an interval of follow-up and the patient's fate at the end of this interval. This fate is a dichotomous outcome such as vital status or the occurrence of some event. Survival models are discussed in Chapter 6 and 7 (see also Table A.3).
- **Rates** Sometimes data are available on groups of patients who share specific risk factors. For each group we are provided the rate at which some event occurs or the number of events observed in a specified number of patient–years of follow-up. If the event rate is rare, then these data are usually analyzed with Poisson regression models. They are discussed in Chapters 8 and 9 (see also Table A.4).

### 1.5.2. Models with multiple responses per patient

It is common for multiple observations to be made on the same patient at different times. The analysis of such data is complicated by the fact that observations on the same subject are likely to be correlated. Models for such data are often referred to as **repeated measures** models or models for **longitudinal data.** This text provides a brief introduction to the analysis of such data. The simplest approach is called **response feature** analysis or **two-staged** analysis. The basic idea is to derive a single statistic from each patient's response values that captures the most biologically important aspect of her overall response. This statistic is then analyzed as a single response measure using a fixed-effects model. We illustrate this approach in Chapter 11.

There are a number of very sophisticated methods for analyzing repeated measures data that model the correlation structure of the multiple responses on each subject. One of these is **generalized estimating equations** analysis, which we introduce in Chapter 11. The most common types of response variables in these analyses are either continuous or dichotomous (see Table A.5).

## 1.6. Additional reading

At the end of each chapter I have referenced textbooks that cover additional material that may be of interest to readers. I have selected texts that I have found helpful in writing this book or that may appeal to readers with varying levels of mathematical and statistical backgrounds. These references are by no means exhaustive. There are many other excellent texts that cover the same material that are not listed here.

Katz (2006) and

Pagano and Gauvreau (2000) are excellent all round introductory texts on biostatistics.

Armitage et al. (2002) is another well written introductory text. It covers some material in greater detail than Katz (2006) or Pagano and Gauvreau (2000).

Gordis (2004) is an excellent introductory text in epidemiology.

Rothman and Greenland (1998) is a more advanced epidemiology text. It has an excellent section on the definition of confidence intervals and on the foundations of statistical inference as they apply to epidemiology.

Cleveland (1993) is an excellent text on graphical methods for analyzing data.

Stata (2007) is available with excellent paper documentation and good on-line documentation. I recommend their paper documentation for anyone who can afford it. I particularly recommend their *Getting Started with Stata* manual which can be purchased separately from their other documentation.

Bernard et al. (1997) conducted a randomized clinical trial of ibuprofen in patients with sepsis. We use data from this study to illustrate a number of important methods for analyzing medical data.

Brent et al. (1999) studied patients with ethylene glycol poisoning. We use data from this study to illustrate elementary methods of analyzing bivariate data.

Student (1908) is the original reference on *t* tests. It was written by W. S. Gosset under the pen name "Student" because his employer, an Irish brewer, did not allow its employees to publish under their own names.

Satterthwaite (1946) is the original reference for the *t* test with unequal variances.

## 1.7. Exercises

The following questions relate to the *1.4.11.Sepsis.dta* data set from my web site, which you should download onto your computer.

1 List the names and labels of all variables in the *1.4.11.Sepsis.dta* data set.

2 What are the numeric values of the *race* variable? Which races do these numeric codes represent? Can you answer this question without opening the data editor?

3 List the APACHE score and baseline temperature of the six patients with the lowest APACHE scores. List the APACHE score, fate, and ID number of all black patients whose APACHE score is 35 or greater.
4 Draw dot plots of baseline temperature in black and white patients. Draw these plots on a single graph. Do not include people of other races. Where does Stata obtain the title of the *y*-axis of your dot plot?
5 Draw box plots of temperature at two hours in treated and untreated patients.
6 Consider treated patients whose race is recorded as "other". Test whether these patients' baseline temperature is significantly different from their temperature after two hours. What is the *P*-value associated with this test? How many degrees of freedom does it have? What is a 95% confidence interval for the true change in temperature among this group of subjects?
7 Test whether baseline APACHE score is different in treated and untreated patients. How many degrees of freedom does it have? What is the *P*-value associated with this test? What is a 95% confidence interval for the true difference in APACHE score between treated and untreated patients? Why is this test important in a clinical trial of the efficacy of ibuprofen in septic patients?

2

# Simple linear regression

In this chapter, we are concerned with data where we observe two continuous variables on each patient. Each variable is measured once per subject, and we wish to model the relationship between these variables. Figure 2.1 shows a scatter plot of such data in which plasma glycolate levels are plotted against arterial pH in 18 patients with ethylene glycol poisoning (Brent et al. 1999, see also Section 1.2.9). This plot shows an overall trend of decreasing glycolate levels with increasing arterial pH. Moreover, this relationship appears to be linear. That is, it can be approximated by a straight line. Simple linear regression is used to model data where there is an approximately linear relationship between two continuous variables and we wish to predict the value of one of these variables given the other. Before explaining how to do this we need to introduce a few additional concepts and statistics.

## 2.1. Sample covariance

Figure 2.1 shows the scatter plot of plasma glycolate vs. arterial pH in patients with ethylene glycol poisoning (see Section 1.2.9). These variables are negatively correlated in that the glycolate levels tend to decrease with increasing pH. Note, however, that there is some individual variation in this relationship, with different glycolate levels in patients with similar pH levels. In Figure 2.2 the sample mean glycolate and pH values are indicated by the horizontal and vertical lines at $\bar{y} = 90.44$ and $\bar{x} = 7.21$, respectively. Dashed lines show the glycolate and pH residuals for three of these patients. For example, one of the patients has glycolate and pH values of 265.24 and 6.88, respectively. The glycolate and pH residuals for this patient are $265.24 - 90.44 = 174.8$ and $6.88 - 7.21 = -0.33$. The product of these residuals is $174.8 \times (-0.33) = -57.7$. If we divide Figure 2.2 into four quadrants defined by the two sample means, then all observations in the upper left or lower right quadrants will have a product of residuals that is negative. All observations in the lower left and upper right quadrants will have a positive product of residuals. Since glycolate levels tend to fall with increasing pH levels, most observations are in the upper left or lower right quadrants

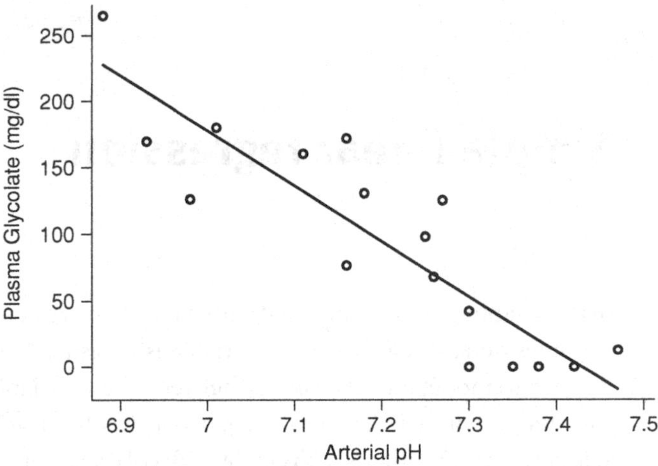


Figure 2.1 Scatter plot of plasma glycolate vs. arterial pH in patients with ethylene glycol poisoning. In simple linear regression we derive a straight line that estimates the expected plasma glycolate for patients with a specified arterial pH level (Brent et al., 1999).

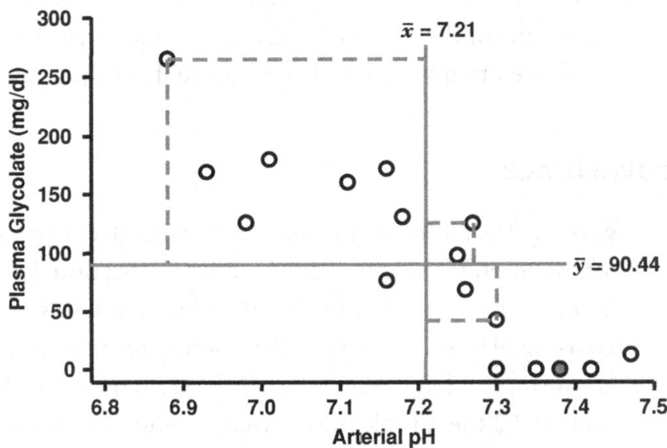


Figure 2.2 Scatter plot of plasma glycolate vs. arterial pH in patients with ethylene glycol poisoning. The dashed lines show the glycolate and pH residuals for three patients (Brent et al., 1999).

and have a negative product of residuals. For this reason the sum of these products, $\sum (x_i - \bar{x})(y_i - \bar{y})$, will be negative. The **sample covariance** is

$$s_{xy} = \sum (x_i - \bar{x})(y_i - \bar{y})/(n - 1), \tag{2.1}$$

which can be thought of as the average product of residuals. In the poison example, there are $n = 18$ patients, and the sample covariance is

$s_{xy} = -211.26/17 = -12.43$. Note that if there is no relationship between values of the two variables then there will be roughly equal numbers of observations in the four quadrants. In this case, the sum of products of residuals will tend to cancel each other out, giving a small sample covariance. If there is a positive relationship between $x_i$ and $y_i$ then most observations will lie in the lower left or upper right quadrants and $s_{xy}$ will be positive.

## 2.2. Sample correlation coefficient

It is often useful to be able to quantify the extent to which one variable can be used to predict the value of another. The sample covariance measures this relationship to some extent but is also affected by the variability of the observations. A better measure of this association is the sample correlation coefficient, which is adjusted for the variability of the two variables. If $s_x$ and $s_y$ denote the standard deviations of $x_i$ and $y_i$, then

$$r = \frac{s_{xy}}{s_x s_y} \tag{2.2}$$

is the **sample correlation coefficient** between $x_i$ and $y_i$. In the poison example $s_x = 0.1731$, $s_y = 80.58$, and $r = -12.43/(0.1731 \times 80.58) = -0.891$. The correlation coefficient can take values from $-1$ to 1; $r = 1$ implies that the points of a scatter plot of $x_i$ and $y_i$ fall on a straight line with a positive slope; $r = 0$ implies no linear relationship between $x_i$ and $y_i$ while $r = -1$ implies a strict linear relationship with negative slope. The closer $r$ is to $\pm 1$ the more accurately the values of one variable can be predicted by a linear function of the other (see Figure 2.3).

## 2.3. Population covariance and correlation coefficient

Suppose that two variables $x$ and $y$ describe attributes of members of some target population. Let $\mu_x$, $\mu_y$, $\sigma_x$, and $\sigma_y$ denote the population means and standard deviations for these variables. Then a patient with variable values $x_i$ and $y_i$ will have a residual product equal to $(x_i - \mu_x)(y_i - \mu_y)$. The **population covariance**, $\sigma_{xy}$, is the mean residual product for all members of the population. If we observe $x_i$ and $y_i$ on an unbiased sample of $n$ patients from the target population, then

$$\mathrm{E}[s_{xy}] = \sigma_{xy}. \tag{2.3}$$

The reason why the denominator of $s_{xy}$ in Equation (2.1) is $n - 1$ rather than $n$ is to make Equation (2.3) true.

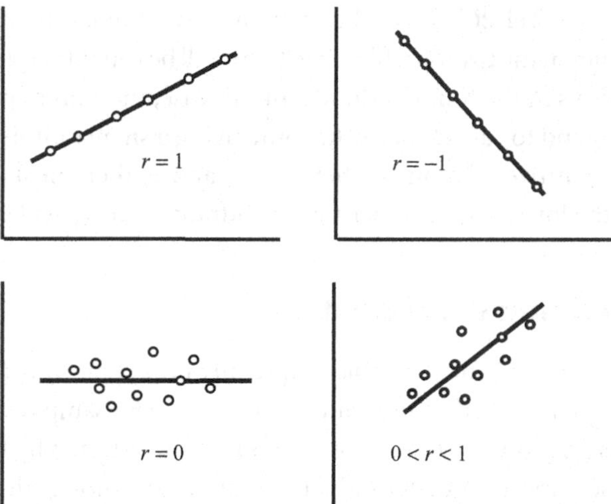


Figure 2.3 Correlation coefficients for four different scatter plots. The closer the points are to lying on a straight line, the closer $r$ is to 1 or −1.

The **population correlation coefficient** is $\rho = \sigma_{xy}/(\sigma_x \sigma_y)$, which is estimated by the sample correlation coefficient $r$. The key difference between $\rho$ and $r$ and $s_{xy}$ and $\sigma_{xy}$ is that $\rho$ and $\sigma_{xy}$ are unknown parameters of the target population while $r$ and $s_{xy}$ are known statistics that are calculated from a sample. We will often omit the adjective "population" or "sample" when it is clear from the context whether we are talking about a known statistic or an unknown parameter.

The population correlation coefficient also lies between $\pm 1$. Variables are said to be positively or negatively **correlated** if $\rho$ is positive or negative. Normally distributed variables are said to be **independent** if $\rho = 0$. In this case knowing the value of one variable for a patient tells us nothing about the likely value of the other.

## 2.4. Conditional expectation

Suppose that $x$ and $y$ are variables that can be measured on patients from some population. We observe an unbiased, mutually independent sample of patients from this population. Let $x_i$ and $y_i$ be the values of $x$ and $y$ for the $i^{\text{th}}$ patient in this sample. The expected value of $y_i$, denoted $\text{E}[y_i]$, is the average value of $y$ in the population. The **conditional expectation** of $y_i$ given $x_i$ is the average value of $y$ in the subpopulation whose value of $x$ equals $x_i$. We denote this conditional expectation $\text{E}[y_i \mid x_i]$. For example, suppose that half of a population are men, and that $x = 1$ for men and $x = 2$ for women. Let $y$ denote a subject's weight. Suppose that the average weight of men and women in the population is 80 and 60 kg, respectively. Then $\mathrm{E}[y_i \mid x_i = 1] = 80$ is the expected weight of the $i^{\text{th}}$ sampled subject given that he is a man. $\mathrm{E}[y_i \mid x_i = 2] = 60$ is the expected weight of $i^{\text{th}}$ sampled subject given that she is a woman, and $\mathrm{E}[y_i] = 70$ is the expected weight of the $i^{\text{th}}$ subject without considering his or her sex.

## 2.5. Simple linear regression model

There is often an approximately linear relationship between variables from a population. Simple linear regression allows us to quantify such relationships. As with most inferential statistics, we first assume a statistical model for the data and then estimate the parameters of the model from an unbiased sample of observations. Suppose that we observe an unbiased sample of $n$ patients from a population, with $x_i$ and $y_i$ representing the values of two variables measured on the $i^{\text{th}}$ patient. The **simple linear regression model** assumes that

$$y_i = \alpha + \beta x_i + \varepsilon_i, \tag{2.4}$$

where

(i) $\alpha$ and $\beta$ are unknown parameters of the population,

(ii) $\varepsilon_i$ has a normal distribution with mean 0 and standard deviation $\sigma$, and

(iii) the values of $\varepsilon_i$ are mutually independent.

That is, the value of $\varepsilon_i$ for any one patient is unaffected by the values of any other. $\varepsilon_i$ is called the **error** for the $i^{\text{th}}$ patient; $\sigma$ and $\sigma^2$ are called the **error standard deviation** and **error variance**, respectively.

It can be shown for any statistics $u$ and $v$ and any constant $c$ that $\mathrm{E}[u + v] = \mathrm{E}[u] + \mathrm{E}[v]$, $\mathrm{E}[cu] = c\mathrm{E}[u]$ and $\mathrm{E}[c] = c$. Suppose that we hold $x_i$ fixed. That is, we restrict our attention to a subpopulation of patients with a specific value of $x_i$. Then the expected value of $y_i$ given $x_i$ for this subpopulation is

$$\begin{aligned} \mathrm{E}[y_i \mid x_i] &= \mathrm{E}[\alpha + \beta x_i \mid x_i] + \mathrm{E}[\varepsilon_i \mid x_i] = \alpha + \beta x_i + 0 \\ &= \alpha + \beta x_i. \end{aligned} \tag{2.5}$$

Thus, the expected value of $y_i$ given $x_i$ is $\mathrm{E}[y_i \mid x_i] = \alpha + \beta x_i$, and the response $y_i$ equals the sum of a deterministic linear component $\alpha + \beta x_i$ plus

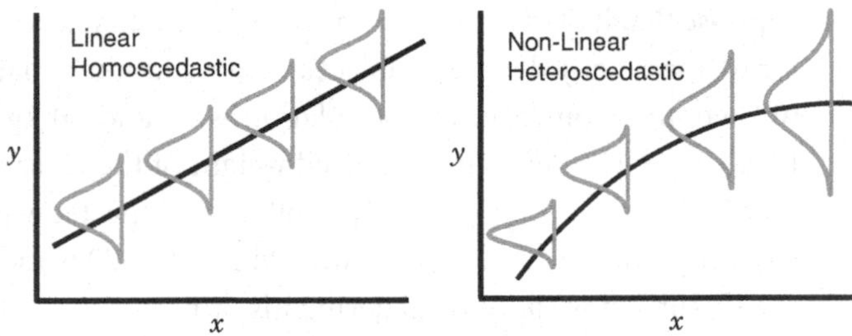


Figure 2.4 Schematic diagrams depicting a simple linear model (left) and a non-linear model with heteroscedastic errors (right). The linear model assumes that the expected value of $y$ given $x$ is a linear function of $x$ and that the error terms are independent and have a constant standard deviation.

a random error component $\varepsilon_i$. Two explicit assumptions of the model are that the expected response $y_i$ is a linear function of $x_i$ and that the standard deviation of $\varepsilon_i$ is a constant that does not depend on $x_i$. Models that have the latter property are called **homoscedastic**. The left panel of Figure 2.4 shows a schematic representation of the linear model. The expected value of $y$ given $x$ is represented by the straight line while the homoscedastic errors are indicated by identical normal probability density functions. The right panel of Figure 2.4 violates the linear model in that the expected value of $y$ is a non-linear function of $x$, and $y$ has **heteroscedastic** error terms whose standard error increases with increasing $x$.

## 2.6. Fitting the linear regression model

Let us return to the ethylene glycol poisoning example introduced in Section 1.2.9. We wish to fit the linear model $E[y_i \mid x_i] = \alpha + \beta x_i$, where $E[y_i \mid x_i]$ is the expected glycolate value of a patient whose arterial pH is $x_i$. Let $a$ and $b$ be estimates of $\alpha$ and $\beta$. Then $\hat{y}_i = a + bx_i$ is an estimate of $E[y_i \mid x_i]$. The **residual** of $y_i$ given $x_i$ is $y_i - \hat{y}_i$, the difference between the observed value of $y_i$ and its estimated expected value. The dotted lines in Figure 2.5 show these residuals for six of these study subjects. A line that gives a good fit to the data will come as close to as many of the observations as possible. For this reason, we choose as our estimates of $\alpha$ and $\beta$ those values of $a$ and $b$ that minimize the sum of squared residuals for all patients in the observed sample. It can be shown that these estimates are

$$b = rs_y/s_x \tag{2.6}$$

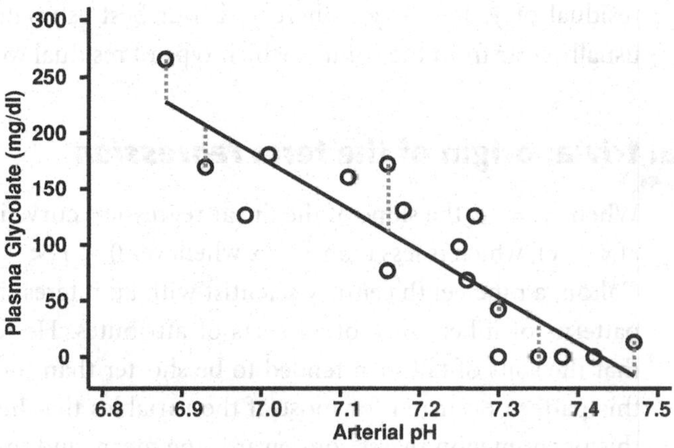


Figure 2.5 The estimated linear regression line is chosen so as to minimize the sum of squared residuals between the observed and expected values of the $y$ variable. The gray dotted lines show the lengths of six of these residuals.

and

$$a = \bar{y} - b\bar{x}. \tag{2.7}$$

The statistic

$$\hat{y}[x] = a + bx \tag{2.8}$$

is called the **least squares estimate** of $\alpha + \beta x$, and Equation (2.8) defines the **linear regression line** of $y_i$ against $x_i$. It can also be shown that $\hat{y}_i = \hat{y}[x_i]$ is an unbiased estimate of $\alpha + \beta x_i$. Substituting Equation (2.7) into Equation (2.8) gives us $\hat{y}[x] - \bar{y} = b(x - \bar{x})$. Hence, the linear regression line always passes through the point $(\bar{x}, \bar{y})$. Since $b = rs_y/s_x$ the slope of the regression line approaches zero as $r$ approaches zero. Thus, if $x$ and $y$ are independent and $n$ is large then $r$ will be very close to zero since $r \cong \rho = 0$, and the regression line will be approximately $\hat{y}(x) = \bar{y}$. This makes sense since if $x$ and $y$ are independent then $x$ is of no value in predicting $y$. On the other hand, if $r = 1$, then the observations lie on the linear regression line (all the residuals are zero). The slope of this line equals $s_y/s_x$, which is the variation of $y_i$ relative to the variation of $x_i$.

Note that we have used the term *residual* in two slightly different ways. In general, the residual for an observation is the difference between the observation and its estimated expected value. When we are looking at a single variable $y_i$ the residual of $y_i$ is $y_i - \bar{y}$, since $\bar{y}$ is our best estimate of $E[y_i]$. This is the definition of residual that we have used before this section. When we have two variables and wish to predict $y_i$ in terms of $x_i$ then the residual of $y_i$ is $y_i - \hat{y}_i$, where $\hat{y}_i$ is our best estimate of $\mathrm{E}[y_i \mid x_i]$. It is usually clear from the context which type of residual we are talking about.

## 2.7. Historical trivia: origin of the term *regression*

When $s_y = s_x$, the slope of the linear regression curve is $r$ and $\hat{y}[x] - \bar{y} = r(x - \bar{x})$, which is less than $x - \bar{x}$ whenever $0 < r < 1$ and $x > \bar{x}$. Francis Galton, a nineteenth century scientist with an interest in eugenics, studied patterns of inheritance of all sorts of attributes. He found, for example, that the sons of tall men tended to be shorter than their fathers, and that this pattern occurred for most of the variables that he studied. He called this phenomenon regression towards the mean, and the origin of the term *linear regression* is from his work. Regression towards the mean will be observed whenever the linear model is valid, the correlation between $x$ and $y$ is between −1 and 1, and the standard deviations of the $x$ and $y$ variables are equal. Had he run his regressions the other way he would have also discovered that the fathers of tall men tend to be shorter than their sons.

Note that the regression line of $x$ on $y$ is not the inverse of the regression line of $y$ on $x$ unless $r = \pm 1$. The reason for this asymmetry is that when we regress $y$ on $x$ we are minimizing the squared residuals of $y$ compared with $\hat{y}[x]$ while when we regress $x$ on $y$ we are minimizing the squared residuals of $x$ compared with $\hat{x}[y]$. Figure 2.6 shows the linear regression lines of $y$ on $x$ and $x$ on $y$ for a positively correlated set of data.

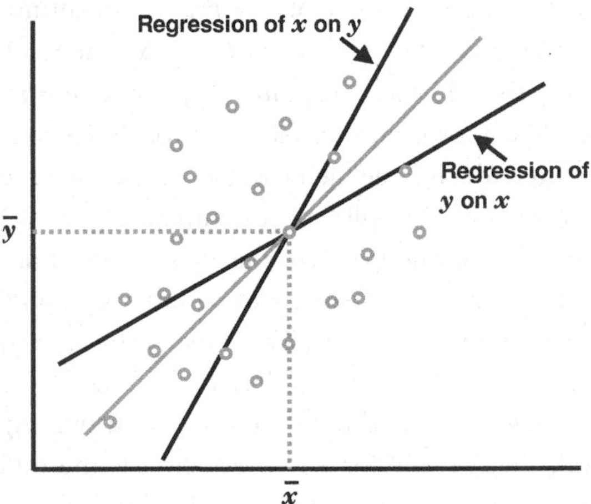


Figure 2.6 Plot of linear regression lines of $y$ on $x$ and $x$ on $y$ for a positively correlated set of data. These plots are not inverses of each other because of the presence of the correlation coefficient in Equation (2.6).

## 2.8. Determining the accuracy of linear regression estimates

In the linear regression model, the error term $\varepsilon_i$ has a normal distribution with mean 0 and standard deviation $\sigma$. We estimate the error variance $\sigma^2$ by

$$s^2 = \sum (y_i - \hat{y}_i)^2/(n-2). \qquad (2.9)$$

The denominator of Equation (2.9) is reduced by two in order to make $s^2$ an unbiased estimate of $\sigma^2$. For large $n$, $s^2$ is very close to the average squared residual of $y_i$. This statistic, $s^2$, is often called the **mean squared error**, or **MSE**; $s$ is called the **root MSE**.

The variance of $b$ can be shown to be

$$\sigma^2 \Big/ \sum (x_i - \bar{x})^2 \qquad (2.10)$$

and the standard error of $b$ is

$$\sigma \Big/ \sqrt{\sum (x_i - \bar{x})^2} = \sigma/(s_x\sqrt{n-1}). \qquad (2.11)$$

This implies that the precision with which we can estimate $b$

(i) decreases as $\sigma$, the standard deviation of $\varepsilon_i$, increases,

(ii) increases as the square root of the sample size increases, and

(iii) increases as the estimated standard deviation of the $x$ variable increases.

The reason why $s_x$ appears in Equation (2.11) can be explained intuitively by looking at Figure 2.7. The panels on this figure depict linear regression models with identical values of $\alpha$ and $\beta$ (indicated by black lines), identical values of $\sigma$, and identical sample sizes. They differ in that the range of the

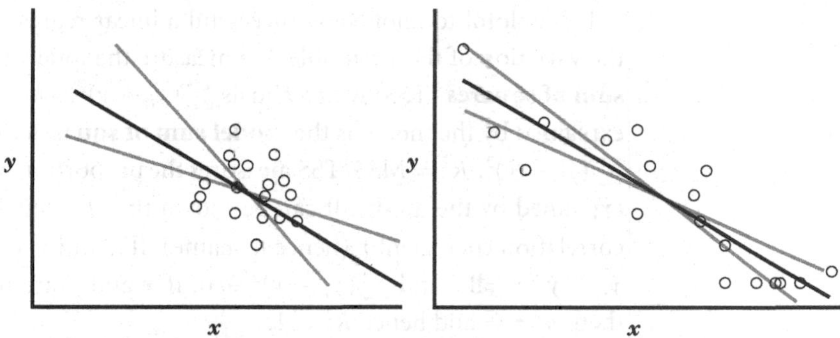


Figure 2.7 The standard error of $b$ is affected by the range of the observed values of $x$ as well as by the sample size and error standard deviation $\sigma$. In both panels of this figure, the regression lines, error standard deviations and sample sizes are identical. They differ in that the range of the $x$ values is greater in the right panel than in the left. This greater variation allows us to estimate the slope parameter with greater precision in the right panel.

$x$ variable in the left panel is less than that on the right. This implies that $s_x$ is smaller for the data in the left panel than it is in the right. The gray lines denote possible estimates of $\alpha + \beta x$ that are compatible with the data. Note that the small range of $x$ in the left panel makes the data compatible with a larger range of slope estimates than is the case for the right panel.

An unbiased estimate of the variance of $b$ is

$$\mathrm{var}[b] = s^2 / \sum (x_i - \bar{x})^2. \tag{2.12}$$

We estimate the standard error of $b$ to be

$$\mathrm{se}[b] = s/(s_x\sqrt{n-1}). \tag{2.13}$$

Under the null hypothesis that $\beta = 0$,

$$b/\mathrm{se}[b] \tag{2.14}$$

has a $t$ distribution with $n - 2$ degrees of freedom. We can use Equation (2.14) to test this null hypothesis. A 95% confidence interval for $\beta$ is given by

$$b \pm t_{n-2,0.025}\mathrm{se}[b]. \tag{2.15}$$

The variance of $a$ is estimated by

$$\mathrm{var}[a] = \frac{s^2}{n} + \bar{x}^2\,\mathrm{var}[b], \tag{2.16}$$

and $a/\sqrt{\mathrm{var}[a]}$ has a $t$ distribution with $n - 2$ degrees of freedom under the null hypothesis that $a = 0$.

It is helpful to know how successful a linear regression is in explaining the variation of the $y$ variable. We measure the total variation by the **total sum of squares** (TSS) which equals $\sum (y_i - \bar{y})^2$. The analogous variation explained by the model is the **model sum of squares** (MSS), which equals $\sum (\hat{y}_i - \bar{y})^2$. $R^2 = \mathrm{MSS}/\mathrm{TSS}$ measures the proportion of the total variation explained by the model. It can be shown that $R^2$ equals the square of the correlation coefficient $r$ (hence its name). If $x$ and $y$ are independent then $\hat{y}_i \cong \bar{y}$ for all $i$ and $\sum (\hat{y}_i - \bar{y})^2 \cong 0$. If $x$ and $y$ are perfectly correlated, then $y_i = \hat{y}_i$ and hence $R^2 = 1$.

## 2.9. Ethylene glycol poisoning example

For the poison data discussed in Section 1.2.9 and throughout this chapter we have that $n = 18$, $\bar{x} = 7.210\,56$, $\bar{y} = 90.44$, $s_x = 0.173\,05$, $s_y = 80.584\,88$ and $r = -0.891\,12$. Hence, Equations (2.6) and (2.7) give that $b = rs_y/s_x$

$= -0.891\,12 \times 80.584\,88/0.173\,05 = -414.97$ and $a = \bar{y} - b\bar{x} = 90.44 - (-414.97 \times 7.210\,56) = 3082.6$. The estimate of $\sigma$ is

$$s = \sqrt{\sum (y_i - \hat{y}_i)^2/(n-2)} = 37.693. \tag{2.17}$$

The estimated standard error of $b$ is

$$\text{se}[b] = s/(s_x\sqrt{n-1}) = 37.693/(0.173\,05\sqrt{18-1}) = 52.83. \tag{2.18}$$

To test the null hypothesis that $\beta = 0$ we calculate $t = b/\text{se}[b] = -414.97/52.83 = 7.85$, which has a $t$ distribution with 16 degrees of freedom ($P < 0.0005$). Hence, we can accept the alternative hypothesis that glycolate levels fall with increasing pH. Now $t_{16,0.025} = 2.12$. Therefore, a 95% confidence interval for $b$ is $b \pm t_{n-2,0.025}\,\text{se}(b) = -414.97 \pm t_{16,0.025} \times 52.83 = -414.97 \pm 2.12 \times 52.83 = (-527, -303)$.

## 2.10. 95% confidence interval for $y[x] = \alpha + \beta x$ evaluated at $x$

Let $y[x] = \alpha + \beta x$ be the expected value of $y$ given $x$. Then $y[x]$ is estimated by $\hat{y}[x] = a + bx$. The expected value of $\hat{y}[x]$ given $x$ is $\text{E}[\hat{y}[x] \mid x] = y[x]$ and the estimated variance of $\hat{y}[x]$ given $x$ is

$$\text{var}[\hat{y}[x] \mid x] = (s^2/n) + (x - \bar{x})^2\,\text{var}[b]. \tag{2.19}$$

Since the regression line goes through the point $(\bar{x}, \bar{y})$, we have that $\hat{y}[\bar{x}] = \bar{y}$ and Equation (2.19) reduces to $s^2/n$ when $x = \bar{x}$. The farther $x$ is from $\bar{x}$ the greater the variance of $\hat{y}[x]$ and the greater the influence of var$[b]$ in determining this variance. This reflects the fact that errors in the estimate of $\beta$ are amplified as $x$ moves away from $\bar{x}$. The 95% confidence interval for $\hat{y}[x]$ is

$$\hat{y}[x] \pm t_{n-2,0.025}\sqrt{\text{var}[\hat{y}[x] \mid x]}. \tag{2.20}$$

For example, suppose that we wanted to estimate a 95% confidence interval for the expected glycolate level of patients with an arterial pH of 7.0 who have been poisoned by ethylene glycol. Then $\hat{y}[7.0] = a + 7.0b = 3082.6 - 7.0 \times 414.97 = 177.81$, $\text{var}[\hat{y}[7.0] \mid x = 7] = [s^2/n] + (7.0 - \bar{x})^2\,\text{var}[b] = 37.693^2/18 + (7.0 - 7.210\,56)^2 \times 52.83^2 = 202.7$ and a 95% confidence interval for $\hat{y}(7.0)$ is $177.81 \pm 2.12\sqrt{202.7} = (148, 208)$. Figure 2.8 shows a plot of Equation (2.8) for the poison data with a shaded 95% confidence band defined by Equation (2.20). Note that these confidence limits indicate the plausible degree of error in our estimate of the regression line $y[x] = \alpha + \beta x$. They do not

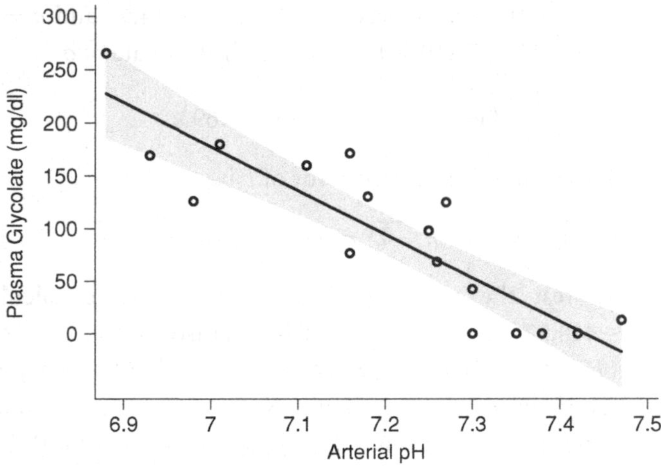


Figure 2.8 This graph shows the estimated linear regression line of plasma glycolate against arterial pH (Brent et al., 1999). The gray band in this graph shows the 95% confidence intervals for the expected glycolate response $E[\hat{y}(x) \mid x] = \alpha + \beta x$.

indicate the likely range of the observed values of $y_i$, and indeed the observations for half of the patients lie outside these bounds. Note also that the linear regression model assumptions are false for larger pH values since the glycolate values cannot be less than zero. Nevertheless, the overall fit of the data to this linear model appears to be excellent.

## 2.11. 95% prediction interval for the response of a new patient

Sometimes we would like to predict the likely range of response for a new patient given her value of the $x$ variable. Under the linear model we can write her response as $y[x] = \alpha + \beta x + \varepsilon_i \cong \hat{y}[x] + \varepsilon_i$. It can be shown for any two independent variables $u$ and $v$ with variances $\sigma_u^2$ and $\sigma_v^2$ that the variance of $u + v$ is $\sigma_u^2 + \sigma_v^2$. Hence $\mathrm{var}[y \mid x] \cong \mathrm{var}[\hat{y}[x] \mid x] + \mathrm{var}[\varepsilon_i] = \mathrm{var}[\hat{y}(x) \mid x] + \sigma^2$, and a **95% prediction interval** for $y$ can be estimated by

$$\hat{y}[x] \pm t_{n-2,0.025}\sqrt{\mathrm{var}[\hat{y}[x] \mid x] + s^2}. \qquad (2.21)$$

That is, the probability that her response will lie in the interval given by Equation (2.21) is 0.95. For example, suppose that a new patient poisoned with ethylene glycol has an arterial pH of 7.0. Then $\hat{y}[7.0] = 177.81$, $\mathrm{var}[\hat{y}[7.0] \mid x = 7] = 202.7$, $s = 37.693$ and a 95% prediction interval for

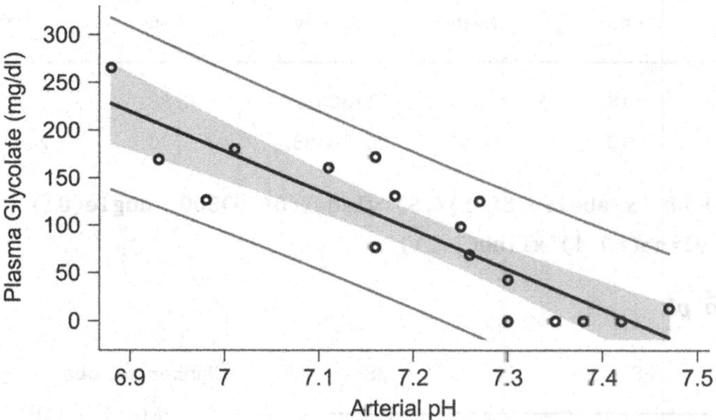


Figure 2.9 The gray lines on this graph show 95% prediction intervals for the plasma glycolate levels of new patients based on the data from Brent et al. (1999).

$y$ at $x = 7.0$ is $177.81 \pm 2.12\sqrt{202.7 + 37.693^2} = (92.4, 263)$. In Figure 2.9 the gray lines show the 95% prediction intervals for new patients poisoned by ethylene glycol. Note that we can make the 95% confidence interval for $\hat{y}[x]$ as narrow as we want by choosing a sufficiently large sample size. The lower limit on the width of the 95% prediction interval for new observations, however, is constrained by the standard deviation of $\varepsilon_i$ for individual observations.

## 2.12. Simple linear regression with Stata

The following log file and comments illustrates how to use Stata to perform the calculations discussed in the previous sections.

```
. *   2.12.Poison.log
. *
. *  Calculate the mean plasma glycolate and arterial pH levels for
. *  the ethylene glycol poisoning data of Brent et al. (1999).
. *  Regress glycolate levels against pH.  Draw a scatter plot of
. *  glycolate against pH.  Plot the linear regression line on this
. *  scatter plot together with the 95% confidence limits for this
. *  line and the 95% prediction intervals for new patients.
. *
. use C:\WDDtext\2.12.Poison.dta, clear                                   1

. summarize ph glyco
```

```
    Variable |       Obs        Mean    Std. Dev.       Min        Max
-------------+--------------------------------------------------------
          ph |        18    7.210556    .1730512       6.88       7.47
       glyco |        18       90.44    80.58488          0     265.24

. scatter glyco ph, xlabel(6.8(.1)7.5) ylabel(0(50)300, angle(0))      2
>   symbol(Oh) yline(90.4) xline(7.21)                                 3

. regress glyco ph                                                     4

      Source |       SS       df       MS              Number of obs =      18      5
-------------+------------------------------           F(  1,    16) =   61.70
       Model |  87664.6947     1  87664.6947           Prob > F      =  0.0000      6
    Residual |  22731.9877    16  1420.74923           R-squared     =  0.7941      7
-------------+------------------------------           Adj R-squared =  0.7812
       Total |  110396.682    17  6493.9225            Root MSE      =  37.693      8

------------------------------------------------------------------------------
       glyco |      Coef.   Std. Err.      t    P>|t|     [95% Conf. Interval]
-------------+----------------------------------------------------------------
          ph |  -414.9666   52.82744    -7.86   0.000    -526.9558   -302.9775    9
       _cons |    3082.58   381.0188     8.09   0.000     2274.856    3890.304    10
------------------------------------------------------------------------------

. predict yhat, xb                                                     11

. scatter glyco  ph || line yhat ph                                    12
>     , ylabel(0(50)250) xlabel(6.9(.1)7.5)                            13
>       ytitle(Plasma Glycolate (mg/dl)) legend(off)                   14

. *
. *  The preceding graph could also have been generated without
. *  explicitly calculating yhat as follows.
. *
. scatter glyco ph || lfit glyco ph                                    15
>     , ylabel(0(50)250) xlabel(6.9(.1)7.5)
>       ytitle(Plasma Glycolate (mg/dl)) legend(off)

. *
. *  Add 95% confidence interval bands to the preceding graph.
. *
. twoway lfitci  glyco ph || scatter glyco ph                          16
```

```
>      , ylabel(0(50)300) xlabel(6.9 (.1) 7.5)
>        ytitle(Plasma Glycolate (mg/dl)) legend(off)

. *
. *  Add 95% prediction interval bands to the preceding graph.
. *
. twoway lfitci glyco ph
>      , stdf ciplot(rline) color(gray) lwidth(medthick)          17
>      || lfitci glyco ph, lpattern(solid)                        18
>      || scatter glyco ph
>      , ylabel(0(50)300) xlabel(6.9 (.1) 7.5)
>        ytitle(Plasma Glycolate (mg/dl)) legend(off)
```

**Comments**

1 The *2.12.Poison.dta* data set contains the plasma glycolate and arterial pH levels of 18 patients admitted for ethylene glycol poisoning. These levels are stored in variables called *glyco* and *ph*, respectively. The *clear* option of the *use* command deletes any data that may have been in memory when this command was given.

2 This *scatter* command draws a scatter plot of *glyco* by *ph*. The options following the comma improve the visual appearance of the scatter plot. The *xlabel* option labels the $x$-axis from 6.8 to 7.5 in even increments 0.1 units apart. Similarly, the *ylabel* option labels the $y$-axis from 0 to 300. The *angle(0)* suboption of the *ylabel* option orients these labels parallel to the $x$-axis (*angle(0)* means that the angle between the orientation of the text and the $x$-axis is zero degrees). This suboption must be used if you want the $y$-axis labels to have this orientation and you are using Stata's default scheme (see Section 1.3.6).

3 Stata commands can often be too long to fit on a single line of a log file or the Command window. When this happens the command wraps onto the next line. A ">" symbol at the beginning of a line indicates the continuation of the preceding command rather than the start of a new one. On the command line you cannot control when the line breaks occur. In this text I have placed the line breaks to increase legibility of the commands. This line, and the next, contain options that affect the appearance of the preceding graph.

The *symbol(Oh)* option causes the plot symbol to be a large open circle. This option must be used if you want an open plot symbol and you are using the default Stata scheme (see Section 1.3.6). The *xline* and *yline* options draw vertical and horizontal lines at $x = 7.21$ and $y = 90.4$

respectively. The default titles of the *x*- and *y*-axes are labels assigned to the *ph* and *glyco* variables in the *Poison.dta* data set.

The resulting graph is similar to Figure 2.2. (In this latter figure I used a graphics editor to annotate the mean glycolate and pH values and to indicate the residuals for three data points.) The point-and-click version of this command is Graphics ▶ Twoway graph (scatter plot, line etc) ⌋Plots⌊ [Create] ⌋Plot⌊ ┌ Plot type: (scatter plot) — Y variable: *glyco* , X variable: *ph* [Marker properties] ⌋Main⌊ ┌ Marker properties — Symbol: *Hollow Circle* ⌋ [Accept] ⌋ [Accept] ⌋Y axis⌊ [Major tick/label properties] ⌋Rule⌊ ┌ Axis rule — ⦿ Range/Delta , *0* Minimum value , *300* Maximum value , *50* Delta ⌋ ⌋Labels⌊ ┌ Labels — Angle: *0* ⌋ [Accept] [Reference lines] ┌ [✓] Add lines to graph at specified y axis values: *90.4* [Accept] ⌋X axis⌊ [Major tick/label properties] ⌋Rule⌊ ┌ Axis rule — ⦿ Range/Delta , *6.8* Minimum value , *7.5* Maximum value , *.1* Delta ⌋ [Accept] [Reference lines] ┌ [✓] Add lines to graph at specified x axis values: *7.21* [Accept] [Submit].

The *scatter* command is a particular case of the *graph twoway* command, which draws many different types of plots of one variable against another. The commands

```
graph twoway scatter yvar xvar
twoway scatter yvar xvar
```

and

```
scatter yvar xvar
```

are all equivalent. Stata permits the words *graph twoway* to be omitted from the *scatter* command.

4 This command performs a linear regression of *glyco* against *ph*. That is, we fit the model $E[glyco \mid ph] = \alpha + \beta \times ph$ (see Equation 2.5). The most important output from this command has been highlighted and is defined below. The point-and-click version of this command is Statistics ▶ Linear models and related ▶ Linear regression ⌋Model⌊ Dependent Variable: *glyco* , Independent variables: *ph* [Submit].

5 The number of patients $n = 18$.

6 The model sum of squares is MSS = 87 664.6947.

7 $R^2 = \text{MSS}/\text{TSS} = 0.7941$. Hence 79% of the variation in glycolate levels is explained by this linear regression.

8 The root MSE is $s = 37.693$ (see Equation 2.9). The total sum of squares is TSS = 110 396.682.

9 The slope estimate of $\beta$ for this linear regression is $b = -414.9666$ (see Equation 2.6). The estimated standard error of $b$ is $\text{se}[b] = 52.827\,44$ (see Equation 2.13). The $t$ statistic to test the null hypothesis that $\beta = 0$ is $t = b/\text{se}[b] = -7.86$ (see Equation 2.14). The $P$-value associated with this statistic is less than 0.0005. The 95% confidence interval for $\beta$ is (–526.9558, –302.9775) (see Equation 2.15).

10 The $y$ intercept estimate of $\alpha$ for this linear regression is $a = 3082.58$ (see Equation 2.7).

11 The *predict* command can estimate a variety of statistics after a regression or other estimation command. (Stata refers to such commands as post-estimation commands.) The *xb* option causes a new variable (in this example *yhat*) to be set equal to each patient's expected plasma glycolate level $\hat{y}[x] = a + bx$; in this equation, $x$ is the patient's arterial pH and $a$ and $b$ are the parameter estimates of the linear regression (see also Equation 2.8). The equivalent point-and-click command is Statistics ▶ Postestimation ▶ Predictions, residuals, etc. Main New variable name: *yhat* Submit.

12 This command overlays a line plot of *yhat* against *ph* on a scatter plot of *glyco* against *ph*. In a line plot the individual points defined by each patient's values of the $x$ and $y$ variables are joined by a straight line. These points are joined in the same order that they are found in the data set. The two vertical bars indicate that both plots are to be drawn on the same graph. The net effect of this command is to produce a scatter plot of glycolate against pH together with a straight line indicating the expected glycolate levels as a function of pH. The resulting graph is shown in Figure 2.1.

13 Note that in Figure 2.1 the labels on the $y$-axis have a horizontal orientation even though I did not specify an *angle(0)* suboption on the *ylabel* option. This is because the figures in this text were generated using a Stata scheme that is given on my web page. In this scheme, the default orientation of $y$-axis labels is horizontal. In the standard Stata schemes, this orientation is parallel to the $y$-axis. If you are using a standard Stata scheme and you wish a horizontal orientation for your $y$-axis labels you need to specify the *angle(0)* suboption. Another difference between my schemes and the standard Stata schemes is that my default plot symbol for small graphs is the large open circle used in Figure 2.1, while the

standard Stata schemes use a solid circle. To implement large open circle symbols using a standard Stata scheme you must use the *symbol(Oh)* option. (Small open circles are implemented with the *symbol(oh)* option.) A strength of Stata is that it is very easy to create your own schemes. This means that if you are using the same options in many graphs it may make more sense to specify them once in a scheme than repeatedly in all of your graphs. See Section 1.3.6 for additional information.

14 The *ytitle* option gives a title to the *y*-axis. By default Stata provides a figure legend whenever more than one plot is drawn on the same graph. This legend is deleted by the *legend(off)* option.

Stata remembers the last point-and-click command that you gave of a given type. This allows us to modify old commands to create new ones. If we have already given the point-and-click commands in Comment 3 we can modify this command to create Figure 2.1 by overlaying the regression line on the previously created scatter plot, adding a title to the *y*-axis, changing the range of the *y*-variable, and removing the horizontal and vertical reference lines. This is done as follows: Graphics ► Twoway graph (scatter plot, line etc) ⌋ Plots ⌊ [Create] ⌋ Plot ⌊ ┌ Choose a plot category and type — Basic plots: (select type) *Line* ⌋ ┌ Plot type: (line plot) — Y variable: *yhat* , X variable: *ph* ⌋ [Accept] ⌋ Y axis ⌊ Title: *Plasma Glycolate (mg/dl)* [Major tick/label properties] ⌋ Rule ⌊ ┌ Axis rule — *250* Maximum value ⌋ [Accept] [Reference lines] ┌ ☐ Add lines to graph at specified y axis values: [Accept] ⌋ X axis ⌊ [Reference lines] ┌ ☐ Add lines to graph at specified y axis values: [Accept] ⌋ Legend ⌊ ┌ Legend behavior — ⦿ Hide legend ⌋ [Submit].

15 The *lfit* command is another component of the twoway graph command. This command regresses *glyco* against *ph* and draws the linear regression line. You do not need to explicitly run the *regress* command or calculate *yhat*. The point-and-click equivalent command is identical to the one given above except that the overlayed plot (Plot 2) is specified by [Create] ⌋ Plot ⌊ ┌ Choose a plot category and type — ⦿ Fit plots ⌋ ┌ Plot type: (linear prediction plot) — Y variable: *glyco* , X variable: *ph* ⌋ [Accept].

16 The *lfitci* command plots the same linear regression line as the *lfit* command. In addition, it calculates the 95% confidence band for this line

using Equation (2.20). By default, this band is shown as a shaded region. A scatter plot is overlayed on top of the *lfitci* plot. Overlayed plots are drawn in the order that they are specified. Hence, it is important that the *lfitci* plot precede the scatter plot so that the former does not mask any of the scatter plot observations. When the *lfitci* command is given first as in this example, *lfitci* must be preceded by the word *twoway*. This command generates Figure 2.8. If we have already created Figure 2.1 with the point-and-click interface then the point-and-click command for Figure 2.8 is Graphics ▶ Twoway graph (scatterplot, line etc) ⌋ Plots ⌊ Plot definitions: *Plot 1* [Edit] ⌋ Plot ⌊ ⌜ Choose a plot category and type — ⊙ Fit plots, Fit plots: (select type) *Linear prediction w/CI* ⌟ ⌜ Plot type: (linear prediction plot with confidence intervals) — Y variable: *glyco* , X variable: *ph* ⌟ [Accept] Plot definitions: *Plot 2* [Edit] ⌋ Plot ⌊ ⌜ Choose a plot category and type — ⊙ Basic plots ⌟ ⌜ Plot type: (scatter plot) — Y variable: *glyco* , X variable: *ph* ⌟ [Accept] ⌋ Y axis ⌊ [Major tick/label properties] ⌋ Rule ⌊ ⌜ Axis rule — *300* Maximum value ⌟ [Accept] [Submit].

17 The *stdf* option causes the *lfitci* command to draw the 95% prediction (forecast) interval for the response of a new patient; *ciplot(rline)* causes this interval to be denoted by two lines rather than a shaded region; *color(gray)* and *lwidth(medthick)* specify that these lines are gray and of medium thickness, respectively.

This command creates a graph that is similar to Figure 2.9. The *color* option can also be used to select the color or plot-symbols or shaded regions. The equivalent point-and-click command that adds these forecast intervals to the graph generated by the previous point-and-click command is Graphics ▶ Twoway graph (scatter plot, line etc) ⌋ Plots ⌊ [Create] ⌋ Plot ⌊ ⌜ Choose a plot category and type — ⊙ Fit plots, Fit plots: (select type) *Linear prediction w/CI* ⌟ ⌜ Plot type: (linear prediction plot with confidence intervals) — Y variable: *glyco* , X variable: *ph* [Options] ⌋ Main ⌊ ⌜ Basis for confidence intervals — ⊙ Confidence interval for an individual forecast ⌟ ⌜ Plots — Plot type of CI: *Range line* [Line properties] ⌜ Color: *Gray* , Width: *Medium thick* [Accept] ⌟ [Accept] ⌟ [Accept] [Submit].

18 This *lpattern(solid)* option draws a solid black line for the regression curve. In overlayed two-way graphs like this one, the default colors and patterns of lines are determined by the Stata scheme that is in effect when the command is given. Stata schemes assign default options to plots in the order that they are given. In this graph the first two plots are for the prediction interval and the regression line of the first *lfitci* command. The third plot is the regression line from the second *liftci* command. In the *WDDtext* schemes used in this text the default patterns for the first two plots are solid and the third plot is a dashed line. I have used the *lpattern(solid)* option here to override this default pattern.

## 2.13. Lowess regression

Linear regression is a useful tool for describing a relationship that is linear, or approximately linear. It has the disadvantage that the linear relationship is assumed a priori. It is often useful to fit a line through a scatter plot that does not make any model assumptions. One such technique is **lowess regression**, which stands for locally weighted scatter plot smoothing (Cleveland, 1993). The idea is that each observation $(x_i, y_i)$ is fitted to a separate linear regression line based on adjacent observations. These points are weighted so that the farther away the $x$ value is from $x_i$, the less effect it has on determining the estimate of $\hat{y}_i$. The proportion of the total data set that is considered for each estimate $\hat{y}_i$ is called the **bandwidth**. In Stata, the default bandwidth is 0.8, which works well for midsize data sets. For large data sets a bandwidth of 0.3 or 0.4 usually works best; a bandwidth of 0.99 is recommended for small data sets. The wider the bandwidth the smoother the regression curve. Narrow bandwidths produce curves that are more sensitive to local perturbations in the data. Experimenting with different bandwidths helps to find a curve that is sensitive to real trends in the data without being unduly affected by random variation. The lowess method is computationally intensive on large data sets. Reducing the bandwidth will reduce the time needed to derive these curves.

The black curve in Figure 2.10 shows a lowess regression curve for the ethylene glycol poisoning data. It was drawn with a bandwidth of 0.99. The gray line in this graph marks the least squares linear regression line. These two curves are similar for pHs lower than 7.4. There is evidence of a mild departure from the linear model for the larger pH values that are associated with glycolate values at, or near, zero.

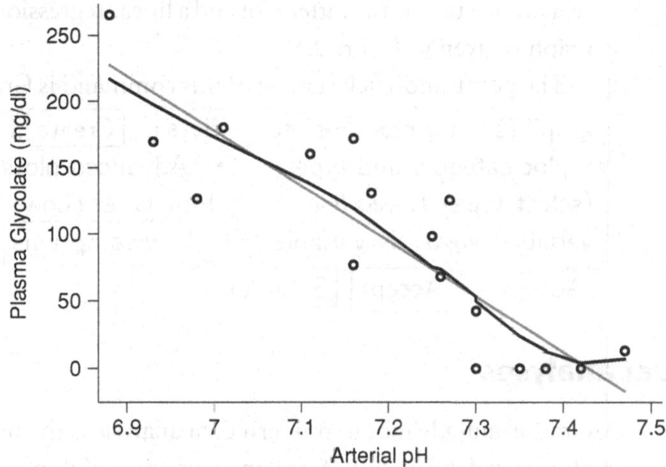


Figure 2.10 The black line shows the lowess regression curve for the ethylene glycol poisoning data (Brent et al., 1999). This curve closely approximates the linear regression curve over most of the observed range of arterial pH.

## 2.14. Plotting a lowess regression curve in Stata

The *2.12.Poison.log* file that was started in Section 2.12 continues as follows.

```
. *
. *  Derive a lowess regression curve for the ethylene glycol
. *  poisoning data using a bandwidth of 0.99.  Plot this curve
. *  together with the linear regression line and a scatterplot of
. *  plasma glycolate by arterial pH levels.
. *
. twoway lfit glyco ph, lcolor(gray)
>      || scatter glyco ph
>      || lowess glyco ph, bwidth(.99) lpattern(solid)                1
>     , xlabel(6.9 (.1) 7.5) ylabel(0(50)250)
>       ytitle(Plasma Glycolate (mg/dl)) legend(off)

. log close
```

**Comment**

1 Another type of graph generated by the *twoway* command is the lowess regression curve. The command on this line generates a lowess plot of *glyco* versus *ph*. The default bandwidth for lowess regression is 0.8. To use a different bandwidth add the *bwidth(#)* option, where # is a number greater than zero and less than one. In this example I have chosen a bandwidth of 0.99. The complete *twoway* command in this example overlays a lowess

regression curve on a scatter plot and a linear regression line. The resulting graph is given in Figure 2.10.

The point-and-click version of this command is Graphics ▶ Twoway graph (scatter plot, line etc) ⌋ Plots ⌊ [Create] ⌋ Plot ⌊ ⌈ Choose a plot category and type — ⦿ Advanced plots, Advanced plots: (select type) *Lowess line* ⌋ ⌈ Plot type: (Lowess line plot) — Y variable: *glyco* , X variable: *ph* [Lowess options] ⌈ *.99* Bandwidth [Accept] ⌋ [Accept] [Submit].

## 2.15. Residual analyses

An important advance in modern data analysis is the use of computers for exploratory data analysis. Such analyses are useful in determining whether a given model is appropriate for a given data set or whether specific observations are having excessive influence on the conclusions of our analyses. One of these techniques is residual analysis. In linear regression the residual for the $i^{th}$ patient is $e_i = y_i - \hat{y}_i$ (see Section 2.6). Figure 2.11 shows a linear regression of systolic blood pressure (SBP) against body mass index (BMI) for 25 patients from the Framingham Heart Study (Levy, 1999). The solid line shows the estimated expected SBP derived from all 25 patients.

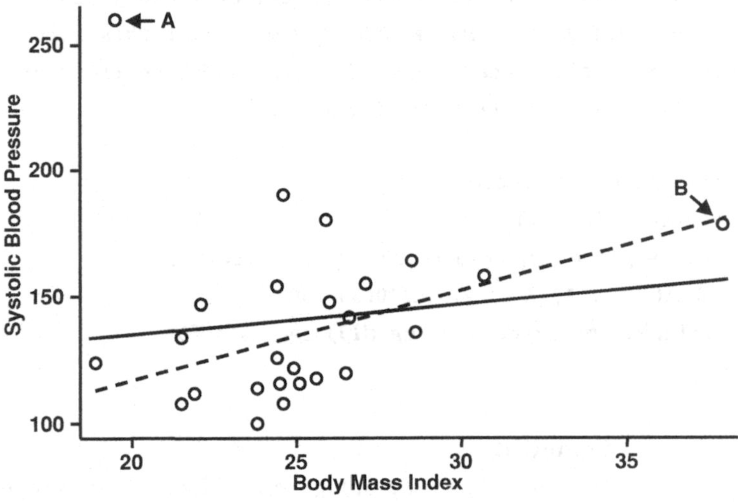


Figure 2.11 Regression of systolic blood pressure against body mass index. The solid line includes all patients in the regression. The dashed line excludes Patient A. Patient A exerts a large influence on the regression line. Patients A and B both have high leverage because they are both far from the mean body mass index. However, Patient B has little influence because her systolic blood pressure falls near the regression line.

Note that patient A has an observed SBP of 260 and an expected SBP of 134 giving a very large residual 260−134 = 126. If we delete this patient from the analysis the regression line shifts to the dashed line in Figure 2.11. The solid and dashed lines in this figure have slopes of 1.19 and 3.53, respectively. Thus, the deletion of this single data point causes a three-fold increase in the regression slope. This data point is said to have great **influence** on our slope estimate. The reason for this is partly because of the large residual and partly because the patient's BMI is fairly far from the mean BMI value. Recall that the regression line is fitted by minimizing the sum of the squared residuals. Rotating the dashed line in a clockwise direction towards the solid line reduces the squared residual for patient A more than it increases the squared residuals for all other patients.

The potential for an independent variable value to influence the results is quantified by its **leverage**, which is given by the formula

$$h_j = \frac{1}{n} + \frac{(\bar{x} - x_j)^2}{\sum_i (\bar{x} - x_i)^2}. \qquad (2.22)$$

The leverage is minimized when $\bar{x} = x_j$, in which case $h_j = 1/n$. A large residual with little leverage will have little effect on the parameter estimates, particularly if the sample size, $n$, is large. It can be shown that $h_j$ always lies between $1/n$ and 1. Data points with high leverage will have great influence if the associated residual is large. In Figure 2.11 patient B has high leverage but little influence since the regression lines pass near the data point. This is particularly true of the regression in which patient A is omitted. Note that the leverage is determined entirely by the values of the $x$ variable and is not affected by the $y$ variable.

We can rewrite Equation (2.19) using Equation (2.22) as

$$\text{var}[\hat{y}_i \mid x_i] = s^2 h_i. \qquad (2.23)$$

Hence, an alternative definition of $h_i$ is that it is the variance of $\hat{y}_i$ given $x_i$ expressed in units of $s^2$. If $x$ is the covariate of a new patient with leverage $h$ then the estimated variance of her predicted response $y$ given $x$ is

$$\text{var}[y \mid x] = s^2(h + 1). \qquad (2.24)$$

Thus, we can rewrite the 95% prediction interval for $y$ (Equation (2.21)) as

$$\hat{y}[x] \pm t_{n-2,0.025}(s\sqrt{h+1}). \qquad (2.25)$$

We will discuss the concepts of influence and leverage in greater detail in the next chapter.

The variance of the residual $e_i$ is

$$\text{var}[e_i] = s^2(1 - h_i). \qquad (2.26)$$

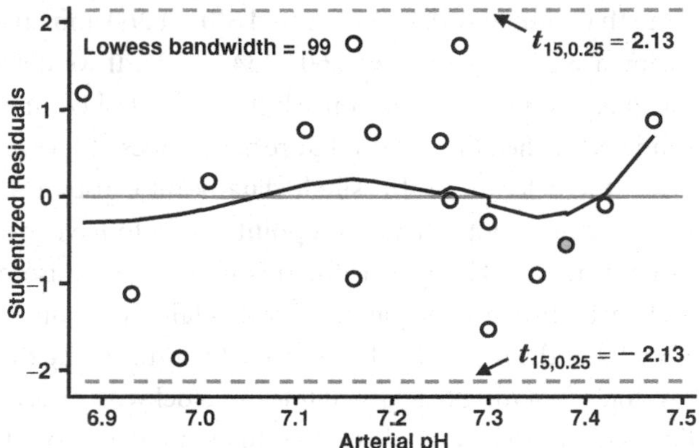


Figure 2.12 Scatter plot of studentized residuals against arterial pH for the linear regression performed in Section 2.9. A lowess regression is fitted to these residuals.

Note that high leverage reduces the variance of $e_i$ because the data point tends to pull the regression line towards it, thereby reducing the variation of the residual. (In the extreme case when $h_i = 1$ the regression line always goes through the $i^{\text{th}}$ data point giving a residual of zero. Hence the variance of $e_i$ also equals zero.) Dividing $e_i$ by its standard deviation gives the **standardized residual** for the $i^{\text{th}}$ patient, which is

$$z_i = e_i/(s\sqrt{1 - h_i}). \tag{2.27}$$

Large standardized residuals identify values of $y_i$ that are outliers and are not consistent with the linear model. A problem with Equation (2.27) is that a single large residual can inflate the value of $s^2$, which in turn will decrease the size of the standardized residuals. To avoid this problem, we usually calculate **the studentized residual**

$$t_i = e_i/(s_{(i)}\sqrt{1 - h_i}), \tag{2.28}$$

where $s_{(i)}$ denotes the root MSE estimate of $\sigma$ with the $i^{\text{th}}$ case deleted ($t_i$ is sometimes referred to as the **jackknife residual**). If the linear model is correct, then $t_i$ should have a $t$ distribution with $n - 3$ degrees of freedom. Plotting these residuals against $x_i$ is useful for assessing the homoscedasticity assumption and detecting departures from linearity. Figure 2.12 shows a plot of studentized residuals against pH values for the linear regression performed in Section 2.9. A lowess regression curve of the studentized residuals against pH is also plotted. This curve should be flat and close to zero when the regression is from a large data set in which the linear model is valid. Dashed horizontal lines are drawn at $\pm t_{n-3,0.25} = \pm t_{15,0.25} = \pm 2.13$; if the model is correct 95% of the residuals should lie between these dotted lines. This is, in fact, the case and there is no obvious pattern in the distribution of the residuals. The variation of the residuals does not appear to vary with pH and the lowess regression curve is fairly flat and close to zero. Hence, this graph suggests that the linear regression model is appropriate for these data.

It is always a good idea to double check data points with large studentized residuals. They may indicate data errors or some anomaly in the way the experiment was conducted. If the data point is valid but has high influence you may wish to report your findings both with and without this data point included in the analysis.

## 2.16. Studentized residual analysis using Stata

The following log file and comments illustrate a residual analysis of the ethylene glycol poison data.

```
. *  2.16.Poison.log
. *
. *  Perform a residual analysis of the linear regression of plasma
. *  glycolate against arterial pH from the poison data set
. *  (Brent et al. 1999).
. *
. use C:\WDDtext\2.12.Poison.dta, clear

. regress glyco ph
                                        Output omitted. See Section 2.12

. predict residual, rstudent                                           1

. display _N                                                           2

18

. display invttail(_N-3,.025)                                          3

2.1314495

. scatter residual ph || lowess residual ph, bwidth(.99)               4
>     , yscale(range(-2.13 2.13))  xlabel(6.9 (.1)7.5)                 5
>       yline(-2.13 2.13, lcolor(gray) lpattern(dash))                 6
>       yline(0, lcolor(gray)) legend(off)

. log close
```

**Comments**

1 The *rstudent* option of the *predict* command causes studentized residuals to be derived and stored in the specified variable – in this case *residual.* The equivalent point-and-click command is Statistics ▶ Postestimation ▶ Predictions, residuals, etc ⌡Main⌊ New variable name: *residual* ┌ Produce: — ⊙ Studentized residuals ┘ [Submit].

2 The *display* command calculates and displays a numeric expression or constant. *_N* denotes the number of observations in the data set, which in this example is 18.

3 The Stata function *invttail*($n$, $1 - \alpha$) calculates a critical value of size $\alpha$ for a $t$ distribution with $n$ degrees of freedom. Thus, $invttail(\_N - 3, 0.025) = invttail(15, 0.025) = t_{15,0.025} = 2.131\,449\,5$. If the linear model is correct 95% of the studentized residuals should lie between $\pm 2.13$.

4 This command draws a graph that is similar to Figure 2.12. In this figure, some annotation has been added using a graphics editor.

5 This *yscale* option forces the $y$-axis to extend from $-2.13$ to 2.13 in spite of the fact that none of the residuals have a magnitude that is this large.

6 The *yline* options on this and the next line draw horizontal lines at $-2.13$, 0 and 2.13. They are colored gray by the *lcolor(gray)* suboption. The *lpattern(dash)* suboption causes the upper and lower lines to be dashed. Note that a comma is needed between 2.13 and *lcolor(gray)* to distinguish values at which lines are drawn from the suboptions that specify the color and pattern of these lines. The point-and-click equivalent commands for these *yscale* and *yline* commands are given on the *Y axis* tab of the *Twoway* dialog box as follows: ⌡Y axis⌊ [Axis scale properties] ┌ ┌ [✓] Extend range of axis scale — Lower limit *-2.13* , Upper limit: *2.13* , ┘ [Accept] [Reference lines] ┌ [✓] Add lines to graph at specified y axis values: *-2.13 0 2.13* , Pattern *Dash* , Color *Gray* [Accept] [Submit]. Note that this dialog box is unable to create horizontal lines with multiple colors or patterns. To do this, you must enter multiple *yline* options in the command window as is illustrated above.

## 2.17. Transforming the $x$ and $y$ variables

### 2.17.1. Stabilizing the variance

Suppose that we regress $y$ against $x$, and then perform a residual plot as in Section 2.15. If this plot shows evidence of heteroscedasticity we can sometimes rectify the problem by transforming the $y$ variable. If the residual standard deviation appears to be proportional to the expected value $\hat{y}_i$, try using a **logarithmic transformation**. That is, try the model

$$\log[y_i] = \alpha + \beta x_i + \varepsilon_i. \tag{2.29}$$

If the residual variance is proportional to the expected value $\hat{y}_i$, then the **square root transform**

$$\sqrt{y_i} = \alpha + \beta x_i + \varepsilon_i \tag{2.30}$$

will stabilize the variance. Note, however, that transforming the $y$ variable affects the shape of the curve $\log[\hat{y}[x]]$ as well as the residual standard deviation. Hence, if the relationship between $x$ and $y$ is linear but the residual standard deviation increases with $\hat{y}_i$, then Equation (2.29) may stabilize the residual variance but impose an invalid non-linear relationship between $E[y_i]$ and $x_i$. In this case we can transform the data to stabilize the residual variance and then use a restricted cubic spline regression model. We will discuss how to do this in Sections 3.24 and 3.25. Other non-linear regression methods that can be used are discussed by Hamilton (1992) and Draper and Smith (1998).

### 2.17.2. Correcting for non-linearity

Figure 2.13 shows four common patterns on non-linearity between $x$ and $y$ variables. If $x$ is positive, then models of the form

$$y_i = \alpha + \beta(x_i)^p + \varepsilon_i, \tag{2.31}$$

$$y_i = \alpha + \beta \log[x_i] + \varepsilon_i, \text{ or} \tag{2.32}$$

$$y_i = \alpha + \beta \sqrt[p]{x_i} + \varepsilon_i \tag{2.33}$$

should be considered for some $p > 1$. Data similar to panels A and B of this figure may be modeled with Equation (2.31). Data similar to panels C and D may be modeled with Equation (2.32) or (2.33). The best value of $p$ is found empirically. Alternatively, data similar to panels A or C may be modeled with

$$\log[y_i] = \alpha + \beta x_i + \varepsilon_i \tag{2.34}$$

or

$$\sqrt[p]{y_i} = \alpha + \beta x_i + \varepsilon_i. \tag{2.35}$$

Data similar to panels B or D may be modeled with

$$y_i^p = \alpha + \beta x_i + \varepsilon_i. \tag{2.36}$$

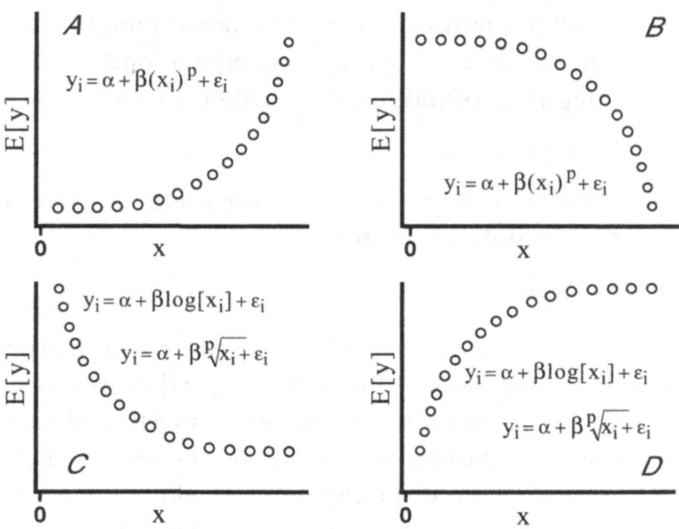


Figure 2.13 Transforms to consider to achieve a linear relationship between $\text{E}[y_i]$ and either $\log[x_i]$, $(x_i)^p$, or $\sqrt[p]{x_i}$. We choose a constant $p > 1$ that gives the best linear relationship for the transformed data.

These models may correctly model the relationship between $x$ and $y$ but introduce heteroscedasticity in the model errors. In this case non-linear regression methods should be used (see Sections 3.24 and 3.25).

Data transformations can often lead to more appropriate statistical models. In most cases, however, the results of our analyses should be presented in terms of the untransformed data. It is important to bear in mind that the ultimate purpose of statistics in biomedical research is to help clinicians and scientists communicate with each other. For this reason, results should be presented in a way that will be easily understood by readers who do not necessarily have strong backgrounds in biostatistics.

### 2.17.3. Example: research funding and morbidity for 29 diseases

Gross et al. (1999) studied the relationship between NIH research funding in 1996 for 29 different diseases and disability-adjusted person–years of life lost due to these illnesses. Scatter plots of these two variables are shown in the panels of Figure 2.14. Panel A shows the untransformed scatter plot. Funding for AIDS was 3.7 times higher than for any other disease, which makes the structure of the data hard to see. Panel B is similar to panel A except the AIDS observation has been deleted and the $y$-axis has been rescaled. This scatter plot has a concave shape similar to panel D of Figure 2.13, which suggests

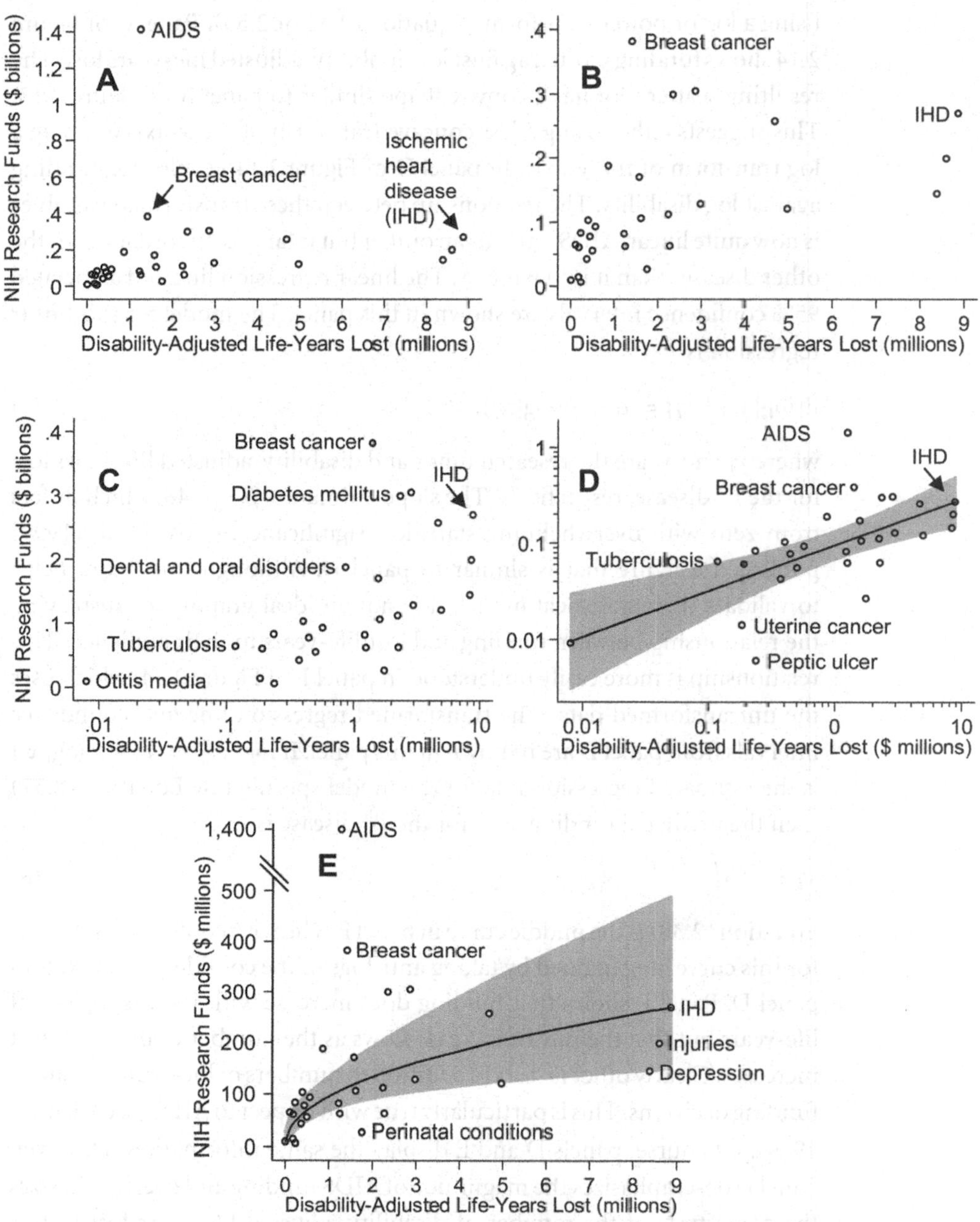


Figure 2.14 Scatter plots of NIH funding in 1996 against disability-adjusted life-years lost for 29 diseases (Gross et al., 1999). The $x$- and $y$-axes of these variables are plotted on either linear or logarithmic scales. The relationship between log funds and log life-years in panel D is reasonably linear. The black lines in panels D and E estimate the expected funding under this model. The gray bands give the 95% confidence intervals for these curves.

using a log or power transform (Equations 2.32 or 2.33). Panel C of Figure 2.14 shows funding plotted against log disability-adjusted life-years lost. The resulting scatter plot has a convex shape similar to panel A of Figure 2.13. This suggests either using a less concave transform of the $x$-axis or using a log transform of the $y$-axis. In panel D of Figure 2.14 we plot log funding against log disability. The relationship between these transformed variables is now quite linear. AIDS remains an outlier but is far less discordant with the other diseases than it is in panel A. The linear regression line and associated 95% confidence intervals are shown in this panel. The model for this linear regression is

$$E[\log[y_i] \mid x_i] = \alpha + \beta \log[x_i], \tag{2.37}$$

where $y_i$ and $x_i$ are the research funds and disability-adjusted life-years lost for the $i^{\text{th}}$ disease, respectively. The slope estimate is $\beta = 0.48$, which differs from zero with overwhelming statistical significance. Gross et al. (1999) published a figure that is similar to panel D. Although this figure helps to validate their statistical model, it is not an ideal graphic for displaying the relationship between funding and lost life-years to their audience. This relationship is more easily understood in panel E of Figure 2.14, which uses the untransformed data. The transformed regression line and confidence intervals from panel D are redrawn in this panel. If $\log[\hat{y}_i] = a + b\log[x_i]$ is the estimated regression line for the model specified by Equation (2.37) then the predicted funding level for the $i^{\text{th}}$ disease is

$$\hat{y}_i = e^a x_i^b. \tag{2.38}$$

Equation (2.38) is the middle curve in panel E. The 95% confidence intervals for this curve are obtained by taking anti-logs of the confidence intervals in panel D. Panel E shows that funding does increase with increasing loss of life-years but that the rate of increase slows as the number of life-years lost increases. Clearly other factors in addition to numbers of life-years lost affect funding decisions. This is particularly true with respect to AIDS (see Varmus, 1999). Of course, panels D and E display the same information. However, panel D de-emphasizes the magnitude of AIDS funding and overemphasizes the magnitude of the number of disability-adjusted life-years lost to this disease.

## 2.18. Analyzing transformed data with Stata

The following log file illustrates how data may be transformed to obtain data that are appropriate for linear regression.

```
. *  2.18.Funding.log
. *
. *  Explore the relationship between NIH research funds and
. *  disability-adjusted life-years lost due to the 29 diseases
. *  discussed by Gross et al. (1999).  Look for transformed values
. *  of these variables that are linearly related.
. *  Perform a linear regression on these transformed variables.
. *  Replot this regression line as a function of the untransformed
. *  variables.
. use C:\WDDtext\2.18.Funding.dta, clear                                1

. scatter dollars disabil, ylabel(0(.2)1.4) xlabel(0(1)9)                2
> xsize(2.7) ysize(1.964) scale(1.5)                                     3

. scatter dollars disabil if dollars < 1                                 4
>     , ylabel(0(.1).4) ymtick(.05(.1).35) xlabel(0(1)9)                 5
>     xsize(2.7) ysize(1.964) scale(1.5)

. scatter dollars disabil if dollars < 1                                 6
>     , ylabel(0(.1).4) ymtick(.05(.1).35)
>       xscale(log) xlabel(0.01 0.1 1 10)                                7
>       xmtick(.02 (.01) .09 .2 (.1) .9 2 (1) 9)                         8
>       xsize(2.7) ysize(1.964) scale(1.5)

. generate logdis = log(disabil)

. generate logdol = log(dollars)

. regress logdol logdis                                                  9

      Source |       SS       df       MS              Number of obs =      29
-------------+------------------------------           F(  1,    27) =   18.97
       Model |  14.8027627     1  14.8027627           Prob > F      =  0.0002
    Residual |  21.0671978    27  .780266584           R-squared     =  0.4127
-------------+------------------------------           Adj R-squared =  0.3909
       Total |  35.8699605    28  1.28107002           Root MSE      =  .88333

------------------------------------------------------------------------------
      logdol |      Coef.   Std. Err.      t    P>|t|     [95% Conf. Interval]
-------------+----------------------------------------------------------------
      logdis |   .4767575    .109458     4.36   0.000     .2521682    .7013468   10
       _cons |  -2.352205   .1640383   -14.34   0.000    -2.688784   -2.015626
------------------------------------------------------------------------------
```

```
. predict yhat,xb

. predict stdp, stdp                                                         11

. generate ci_u = yhat +invttail(_N-2,.025)*stdp                             12

. generate ci_l = yhat -invttail(_N-2,.025)*stdp

. sort logdis                                                                13

. twoway rarea ci_u ci_l logdis, color(gs14)                                 14
>       || line yhat logdis
>       || scatter logdol logdis
>       , ylabel(-4.61 "0.01" -2.3 "0.1" 0 "1")                              15
>         ymtick(-4.61 -3.91 -3.51 -3.22 -3.00 -2.81 -2.66 -2.53             16
>         -2.41 -2.3 -1.61 -1.2 -.92 -.69 -.51 -.36 -.22 -.11 0)
>         xtitle(Disability-Adjusted Life-Years Lost ($ millions))           17
>         xlabel(-4.61 "0.01" -2.3 "0.1" 0 2.3 "10")
>         xmtick(-2.3 -1.61 -1.2 -.92 -.69 -.51 -.36 -.22 -.11
>         0 .69 1.1 1.39 1.61 1.79 1.95 2.08 2.2 2.3) legend(off)
>         xsize(2.7) ysize(1.964) scale(1.5)

. generate yhat2 = exp(yhat)                                                 18

. generate ci_u2 = exp(ci_u)

. generate ci_l2 = exp(ci_l)

. twoway  rarea ci_u2 ci_l2 disabil, color(gs14)                             19
>       || line yhat2 disabil
>       || scatter dollars disabil
>       , ytitle(NIH Research Funds ($ Billions))
>         ylabel(0(.2)1.4) ymtick(.1(.2)1.3) xlabel(0(1)9)
>         xsize(2.7) ysize(1.964) scale(1.5) legend(off)

. twoway rarea ci_l2 ci_u2 disabil, color(gs14)
>       || line yhat2 disabil, sort                                          20
>       || scatter dollars disabil if dollars < 1
>       , ytitle(NIH Research Funds (it $ Billions))                         21
>         ylabel(0 (.1) .5) xlabel(0 (1) 9) legend(off)
>         xsize(2.7) ysize(1.964) scale(1.5)

. log close
```

**Comments**

1 This data set is from Table 1 of Gross et al. (1999). It contains the annual allocated NIH research funds in 1996 and disability-adjusted life-years lost for 29 diseases. These two variables are denoted *dollars* and *disabil* in this data set, respectively.

2 This command produces a scatter plot that is similar to panel A of Figure 2.14. In this figure the annotation of individual diseases was added with a graphics editor.

3 We want this to be one of the five panels in Figure 2.14. This requires that the size of the panel be smaller and the relative size of text be larger than Stata's default values. The *xsize* and *ysize* options specify the size of the width and height of the graph in inches, respectively; *scale(1.5)* specifies that the size of all text, marker-symbols and line widths be increased by 50% over their default values.

4 AIDS was the only disease receiving more than one billion dollars. The *if dollars < 1* qualifier restricts this graph to diseases with less than one billion dollars in funding and produces a graph similar to panel B of Figure 2.14.

5 The *ymtick* option draws tick marks on the *y*-axis at the indicated values. These tick marks are shorter than the ticks used for the axis labels. The *ytick* option works the same way as the *ymtick* option except that the tick lengths are the same as those of the *ylabel* command.

6 This command produces a graph similar to panel C of Figure 2.14. The equivalent point-and-click command is Graphics ▶ Twoway graph (scatter plot, line etc) ⌋Plots⌊ [Create] ⌋Plot⌊ ⌜ Plot type: (scatter plot) — Y variable: *dollars* , X variable: *disabil* ⌋ ⌋if/in⌊ ⌜ Restrict observations — If: (expression) *dollars < 1* ⌋ [Accept] ⌋Y axis⌊ [Major tick/label properties] ⌋Rule⌊ ⌜ Axis rule — ⊙ Range/Delta , *0* Minimum value , *.4* Maximum value , *.1* Delta ⌋ [Accept] [Minor tick/label properties] ⌋Rule⌊ ⌜ Axis rule — ⊙ Range/Delta , *.05* Minimum value , *.35* Maximum value , *.05* Delta ⌋ [Accept] ⌋X axis⌊ [Major tick/label properties] ⌋Rule⌊ ⌜ Axis rule — ⊙ Custom , Custom rule: *0.01 0.1 1 10* ⌋ [Accept] [Minor tick/label properties] ⌋Rule⌊ ⌜ Axis rule — ⊙ Custom , Custom rule: *.02(.01).09 .2(.1).9 2(1)9* ⌋ [Accept] [Axis scale properties] ⌜ ☑ Use logarithmic scale [Accept] ⌋Overall⌊ ⌜ Graph size — Width: (inches) *2.7* ,

Height: (inches) *1.964* ⌋ ⌈ ☑ Scale text, markers, and lines — Scale multiplier: *1.5* ⌋ Submit.

7 We plot *disabil* on a logarithmic scale using the *xscale(log)* option.

8 The minor tick marks of this *xmtick* option are specified to be from 0.02 to 0.09 in units of 0.01, from 0.2 to 0.9 in units of 0.1 and from 2 to 9 in integer units. The *xmtick* and *xtick* options have the same effects on the *x*-axis that the *ymtick* and *ytick* options have on the *y*-axis.

9 This command fits the regression model of Equation (2.37).

10 The slope of the regression of log funding against log life-years lost is 0.4768. The $P$-value associated with the null hypothesis that $\beta = 0$ is $< 0.0005$.

11 This predict command defines *stdp* to be the standard error of the expected value of *logdol* from the preceding linear regression (i.e. *stdp* is the standard error of *yhat*). The option *stdp* specifies that this standard error is to be calculated. We have also used *stdp* as the name of this variable.

12 The variables *ci_u* and *ci_l* give the 95% confidence interval for *yhat* using Equation 2.20. In Section 2.12 we used the *lfit* and *lfitci* commands to derive and plot this interval for us. Although we could have done this here as well we will need the variables *ci_u* and *ci_l* to derive the confidence band of Panel E in Figure 2.14.

13 This command sorts the data set in ascending order by *logdis*. The equivalent point-and-click command is Data ► Sort ► Ascending sort ⌈ Variables: *treat* Submit.

Stata needs the data set to be sorted by the *x*-variable whenever a non-linear line is plotted.

14 This plot is similar to Panel D of Figure 2.14. The *rarea* command shades the region between *ci_u* and *ci_l* over the range of values defined by *logdis*. The option *color(gs14)* shades this region gray. Stata provides 15 different shades of gray named *gs1*, *gs2*, . . . , *gs15*. The higher the number the lighter the shade of gray; *gs0* is black and *gs16* is white. This option may also be used to color plot-symbols and lines. The point-and-click version of this command is similar to that given above. The *rarea* plot is specified on the *Plots* tab of the *twoway–Twoway graphs* dialogue box as Create ⌋ Plot ⌊ ⌈ Choose a plot category and type — ⦿ Range plots , Range plots: (select type) *Range area* ⌋ ⌈ Plot type: (range plot with area shading) — Y1 variable: *ci_u2* , X variable: *disabil* , Y2 variable: *ci_l2* ⌋ Accept.

15 In Panel D of Figure 2.14 the $y$-axis is labeled in billions of dollars. In this graph command, the $y$-variable is *logdol*, which is the logarithm of *dollars*. This *ylabel* option places the labels 0.01, 0.1 and 1 at the values of *logdol* of −4.61, −2.3 and 0, respectively. (Note that $\log[0.01] = -4.61$, $\log[0.1] = -2.3$ and $\log[1] = 0$.) This syntax may also be used to label the $x$-axis with the *xlabel* option.

16 The tick marks specified for *logdis* by this *ymtick* command are equal to the logarithms of the tick marks for *disabil* in Panel B. Compare this option with that described in Comment 8 when we were also using the *xscale(log)* option. Tick marks may be specified as a list of values, as is illustrated here, for the *ymtick, ytick, ylabel, xmtick, xtick,* and *xlabel* commands.

17 In the previous graphs in this example the title of the $x$-axis was taken from the variable label of the $x$-variable in the database. Here, the $x$-variable is *logdis* and we have not given it a label. For this reason we title the $x$-axis explicitly with a *xtitle* option.

18 The variable *yhat2* equals the left-hand side of Equation (2.38); *ci_u2* and *ci_l2* give the upper and lower bounds of the 95% confidence interval for *yhat2*. In Stata and this text, $\exp[x]$ denotes $e$ raised to the power $x$, where $e$ is the base of the natural logarithm.

19 This graph plots funding against life-years lost. The regression curve and 95% confidence intervals are shown.

20 This *line* command plots *yhat2* against *logdis*. The *sort* option sorts the data by the $x$-variable prior to drawing the graph. In this example, this option is not needed since we have already sorted the data by *logdis*. If the data had not been sorted in this way, and we had not used the *sort* option, then straight lines would have been drawn between consecutive observations as listed in the data set. This often produces a garbled graph that looks nothing like the intended line plot.

21 Deleting AIDS (diseases with dollars $\geq 1$) permits using a more narrow range for the $y$-axis. The resulting graph is similar to panel E of Figure 2.14. In panel E, however, the $y$-axis is expressed in millions rather than billions and a graphics editor has been used to break the $y$-axis and add the data for AIDS.

## 2.19. Testing the equality of regression slopes

Consider the relationship between systolic blood pressure (SBP) and body mass index (BMI) in men and women. Suppose that we have data on samples of $n_1$ men and $n_2$ women. Let $x_{i1}$ and $y_{i1}$ be the SBP and BMI for the $i^{\text{th}}$

man and let $x_{i2}$ and $y_{i2}$ be similarly defined for the $i^{\text{th}}$ woman. Let

$$y_{i1} = \alpha_1 + \beta_1 x_{i1} + \varepsilon_{i1} \text{ and}$$
$$y_{i2} = \alpha_2 + \beta_2 x_{i2} + \varepsilon_{i2}$$

be linear models of the relationship between SBP and BMI in men and women, where $\varepsilon_{i1}$ and $\varepsilon_{i2}$ are normally distributed error terms with mean 0 and standard deviation $\sigma$. It is of interest to know whether the rate at which SBP increases with increasing BMI differs between men and women. That is, we wish to test the null hypothesis that $\beta_1 = \beta_2$. To test this hypothesis we first perform separate linear regressions on the data from the men and women. Let $a_1$, $b_1$, and $s_1^2$ estimate the $y$-intercept, slope, and error variance for the men and let $a_2$, $b_2$, and $s_2^2$ be similarly defined for the women. Let $\hat{y}_{i1} = a_1 + b_1 x_{i1}$ and $\hat{y}_{i2} = a_1 + b_2 x_{i2}$. Then a pooled estimate of the error variance $\sigma^2$ is

$$\begin{aligned} s^2 &= \left( \sum_{i=1}^{n_1} (y_{i1} - \hat{y}_{i1})^2 + \sum_{i=1}^{n_2} (y_{i2} - \hat{y}_{i2})^2 \right) \Big/ (n_1 + n_2 - 4) \\ &= \left( s_1^2(n_1 - 2) + s_2^2(n_2 - 2) \right) / (n_1 + n_2 - 4). \end{aligned} \tag{2.39}$$

The variance of the slope difference is

$$\mathrm{var}[b_1 - b_2] = s^2 \left( 1 \Big/ \sum_{i=1}^{n_1} (x_{i1} - \bar{x}_1)^2 + 1 \Big/ \sum_{i=1}^{n_2} (x_{i2} - \bar{x}_2)^2 \right). \tag{2.40}$$

But

$$\mathrm{var}[b_1] = s_1^2 \Big/ \sum_{i=1}^{n_1} (x_{i1} - \bar{x}_1)^2$$

and hence

$$\sum_{i=1}^{n_1} (x_{i1} - \bar{x}_1)^2 = s_1^2 / \mathrm{var}[b_1].$$

This allows us to rewrite Equation (2.40) as

$$\mathrm{var}[b_1 - b_2] = s^2 \left( \mathrm{var}[b_1]/s_1^2 + \mathrm{var}[b_2]/s_2^2 \right). \tag{2.41}$$

Under the null hypothesis that $\beta_1 = \beta_2$,

$$t = (b_1 - b_2) / \sqrt{\mathrm{var}[b_1 - b_2]} \tag{2.42}$$

has a $t$ distribution with $n_1 + n_2 - 4$ degrees of freedom. A 95% confidence interval for $\beta_1 - \beta_2$ is

$$(b_1 - b_2) \pm t_{n_1+n_2-4,\, 0.05} \sqrt{\mathrm{var}[b_1 - b_2]}. \tag{2.43}$$

**Table 2.1.** Results of linear regressions of log systolic blood pressure against log body mass index in men and women from the Framingham Heart Study (Levy, 1999)

| Sex | $i$ | Number of subjects $n_i$ | $y$ intercept $a_i$ | Slope $b_i$ | MSE $s_i^2$ | se$[b_i]$ | var$[b_i]$ |
|---|---|---|---|---|---|---|---|
| Men | 1 | 2047 | 3.988 043 | 0.272 646 | 0.018 778 8 | 0.023 215 2 | 0.000 538 9 |
| Women | 2 | 2643 | 3.593 017 | 0.398 595 | 0.026 116 7 | 0.018 546 4 | 0.000 344 0 |

### 2.19.1. Example: the Framingham Heart Study

The Framingham Heart Study (Levy, 1999) has collected cardiovascular risk factor data and long-term follow-up on almost 5000 residents of the town of Framingham, Massachusetts. They have made available a didactic data set from this study that includes baseline systolic blood pressure (SBP) and body mass index (BMI) values on $n_1 = 2047$ men and $n_2 = 2643$ women (see also Section 3.11). Table 2.1 summarizes the results of two separate linear regressions of log[SBP] against log[BMI] in men and women from this data set. The observed rate at which log[SBP] increases with increasing log[BMI] in men is $b_1 = 0.272\,646$ mm Hg per unit of BMI (kg/m$^2$). This is appreciably less than the corresponding rate of $b_2 = 0.398\,595$ in women.

Figure 2.15 shows scatter plots of log[SBP] vs. log[BMI] in men and women together with lines depicting the expected log[SBP] from these linear regressions. The regression line for women (dashed line) is also superimposed on the scatter plot for men to provide an indication of the magnitude of the slope difference.

Substituting these values into Equations (2.39) and (2.41) gives

$$\begin{aligned} s^2 &= (0.018\,778\,8 \times (2047 - 2) + 0.026\,116\,7 \times (2643 - 2))/ \\ &\quad (2047 + 2643 - 4) \\ &= 0.022\,91 \text{ and var } [b_1 - b_2] \\ &= 0.022\,91 \times ((0.000\,538\,9/0.018\,778\,8) + (0.000\,344\,0/0.026\,116\,7)) \\ &= 0.000\,959. \end{aligned}$$

Therefore, a $t$ statistic (Equation (2.42)) to test the equality of these slopes is $t = (0.272\,646 - 0.398\,595)/\sqrt{0.000\,959} = -4.07$ with 4686 degrees of freedom. The $P$ value associated with this test is $P = 0.000\,05$. A 95% confidence interval for $\beta_1 - \beta_2$ (Equation (2.43)) is $0.272\,646 - 0.398\,595 \pm t_{4686,0.025}\sqrt{0.000\,959} = -0.126 + 1.96 \times 0.0310 = (-0.19, -0.065)$. This test allows us to conclude with great confidence that the difference in slopes between men and women in these regressions is not due to chance variation. Whether this difference is due to an inherent difference between

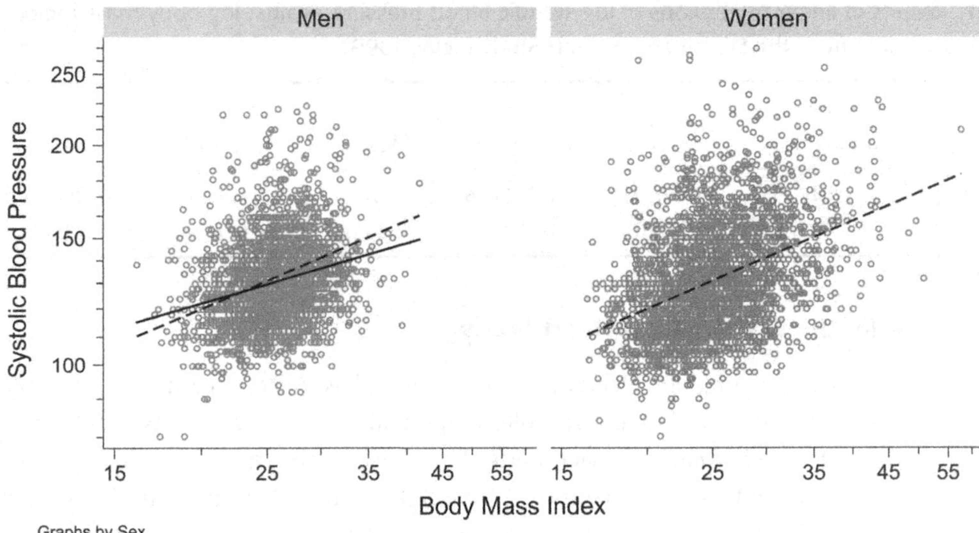


Figure 2.15 Linear regressions of log systolic blood pressure against log body mass index in men and women from the Framingham Heart Study (Levy, 1999). The regression line for women (dashed line) has been superimposed over the corresponding line for men (solid line).

men and women or is due to confounding with other variables remains to be determined. It is worth noting, however, that these differences are clinically appreciable. A man with a BMI of 35 will have an expected SBP of $\exp[3.988 + 0.2726 \times \log[35]] = 142$ mm Hg. The corresponding expected SBP for a woman with this BMI is $\exp[3.593 + 0.3986 \times \log[35]] = 150$ mm Hg.

## 2.20. Comparing slope estimates with Stata

The following log file and comments illustrate how to perform the calculations and draw the graphs from the preceding section using Stata.

```
. *  2.20.Framingham.log
. *
. *  Regression of log systolic blood pressure against log body mass
. *  index at baseline in men and women from the Framingham Heart
. *  Study.
. *
. use C:\WDDtext\2.20.Framingham.dta, clear                          1

. generate logsbp = log(sbp)                                           2
```

```
. generate logbmi = log(bmi)
(9 missing values generated)

. codebook sex
```

3

Output omitted

```
           tabulation:  Freq.   Numeric  Label
                         2049         1  Men
                         2650         2  Women

. regress logsbp logbmi if sex == 1
```

4

```
      Source |       SS       df       MS              Number of obs =    2047
-------------+------------------------------           F(  1,  2045) =  137.93
       Model |  2.5901294     1  2.5901294             Prob > F      =  0.0000
    Residual | 38.4025957  2045  .018778775            R-squared     =  0.0632
-------------+------------------------------           Adj R-squared =  0.0627
       Total | 40.9927251  2046  .020035545            Root MSE      =  .13704

------------------------------------------------------------------------------
      logsbp |      Coef.   Std. Err.      t    P>|t|     [95% Conf. Interval]
-------------+----------------------------------------------------------------
      logbmi |    .272646   .0232152    11.74   0.000     .2271182    .3181739
       _cons |   3.988043   .0754584    52.85   0.000      3.84006    4.136026
------------------------------------------------------------------------------

. predict yhatmen, xb
```

5

```
(9 missing values generated)

. regress logsbp logbmi if sex == 2
```

6

```
      Source |       SS       df       MS              Number of obs =    2643
-------------+------------------------------           F(  1,  2641) =  461.90
       Model | 12.0632111     1  12.0632111            Prob > F      =  0.0000
    Residual | 68.9743032  2641  .026116737            R-squared     =  0.1489
-------------+------------------------------           Adj R-squared =  0.1485
       Total | 81.0375143  2642  .030672791            Root MSE      =  .16161

------------------------------------------------------------------------------
      logsbp |      Coef.   Std. Err.      t    P>|t|     [95% Conf. Interval]
-------------+----------------------------------------------------------------
      logbmi |   .3985947   .0185464    21.49   0.000     .3622278    .4349616
       _cons |   3.593017   .0597887    60.10   0.000     3.475779    3.710254
------------------------------------------------------------------------------
```

```
. predict yhatwom, xb
(9 missing values generated)

. sort logbmi

. *
. * Scatter plots of SBP by BMI for men and women. The estimated
. * expected SBP is shown for each gender on these plots. The
. * expected SBP is shown for both genders on the male scatter
. * plot. Both SBP and BMI are plotted on a log scale.
. *
. scatter logsbp logbmi , color(gray)                                  7
>     || line yhatmen logbmi if sex == 1, lwidth(medthick)             8
>     || line yhatwom logbmi, lwidth(medthick) lpattern(dash)          9
>     , by(sex, legend(off)) ytitle(Systolic Blood Pressure)           10
>       xsize(5.4) ylabel( 4.61 "100"  5.01 "150"  5.3 "200"
>       5.52 "250") ymtick(4.38 4.5 4.7 4.79 4.87 4.94 5.08
>       5.14 5.19 5.25 5.35 5.39 5.43 5.48 5.56 5.60)
>       xtitle(Body Mass Index) xlabel( 2.71 "15" 3.22 "25"
>       3.56 "35" 3.81 "45" 4.01 "55")
>       xmtick(3.0 3.22 3.4 3.56 3.69 3.91 4.01 4.09)

. scalar s2 = (.018778775 *2045 + 0.026116737*2641)                    11
>                  /(2047 + 2643 - 4)

. scalar varb_dif =                                                    12
>        s2 *(0.0232152^2/ 0.018778775 +0.0185464^2/0.026116737)

. scalar t =  (0.272646 - 0.3985947)/sqrt(varb_dif)                    13

. scalar ci95_lb =  (0.272646 - 0.3985947)                             14
>        - invttail(4686,.025)*sqrt(varb_dif)

. scalar ci95_ub = (0.272646 - 0.3985947)
>        + invttail(4686,.025)*sqrt(varb_dif)

. display  "s2 = " s2 ", varb_dif = " varb_dif ", t = " t              15

s2 = .0229144, varb_dif = .00095943, t = -4.0661848

. display  "ci95_lb = " ci95_lb  ", ci95_ub = " ci95_ub

ci95_lb = -.18667361, ci95_ub = -.06522379

. display 2*ttail(4686,abs(t))                                         16
.00004857
. log close
```

**Comments**

1 This data set contains long-term follow-up on 4699 people from the town of Framingham. In this example, we focus on three variables collected at each patient's baseline exam: *sbp*, *bmi*, and *sex*. The variable *sbp* records systolic blood pressure in mm Hg; *bmi* records body mass index in kg/m$^2$.

2 An exploratory data analysis (not shown here) indicates that the relationship between log[*sbp*] and log[*bmi*] comes closer to meeting the assumptions of a linear model than does the relationship between *sbp* and *bmi*.

3 There are 2049 men and 2650 women in this data set; *sex* is coded 1 or 2 for men or women, respectively.

4 This regression command is restricted to records where *sex == 1* is true. That is, to records of men. The statistics from this regression that are also in Table 2.1 are highlighted. Two of the 2049 men in this data set are missing values for either *sbp* or *bmi*, giving a total of 2047 observations in the analysis.

5 The variable *yhatmen* contains the expected value of each man's log[*sbp*] given his body mass index. These expected values are based on the regression of *logsbp* against *logbmi* among men. There are nine subjects with missing values of *logbmi* (two men and seven women). The variable *yhatmen* is missing for these people. Note that this *predict* command defines *yhatmen* for all subjects including women. The command *predict yhatmen if sex == 1, xb* would have defined *yhatmen* for men only.

6 This regression of *logsbp* against *logbmi* is restricted to women with non-missing values of *sbp* and *bmi*.

7 This command generates Figure 2.15. We distinguish between the regression lines for women and men by using a dashed line for women.

8 We plot the expected SBP for both men and women on the scatter plot for men in order to make the difference in the slopes of these lines visually apparent. This *line* command plots the expected SBP for men on the male scatter plot. The *if sex == 1* qualifier prevents this curve from being replicated on the female scatter plot.

9 Plot the expected SBP for women on both the male and female scatter plots. The *lpattern(dash)* and *lwidth(medthick)* option chooses dashed lines of medium thickness for these curves.

10 This *by(sex, legend(off))* option causes separate graphs to be plotted for each gender (i.e. for each distinct value of *sex*) By default, a legend is generated whenever a *by* option is used. Here, this legend is

suppressed by the *legend(off)* suboption. A point-and-click command that is similar to this one is Graphics ▶ Twoway graph (scatter plot, line etc) ⌋Plots⌊ [Create] ⌋Plot⌊ ⌈ Plot type: (scatter plot) — Y variable: *logsbp* , X variable: *logbmi* [Marker properties] ⌋Main⌊ ⌈ Marker properties — Color: *Gray* ⌋ [Accept] ⌋ [Accept] [Create] ⌋Plot⌊ ⌈ Choose a plot category and type — Basic plots: (select type) *Line* ⌋ ⌈ Plot type: (line plot) — Y variable: *yhatmen* , X variable: *logbmi* [Line properties] ⌈ Width: *Medium thick* [Accept] ⌋ ⌋if/in⌊ ⌈ Restrict observations — If: (expression) *sex == 1* ⌋ [Accept] [Create] ⌋Plot⌊ ⌈ Choose a plot category and type — Basic plots: (select type) *Line* ⌋ ⌈ Plot type: (line plot) — Y variable: *yhatwom* , X variable: *logbmi* [Line properties] ⌈ Width: *Medium thick* , Pattern: *Dash* [Accept] ⌋ [Accept] ⌋Y axis⌊ Title: *Systolic Blood Pressure* [Major tick/label properties] ⌋Rule⌊ ⌈ Axis rule — ⊙ Custom , *4.61 "100" 5.01 "150" 5.3 "200" 5.52 "250"* ⌋ [Accept] ⌋X axis⌊ Title: *Body Mass Index* [Major tick/label properties] ⌋Rule⌊ ⌈ Axis rule — ⊙ Custom ,*2.71 "15" 3.22 "25" 3.56 "35" 3.81 "45" 4.01 "55"* ⌋ [Accept] ⌋Legend⌊ ⌈ Legend behavior — ⊙ Hide legend ⌋ ⌋Overall⌊ ⌈ Graph size — Width: (inches) *5.4* ⌋ ⌋by⌊ ⌈ [✓] Draw subgraphs for unique values of variables — Variables: *sex* ⌋ [Submit].

11 This command defines *s2* to be a scalar that equals $s^2$ in Equation (2.39). Scalars are kept in memory until they are dropped or the Stata session ends. They may be used like conventional variables in Stata commands such as *generate, rename,* or *display.* If we had used the *generate* command to define *s2* then *s2* would be a variable in the data file that contained the same constant value for each observation.

12 This command defines *varb_dif* to equal $\text{var}[b_1 - b_2]$ in Equation (2.41).

13 This is the $t$ statistic given in Equation (2.42). The function *sqrt(x)* calculates the square root of $x$.

14 The next two lines calculate the lower and upper bounds of the 95% confidence interval given in Equation (2.43).

15 The next two *display* commands list the values of *s2, varb_dif, t, ci95_lb* and *ci95_ub*. Note that these values agree with those given for $s^2$, $\text{var}[b_1 - b_2]$ and $(b_1 - b_2) \pm t_{n_1+n_2-4,\,0.025}\sqrt{\text{var}(b_1 - b_2)}$ in the example from Section 2.19.1. The *display* command can calculate a number of expressions, which may be separated by quoted text-strings to improve legibility, as is illustrated here.

16 The function *ttail(df, t)* gives the probability that a $t$ statistic with *df* degrees of freedom is greater than $t$. The function *abs(t)* gives the absolute value of $t$. Hence *2*ttail(4686, abs(t))* gives the two-sided $P$-value associated with a $t$ statistic with 4686 degrees of freedom. In this example, $t = -4.07$, giving $P = -0.000\,05$.

## 2.21. Density-distribution sunflower plots

The scatter plot is a powerful and ubiquitous graphic for displaying bivariate data. These plots, however, become difficult to read when the density of points in a region becomes high enough to obscure individual plot symbols (see Figure 2.15). One solution to this problem is the density-distribution sunflower plot (Dupont and Plummer, 2005). An example of such a plot displaying the relationship between diastolic blood pressure and body mass index from the Framingham Heart Study (Levy, 1999) is illustrated in Figure 2.16. In a **density-distribution sunflower plot** the $x$–$y$ plane is subdivided into a lattice of small regular hexagonal bins. These bins are classified as being low-density, medium-density or high-density depending on the number of observations they contain. Individual observations are plotted in low-density bins while light and dark sunflowers are plotted in medium- and high-density bins, respectively. A sunflower is a number of short line segments, called petals, that radiate from a central point (Cleveland and McGill, 1984). In a light sunflower each petal represents one observation, while in a dark sunflower, each petal represents multiple observations. A key on the graph specifies the number of observations represented by each dark sunflower petal. By selecting appropriate colors and sizes for the light and dark sunflowers, plots can be obtained that give both the overall sense of the data distribution and the number of data points in any given region. The viewer can ascertain the exact location of observations in low-density bins, the exact number of observations in medium-density bins, and the approximate number of observations in high-density bins. Figure 2.16 gives a good sense of the distribution of the observations in the central portion of the graph. In contrast, the central regions of the scatter plots in Figure 2.15

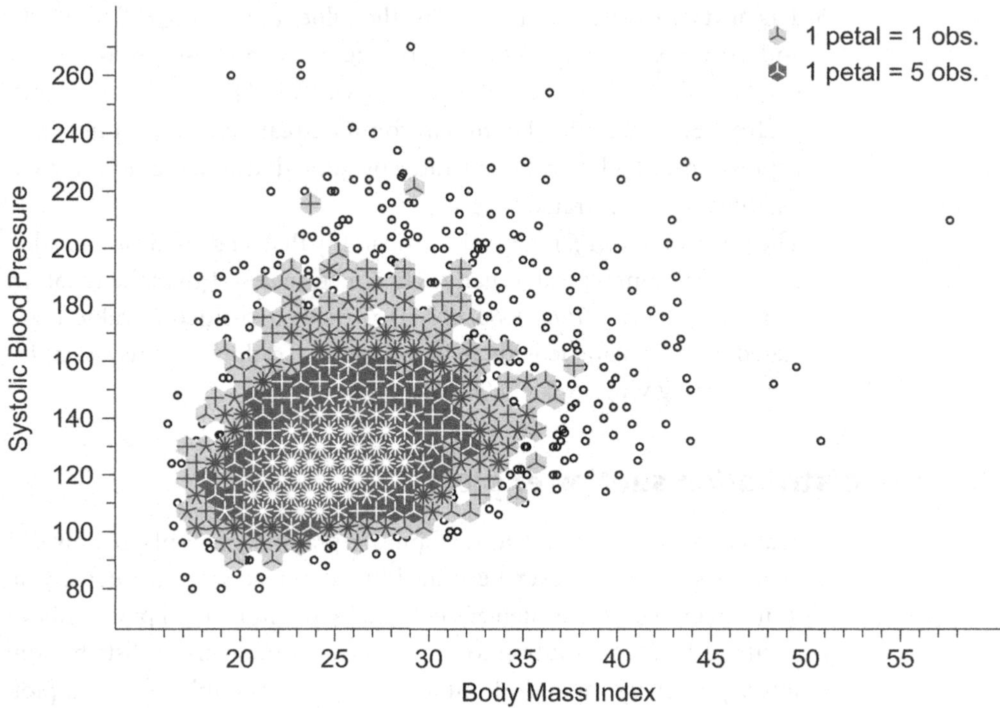


Figure 2.16 A density-distribution sunflower plot of systolic blood pressure versus body mass index from the Framingham Heart Study. In this figure, the $x$–$y$ plane is divided into regular hexagonal bins of width 1.0 kg/m$^2$. Individual observations are depicted by black circles at their exact location as long as there are less than three observations per bin. Observations in bins with higher densities are represented by light or dark sunflowers. Light sunflowers are gray with light gray backgrounds and represent one observation for each petal. Dark sunflowers are white with dark gray backgrounds and represent five observations per petal. This plot conveys the density distribution of the observations while also allowing the reader to determine the number of observations in any region with considerable precision.

are uniformly gray due to the overstriking of many hundreds of observations. Additional details on the use of these graphs are given in Dupont and Plummer (2005).

## 2.22. Creating density-distribution sunflower plots with Stata

The following log file and comments illustrates how Figure 2.16 was created.

```
. *  2.22.Framingham.log
. *
. *  Illustrate Density Distribution Sunflower Plots.
. *  Graph systolic blood pressure against body mass
. *  index at baseline for patients in the Framingham
. *  Heart Study.
. *
. use C:\WDDtext\2.20.Framingham.dta, clear

. sunflower sbp bmi                                                        1
>     , binwidth(1) ylabel(80 (20) 260)                                    2
>       ymtick(90(10)270) xlabel(20 (5) 55) xmtick(16 (1) 58)
>       legend(ring(0) position(2) cols(1) order(2 3)) scale(0.8)         3
Bin width          =          1
Bin height         =    7.55828                                            4
Bin aspect ratio   =    6.54567
Max obs in a bin   =         69
Light              =          3                                            5
Dark               =         13
X-center           =       25.2
Y-center           =        130
Petal weight       =          5                                            6
```

| flower type | petal weight | No. of petals | No. of flowers | estimated obs. | actual obs. |
|---|---|---|---|---|---|
| none | | | | 246 | 246 |
| light | 1 | 3 | 23 | 69 | 69 |
| light | 1 | 4 | 34 | 136 | 136 |
| light | 1 | 5 | 17 | 85 | 85 |
| light | 1 | 6 | 14 | 84 | 84 |
| light | 1 | 7 | 18 | 126 | 126 |
| light | 1 | 8 | 9 | 72 | 72 |
| light | 1 | 9 | 5 | 45 | 45 |
| light | 1 | 10 | 5 | 50 | 50 |
| light | 1 | 11 | 7 | 77 | 77 |
| light | 1 | 12 | 7 | 84 | 84 |
| dark | 5 | 3 | 23 | 345 | 338 |
| dark | 5 | 4 | 18 | 360 | 355 |
| dark | 5 | 5 | 9 | 225 | 224 |

7

```
  dark        5        6       13       390       381
  dark        5        7       12       420       424
  dark        5        8        6       240       237
  dark        5        9        4       180       177
  dark        5       10        7       350       350
  dark        5       11        7       385       384
  dark        5       12        7       420       420
  dark        5       13        4       260       257
  dark        5       14        1        70        69
--------------------------------------------------------
                                       4719      4690

. log close
```

**Comments**

1 This command produces the density-distribution sunflower plot of *sbp* vs *bmi* shown in Figure 2.16.

2 This *binwidth(1)* option specifies the width of the hexagonal bins will be 1.0 kg/m$^2$. That is, this width is specified in the units of the $x$-axis. The default bin width is determined by a formula given in the online documentation. Most of the standard graph options may be used with the *sunflower* command.

Like all Stata graphs, the default colors used by the *sunflower* command are determined by the Stata scheme in effect when the command is given. I have used the WDDtext schemes to produce this and other graphs in this text (see Section 1.3.6). Other schemes will use other colors for light and dark sunflowers. The sunflower command also has options that permit you to make explicit choices for your sunflower colors. For example, the options *lflcolor(gray) lbcolor(green) dflcolor(black) dbcolor(orange)* would produce light sunflowers with gray petals on green backgrounds and dark sunflowers with black petals on orange backgrounds. Type *help sunflower* from the Stata Command window for additional details on sunflower options.

3 By default, the legend of Stata graph commands is placed below the graph. Often, as in Figure 2.16, we can save space by putting the legend within the region defined by the $x$- and $y$-axes. This *legend* option places the legend in the upper right-hand corner of Figure 2.16; *ring(0)* places the legend within the region defined by the $x$- and $y$-axes. The suboption *position(2)* places the legend at 2 o'clock on the graph. That is, it gives the legend position in terms of an analog clock-face; *position(1)* and *position(2)* both

place the legend in the upper right-hand corner, *position(9)* places it on the left in the middle of the *y*-axis, etc. By default, a *sunflower* plot produces three legend keys: the low-density plot symbol, which has the *y*-variable label, and keys explaining the light and dark sunflowers. The suboption *cols(1)* places these keys in a single column. I do not find the first default key to be terribly useful, and have deleted it from Figure 2.16. This is done with the *order* suboption; *order(2 3)* specifies that only the second and third keys are to be shown. The order that these keys are to be listed are the second key followed by the third. In a sunflower plot these keys are the light and dark sunflower keys, respectively.

The equivalent point-and-click command is Graphics ▶ Smoothing and densities ▶ Density-distribution sunflower plot ⌋Main⌊ Y variable: *sbp*, X Variable: *bmi* ⌋Bins / Petals⌊ ⌜ Bins — Bin width: *1* ⌋ ⌋Y axis⌊ [Major tick/label properties] ⌋Rule⌊ ⌜ Axis rule — ⦿ Range/Delta , *80* Minimum value , *260* Maximum value , *20* Delta ⌋ [Accept] [Minor tick/label properties] ⌋Rule⌊ ⌜ Axis rule — ⦿ Range/Delta , *90* Minimum value , *270* Maximum value , *10* Delta ⌋ [Accept] ⌋X axis⌊ [Major tick/label properties] ⌋Rule⌊ ⌜ Axis rule — ⦿ Range/Delta , *20* Minimum value , *55* Maximum value , *5* Delta ⌋ [Accept] [Minor tick/label properties] ⌋Rule⌊ ⌜ Axis rule — ⦿ Range/Delta , *16* Minimum value , *58* Maximum value , *1* Delta ⌋ [Accept] ⌋Legend⌊ ⌜ [✓] Override default keys — Specify order of keys and optionally change labels: *2 3* ⌋ [Organization / Appearance] ⌋Organization⌊ ⌜ Organization — Rows/Columns: *Columns* ⌋ [Accept] [Placement] ⌜ Position: *2 o'clock* , [✓] Place legend inside plot region [Accept] ⌋Overall⌊ ⌜ [✓] Scale text, markers, and lines — Scale Multiplier: *0.8* ⌋ [Submit].

4 The bin height is calculated by the program and is given in the units of the *y*-axis (in this case mm Hg.) It is chosen to make the bin shapes regular hexagons.

5 By default, the minimum number of observations in light and dark sunflower bins is 3 and 13, respectively. These values may be changed with the light and dark options; *light(5) dark(15)* would set these thresholds to 5 and 15, respectively.

6 Each dark sunflower petal represents five observations. By default, this number is chosen so that the maximum number of petals on a dark sunflower is 14. This number can be set explicitly with the *petalweight* option; *petalweight(10)* specifies that each dark sunflower petal will represent ten observations.

7 This table specifies the number of light and dark sunflowers with different petal counts and the estimated and actual number of observations represented by the plot.

## 2.23. Additional reading

Armitage et al. (2002) and

Pagano and Gauvreau (2000) provide excellent introductions to simple linear regression. The approach to testing the equality of two regression slopes described in Section 2.19 is discussed in greater detail by Armitage et al. (2002).

Cleveland (1993) discusses lowess regression along with other important graphical techniques for data analysis.

Hamilton (1992) provides a brief introduction to non-linear regression.

Draper and Smith (1998) provide a more thorough and more mathematically advanced discussion of non-linear regression.

Cleveland (1979) is the original reference on lowess regression.

Levy (1999) provides a review of the research findings of the Framingham Heart Study.

Framingham Heart Study (1997) provides the 40 year follow-up data from this landmark study. The didactic data set used in this text is a subset of the 40 year data set that is restricted to patients who were free of coronary heart disease at the time of their baseline exam.

Brent et al. (1999) studied patients with ethylene glycol poisoning. We used data from this study to illustrate simple linear regression.

Gross et al. (1999) studied the relationship between research funding and disability-adjusted life-years lost due to 29 diseases. We used data from this study to illustrate data transformations in linear regression.

Varmus (1999) discussed NIH policy towards research funding.

Dupont and Plummer (2005) discuss density-distribution sunflower plots and provide additional information on producing these graphs in Stata.

Cleveland and McGill (1984) is the original reference on sunflower plots.

Carr et al. (1987) introduced new ideas for the display of high-density bivariate data. The density-distribution sunflower plot uses ideas published by Cleveland and McGill (1984) and Carr et al. (1987).

## 2.24. Exercises

Eisenhofer et al. (1999) investigated the use of plasma normetanephrine and metanephrine for detecting pheochromocytoma in patients with von Hippel–Lindau disease and multiple endocrine neoplasia type 2. The *2.ex.vonHippelLindau.dta* data set contains data from this study on 26 patients with von Hippel–Lindau disease and nine patients with multiple endocrine neoplasia. The variables in this data set are

$$disease = \begin{cases} 0: & \text{patient has von Hippel–Lindau disease} \\ 1: & \text{patient has multiple endocrine neoplasia type 2} \end{cases}$$

*p_ne* = plasma norepinephrine (pg/ml)
*tumorvol* = tumor volume (ml).

1 Regress plasma norepinephrine against tumor volume. Draw a scatter plot of norepinephrine against tumor volume together with the estimated linear regression curve. What is the slope estimate for this regression? What proportion of the total variation in norepinephrine levels is explained by this regression?

2 Calculate the studentized residuals for the regression in question 1. Determine the 95% prediction interval for these residuals. Draw a scatter plot of these residuals showing the 95% prediction interval and the expected residual values. Comment on the adequacy of the model for these data.

3 Plot the lowess regression curve for norepinephrine against tumor volume. How does this curve differ from the regression curve in Exercise 1?

4 Experiment with different transformations of norepinephrine and tumor volume. Find transformations that provide a good fit to a linear model.

5 Regress the logarithm of norepinephrine against the logarithm of tumor volume. Draw a scatter plot of these variables together with the linear regression line and the 95% confidence intervals for this line. What proportion of the total variation in the logarithm of norepinephrine levels is explained by this regression? How does this compare with your answer to Question 1?

6 Using the model from Question 5, what is the predicted plasma norepinephrine concentration for a patient with a tumor volume of 100 ml? What is the 95% confidence interval for this concentration? What would be the 95% prediction interval for a new patient with a 100 ml tumor?

7 Calculate the studentized residuals for the regression in Question 5. Determine the 95% prediction interval for these residuals. Draw a scatter plot of these residuals showing the 95% prediction interval and the expected residual values. Include the lowess regression curve of these residuals against tumor volume on your graph. Contrast your answer to that for Question 2. Which model provides the better fit to the data?

8 Perform separate linear regressions of log norepinephrine against log tumor volume in patients with von Hippel–Lindau disease and in patients with multiple endocrine neoplasia. What are the slope estimates for these two diseases? Give 95% confidence intervals for these slopes. Test the null hypothesis that these two slope estimates are equal. What is the 95% confidence interval for the difference in slopes for these diseases?

The following exercises concern the Framingham Heart Study data set *2.20.Framingham.dta.*

9 Evaluate the relationship between systolic blood pressure (SBP) and body mass index (BMI). Do these variables meet the assumptions of a linear model? If not, explore different transformations of these two variables that will result in variables that come closer to meeting the linear model assumptions.

10 Replicate the regressions of log[SBP] against log[BMI] for men and women in Section 2.20. What are the predicted SBPs for men and women with a BMI of 40? Do you think that the difference between these two blood pressures is clinically significant?

11 Plot the predicted SBPs in men and women as a function of BMI. Plot the 95% confidence intervals for these predicted values.

12 Draw a density-distribution sunflower plot of log diastolic blood pressure against serum cholesterol. Draw a scatter plot of these same two variables. What does the sunflower plot tell you about the joint distribution of these two variables that the scatter plot does not? Draw your sunflower plot with different bin widths. What are the pros and cons of larger vs. smaller bin widths?

The following question is for those who would like to sharpen their intuitive understanding of simple linear regression.

13 When a data point has leverage $h_i = 1$, the regression line always goes through the data point. Can you construct an example where this happens? Enter your example into Stata and confirm that $h_i = 1$ for your designated data point. (Hint: this is not a math question. All you need to remember is that the regression line minimizes the sum of squares of the residuals. By experimenting with different scatter plots, find a set of $x$ values for which the sum of squared residuals is always minimized by having a zero residual at your designated data point.)

# 3

# Multiple linear regression

In simple linear regression we modeled the value of a response variable as a linear function of a single covariate. In multiple linear regression we expand on this approach by using two or more covariates to predict the value of the response variable.

## 3.1. The model

It is often useful to predict a patient's response from multiple explanatory variables. The simple linear regression Model (2.4) can be generalized to do this as follows. Suppose we have observations on $n$ patients. The **multiple linear regression model** assumes that

$$y_i = \alpha + \beta_1 x_{i1} + \beta_2 x_{i2} + \cdots + \beta_k x_{ik} + \varepsilon_i, \tag{3.1}$$

where

$\alpha, \beta_1, \beta_2, \ldots, \beta_k$ are unknown parameters,

$x_{i1}, x_{i2}, \ldots, x_{ik}$ are the values of known variables measured on the $i^{\text{th}}$ patient,

$\varepsilon_i$ has a normal distribution with mean 0 and standard deviation $\sigma$,

$\varepsilon_1, \varepsilon_2, \ldots, \varepsilon_n$ are mutually independent, and

$y_i$ is the value of the response variable for the $i^{\text{th}}$ patient.

We usually assume that the patient's response $y_i$ is causally related to the variables $x_{i1}, x_{i2}, \ldots, x_{ik}$ through the model. These latter variables are called **covariates** or **explanatory variables**; $y_i$ is called the **dependent** or **response variable.** The model parameters are also called **regression coefficients.**

Multiple linear regression is often useful when we wish to improve our ability to predict a response variable and we have several explanatory variables that affect the patient's response.

## 3.2. Confounding variables

A **confounding variable** is one of little immediate interest that is correlated with the risk factor and is independently related to the outcome variable of interest. For example, blood pressure and body mass index (BMI) both tend to increase with age. Also, blood pressure and BMI are positively correlated. If we select a stout and lean subject at random from a population, the stout person is likely to be older than the lean subject and this difference in age will account for some of their difference in blood pressure. If we are interested in the effect of BMI per se on blood pressure we must adjust for the effect of age on the relationship between these two variables. We say that age confounds the effect of BMI on blood pressure. One way to adjust for age is to compare BMI and blood pressure in a sample of patients who are all the same age. It may, however, be difficult to find such a sample and the relationship between BMI and blood pressure may be different at different ages. Another approach is through multiple linear regression. The interpretation of $\beta_1$ in Equation (3.1) is that it estimates the rate of change in $y_i$ with $x_{i1}$ among patients with identical values of $x_{i2}, x_{i3}, \ldots, x_{ik}$. To see this more clearly, suppose that we have two covariates $x_{i1}$and $x_{i2}$. Let $\alpha = 0$, $\beta_1 = 1$, $\beta_2 = 2$ and $\varepsilon_i = 0$ for all $i$ (i.e., $\sigma = 0$). Then Equation (3.1) reduces to $y_i = x_{i1} + 2x_{i2}$. Figure 3.1 shows a sample of values that fit this model in which $x_{i1}$ and $x_{i2}$ are positively correlated. Note that the values of $y_i$ increase from 0 to 4 as $x_{i2}$ increases from 0 to 1. Hence, the slope of the simple regression curve of $y_i$ against $x_{i2}$ is 4. However, when $x_{i1}$ is held constant, $y_i$ increases from $x_{i1}$ to $x_{i1} + 2$ as $x_{i2}$ increases from 0 to 1. Hence, the rate at which $y_i$ increases with $x_{i2}$ adjusted for $x_{i1}$ is $\beta_2 = 2$.

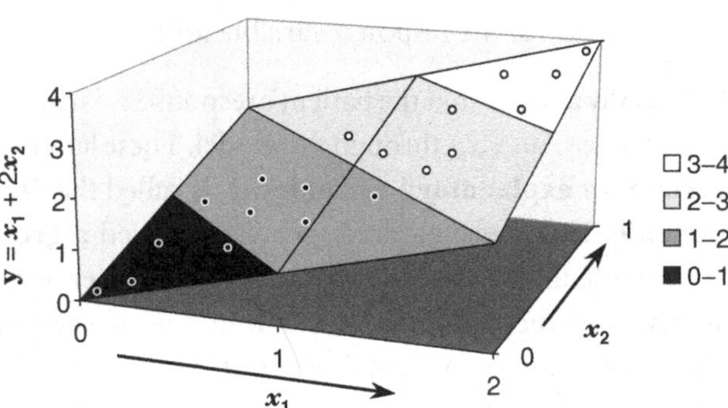


Figure 3.1 This graph shows points on the plane defined by the equation $y = x_1 + 2x_2$. The rate at which $y$ increases with increasing $x_2$ is 2 when $x_1$ is held constant and equals 4 when $x_2$ is not.

## 3.3. Estimating the parameters for a multiple linear regression model

Let $\hat{y}_i = a + b_1 x_{i1} + b_2 x_{i2} + \cdots + b_k x_{ik}$ be an estimate of $y_i$ given $x_{i1}, x_{i2}, \ldots, x_{ik}$. We choose our estimates of $a, b_1, \ldots, b_k$ to be those values that minimize the sum of squared residuals $\sum (y_i - \hat{y}_i)^2$. These values are said to be the **least squares estimates** of $\alpha, \beta_1, \beta_2, \ldots,$ and $\beta_k$. This is precisely analogous to what we did in Section 2.6 for simple linear regression, but now there are $k$ covariates instead of 1. When there are just two covariates the observations $\{(x_{i1}, x_{i2}, y_i) : i = 1, \ldots, n\}$ can be thought of as a cloud of points in three dimensions. The estimates $\hat{y}_i = a + b_1 x_{i1} + b_2 x_{i2}$ all lie on a plane that bisects this cloud (see Figure 3.1). The **residual** $y_i - \hat{y}_i$ is the vertical distance between the observation $y_i$ and this plane. We choose the values of $a$, $b_1$, and $b_2$ that give the plane that minimizes the sum of squares of these vertical distances. When the points all lie on the same plane (as in Figure 3.1) the values of $a$, $b_1$ and $b_2$ that define this plane give residuals that are all zero. These values are our least squares estimates of $\alpha$, $\beta_1$ and $\beta_2$, since they give a sum of squared residuals that equals zero.

## 3.4. $R^2$ statistic for multiple regression models

As in simple linear regression, the total variation of the dependent variable is measured by the total sum of squares (TSS), which equals $\sum (y_i - \bar{y})^2$. The variation explained by the model, the model sum of squares (MSS), equals $\sum (\hat{y}_i - \bar{y})^2$. The proportion of the variation explained by the model is $R^2 = \text{MSS}/\text{TSS}$. This is the same formula given in Section 2.8 for simple linear regression. This statistic is a useful measure of the explanatory power of the model. It is also equal to the square of the correlation coefficient between $y_i$ and $\hat{y}_i$.

## 3.5. Expected response in the multiple regression model

Let $\mathbf{x}_i = (x_{i1}, x_{i2}, \ldots, x_{ik})$ be a compact way of denoting the values of all of the covariates for the $i^{\text{th}}$ patient. Then, if the model is true, it can be shown that the expected value of both $y_i$ and $\hat{y}_i$ given her covariates is

$$\text{E}[y_i \mid \mathbf{x}_i] = \text{E}[\hat{y}_i \mid \mathbf{x}_i] = \alpha + \beta_1 x_{i1} + \beta_2 x_{i2} + \cdots + \beta_k x_{ik}. \tag{3.2}$$

We estimate the expected value of $y_i$ among subjects whose covariate values are identical to those of the $i^{\text{th}}$ patient by $\hat{y}_i$. The equation

$$\hat{y}_i = a + b_1 x_{i1} + b_2 x_{i2} + \cdots + b_k x_{ik} \tag{3.3}$$

may be rewritten

$$\hat{y}_i = \bar{y} + b_1(x_{i1} - \bar{x}_1) + b_2(x_{i2} - \bar{x}_2) + \cdots + b_k(x_{ik} - \bar{x}_k). \tag{3.4}$$

Thus $\hat{y}_i = \bar{y}$ when $x_{i1} = \bar{x}_1, x_{i2} = \bar{x}_2, \ldots,$ and $x_{ik} = \bar{x}_k$.

## 3.6. The accuracy of multiple regression parameter estimates

In Equation (3.1) the error term $\varepsilon_i$ has a variance of $\sigma^2$. We estimate this variance by

$$s^2 = \sum (y_i - \hat{y}_i)^2/(n - k - 1). \tag{3.5}$$

As was the case with simple linear regression, you can think of $s^2$ as being the average squared residual as long as $n$ is much larger than $k + 1$. It is often called the **mean squared error** (MSE). It can be shown that the expected value of $s^2$ is $\sigma^2$. The standard deviation $\sigma$ is estimated by $s$ which is called the **root MSE**.

The standard errors of the parameter estimates $a, b_1, b_2, \ldots, b_k$ are estimated by formulas of the form

$$\text{se}[b_j] = s/f_j[\{x_{ij} : i = 1, \ldots, n; j = 1, \ldots, k\}], \tag{3.6}$$

where $f_j[\{x_{ij} : i = 1, \ldots, n; j = 1, \ldots, k\}]$ is a complicated function of all of the covariates on all of the patients. Fortunately, we do not need to spell out this formula in detail as statistical software can derive it for us. The important thing to remember about Equation (3.6) is that the standard error of $b_j$ increases as $s$, the standard deviation of the residuals, increases, and decreases as the dispersion of the covariates increases. Equation (3.6) is a generalization of Equation (2.13), which gives the standard error of the slope coefficient for the simple linear regression model.

Under the null hypothesis that $\beta_j = 0$,

$$b_j/\text{se}[b_j] \tag{3.7}$$

has a $t$ distribution with $n - k - 1$ degrees of freedom. That is, the number of degrees of freedom equals $n$, the number of patients, minus $k + 1$, the number of parameters in the model. We can use Equation (3.7) to test this null hypothesis. A 95% confidence interval for $\beta_j$ is given by

$$b_j \pm t_{n-k-1,0.025} \times \text{se}[b_j]. \tag{3.8}$$

## 3.7. Hypothesis tests

If $\beta_1 = \beta_2 = \cdots = \beta_k = 0$ then $\mathrm{E}[y_i \mid \mathbf{x}_i] = \alpha$ and the values of the covariates have no influence on the value of the outcome variable. Testing the hypothesis that $y_i$ is unaffected by $\mathbf{x}_i$ is equivalent to testing the null hypothesis that $\beta_1 = \beta_2 = \cdots = \beta_k = 0$. Let the mean sum of squares due to the model (MSM) = MSS/$k$. Then if this null hypothesis is true the ratio MSM/MSE has a known distribution, called an $F$ distribution. The $F$ distributions are a family whose shapes are determined by two integer parameters called degrees of freedom. An $F$ distribution with $n_1$ and $n_2$ degrees is denoted $F_{n_1,n_2}$. If the null hypothesis is false then MSM will be large relative to MSE. Hence, large values of MSM/MSE will lead to rejection of the null hypothesis that the $\beta$ parameters are all simultaneously zero. The $P$-value associated with this hypothesis is

$$P = \Pr\left[\mathrm{MSM/MSE} > F_{k,n-k-1}\right]. \tag{3.9}$$

Sometimes we will wish to test the null hypothesis that some subset of the $\beta$ parameters are simultaneously zero. If there are $q$ such parameters $\beta_{(1)}, \ldots, \beta_{(q)}$ then under the null hypothesis that $\beta_{(1)} = \beta_{(2)} = \cdots = \beta_{(q)} = 0$ we can derive an $F$ statistic with $q$ and $n - k - 1$ degrees of freedom. If we denote this statistic by $f$ then the $P$ value associated with this null hypothesis is

$$P = \Pr\left[f > F_{q,n-k-1}\right]. \tag{3.10}$$

The statistic $f$ is a function of the $q$ beta parameter estimates, the estimated variances of the model's parameters, and the estimated covariances of all possible pairs of parameter estimates. It is easily calculated by statistical software packages like Stata. When $q = k$ we are testing whether all of the $\beta$ parameters are zero and $f$ = MSM/MSE. Hence, Equation (3.9) is a special case of Equation (3.10).

## 3.8. Leverage

Many of the concepts and statistics that we introduced for simple linear regression have counterparts in multiple linear regression. One of these is leverage. The **leverage** $h_i$ is a measure of the potential ability of the $i^{\text{th}}$ patient to influence the parameter estimates. Patients with high leverage will have an appreciable influence on these estimates if the residual $e_i = y_i - \hat{y}_i$ is large. The formula for $h_i$ is a complex function of the covariates

$\{x_{ij} : i = 1, \ldots, n; j = 1, \ldots, k\}$ but does not involve the response values $\{y_i : i = 1, \ldots, n\}$. It can be shown that $1/n \leq h_i \leq 1$. A leverage greater than 0.2 is generally considered to be large. Leverage is easily calculated by any modern statistical software package.

The variance of $\hat{y}_i$, given all of the covariates $\mathbf{x}_i$ for the $i^{\text{th}}$ patient, is estimated by

$$\text{var}[\hat{y}_i \mid \mathbf{x}_i] = s^2 h_i. \tag{3.11}$$

Hence $h_i$ can also be thought of as the variance of $\hat{y}_i$ given $\mathbf{x}_i$ expressed in units of $s^2$. Note that Equation (3.11) is analogous to Equation (2.23) for simple linear regression.

## 3.9. 95% confidence interval for $\hat{y}_i$

It can be shown that $(\hat{y}_i - \text{E}[y_i \mid \mathbf{x}_i])/\sqrt{\text{var}[\hat{y}_i \mid \mathbf{x}_i]}$ has a $t$ distribution with $n - k - 1$ degrees of freedom. From Equation (3.11) we have that the standard error of $\hat{y}_i$ given this patient's covariates is $s\sqrt{h_i}$. Hence, the 95% confidence interval for $\hat{y}_i$ is

$$\hat{y}_i \pm t_{n-k-1,0.025}(s\sqrt{h_i}). \tag{3.12}$$

## 3.10. 95% prediction intervals

Suppose that a new patient has covariates $x_1, x_2, \ldots, x_k$, which we will denote by $\mathbf{x}$, and leverage $h$. Let $\hat{y}[\mathbf{x}] = a + b_1x_1 + b_2x_2 + \cdots + b_kx_k$ be her estimated expected response given these covariates. Then the estimated variance of her predicted response $y$ is

$$\text{var}[y \mid \mathbf{x}] = s^2(h + 1), \tag{3.13}$$

and a 95% prediction interval for $y$ is

$$\hat{y}[\mathbf{x}] \pm t_{n-k-1,0.025}(s\sqrt{h+1}). \tag{3.14}$$

Equations (3.11), (3.13), and (3.1) are precisely analogous to Equations (2.23), (2.24) and (2.25) for simple linear regression.

## 3.11. Example: the Framingham Heart Study

The Framingham Heart Study (Levy, 1999) has collected long-term follow-up and cardiovascular risk factor data on almost 5000 residents of the town of Framingham, Massachusetts. Recruitment of patients started in 1948. At the time of the baseline exams there were no effective treatments for hypertension. I have been given permission to use a subset of the 40-year data from this study in this text (Framingham Heart Study, 1997). We will refer to this subset as the Framingham Heart Study didactic data set. It consists of data on 4699 patients who were free of coronary heart disease at their baseline exam. At this exam, the following variables were recorded on each patient. The Stata names for these variables are given in the first column below:

*sbp* = systolic blood pressure (SBP) in mm Hg,
*dbp* = diastolic blood pressure (DBP) in mm Hg,
*age* = age in years,
*scl* = serum cholesterol (SCL) in mg/100 ml,
*bmi* = body mass index (BMI) = weight/height$^2$ in kg/m$^2$,
*sex* = gender coded as $\begin{cases} 1\text{: if subject is male} \\ 2\text{: if subject is female,} \end{cases}$
*month* = month of year in which baseline exam occurred, and
*id* = a patient identification variable (numbered 1 to 4699).

Follow-up information on coronary heart disease is also provided:

*followup* = the subject's follow-up in days, and

$$chdfate = \begin{cases} 1\text{: if the patient develops CHD at the end of follow-up} \\ 0\text{: otherwise.} \end{cases}$$

In Section 2.19.1 we showed that the rate at which SBP increased with BMI was greater for women than for men. In this example, we will explore this relationship in greater detail, and will seek to build a multiple linear regression model that adequately explains how SBP is affected by the other variables listed above. Although we usually have hypotheses to test that were postulated in advance of data collection, there is almost always an exploratory component to the modeling of a multivariate data set. It is all too easy to force an inappropriate model on the data. The best way to avoid doing this is to become familiar with your data through a series of analyses of increasing complexity and to do residual analyses that will identify individual patients whose data may result in misleading conclusions.

### 3.11.1. Preliminary univariate analyses

We first perform separate simple linear regressions of SBP on each of the continuous covariates: age, BMI, and serum cholesterol. Residual analyses should be performed and the variables should be transformed if appropriate

**Table 3.1.** Summary of results of three separate simple linear regressions of log systolic blood pressure against log body mass index, age, and log serum cholesterol

| Model | Slope coefficient | $t$ | $P$-value | 95% confidence interval | $R^2$ |
|---|---|---|---|---|---|
| $\log[sbp_i] = \alpha + \beta \times \log[bmi_i]$ | 0.355 | 24.7 | $< 0.0005$ | 0.33–0.38 | 0.12 |
| $\log[sbp_i] = \alpha + \beta \times age_i$ | 0.007 52 | 29.6 | $< 0.0005$ | 0.0070–0.0080 | 0.16 |
| $\log[sbp_i] = \alpha + \beta \times \log[scl_i]$ | 0.196 | 16.3 | $< 0.0005$ | 0.17–0.22 | 0.05 |

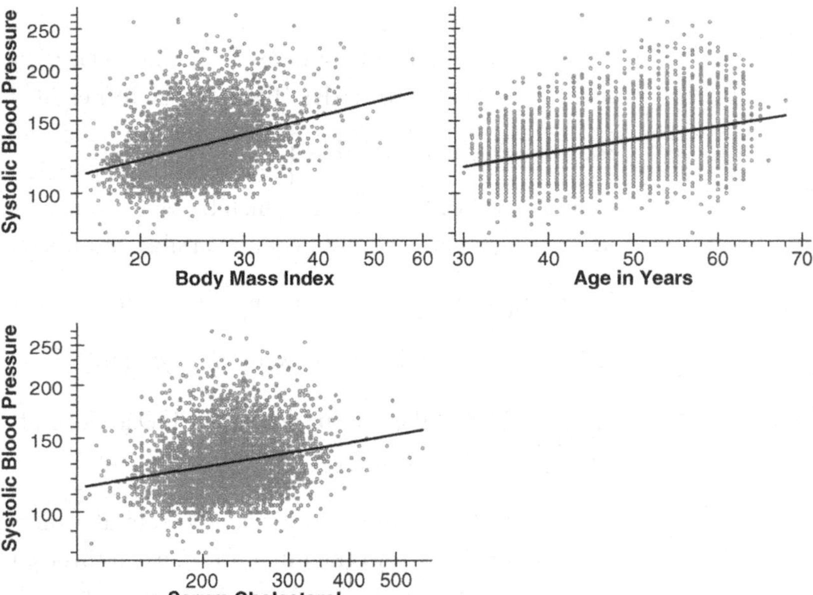


Figure 3.2 Simple linear regressions of log systolic blood pressure against log body mass index, age, and log serum cholesterol. These data are from the Framingham Heart Study (Levy, 1999). All measurements were taken at each subject's baseline exam.

(see Sections 2.15–2.18). These analyses indicate that reasonable linear fits can be obtained by regressing log SBP against log BMI, log SBP against age, and log SBP against log SCL. Table 3.1 summarizes the results of these simple linear regressions. Figure 3.2 shows the corresponding scatter plots and linear regression lines. These univariate regressions show that SBP is related to age and SCL as well as BMI. Although the statistical significance of the slope coefficients is overwhelming, the $R^2$ statistics are low. Hence, each of these risk factors individually only explain a modest proportion of the total variability in systolic blood pressure. By building a multivariate model of these variables we seek to achieve a better understanding of the relationship between these variables.

Note that the importance of a parameter depends not only on its magnitude but also on the range of the corresponding covariate. For example, the age coefficient is only 0.007 52 as compared with 0.355 and 0.196 for log[BMI] and log[SCL]. However, the range of age is from 30 to 68 as compared with 2.79–4.05 for log[BMI] and 4.74–6.34 for log[SCL]. The large age range increases the variation in log[SBP] that is associated with age. In fact, age explains more of the variation in log[SBP] (has a higher $R^2$ statistic) than either of the other two covariates.

Changing the units of measurement of a covariate can have a dramatic effect on the size of the slope estimate, but no effect on its biologic meaning. For example, suppose we regressed blood pressure against weight in grams. If we converted weight from grams to kilograms we would increase the magnitude of the slope parameter by 1000 and decrease the range of observed weights by 1000. The appearance of the plotted regression line and the statistical significance of the regression analysis would be unchanged.

## 3.12. Scatter plot matrix graphs

Another useful exploratory graphic is the scatter plot matrix, which consists of all possible scatter plots of the specified variables. Such graphs can be effective at showing the interrelationships between multiple variables observed on a sample of patients. Figure 3.3 shows such a plot for log[SBP], log[BMI], age, and log[SCL] from the Framingham Heart Study. The graph is restricted to women recruited in January to reduce the number of data points and allow individual patient values to be discernible.

### 3.12.1. Producing Scatter Plot Matrix Graphs with Stata

The following log file and comments illustrate how to produce a scatter plot matrix graph with Stata.

```
. *  3.12.1.Framingham.log
. *
. *  Plot a scatterplot matrix of log(sbp), log(bmi), age and
. *  log(scl) for women from the Framingham Heart Study who
. *  were recruited in January.
. *
. use C:\WDDtext\2.20.Framingham.dta
```

```
. generate logsbp = log(sbp)

. label variable logsbp "Log Systolic Blood Pressure"                    1

. generate logbmi = log(bmi)
(9 missing values generated)

. label variable logbmi "Log Body Mass Index"

. generate logscl = log(scl)
(33 missing values generated)

. label variable logscl "Log Serum Cholesterol"

. graph matrix logsbp logbmi age logscl if month==1 & sex==2             2
```

**Comments**

1 This command adds "Log Systolic Blood Pressure" as a label to the variable *logsbp*. This label will be used as the axis title in plots that show *logdis* on

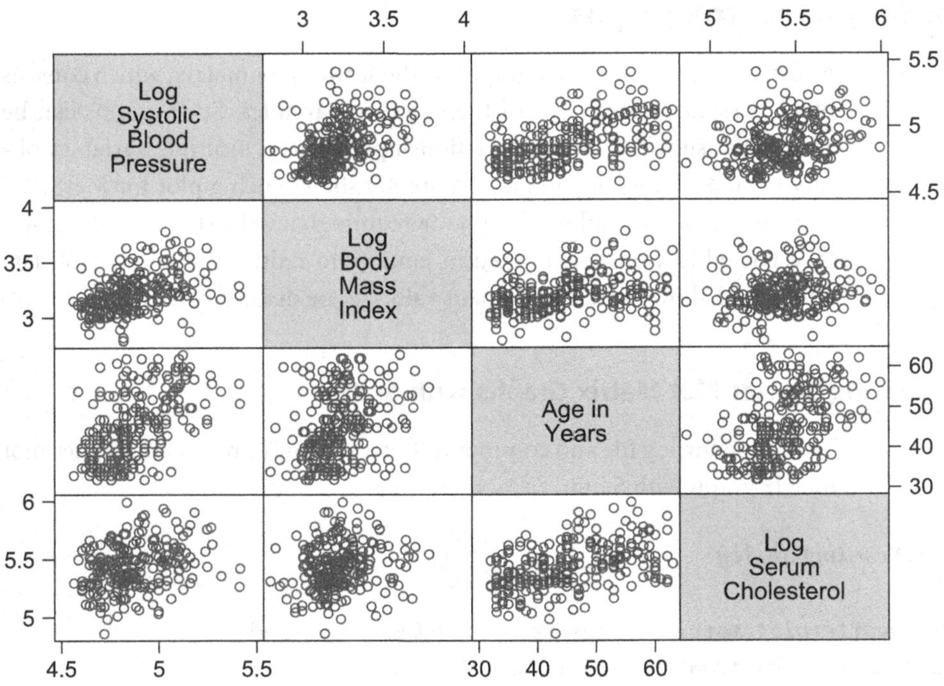


Figure 3.3 Scatter plot matrix of data from women recruited into the Framingham Heart Study during one month. This graph shows all possible scatter plots of the specified variables.

either the $x$- or the $y$-axis and in the output from various Stata commands. The equivalent point-and-click command is Data ▶ Labels ▶ Label variable ⌜ Variable: *logbmi* , New variable label: (may be up to 80 characters) *Log Systolic Blood Pressure* Submit

2 This *graph matrix* command generates a scatter plot matrix for *logsbp, logbmi, age,* and *logscl.* The *if* clause restricts the graph to women (*sex* == *2*) who entered the study in January (*month* == *1*). The equivalent point-and-click command is Graphics ▶ Scatter plot matrix Main Variables: *logsbp logbmi age logscl* if/in ⌜ Restrict observations — If: (expression) *month == 1 & sex == 2* Submit

## 3.13. Modeling interaction in multiple linear regression

### 3.13.1. The Framingham example

Let $\mathbf{x}_i = (logbmi_i, age_i, logscl_i, sex_i)$ denote the covariates for log[BMI], age, log[SCL], and sex for the $i^{\text{th}}$ patient. Let $logsbp_i$ denote his or her log[SBP]. The first model that comes to mind for regressing log[SBP] against these covariates is

$$\begin{aligned} \mathrm{E}[logsbp_i \mid \mathbf{x}_i] = \alpha + \beta_1 \times logbmi_i + \beta_2 \times age_i \\ + \beta_3 \times logscl_i + \beta_4 \times sex_i. \end{aligned} \tag{3.15}$$

A potential weakness of this model is that it implies that the effects of the covariates on $logsbp_i$ are additive. To understand what this means consider the following. Suppose we look at patients with identical values of $age_i$ and $logscl_i$. Then for these patients $\alpha + \beta_2 \times age_i + \beta_3 \times logscl_i$ will equal a constant and Model (3.15) implies that

$$\mathrm{E}[logsbp_i \mid \mathbf{x}_i] = \text{constant} + \beta_1 \times logbmi_i + \beta_4 \tag{3.16}$$

for men, and

$$\mathrm{E}[logsbp_i \mid \mathbf{x}_i] = \text{constant} + \beta_1 \times logbmi_i + 2\beta_4 \tag{3.17}$$

for women (recall that the covariate $sex_i$ takes the values 1 and 2 for men and women, respectively). Subtracting Equation (3.16) from Equation (3.17) gives that the difference in expected log[SBP] for men and women with identical BMIs is $\beta_4$. Hence, the $\beta_4$ parameter allows men and women with the same BMI to have different expected log[SBP]s. However, the slope of the $logsbp_i$ vs. $logbmi_i$ relationship for both men and women is $\beta_1$. Our analysis

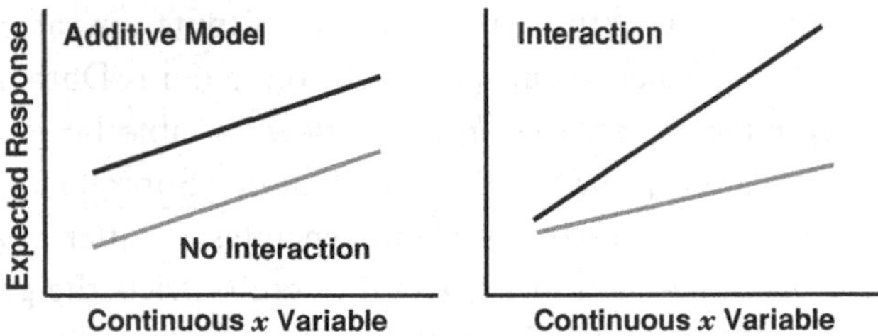


Figure 3.4 Effect of a dichotomous and a continuous covariate on expected patient response. On the left the dichotomous variable (black and gray lines) does not interact with the continuous variable ($x$-axis) giving parallel regression lines. On the right the two variables interact and the effect of the dichotomous variable is much greater for large values of $x$ than for small values.

in Section 2.19.1 indicated, however, that this slope is higher for women than for men. This is an example of what we call **interaction**, in which the effect of one covariate on the dependent variable is influenced by the value of a second covariate. Models such as (3.15) are said to be **additive** in that the joint effect of any two covariates equals the sum of the individual effects of these covariates. Figure 3.4 illustrates the difference between additive and interactive models. In the additive model, the regression lines for, say, men and women are parallel; in the model with interaction they diverge.

We need a more complex model to deal with interaction. In the Framingham example let

$$woman_i = sex_i - 1. \tag{3.18}$$

Then

$$woman_i = \begin{cases} 1\text{: if } i^{\text{th}} \text{ subject is female,} \\ 0\text{: if } i^{\text{th}} \text{ subject is male.} \end{cases} \tag{3.19}$$

Consider the model

$$\begin{aligned} \text{E}[logsbp_i \mid \mathbf{x}_i] = \alpha + \beta_1 \times logbmi_i + \beta_2 \times woman_i \\ + \beta_3 \times logbmi_i \times woman_i. \end{aligned} \tag{3.20}$$

In this and subsequent models, $\mathbf{x}_i$ represents the values of all of the model's covariates for the $i^{\text{th}}$ patient, in this case $logbmi_i$ and $woman_i$. Model (3.20) reduces to

$$\text{E}[logsbpi_i \mid \mathbf{x}_i] = \alpha + \beta_1 \times logbmi_i \tag{3.21}$$

for men and

$$\text{E}[logsbpi_i \mid \mathbf{x}_i] = \alpha + (\beta_1 + \beta_3) \times logbmi_i + \beta_2 \tag{3.22}$$

for women. Hence, the regression slopes for men and women are $\beta_1$ and $\beta_1 + \beta_3$, respectively. The parameter $\beta_3$ is the difference in slopes between men and women.

## 3.14. Multiple regression modeling of the Framingham data

In Section 2.19.1 we showed that there was a significant difference between the slopes of the simple linear regressions of log[SBP] against log[BMI] in men and women. A reasonable approach to multiple regression modeling of these data is to regress log[SBP] against log[BMI], sex, age, log[SCL], and the interaction of sex with log[BMI], age, and log[SCL]. That is, we consider the model

$$\begin{aligned} \mathrm{E}[\log[sbp_i] \mid \mathbf{x}_i] = \alpha &+ \beta_1 \times \log[bmi_i] + \beta_2 \times age_i + \beta_3 \times \log[scl_i] \\ &+ \beta_4 \times woman_i + \beta_5 \times woman_i \times \log[bmi_i] \\ &+ \beta_6 \times woman_i \times age_i \\ &+ \beta_7 \times woman_i \times \log[scl_i]. \end{aligned} \tag{3.23}$$

The estimates of the regression coefficients from Model (3.23) are given in Table 3.2. The covariate associated with each coefficient is given in the left-most column of this table. The *P*-values correspond to the test of the null hypothesis that the true values of these parameters are zero. The $R^2$ value for this model is 0.2550, which is about twice the $R^2$ from the simple linear

**Table 3.2.** Parameter estimates from Models (3.23), (3.24), and (3.25) for analyzing the Framingham Heart Study baseline data (Levy, 1999)

| | Model (3.23) | | | Model (3.24) | | | Model (3.25) | | |
|---|---|---|---|---|---|---|---|---|---|
| Covariate | Parameter | Parameter estimate | *P*-value | Parameter | Parameter estimate | *P*-value | Parameter | Parameter estimate | *P*-value |
| 1 | $\alpha$ | 3.5494 | <0.0005 | $\alpha$ | 3.5726 | < 0.0005 | $\alpha$ | 3.5374 | <0.0005 |
| $\log[bmi_i]$ | $\beta_1$ | 0.2498 | <0.0005 | $\beta_1$ | 0.2509 | < 0.0005 | $\beta_1$ | 0.2626 | <0.0005 |
| $age_i$ | $\beta_2$ | 0.0035 | <0.0005 | $\beta_2$ | 0.0035 | < 0.0005 | $\beta_2$ | 0.0035 | <0.0005 |
| $\log[scl_i]$ | $\beta_3$ | 0.0651 | <0.0005 | $\beta_3$ | 0.0601 | < 0.0005 | $\beta_3$ | 0.0596 | <0.0005 |
| $woman_i$ | $\beta_4$ | −0.2292 | 0.11 | $\beta_4$ | −0.2715 | 0.004 | $\beta_4$ | −0.2165 | <0.0005 |
| $woman_i \times \log[bmi_i]$ | $\beta_5$ | 0.0189 | 0.52 | $\beta_5$ | 0.0176 | 0.55 | | | |
| $woman_i \times age_i$ | $\beta_6$ | 0.0049 | <0.0005 | $\beta_6$ | 0.0048 | < 0.0005 | $\beta_5$ | 0.0049 | <0.0005 |
| $woman_i \times \log[scl_i]$ | $\beta_7$ | −0.0090 | 0.70 | | | | | | |

regression of log[$sbp$] against log[$bmi$]. Hence, Model (3.23) explains 25.5% of the variation in log[SBP]. We seek the simplest model that satisfactorily explains the data. The estimate of coefficient $\beta_7$ is very small and has a non-significant $P$-value of 0.70. This $P$-value is larger than any of the other parameter $P$-values in the model. Hence, the $woman_i \times \log(scl_i)$ interaction term is not contributing much to our ability to predict log[SBP]. Dropping this interaction term from the model gives

$$\begin{aligned} \mathrm{E}[\log[sbp_i] \mid \mathbf{x}_i] = {} & \alpha + \beta_1 \times \log[bmi_i] + \beta_2 \times age_i + \beta_3 \times \log[scl_i] \\ & + \beta_4 \times woman_i + \beta_5 \times woman_i \times \log[bmi_i] \\ & + \beta_6 \times woman_i \times age_i. \end{aligned} \tag{3.24}$$

Model (3.24) gives parameter estimates for $\alpha$, log[BMI], age, log[SCL], and sex that are very similar to those of Model (3.23). The $R^2$ is unchanged, indicating that we have not lost any explanatory power by dropping the $woman_i \times \log[scl_i]$ interaction term. Dropping ineffectual terms from the model not only clarifies the relationship between the response variable and the covariates, but also increases the statistical power of our analyses.

In Model (3.24) the $woman_i \times \log[bmi_i]$ interaction term is small and non-significant. Dropping this term gives

$$\begin{aligned} \mathrm{E}[\log[sbp_i] \mid \mathbf{x}_i] = {} & \alpha + \beta_1 \times \log[bmi_i] + \beta_2 \times age_i + \beta_3 \times \log[scl_i] \\ & + \beta_4 \times woman_i + \beta_5 \times woman_i \times age_i. \end{aligned} \tag{3.25}$$

This deletion has little effect on the remaining coefficient estimates, all of which are now highly statistically significant. The $R^2$ statistic is 0.2549, which is virtually unchanged from the previous two models. All of the remaining terms in the model remain highly significant and should not be dropped.

## 3.15. Intuitive understanding of a multiple regression model

### 3.15.1. The Framingham example

When we did simple linear regressions of log[SBP] against log[BMI] for men and women we obtained slope estimates of 0.273 and 0.399 for men and women, respectively. The multiple regression Model (3.25) gives a single slope estimate of 0.2626 for both sexes, but finds that the effect of increasing age on log[SBP] is twice as large in women than men. That is, for women this slope is $\beta_2 + \beta_5 = 0.0035 + 0.0049 = 0.0084$ while for men it is

$\beta_2 = 0.0035$. How reasonable is our model? In Section 3.2 we said that the parameter for a covariate in a multiple regression model measures the slope of the relationship between the response variable and this covariate when all other covariates are held constant. One way to increase our intuitive understanding of the model is to plot separate simple linear regressions of SBP against BMI in groups of patients who are homogeneous with respect to the other variables in the model. Figure 3.5 shows linear regressions of log[SBP] against log[BMI] in subgroups defined by sex and 10-year age groups. These regressions are restricted to subjects whose log[SCL] lies in the inter-quartile range for this variable, which is from 5.28 to 5.42. The vertical and horizontal lines show the mean log[BMI] and log[SBP] in each panel. The black regression lines plot the simple linear regression of log[SBP] against log[BMI] for the patients in each panel. The thick gray lines are drawn through each panel's joint mean value for log[SBP] and log[BMI] and have slope 0.263 (the estimated parameter for log[BMI] from Model (3.25)). A dashed line is also drawn through the joint mean values in the panels for women and has slope 0.399. This is the slope of the simple linear regression of log[SBP] against log[BMI] restricted to women (see Section 2.19.1). Note that the slopes of the black and gray lines are almost identical in all of the panels except for women aged 30–40 and 40–50. For women aged 30–40 the black simple regression slope for this panel is less than both the gray multiple regression slope and the dashed simple regression slope for all women. The gray multiple regression slope comes much closer to the simple regression slope for this panel than does the dashed simple regression line for all women. For women aged 40–50 the simple regression slope exceeds the multiple regression slope and comes close to the dashed line for all women. However, by and large, this figure supports the finding that there is little variation in the rate at which SBP increases with BMI among people of the same sex and similar age and SCL.

The interrelationship between SBP, sex, BMI, and age is better illustrated in Figure 3.6. In this figure SBP and BMI are drawn on a linear scale. In each panel the vertical and horizontal lines mark the mean SBP and BMI for all subjects with the gender and age range specified for the panel. In their thirties men, on average, are fatter than women and have higher systolic blood pressures. The average increase in BMI with increasing age among men, however, is modest. In contrast, the mean BMI increases in women from 23.8 in their thirties to 27.5 in their sixties. This corresponds to an average increase in weight of 9.5 kg (21 lb) for a woman 160 cm (5 ft 3 in) tall. Moreover, SBP increases much faster with age for women than men, and by their sixties, women have a higher mean SBP than their male counterparts.

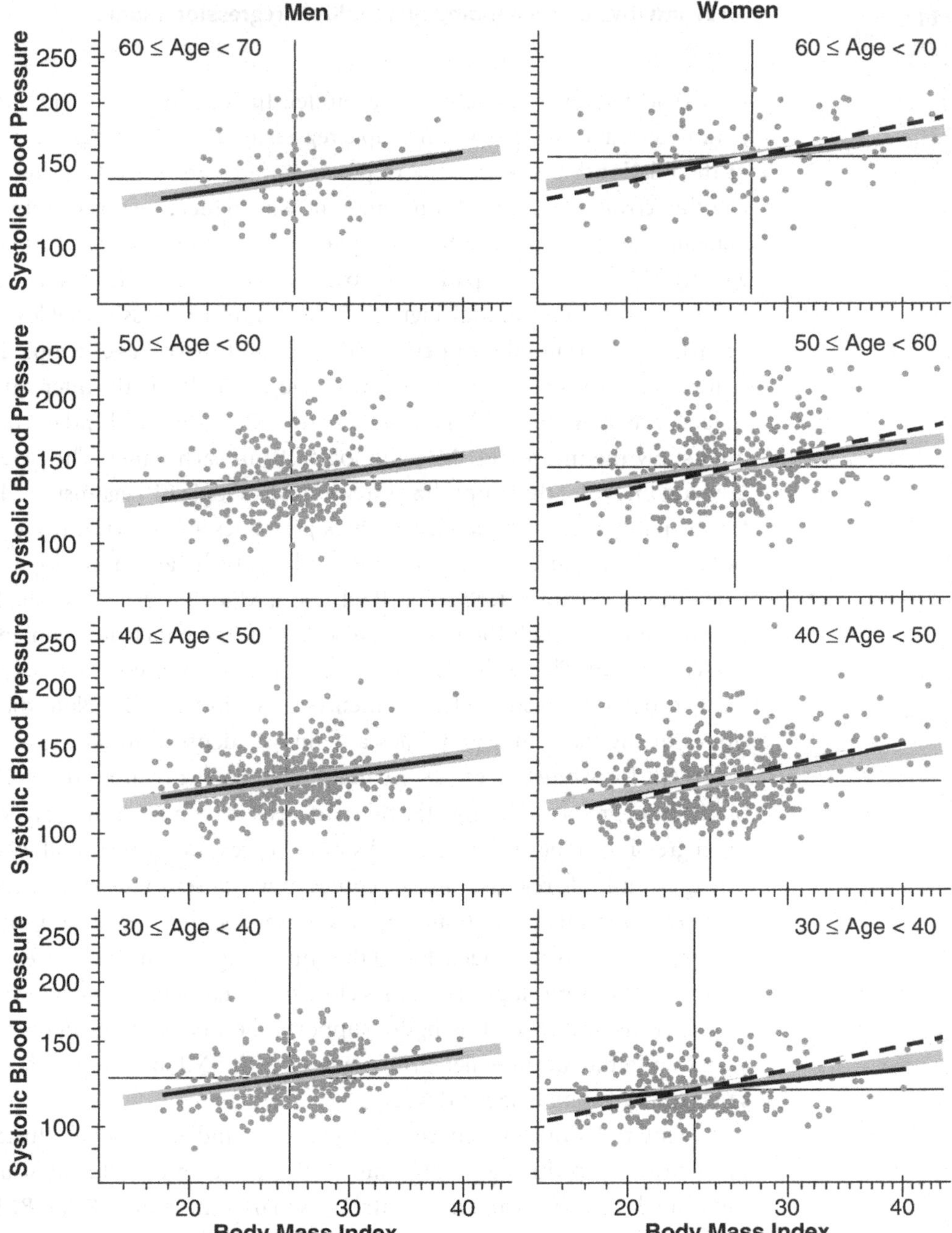


Figure 3.5 The black sloping lines in these panels are simple linear regressions of log systolic blood pressure (SBP) against log body mass index (BMI) in men and women of similar age and serum cholesterol levels (SCL) from the Framingham Heart Study. The thick gray lines have the slope of the log[BMI] parameter in the multiple linear regression Model (3.25). The dashed lines have the slope of the simple linear regression of log[SBP] against log[BMI] among women in this study. This graph confirms the finding of Model (3.25) that the relationship between log[SBP] and log[BMI] is similar among men and women of similar age and SCL levels (see text).

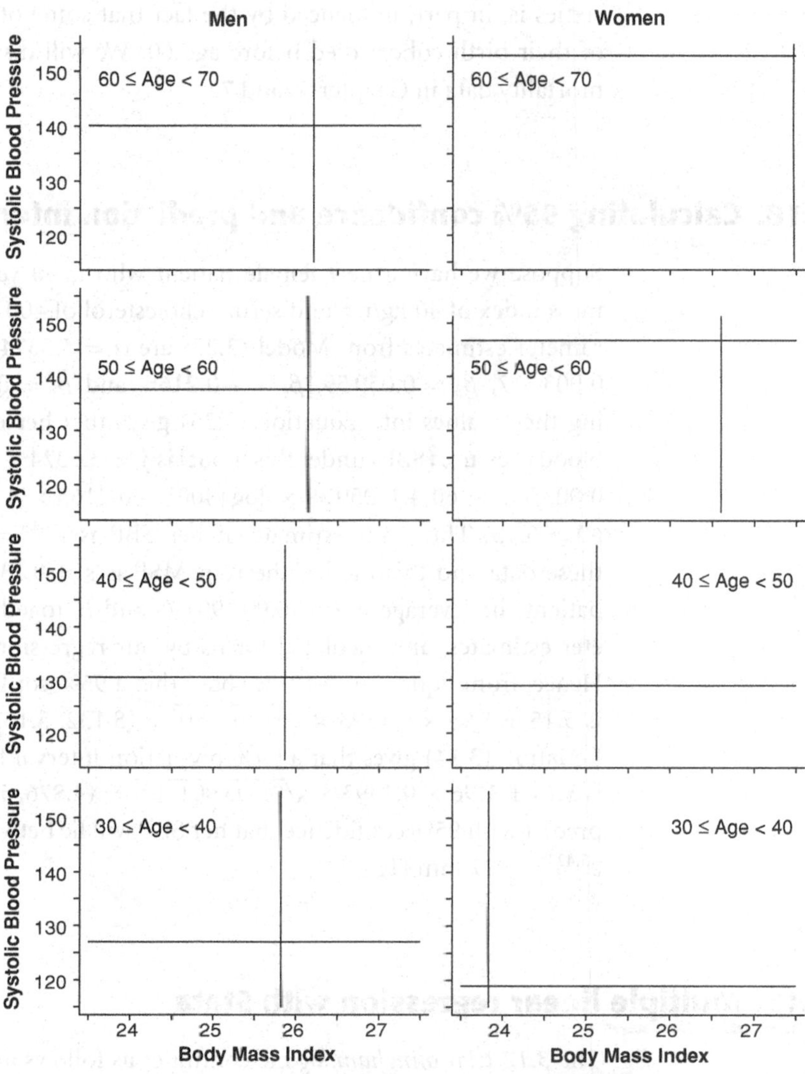


Figure 3.6 The mean systolic blood pressure and body mass index of patients from the Framingham Heart Study are indicated by horizontal and vertical lines in panels defined by age and sex. This figure illustrates the marked interaction between gender, body mass index, and age on systolic blood pressure.

Thus, Figure 3.6 is consistent with our analysis, Model (3.25), which found that there is a pronounced interaction of sex and age on log[SBP] but no evidence of interaction between sex and log[BMI] on log[SBP].

A factor that should be considered in interpreting Figures 3.5 and 3.6 is that these figures do not take differential mortality rates between men and women into account. Hence, the comparatively modest BMI of men in their sixties is, in part, influenced by the fact that some of the fatter members of their birth cohort died before age 60. We will discuss how to analyze mortality data in Chapters 6 and 7.

## 3.16. Calculating 95% confidence and prediction intervals

Suppose we have a new female patient who is 60 years old, has a body mass index of 40 kg/m$^2$ and serum cholesterol of 400 mg/100 ml. The parameter estimates from Model (3.25) are $\alpha = 3.5374$, $\beta_1 = 0.2626$, $\beta_2 = 0.003\,517$, $\beta_3 = 0.059\,59$, $\beta_4 = -0.2165$, and $\beta_5 = 0.004\,862$. Substituting these values into Equation (3.25) gives that her expected log systolic blood pressure (SBP) under this model is $\hat{y} = 3.5374 + 0.2626 \times \log[40] + 0.003\,517 \times 60 + 0.059\,59 \times \log[400] - 0.2165 \times 1 + 0.004\,862 \times 1 \times 60 = 5.15$. Thus, our estimate of her SBP is $e^{5.15} = 172$ mm Hg. For these data and this model, the root MSE is $s = 0.1393$. For this specific patient the leverage is $h = 0.003\,901$ ($s$ and $h$, together with the parameter estimates, are calculated for us by our regression software package). Hence, from Equation (3.12) we have that a 95% confidence interval for $\hat{y}$ is $5.15 \pm 1.96 \times 0.1393 \times \sqrt{0.003\,901} = (5.132, 5.167)$. Substituting into Equation (3.14) gives that a 95% prediction interval for $\hat{y}$ for this patient is $5.15 \pm 1.96 \times 0.1393 \times \sqrt{0.003\,901 + 1} = (4.876, 5.423)$. Hence, we can predict with 95% confidence that her SBP will lie between $e^{4.876} = 131$ and $e^{5.423} = 227$ mm Hg.

## 3.17. Multiple linear regression with Stata

The *3.12.1.Framingham.log* file continues as follows and illustrates how to perform the analyses discussed in Sections 3.14, 3.15, and 3.16.

```
. *
. *  Use multiple regression models to analyze the effects of log(sbp),
. *  log(bmi), age and log(scl) on log(sbp)
. *
. generate woman = sex - 1

. generate wo_lbmi = woman * logbmi
(9 missing values generated)

. generate wo_age  = woman * age
```

```
. generate wo_lscl = woman * logscl

(33 missing values generated)

. regress logsbp logbmi age logscl woman  wo_lbmi wo_age wo_lscl    1
                                            Output omitted. See Table 3.2
. regress logsbp logbmi age logscl woman  wo_lbmi wo_age            2
                                            Output omitted. See Table 3.2
. regress logsbp logbmi age logscl woman  wo_age                    3

      Source |       SS       df       MS              Number of obs =    4658
-------------+------------------------------           F(  5,  4652) =  318.33   4
       Model |  30.8663845     5  6.1732769            Prob > F      =  0.0000   5
    Residual |  90.2160593  4652  .019392962           R-squared     =  0.2549   6
-------------+------------------------------           Adj R-squared =  0.2541
       Total |  121.082444  4657  .026000095           Root MSE      =  .13926

------------------------------------------------------------------------------
      logsbp |      Coef.   Std. Err.      t    P>|t|     [95% Conf. Interval]    7
-------------+----------------------------------------------------------------
      logbmi |    .262647   .0137549    19.09   0.000     .2356808    .2896131
         age |   .0035167   .0003644     9.65   0.000     .0028023    .0042311    8
      logscl |   .0595923   .0114423     5.21   0.000     .0371599    .0820247
       woman |  -.2165261   .0233469    -9.27   0.000    -.2622971   -.1707551
      wo_age |   .0048624   .0004988     9.75   0.000     .0038846    .0058403
       _cons |   3.537356   .0740649    47.76   0.000     3.392153    3.682558    9
------------------------------------------------------------------------------

. *
. * Calculate 95% confidence and prediction intervals for a 60
. * year-old woman with a SCL of 400 and a BMI of 40.
. *
. edit                                                              10

- preserve
- set obs 4700
- replace scl = 400 in 4700
- replace age = 60 in 4700
- replace bmi = 40 in 4700
- replace woman = 1 in 4700
- replace id = 9999 in 4700
-
```

```
. replace logbmi = log(bmi) if id == 9999                                  11

(1 real change made)

. replace logscl = log(scl) if id == 9999

(1 real change made)

. replace wo_age = woman*age if id == 9999

(1 real change made)

. predict yhat,xb                                                          12

(41 missing values generated)

. label variable yhat "Expected log[BMI]"

. predict h, leverage                                                      13

(41 missing values generated)

. predict std_yhat, stdp                                                   14

(41 missing values generated)

. predict std_f, stdf                                                      15

(41 missing values generated)

. generate cil_yhat = yhat - invttail(4658-5-1,.025)*std_yhat              16

(41 missing values generated)

. generate ciu_yhat = yhat + invttail(4658-5-1,.025)*std_yhat

(41 missing values generated)

. generate cil_f = yhat - invttail(4658-5-1,.025)*std_f                    17

(41 missing values generated)

. generate ciu_f = yhat + invttail(4658-5-1,.025)*std_f

(41 missing values generated)

. generate cil_sbpf = exp(cil_f)                                           18

(41 missing values generated)
```

```
. generate ciu_sbpf = exp(ciu_f)

(41 missing values generated)

. list bmi age scl woman logbmi logscl yhat h std_yhat std_f
>     cil_yhat ciu_yhat cil_f ciu_f cil_sbpf ciu_sbpf if id==9999
```
19

| 4700. | bmi | age | scl | woman | logbmi | logscl | yhat | h |
|---|---|---|---|---|---|---|---|---|
| | 40 | 60 | 400 | 1 | 3.688879 | 5.991465 | 5.149496 | .003901 |

| std_yhat | std_f | cil_yhat | ciu_yhat | cil_f | ciu_f |
|---|---|---|---|---|---|
| .0086978 | .13953 | 5.132444 | 5.166547 | 4.875951 | 5.42304 |

| cil_sbpf | ciu_sbpf |
|---|---|
| 131.0987 | 226.5669 |

```
. display invttail(4652,.025)

1.9604741
```

## Comments

1 This command regresses *logsbp* against the other covariates given in the command line. It evaluates Model (3.23). The equivalent point-and-click command is Statistics ▶ Linear models and related ▶ Linear regression ⌋ Model ⌊ Dependent variable: *logsbp*, Independent variables: *logbmi age logscl woman wo_lbmi wo_age wo_lscl* [Submit].

Stata has a powerful syntax for building models with interaction that I will introduce in Section 5.23. For didactic reasons, I have chosen to introduce these models by first calculating the interaction covariates explicitly. However, the Stata syntax for these models, which I will introduce for logistic regression, also works for linear regression models and can appreciably reduce your programming effort.

2 This command evaluates Model (3.24).

3 This command evaluates Model (3.25).

4 The output from the *regress* command for multiple linear regression is similar to that for simple linear regression that was discussed in Section 2.12. The mean sum of squares due to the model (MSM) and the mean squared error (MSE) are 6.173 and 0.019 39, respectively. The $F$ statistic for testing whether all of the $\beta$ parameters are simultaneously zero is $F = 6.173/0.019\,39 = 318.33$.

5 This $F$ statistic is of overwhelming statistical significance indicating that the model covariates do affect the value of log SBP.
6 The $R^2$ statistic = MSS/TSS = 30.866/121.08 = 0.2549. Recall that the MSE equals $s^2$ and is defined by Equation (3.5). Taking the square root of this variance estimate gives the root MSE $s = 0.139\,26$.
7 For each covariate in the model, this table gives the estimate of the associated regression coefficient, the standard error of this estimate, the $t$ statistic for testing the null hypothesis that the true value of the parameter equals zero, the $P$-value that corresponds to this $t$ statistic, and the 95% confidence interval for the coefficient estimate. The coefficient estimates in the second column of this table are also given in Table 3.2 in the second column on the right.
8 Note that although the age parameter estimate is small it is almost ten times larger than its associated standard error. Hence this estimate differs from zero with high statistical significance. The large range of the age of study subjects means that the influence of age on *logsbp* will be appreciable even though this coefficient is small.
9 The estimate of the constant coefficient $\alpha$ is 3.537 356.
10 Typing *edit* opens the Stata Editor window (there is a button on the toolbar that does this as well). This command is similar to the *browse* command in that it shows the data in memory. However, unlike the *browse* command, the *edit* command permits you to modify or enter data in memory. We use this editor here to create a new record with covariates *scl*, *age*, *bmi*, and *women* equal to 400, 60, 40, and 1 respectively. For subsequent manipulation set *id* equal to 9999 (or any other identification number that has not already been assigned).
11 The *replace* command redefines those values of an existing variable for which the *if* command qualifier is true. In this command, *logbmi* is only calculated for the new patient with *id* = 9999. This and the following two statements define the covariates *logbmi*, *logscl*, and *wo_age* for this patient. The equivalent point-and-click command is Data ► Create or change variables ► Change contents of variable ⌋ Main ⌊ Variable: *logsbp* , New contents: *log(sbp)* ⌋ if/in ⌊ ⌈ Restrict to observations — If: (expression) *id == 9999* ⌋ Submit .
12 The variable *yhat* is set equal to $\hat{y}_i$ for each record in memory. That is, *yhat* equals the estimated expected value of *logsbp* for each patient. This includes the new record that we have just created. Note that the regression parameter estimates are unaffected by this new record since it was created after the *regress* command was given.

13 The *leverage* option of this *predict* command creates a new variable called *h* that equals the leverage for each patient. Note that *h* is defined for our new patient even though no value of *logsbp* is given. This is because the leverage is a function of the covariates and does not involve the response variable. The equivalent point-and-click command is Statistics ► Postestimation ► Predictions, residuals, etc ⌋Main⌊ New variable name: *h* ⌌ Produce: — ⦿ Leverage ⌋ [Submit].
Other *predict* options are defined on the *predict* dialog box in a similar way.

14 The *stdp* option sets *std_yhat* equal to the standard error of *yhat*, which equals $s\sqrt{h_i}$.

15 The *stdf* option sets *std_f* equal to the standard deviation of *logsbp* given the patient's covariates. That is, $std\_f = s\sqrt{h_i + 1}$.

16 This command and the next define *cil_yhat* and *ciu_yhat* to be the lower and upper bounds of the 95% confidence interval for *yhat*, respectively. This interval is given by Equation (3.12). Note that there are 4658 patients in our regression and there are 5 covariates in our model. Hence the number of degrees of freedom equals $4658 - 5 - 1 = 4652$.

17 This command and the next define *cil_sbpf* and *ciu_sbpf* to be the lower and upper bounds of the 95% prediction interval for *logsbp* given the patient's covariates. This interval is given by Equation (3.14).

18 This command and the next define the 95% prediction interval for the SBP of a new patient having the specified covariates. We exponentiate the prediction interval given by Equation (3.14) to obtain the interval for SBP as opposed to log[SBP].

19 This command lists the covariates and calculated values for the new patient only (that is, for observations for which $id = 9999$ is true). The highlighted values in the output were also calculated by hand in Section 3.16.

## 3.18. Automatic methods of model selection

In Section 3.14 we illustrated how to fit a multiple regression model by hand. When a large number of covariates are available, it can be convenient to use an automatic model selection program for this task. Please note, however, the caveats given in Section 3.18.5. Mindless use of these programs can result in misleading analyses.

There are four approaches to automatic model selection that are commonly used.

### 3.18.1. Forward selection using Stata

The **forward selection** algorithm involves the following steps:

(i) Fit all possible simple linear models of the response variable against each separate covariate. Select the covariate with the lowest *P*-value and include it in the models of the subsequent steps.

(ii) Fit all possible models with the covariate(s) selected in the preceding step(s) plus one other of the remaining covariates. Select the new covariate that has the lowest *P*-value and add it to all subsequent models.

(iii) Repeat step (ii) to add additional variables, one variable at a time. Continue this process until either none of the remaining covariates has a *P*-value less than some threshold or all of the covariates have been selected.

This algorithm is best understood by working through an example. We do this with the Framingham data using Stata. The *3.12.1.Framingham.log* file continues as follows.

```
. *
. * Repeat the preceding analysis using an automatic forward
. * selection algorithm
. *
. drop if id == 9999                                                    1
(1 observation deleted)

. stepwise, pe(.1): regress logsbp logbmi age logscl woman               2
>       wo_lbmi wo_age wo_lscl
                        begin with empty model
p = 0.0000 <  0.1000  adding   age                                       3
p = 0.0000 <  0.1000  adding   logbmi                                    4
p = 0.0000 <  0.1000  adding   logscl                                    5
p = 0.0005 <  0.1000  adding   wo_age
p = 0.0000 <  0.1000  adding   woman                                     6
```

Output omitted. See Section 3.16

**Comments**

1 This *drop* command deletes all records for which *id* == 9999 is true. In this instance the new patient added in Section 3.17 is deleted. The equivalent point-and-click command is Data ▶ Variable utilities ▶ Keep or drop observations ⌋ Main ⌊ ⌈ Keep or drop observations — ⦿

Drop observations ⌋ ⌈ Observations to drop — If: (expression) *id == 9999* ⌋ [Submit].

2 The *stepwise* prefix specifies that an automatic model selection algorithm is to be used to fit a multiple regression model; *regress* specifies a linear regression model. The response variable is *logsbp*. The covariates to be considered for inclusion in the model are *logbmi*, *age*, *logscl*, *woman*, *wo_lbmi*, *wo_age*, and *wo_lscl*. The *pe*(.1) option sets the significance threshold for entering covariates into the model to be 0.1 (*pe* stands for *P*-value for entry). When this is the only option of the *stepwise* prefix a forward selection method is used. At each step new variables will only be considered for entry into the model if their *P*-value after adjustment for previously entered variables is $< 0.1$. Recall that earlier in the *3.12.1.Framingham.log* file we defined $logbmi = \log[bmi_i]$, $logscl = \log[scl]$, $wo\_lbmi = woman \times \log[bmi]$, $wo\_age = woman \times age$, and $wo\_lscl = woman \times \log[scl]$. The choice of the significance threshold is up to the user. The idea is that we wish to include covariates that may have a real effect on the response variable while excluding those that most likely do not. We could set this value to 0.05, in which case only statistically significant covariates would be included. However, this would prevent us from considering variables that might be important, particularly in combination with other risk factors. A threshold of 0.1 is often used as a reasonable compromise. The equivalent point-and-click command is Statistics ▶ Other ▶ Stepwise estimation ⌋ [Model] ⌊ Command: *regress*, Dependent variable: *logsbp*, Term 1 – variables to be included or excluded together: *logbmi* ⌈ Selection criterion — [✓] Significance level for addition to the model *.1* ⌋ Regression terms: *Term 2*, Term 2 – variables to be included or excluded together: *age*, Regression terms: *Term 3*, Term 3 – variables to ···: *logscl*, Regression terms: *Term 4*, Term 4 ···: *woman*, Regression terms: *Term 5*, Term 5 ···: *wo_lbmi*, Regression terms: *Term 6*, Term 6 ···: *wo_age*, Regression terms: *Term 7*, Term 7 ···: *wo_lscl* [Submit].

3 In the first step the program considers the following simple regression models.

$$E[\log[sbp_i] \mid \mathbf{x}_i] = \alpha + \beta_1 \times \log[bmi_i]$$
$$E[\log[sbp_i] \mid \mathbf{x}_i] = \alpha + \beta_1 \times age_i$$
$$E[\log[sbp_i] \mid \mathbf{x}_i] = \alpha + \beta_1 \times \log[scl_i]$$
$$E[\log[sbp_i] \mid \mathbf{x}_i] = \alpha + \beta_1 \times woman_i$$
$$E[\log[sbp_i] \mid \mathbf{x}_i] = \alpha + \beta_1 \times woman_i \times \log[bmi_i]$$
$$E[\log[sbp_i] \mid \mathbf{x}_i] = \alpha + \beta_1 \times woman_i \times age_i$$
$$E[\log[sbp_i] \mid \mathbf{x}_i] = \alpha + \beta_1 \times woman_i \times \log[scl_i]$$

Of these models, the one with age has the most significant slope parameter. The $P$-value associated with this parameter is $<0.000\,05$, which is also $<0.1$. Therefore, we select *age* for inclusion in our final model and go on to step 2.

4 In step 2 we consider the following models.

$E[\log[sbp_i] \mid \mathbf{x}_i] = \alpha + \beta_1 \times age_i + \beta_2 \times \log[bmi_i]$

$E[\log[sbp_i] \mid \mathbf{x}_i] = \alpha + \beta_1 \times age_i + \beta_2 \times \log[scl_i]$

$E[\log[sbp_i] \mid \mathbf{x}_i] = \alpha + \beta_1 \times age_i + \beta_2 \times woman_i$

$E[\log[sbp_i] \mid \mathbf{x}_i] = \alpha + \beta_1 \times age_i + \beta_2 \times woman_i \times \log[bmi_i]$

$E[\log[sbp_i] \mid \mathbf{x}_i] = \alpha + \beta_1 \times age_i + \beta_2 \times woman_i \times age_i$

$E[\log[sbp_i] \mid \mathbf{x}_i] = \alpha + \beta_1 \times age_i + \beta_2 \times woman_i \times \log[scl_i]$

The most significant new term in these models is $\log[bmi_i]$, which is selected.

5 In step 3 the evaluated models all contain the term $\alpha + \beta_1 \times age_i + \beta_2 \times \log[bmi_i]$. The new covariates that are considered are $\log[scl_i]$, $woman_i$ and the three interaction terms involving $\log[bmi_i]$, $age_i$, and $\log[scl_i]$. The most significant of these covariates is $\log[scl_i]$, which is included in the model.

6 This process is continued until at the end of step 5 we have Model (3.25). In step 6 we consider adding the remaining terms $woman_i \times \log[bmi_i]$ and $woman_i \times \log[scl_i]$. However, neither of these covariates have a $P$-value $<0.1$. For this reason we stop and use Equation (3.25) as our final model. The remaining output is identical to that given in Section 3.17 for this model.

It should also be noted that any stepwise regression analysis is restricted to those patients who have non-missing values for all of the covariates considered for the model. If the final model does not contain all of the considered covariates, it is possible that some patients with complete data for the final model will have been excluded because they were missing values for rejected covariates. When this happens it is a good idea to rerun your final model as a conventional regression analysis in order not to exclude these patients.

### 3.18.2. Backward selection

The **backward selection** algorithm is similar to the forward method except that we start with all the variables and eliminate the variable with the least significance. The data are refitted with the remaining variables and the process is repeated until all remaining variables have a $P$-value below some threshold.

The Stata command to use backward selection for our Framingham example is

```
stepwise, pr(.1): regress logsbp logbmi age logscl
>         woman wo_lbmi wo_age wo_lscl
```

Here *pr(.1)* means that the program will consider variables for removal from the model if their associated *P* value is ≥0.1. If you run this command in this example you will get the same answer as with forward selection, which is reassuring. In general, however, there is no guarantee that this will happen. The logic behind the choice of the removal threshold is the same as for the entry threshold. We wish to discard variables that most likely are unimportant while keeping those that may have a noteworthy effect on the response variable.

### 3.18.3. Forward stepwise selection

The **forward stepwise selection** algorithm is like the forward method except that at each step, previously selected variables whose *P*-value has risen above some threshold are dropped from the model. Suppose that $x_1$ is the best single predictor of the response variable $y$ and is chosen in step 1. Suppose that $x_2$ and $x_3$ are chosen next and together predict $y$ better than $x_1$. Then it may make sense to keep $x_2$ and $x_3$ and drop $x_1$ from the model.

In the Stata this is done by giving the *stepwise* prefix the options *pe pr* and *forward*. For example, commands using the prefix *stepwise, pe(0.1) pr(0.2) forward:* would consider new variables for entry with $P < 0.1$ and previously selected variables for removal with $P \geq 0.2$. In other words the most significant covariate is entered into the model as long as the associated *P*-value is <0.1. Once selected it is kept in the model as long as its associated *P*-value is <0.2.

### 3.18.4. Backward stepwise selection

Backward stepwise selection is similar to the backward selection in that we start with all of the covariates in the model and then delete variables with high *P*-values. It differs from backward selection in that at each step variables that have been previously deleted are also considered for re-entry if their associated *P*-value has dropped to a sufficiently low level. In Stata backward stepwise selection is specified with the *stepwise* prefix using the *pe* and *pr* options. For example, *stepwise, pe(.1) pr(.2):* would consider variables for removal from the model if their $P$-values are $\geq 0.2$, and would reconsider previously deleted variables for re-entry if $P < 0.1$.

### 3.18.5. Pros and cons of automated model selection

Automatic selection methods are fast and easy to use. It is important to bear in mind, however, that if you have a very large number of covariates then some of them are likely to have an unadjusted $P$-value $<0.05$ due to chance alone. Automatic selection methods make it very easy to find such covariates. The spurious significance levels of these covariates are called **multiple comparisons** artifacts, and the problem of finding falsely significant effects in the exploratory analysis of complex data sets is called the multiple comparisons problem. At a minimum, if you are publishing an exploratory analysis of a data set then it is mandatory that you state that your analyses are exploratory (as opposed to hypothesis driven) and that you list all of the covariates that you have considered in your analyses. Using a training set–test set approach or a multiple comparisons adjustment to your $P$-values will reduce the likelihood of false rejection of your null hypotheses.

If you do use these methods, it is a good idea to use more than one to see if you come up with the same model. If, say, the forward and backward methods produce the same model then you have some evidence that the selected model is not an artifact of the selection procedure. A disadvantage of these methods is that covariates are entered or discarded without regard to the biologic interpretation of the model. For example, it is possible to include an interaction term but exclude one or both of the individual covariates that define this interaction. This may make the model difficult to interpret. Fitting models by hand is usually worth the effort.

## 3.19. Collinearity

Multiple linear regression can lead to inaccurate models if two or more of the covariates are highly correlated. To understand this situation, consider predicting a person's height from the lengths of their arms. A simple linear regression of height against either left or right arm length will show that both variables are excellent predictors of height. If, however, we include both arm lengths in the model either we will fail to get unique estimates of the model parameters, or the confidence intervals for these parameters will be very wide. This is because the arm lengths of most people are almost identical, and the multiple regression model seeks to measure the predictive value of the left arm length above and beyond that of the right, and vice versa. That is, the model measures the height versus left arm length slope among people whose right arm lengths are identical. This slope can only be estimated if there is variation in left arm lengths among people with identical right arm lengths. Since this variation is small or non-existent, the model is unable to estimate the separate effects of both left and right arm lengths on height.

This problem is called **collinearity**, and occurs whenever two covariates are highly correlated. When this happens you should avoid putting both variables in the model. Collinearity will also occur when there is a linear relationship between three or more of the covariates. This situation is harder to detect than that of a pair of highly correlated variables. You should be aware, however, that you may have a collinearity problem if adding a covariate to a model results in a large increase in the standard error estimates for two or more of the model parameters. When there is an exact linear relationship between two or more of the covariates, the minimum least squares estimates of the parameters are not uniquely defined. In this situation, Stata will drop one of these covariates from the model. Other software may abort the analysis.

## 3.20. Residual analyses

Residual analyses in multiple linear regression are analogous to those for simple linear regression discussed in Section 2.15. Recall that the residual for the $i^{\text{th}}$ patient is $e_i = y_i - \hat{y}_i$. The variance of $e_i$ is given by $s^2(1 - h_i)$, where $s^2$ is our estimate of $\sigma^2$ defined by Equation (3.5). Dividing $e_i$ by its standard deviation gives the **standardized residual**

$$z_i = e_i/(s\sqrt{1 - h_i}). \tag{3.26}$$

When the influence $h_i$ is large, the magnitude of $e_i$ will be reduced by the observation's ability to pull the expected response $\hat{y}_i$ towards $y_i$. In order to avoid missing large outliers with high influence we calculate the **studentized residual**

$$t_i = e_i/(s_{(i)}\sqrt{1 - h_i}), \tag{3.27}$$

where $s_{(i)}$ is the estimate of $\sigma$ obtained from Equation (3.5) with the $i^{\text{th}}$ case deleted ($t_i$ is also called the **jackknifed residual**). If the multiple linear model is correct, then $t_i$ will have a $t$ distribution with $n - k - 2$ degrees of freedom. It is often helpful to plot the studentized residuals against the expected value of the response variable as a graphical check of the model's adequacy. Figure 3.7 shows such a plot for Model (3.25) of the Framingham data. A lowess regression of the studentized residuals against the expected SBP is also included

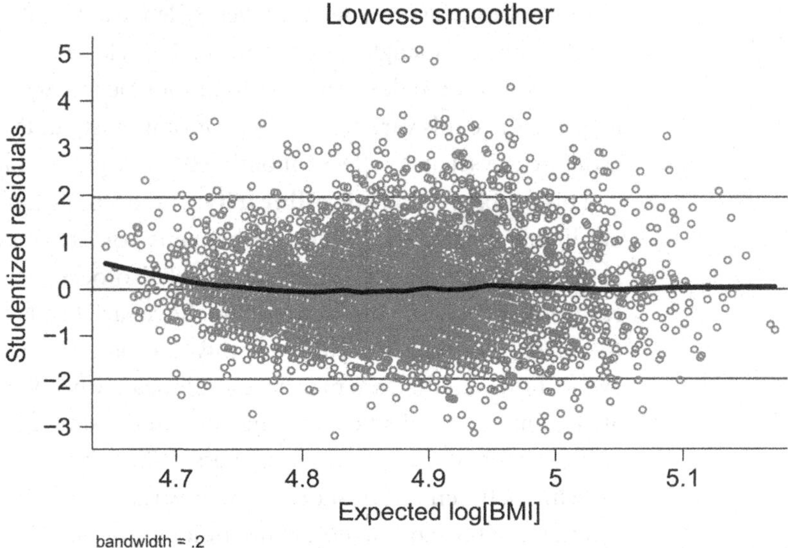


Figure 3.7 **Scatter plot of studentized residuals vs. expected log[SBP] for Model (3.25) of the Framingham Heart Study data. The thick black line is a lowess regression of the studentized residual against the expected log[SBP]. This plot indicates that Model (3.25) provides a good, although not perfect, fit to these data.**

in this graph. If our model fitted perfectly, the lowess regression line would be flat and very close to zero. The studentized residuals would be symmetric about zero, with 95% of them lying between $\pm t_{n-k-2,0.25} = \pm t_{4658-5-2,0.25} = \pm 1.96$. In this example, the residuals are slightly skewed in a positive direction; 94.2% of the residuals lie between ±1.96. The regression line is very close to zero except for low values of the expected log[SBP]. Hence, Figure 3.7 indicates that Model (3.25) fits the data quite well, although not perfectly. The very large sample size, however, should keep the mild departure from normality of our residuals from adversely affecting our conclusions.

It is always a good idea to double-check observations with unusually large studentized residuals. These residuals may be due to coding errors, to anomalies in the way that the experiment was performed or the data were collected, or to unusual attributes of the patient that may require comment when the study is written up for publication.

## 3.21. Influence

We do not want our conclusions to be unduly influenced by any individual unusual patient. For this reason, it is important to know what effect individual subjects have on our parameter estimates. An observation can be very influential if it has both high leverage and a large studentized residual.

### 3.21.1. $\Delta\hat{\beta}$ influence statistic

The $\Delta\hat{\beta}$ **influence statistic** estimates the change in the value of a parameter due to the deletion of a single patient from the analysis. This change is expressed in terms of the parameter's standard error. Specifically, the influence of the $i^{\text{th}}$ patient on the $j^{\text{th}}$ parameter is estimated by

$$\Delta\hat{\beta}_{ij} = (b_j - b_{j(i)})/\text{se}[b_{j(i)}], \tag{3.28}$$

where $b_j$ is the least squares estimate of $\beta_j$ in Equation (3.1), $b_{j(i)}$ is the corresponding estimate of $\beta_j$ with the $i^{\text{th}}$ patient deleted from the analysis, and $\text{se}[b_{j(i)}]$ is an estimate of the standard error of $b_{j(i)}$; this estimate differs slightly from the usual one given with multiple linear regression output in order to reduce the computation time needed to compute $\Delta\hat{\beta}_{ij}$ for every patient in the analysis (Hamilton, 1992). A value of $|\Delta\hat{\beta}_{ij}|$ that is greater than one identifies a single observation that shifts the $j^{\text{th}}$ parameter estimate by more than a standard error. Large values of $\Delta\hat{\beta}_{ij}$ indicate that either special consideration is warranted for the $j^{\text{th}}$ patient or we have built a model that is too complex for our data. Simplifying the regression model will often lead to more robust, although possibly more modest, inferences about our data.

When considering the influence of an individual data point on a specific parameter, it is important to examine the magnitude of the parameter's standard error as well as the magnitude of the $\Delta\hat{\beta}$ statistic. If the standard error is small and the data point does not change the significance of the parameter, then it may be best to leave the data point in the analysis. On the other hand, if the standard error is large and the individual data point changes a small and non-significant parameter estimate into a large and significant one, then we may wish either to drop the data point from the analysis or to choose a simpler model that is less affected by individual outliers. Of course, any time we delete a data point from a published analysis we must make it clear what we have done and why.

### 3.21.2. Cook's distance

Another measure of influence is **Cook's distance**:

$$D_i = \frac{z_i^2 h_i}{(k+1)(1-h_i)}, \tag{3.29}$$

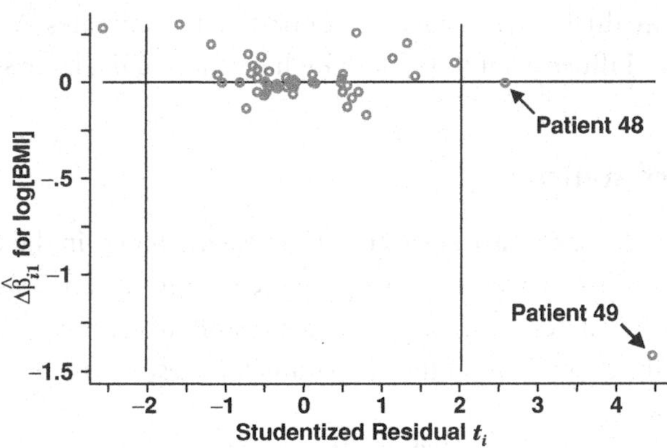


Figure 3.8 Scatter plot of $\Delta\hat{\beta}_{i1}$ versus $t_i$ for 50 Framingham Heart Study patients using Model (3.21). Patient 49 has an enormous studentized residual that has great influence on the log[BMI] parameter. The other patients have little influence on this parameter. Patient 48 has a large residual but virtually no influence due to the low leverage of this observation.

which measures the influence of the $i^{\text{th}}$ patient on all of the regression coefficients taken together (Cook, 1977). Note that the magnitude of $D_i$ increases as both the standardized residual $z_i$ and the leverage $h_i$ increase. Values of $D_i$ that are greater than one identify influential patients. Hamilton (1992) recommends examining patients whose Cook's distance is greater than $4/n$. This statistic can be useful in models with many parameters in that it provides a single measure of influence for each patient. Its major disadvantage is that it is not as easily interpreted as the $\Delta\hat{\beta}$ statistic.

### 3.21.3. The Framingham example

The entire Framingham data set is too large for any individual patient to have substantial influence over the parameters of Model (3.25). To illustrate an analysis of influence, we look at 50 patients from this study. Applying this model to these patients gives an estimate of the log[BMI] coefficient of $b_1 = 0.1659$. Figure 3.8 shows a scatter plot of $\Delta\hat{\beta}_{i1}$ against the studentized residuals $t_i$ for these data. If the model is correct, 95% of these residuals should have a $t$ distribution with $50 - 5 - 2 = 43$ degrees of freedom and lie between $\pm t_{43,0.05} = \pm 2.02$. Three (6%) of these residuals lie outside these bounds. Although this number is consistent with our model, patient 49 has a very large residual, with $t_{49} = 4.46$. (Under our model assumptions, we would only expect to see a residual of this size less than once in every 20 000 patients.) For this patient, $h_{49} = 0.155$ and $\Delta\hat{\beta}_{49,1} = -1.42$. Hence, this patient's very large residual and moderate leverage deflects $b_1$, the log[BMI] coefficient estimate, by 1.42 standard errors. In contrast, for patient 48 we have $t_{48} = 2.58$, $h_{48} = 0.066$ and $\Delta\hat{\beta}_{48,1} = -0.006$. Thus, even though this patient has a large residual, his small leverage results in a trivial influence on the log[BMI] coefficient. If we exclude patient 49 and apply Model (3.25) to the remaining patients, we get an estimate of this coefficient of $b_{1(49)} = 0.3675$ with standard error 0.1489. Note that $(b_1 - b_{1(49)})/\,0.1489 = (0.1659 - 0.3675)/0.1489 = -1.354$, which agrees with $\Delta\hat{\beta}_{49,1}$ to two significant figures. Deleting this single patient raises the estimate of $\beta_1$ by 122%.

The standardized residual for patient 49 is 3.730, and the Cook's distance is

$$D_{49} = \frac{3.730^2 \times 0.1545}{(5+1)\,(1-0.1545)} = 0.424. \qquad (3.30)$$

This value, while less than one, is substantially greater than $4/n = 0.08$. Had we only investigated patients with $D_i > 1$ we would have missed this very influential patient.

Of course, we can always look for influential patients by visually scanning scatter plots of the response variable and each individual covariate (see Figure 2.11). In multivariate analyses, however, it is advisable to look also at the influence statistics discussed above. This is because it is possible for the combined effects of a patient's multiple covariates to have a substantial influence on the parameter estimates without appearing to be an influential outlier on any particular scatter plot.

## 3.22. Residual and influence analyses using Stata

The *3.12.1.Framingham.log* file continues as follows and illustrates how to perform the residual and influence analyses discussed in Section 3.21.3. The output explicitly mentioned in these discussions is highlighted below.

```
. *
. * Draw a scatterplot of studentized residuals against the
. * estimated expected value of logsbp together with the
. * corresponding lowess regression curve.
. *
```

```
. predict t, rstudent                                                          1
(41 missing values generated)

. lowess t yhat, bwidth(0.2) mcolor(gray) lineopts(lwidth(thick))             2
>    ylabel(-3(1)5) yline(-1.96 0 1.96) xlabel(4.7(.1)5.1)

. generate out = abs(t) > 1.96                                                 3

. tabulate out                                                                 4

        out |      Freq.     Percent        Cum.
------------+-----------------------------------
          0 |      4,425       94.17       94.17
          1 |        274        5.83      100.00
------------+-----------------------------------
      Total |      4,699      100.00

. *
. * Perform an influence analysis on patients 2000 through 2050
. *
. keep if id >= 2000 & id <= 2050
(4648 observations deleted)

. regress logsbp logbmi age logscl woman wo_age                                5

      Source |       SS       df       MS              Number of obs =      50
-------------+------------------------------           F(  5,    44) =    2.49
       Model |  .381164541     5  .076232908           Prob > F      =  0.0456
    Residual |  1.34904491    44  .030660112           R-squared     =  0.2203
-------------+------------------------------           Adj R-squared =  0.1317
       Total |  1.73020945    49  .035310397           Root MSE      =   .1751

------------------------------------------------------------------------------
      logsbp |      Coef.   Std. Err.      t    P>|t|     [95% Conf. Interval]
-------------+----------------------------------------------------------------
      logbmi |   .1659182   .1696326     0.98   0.333    -.1759538    .5077902
         age |  -.0006515   .0048509    -0.13   0.894    -.0104278    .0091249
      logscl |   .0983239   .1321621     0.74   0.461    -.1680314    .3646791
       woman |  -.4856951    .294151    -1.65   0.106    -1.078517    .1071272
      wo_age |   .0116644   .0063781     1.83   0.074    -.0011899    .0245187
       _cons |   3.816949   .9136773     4.18   0.000     1.975553    5.658344
------------------------------------------------------------------------------
```

```
. drop  t h                                                          6

. predict h, leverage
(1 missing value generated)

. predict z, rstandard                                               7
(1 missing value generated)

. predict t, rstudent
(1 missing value generated)

. predict deltab1, dfbeta(logbmi)                                    8
(1 missing value generated)

. predict cook, cooksd                                               9
(1 missing value generated)

. display invttail(43,.025)
2.0166922

. label variable deltab1 "Delta Beta for log[BMI]"

. scatter deltab1 t, ylabel(-1.5(.5)0) yline(0)                     10
>    xlabel(-2(1)4) xtick(-2.5(.5)4.5) xline(-2 2)

. sort t

. list id h z t deltab1 cook in  -3/-1                              11
```

| | id | h | z | t | deltab1 | cook |
|---|---|---|---|---|---|---|
| 49. | 2048 | .0655644 | 2.429988 | 2.581686 | -.0063142 | .069052 |
| 50. | 2049 | .1545165 | 3.730179 | 4.459472 | -1.420916 | .423816 |
| 51. | 2046 | . | . | . | . | . |

```
. regress logsbp logbmi age logscl woman wo_age if id != 2049        12
```

| Source | SS | df | MS |
|---|---|---|---|
| Model | .336072673 | 5 | .067214535 |
| Residual | .922432819 | 43 | .021451926 |
| Total | 1.25850549 | 48 | .026218864 |

```
Number of obs =     49
F( 5,    43)  =   3.13
Prob > F      = 0.0169
R-squared     = 0.2670
Adj R-squared = 0.1818
Root MSE      = .14646
```

| logsbp | Coef. | Std. Err. | t | P>\|t\| | [95% Conf. | Interval] |
|---|---|---|---|---|---|---|
| logbmi | .3675337 | .1489199 | 2.47 | 0.018 | .0672082 | .6678592 |
| age | -.0006212 | .0040576 | -0.15 | 0.879 | -.0088042 | .0075617 |
| logscl | .0843428 | .110593 | 0.76 | 0.450 | -.1386894 | .3073749 |
| woman | -.3053762 | .2493465 | -1.22 | 0.227 | -.8082314 | .197479 |
| wo_age | .0072062 | .0054279 | 1.33 | 0.191 | -.0037403 | .0181527 |
| _cons | 3.244073 | .7749778 | 4.19 | 0.000 | 1.681181 | 4.806965 |

```
. display ( .1659182 - .3675337 )/.1489199                                    13
-1.35385

. log close
```

**Comments**

1 The *rstudent* option of the *predict* command defines *t* to equal the studentized residual for each patient.

2 This *lowess* command draws a scatter plot of *t* vs. *yhat* and then overlays a lowess regression curve with bandwidth 0.2 (See Figure 3.7). The *lineopts(lwidth(thick))* option chooses a thick width for the regression line. In Section 2.14 we illustrated how to create a similar plot using the *twoway* command to overlay a lowess curve on a scatter plot. The equivalent point-and-click command is Statistics ► Nonparametric analysis ► Lowess smoothing ⌋Main⌊ Dependent variable: *t*, Independent variable: *yhat* ┌ ☑ Specify the bandwidth — *0.2* Bandwidth ┘ ⌋Plot⌊ [Marker properties] ⌋Main⌊ ┌ Marker properties — Color: *Gray* ┘ [Accept] ⌋Smoothed line⌊ Width: *Thick* ⌋Y axis⌊ [Major tick/label properties] ⌋Rule⌊ ┌ Axis rule — ⦿ Range/Delta , *-3* Minimum value , *5* Maximum value , *1* Delta ┘ [Accept] [Reference lines] ☑ Add lines to graph at specified y axis values: *-1.96 0 1.96* [Accept] ⌋X axis⌊ [Major tick/label properties] ⌋Rule⌊ ┌ Axis rule — ⦿ Range/Delta , *4.7* Minimum value , *5.1* Maximum value , *.1* Delta ┘ [Accept] [Submit].

3 The variable *out* is a logical variable that equals 1 when "abs($t$) > 1.96" is true and equals 0 otherwise. In other words, *out* equals 1 if either $t > 1.96$ or $t < -1.96$, and equals 0 if $-1.96 \le t \le 1.96$.

4 The *tabulate* command lists the distinct values taken by *out*, together with the frequency, percentage, and cumulative percentage of these values. Note that 94.2% of the studentized residuals lie between ±1.96 (see Section 3.20).

5 Apply Model (3.25) to patients with *id* numbers between 2000 and 2050. Note that one patient in this range has a missing serum cholesterol and is excluded from this analysis. Thus, 50 patients are included in this linear regression.

6 The *drop* command deletes the *t* and *h* variables from memory. We do this because we wish to redefine these variables as being the studentized residual and leverage from the preceding linear regression.

7 The *rstandard* option defines *z* to equal the standardized residuals for each patient.

8 The *dfbeta(logbmi)* option defines *deltab1* to equal the $\Delta\hat{\beta}$ influence statistic for the *logbmi* parameter.

9 The *cooksd* option defines *cook* to equal Cook's distance for each patient.

10 This *scatter* command produces a graph that is similar to Figure 3.8.

11 The "*in* –3/–1" command qualifier restricts this listing to the last three records in the file. As the previous command sorted the file by *t*, the records with the three largest values of *t* are listed. Stata sorts missing values after non-missing ones. The last record in the file is for patient 2046. This is the patient with the missing serum cholesterol who was excluded from the regression analysis; *t* is missing for this patient. The two patients with the largest studentized residuals are patients 2048 and 2049 who have residuals $t = 2.58$ and $t = 4.46$, respectively. These patients are referred to as patients 48 and 49 in Section 3.21.3, respectively.

12 Repeat the regression excluding patient 2049. Note the large change in the *logbmi* coefficient that results from deleting this patient (see Section 3.21.3).

13 The difference in the *logbmi* coefficient estimates that result from including or excluding patient 2049 is –1.35 standard errors.

## 3.23. Using multiple linear regression for non-linear models

We often need to model a non-linear relationship between two variables. In Section 2.17 we discussed transforming one or both variables in order to linearize the relationship between these variables. The relationship between the *x* and *y* variables can be too complex for this approach to work. In this case, we often use a multiple linear regression model to obtain a simple

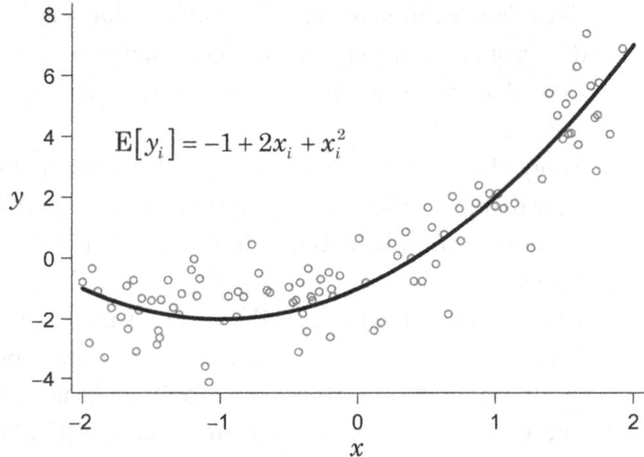


Figure 3.9 This figure illustrates a data set that follows a non-linear quadratic model of the form $\mathrm{E}[y_i] = \alpha + \beta_1 x_i + \beta_2 x_i^2 + \varepsilon_i$. The values of $\alpha$, $\beta_1$, and $\beta_2$ are −1, 2, and 1, respectively.

non-linear one. For example, consider the model

$$\mathrm{E}[y_i] = \alpha + \beta_1 x_i + \beta_2 x_i^2 + \varepsilon_i. \tag{3.31}$$

In this model we have added $x_i^2$ as a second covariate to produce a quadratic relationship between $y$ and $x$. The parameters of this model are $\alpha$, $\beta_1$, and $\beta_2$. Note, that while the relationship between $y$ and $x$ is non-linear, the expected value of $y$ is still a linear function of the model's parameters. Hence, this is a multiple linear regression model that may be analyzed with standard linear regression software. Figure 3.9 shows a data set that was generated with this model using $\alpha = -1$, $\beta_1 = 2$, and $\beta_2 = 1$. This model will perform well when it is correct but will perform poorly for many data sets in which the $x$–$y$ relationship is not quadratic. A quadratic model is particularly problematic if we wish to extrapolate beyond the region where there are many observations. In the next section we will discuss a simple but very powerful and robust approach to using multiple linear regression to model non-linear relationships.

## 3.24. Building non-linear models with restricted cubic splines

Let us consider models of variables $y$ and $x$ in which the expected value of $y$ given $x$ is a function known as a restricted cubic spline (RCS) or as a natural cubic spline. An RCS consists of three or more polynomial line segments. The boundaries of these segments are called knots. Between consecutive

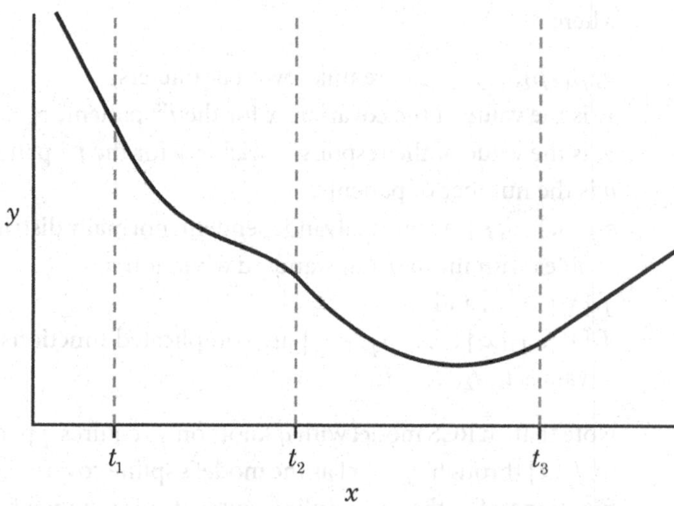


Figure 3.10 **A restricted cubic spline (RCS) consists of three or more polynomial segments. The boundaries of these segments are called knots. Between consecutive knots the curve is a cubic polynomial. The function is a straight line before the first and after the last knot and is continuous and smooth at the knot boundaries. This RCS has three knots at $t_1$, $t_2$, and $t_3$.**

knots the curve is a cubic polynomial. That is, it is a function of the form $\alpha + \beta_1 x + \beta_2 x^2 + \beta_3 x^3$. The function is a straight line before the first and after the last knot and is continuous and smooth at the knot boundaries. (Technically, the first and second derivatives of a RCS are continuous at each knot.) Figure 3.10 shows an example of a RCS with three knots at $t_1$, $t_2$, and $t_3$.

Suppose we have a model in which the expected value of $y$ given $x$ equals a RCS with $q$ knots at $x = t_1, \; t_2, \ldots, t_q$. At first glance, you might think that this model will involve a large number of parameters, since two parameters are required for each of the straight lines at the beginning and end of the model and four parameters are needed for each of the $q - 1$ cubic spline segments between consecutive knots. However, the requirements that the RCS be continuous and smooth places numerous constraints on the values of the parameters. It turns out that a RCS model with $q$ knots can always be written in the form

$$y_i = \alpha + f_1[x_i]\beta_1 + f_2[x_i]\beta_2 + \cdots + f_{q-1}[x_i]\beta_{q-1} + \varepsilon_i \tag{3.32}$$

where

$\alpha, \beta_1, \beta_2, \ldots, \beta_{q-1}$ are unknown parameters,
$x_i$ is the value of the covariate $x$ for the $i^{\text{th}}$ patient,
$y_i$ is the value of the response variable $y$ for the $i^{\text{th}}$ patient,
$n$ is the number of patients,
$\varepsilon_1, \varepsilon_2, \ldots, \varepsilon_n$ are mutually independent, normally distributed random variables with mean 0 and standard deviation $\sigma$,
$f_1[x_i] = x_i$, and
$f_2[x_i], f_3[x_i], \ldots, f_{q-1}[x_i]$ are complicated functions of $x_i$ and the knot values $t_1, t_2, \ldots, t_q$.

Note that an RCS model with $q$ knots only requires $q$ parameters. I will refer to $f_1[x]$ through $f_{q-1}[x]$ as the model's spline covariates. Since they are not functions of $y$ the same spline covariates for $x$ may be used for multiple regressions using different dependent variables. An RCS model is, in fact, a conventional multiple linear regression model. Equation (3.32) is a special case of Equation (3.1) with $k = q - 1$, $x_{i1} = f_1[x_i]$, $x_{i2} = f_2[x_i], \ldots,$ and $x_{ik} = f_{q-1}[x_i]$. Hence, we can use all of the statistical machinery discussed earlier in this chapter to explore the relationship between $x$ and $y$. Equation (3.2) becomes

$$\begin{aligned} \mathrm{E}[y_i|x_i] &= \mathrm{E}[\hat{y}_i|x_i] \\ &= \alpha + \beta_1 f_1[x_i] + \beta_2 f_2[x_i] + \cdots + \beta_{q-1} f_{q-1}[x_i] \end{aligned} \tag{3.33}$$

and Equation (3.3) gives the estimated expected value of $y_i$ to be

$$\hat{y}_i = a + b_1 f_1[x_i] + b_2 f_2[x_i] + \cdots + b_{q-1} f_{q-1}[x_i]. \tag{3.34}$$

Ninety-five percent confidence intervals for $\hat{y}_i$ and prediction intervals for a new response $y$ are given by Equations (3.12) and (3.14), respectively. To test the null hypothesis that there is no relationship between $x$ and $y$ we test the joint null hypothesis that $\beta_1 = \beta_2 = \cdots = \beta_{q-1} = 0$. Since $f_1[x_i] = x_i$, the RCS model reduces to the simple linear model $\mathrm{E}[y] = \alpha + x\beta$ when $\beta_2 = \beta_3 = \cdots = \beta_{q-1} = 0$. Hence, we can test for non-linearity by testing the null hypothesis that $\beta_2 = \beta_3 = \cdots = \beta_{q-1} = 0$. As will be seen in subsequent sections, RCS models not only greatly extend the flexibility of linear regression models but also are very useful in logistic regression and survival analyses.

Another important feature of spline covariates is that $f_2[x] = f_3[x] = \cdots = f_{q-1}[x] = 0$ for all $x < t_1$. In other words, when $x$ is less than the smallest knot, Equation (3.32) reduces to $\mathrm{E}[y] = \alpha + x\beta_1$. This

**Table 3.3.** Default knot locations recommended by Harrell (2001) for RCS models with from three to seven knots.

| Number of knots | Knot locations expressed in percentiles of the $x$ variable | | | | | | |
|---|---|---|---|---|---|---|---|
| 3 | 10 | 50 | 90 | | | | |
| 4 | 5 | 35 | 65 | 95 | | | |
| 5 | 5 | 27.5 | 50 | 72.5 | 95 | | |
| 6 | 5 | 23 | 41 | 59 | 77 | 95 | |
| 7 | 2.5 | 18.33 | 34.17 | 50 | 65.83 | 81.67 | 97.5 |

property can sometimes simplify the calculations of odds ratios and relative risks. We will discuss this further in Chapters 5 and 7 when we apply RCS models to logistic regression and survival analyses.

The algebraic definitions of $f_2[x]$ through $f_{q-1}[x]$ are not very edifying. Interested readers can find them in Harrell (2001) or Durrleman and Simon (1989). The best way to understand RCS models is through the graphic description given in Figure 3.10. The only properties of spline covariates that are important to remember are those listed above. Although they are somewhat tedious to calculate by hand, spline covariates can be calculated by any computer in a twinkling of an eye.

### 3.24.1. Choosing the knots for a restricted cubic spline model

The choice of number of knots involves a trade-off between model flexibility and number of parameters. For most data, a good fit can be obtained with from three to seven knots. Five knots is a good choice when there are at least 100 data points (Harrell, 2001). Using fewer knots makes sense when there are fewer data points. It is important always to do a residual plot or, at a minimum, plot the observed and expected values to ensure that you have obtained a good fit. The linear fits beyond the largest and smallest knots usually track the data well, but are not guaranteed to do so.

Fortunately, RCS models are fairly robust to the precise placements of the knots. Harrell (2001) recommends placing knots at the percentiles of the $x$ variable given in Table 3.3. The basic idea of this table is to place $t_1$ and $t_q$ near the extreme values of $x$ and to space the remaining knots so that the proportion of observations between knots remains constant. When there are fewer than 100 data points Harrell recommends replacing the smallest and largest knots by the fifth smallest and fifth largest observation, respectively.

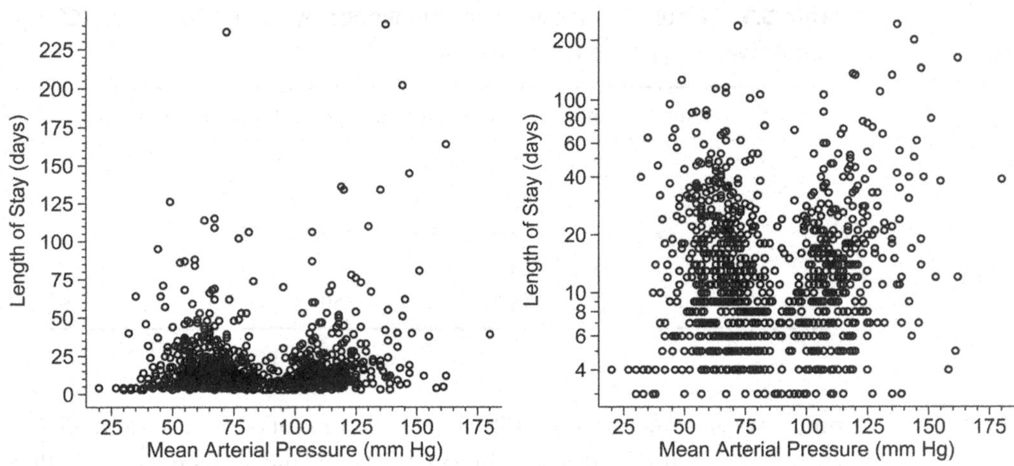


Figure 3.11 Scatter plot of length-of-stay versus mean-arterial-pressure (MAP) in the SUPPORT Study. MAP has a bimodal distribution while length-of-stay is highly skewed. Plotting length-of-stay on a logarithmic scale (right panel) greatly reduces the degree to which this variable is skewed.

## 3.25. The SUPPORT Study of hospitalized patients

The Study to Understand Prognoses Preferences Outcomes and Risks of Treatment (SUPPORT) was a prospective observational study of hospitalized patients (Knaus et al., 1995). Frank E. Harrell, Jr. has posted a random sample of 1000 patients from this study at `biostat.mc.vanderbilt.edu/SupportDesc`. All of these patients were alive on the third day of their hospitalization. My text web site contains the mean-arterial-pressure (MAP), length-of-stay (LOS), and mortal status at discharge on 996 of the patients in this data set. The MAPs on these patients were all measured on their third day. The left panel of Figure 3.11 shows the relationship between length-of-stay and MAP. LOS is highly skewed to the right. The right panel of Figure 3.11 shows these same data with LOS plotted on a logarithmic scale. The relationship between these variables appears to be non-linear: patients with normal blood pressures tend to have the earliest discharges while both hypotensive and hypertensive patients have longer lengths of stay. This relationship cannot be linearized by transforming either or both of these variables but can be effectively modeled using restricted cubic splines.

### 3.25.1. Modeling length-of-stay and MAP using restricted cubic splines

Let $los_i$ and $map_i$ denote the length-of-stay and mean-arterial-pressure of the $i^{th}$ patient from the SUPPORT Study, respectively. We wish to regress

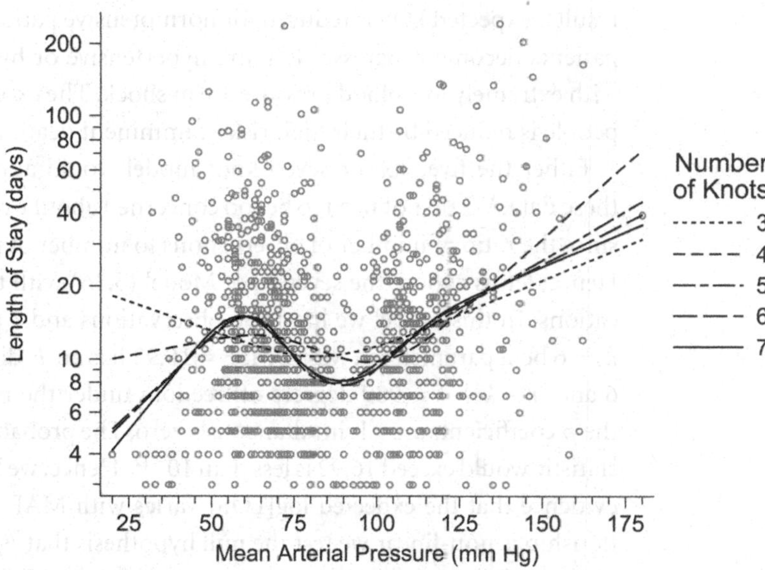


Figure 3.12 Plots of the expected length-of-stay (LOS) versus mean-arterial-pressure for RCS models with from three to seven knots. Models with five, six, and seven knots give very similar results. Both hypertensive and hypotensive patients have increased LOS. Patients in shock have a reduced LOS due to their high risk of imminent in-hospital death.

log[LOS] against MAP using restricted cubic spline (RCS) models with varying numbers of knots. Applying Equation (3.32) gives models of the form

$$\mathrm{E}[\log[los_i] \,|\, map_i] = \alpha + \beta_1 f_1[map_i] + \beta_2 f_2[map_i] + \cdots + \beta_{q-1} f_{q-1}[map_i]\,. \quad (3.35)$$

For example, when there are three knots Equation (3.35) reduces to

$$\mathrm{E}[\log[los_i] \,|\, map_i] = \alpha + \beta_1 f_1[map_i] + \beta_2 f_2[map_i]$$

while when there are seven knots it becomes

$$\mathrm{E}[\log[los_i] \,|\, map_i] = \alpha + \beta_1 f_1[map_i] + \beta_2 f_2[map_i] + \cdots + \beta_6 f_6[map_i]\,. \quad (3.36)$$

Let $\hat{y}_i$ denote the estimated expected value of $\log[los_i]$ under these models as defined by Equation (3.35). Figure 3.12 shows plots of $\hat{y}_i$ versus $x_i$ for models with $k = 3, 4, 5, 6,$ and 7 knots. In these models, I have used the default knot locations given in Table 3.3. Models with 5, 6, and 7 knots all give very similar results. Expected LOS is reduced for normotensive patients and increases as patients become progressively more hypertensive or hypotensive. Patients with extremely low blood pressure are in shock. The expected LOS for these people is reduced by their high risk of imminent death in hospital.

Either the five, six, or seven knot model would appear reasonable for these data. We do not need to be too concerned about overfitting this model since the ratio of number of observations to number of parameters is large. Hence, let us choose the seven knot Model (3.36) with the default knot locations. In this model we have 996 observations and 7 parameters ($\alpha$ plus $k = 6$ beta parameters). MSM/MSE = 16.92 has an $F$ distribution with $k = 6$ and $n - k - 1 = 989$ degrees of freedom under the null hypothesis that the $\beta$ coefficients are all simultaneously zero. The probability that such an $F$ statistic would exceed 16.92 is less than $10^{-17}$. Hence, we have overwhelming evidence that the expected log[LOS] varies with MAP. To test if this relationship is non-linear we test the null hypothesis that $\beta_2 = \beta_3 = \cdots = \beta_6$. Applying Equation (3.10) we derive an $F$ statistic with 5 and 989 degrees of freedom, which equals 18.59. The $P$-value associated with this statistic also indicates overwhelming statistical significance, allowing us to reject the hypothesis that the relationship between log[LOS] and MAP is linear. We next apply Equation (3.36) to derive $\hat{y}_i$, the estimated expected value of the $i^{\text{th}}$ patient's log[LOS]. A 95% confidence interval for this statistic is calculated from Equation (3.12). A plot of $\hat{y}_i$ versus $map_i$ overlayed on a scatter plot of the observations and the 95% confidence interval band is given in the bottom panel of Figure 3.13. Note that this confidence band is very narrow over a range of blood pressures from about 50 to 125 mm Hg. The band widens for blood pressures of patients who are either severely hypotensive or severely hypertensive due to the limited number of observations in these ranges. The top panel of Figure 3.13 is identical to the bottom panel except that the expected log[LOS] and confidence band are based on a model that uses evenly spaced knots. Note that these curves and bands are almost identical. This indicates a strength of RCS models which is that they are usually little affected by the precise knot locations (Harrell, 2001). This is comforting in situations in which the knot values lack any biologic significance and were not predicted in advance of data collection.

An important feature of RCS models is that we can take advantage of all of the model fitting features of powerful software programs for linear regression and related models. For example Figure 3.14 shows a scatter plot of studentized residuals versus MAP. The thick black horizontal curve in the center of the graph is the lowess regression line of these residuals against MAP. The residuals are calculated using Equation (3.27) from Model (3.36)

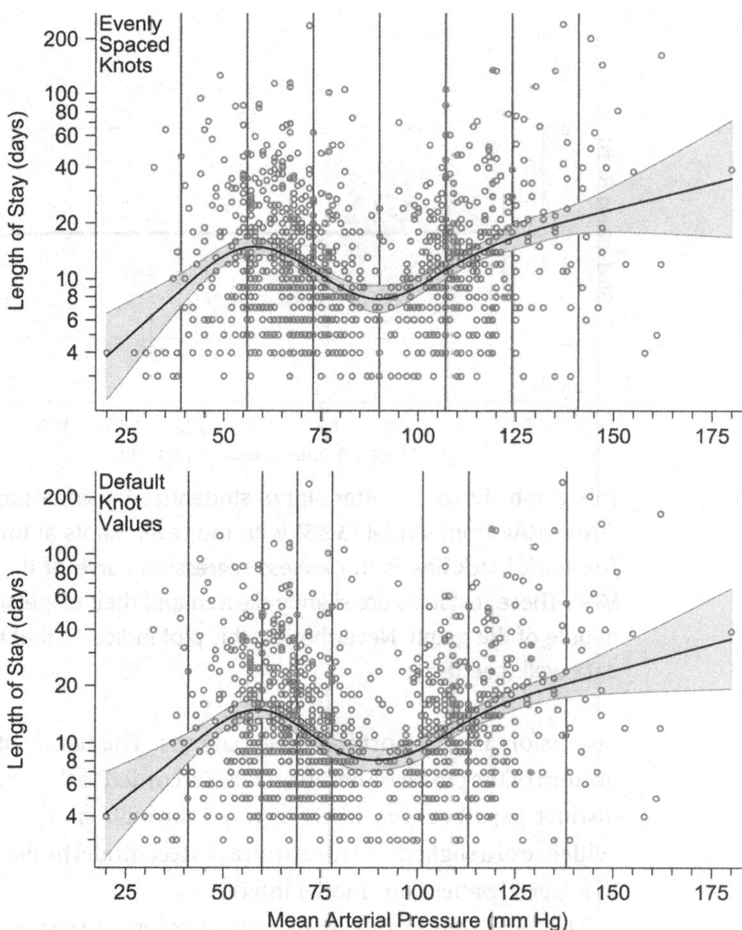


Figure 3.13 Both the top and bottom panels of this figure show the expected LOS from seven-knot RCS models regressing log[LOS] against MAP. The 95% confidence bands for these curves are also shown. The knot locations are indicated by vertical lines. The models differ in that the bottom panel uses knot values from Table 3.3, while the top panel uses evenly spaced knots. The resulting curves and confidence intervals are almost identical. RCS models are not greatly affected by the precise location of their knots.

with default knot values. If the model is correct we would expect the residuals to be symmetric about zero with 5% having an absolute value greater than two. The lowess regression curve should be flat at zero and the dispersion of these residuals should be uniform across the range of values of MAP. Figure 3.14 shows that the model fits well. The lowess regression curve tracks zero very closely and 4.7% of the residuals have absolute values greater than two. The residuals are slightly skewed and there is some evidence of reduced

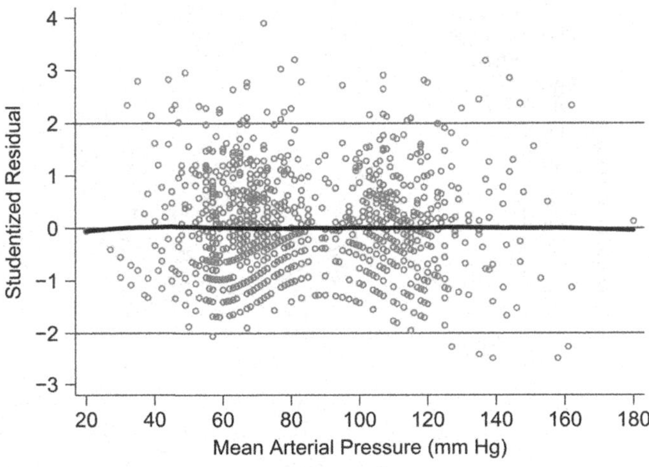


Figure 3.14 This graph shows a scatter plot of studentized residuals against baseline (day three) MAP from Model (3.36) with the seven knots at their default locations. The thick black line is the lowess regression curve of these residuals against MAP. These residuals are slightly skewed and their dispersion is reduced in the middle of the graph. Nevertheless, this plot indicates that this model fits these data well (see text).

dispersion among normotensive patients. The bands of residuals near the bottom of the plot arise because LOS is recorded to the nearest day, producing distinct gaps between LOSs of three through six days. Nevertheless, this evidence of a slight departure from a perfect model fit should not be sufficient to adversely affect our model inferences.

The final step in this analysis is to revert LOS to a linear scale. We do this by exponentiating $\hat{y}_i$ and the associated confidence band. Figure 3.15 shows this curve and confidence band. Because of the extreme dispersion of LOS I have truncated stays greater than 70 days in order for the variation in expected length of stay to be visible. Note that the precision with which we can estimate this expected length of stay for severely hypertensive patients is very poor due to the small number of observations for these patients. For a clinical audience, Figure 3.15 gives a much better impression of how typical length of stay varies with baseline blood pressure than does Figure 3.13. The extent of the variation in lengths of stay is also better depicted in Figure 3.15 than in Figure 3.13.

## 3.25.2. Using Stata for non-linear models with restricted cubic splines

The following log file and comments illustrate how to generate the RCS analyses and graphs discussed in the Section 3.25.

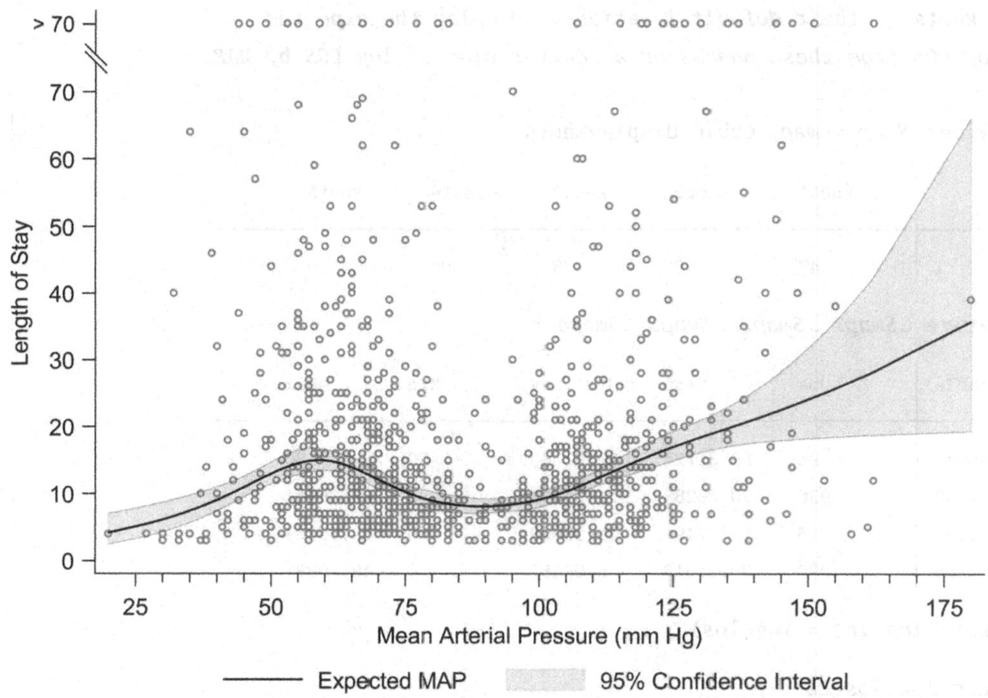


Figure 3.15 Observed and expected length-of-stay of patients in the SUPPORT Study. The gray band gives the 95% confidence interval for the expected length-of-stay. The actual lengths-of-stay for patients who were admitted for more than 70 days are not shown (2.9% of study subjects). This graph is derived from Model (3.36) using the default knot values.

```
. *  3.25.2.SUPPORT.log
. *
. *  Draw scatter plots of length-of-stay (LOS) by mean arterial
. *  pressure (MAP) and log LOS by MAP for the SUPPORT Study data.
. *
. use "C:\WDDtext\3.25.2.SUPPORT.dta" , replace                          1

. scatter los map, xlabel(25 (25) 175) xmtick(20 (5) 180)               2
>     ylabel(0(25)225) ymtick(5(5)240) xsize(2.8)

. scatter los map, xlabel(25 (25) 175) xmtick(20 (5) 180)               3
>     yscale(log) ylabel(4(2)10  20(20)100 200)
>     ymtick(3(1)9 30(10)90) xsize(2.8)

. *
. *  Regress log LOS against MAP using RCS models with from 3 to
```

```
. *   7 knots at their default locations.  Overlay the expected
. *   log LOS from these models on a scatter plot of log LOS by MAP.
. *
. mkspline _Smap = map, cubic displayknots                               4

             |     knot1      knot2      knot3      knot4      knot5
-------------+-------------------------------------------------------
          r1 |        47         66         78        106        129

. summarize _Smap1 _Smap2 _Smap3 _Smap4                                  5

    Variable |       Obs        Mean    Std. Dev.       Min        Max
-------------+--------------------------------------------------------
      _Smap1 |       996    85.31727    26.83566         20        180
      _Smap2 |       996    20.06288    27.34701          0   185.6341
      _Smap3 |       996    7.197497    11.96808          0   89.57169
      _Smap4 |       996    3.121013     5.96452          0   48.20881

. generate log_los = log(los)

. regress log_los _S*                                                    6

      Source |       SS       df       MS              Number of obs =     996
-------------+------------------------------           F(  4,   991) =   24.70
       Model |  60.9019393     4  15.2254848           Prob > F      =  0.0000
    Residual |  610.872879   991  .616420665           R-squared     =  0.0907
-------------+------------------------------           Adj R-squared =  0.0870
       Total |  671.774818   995  .675150571           Root MSE      =  .78512

------------------------------------------------------------------------------
     log_los |      Coef.   Std. Err.      t    P>|t|     [95% Conf. Interval]
-------------+----------------------------------------------------------------
      _Smap1 |   .0296009   .0059566     4.97   0.000      .017912    .0412899
      _Smap2 |  -.3317922   .0496932    -6.68   0.000    -.4293081   -.2342762
      _Smap3 |   1.263893   .1942993     6.50   0.000     .8826076    1.645178
      _Smap4 |  -1.124065   .1890722    -5.95   0.000    -1.495092   -.7530367
       _cons |    1.03603   .3250107     3.19   0.001     .3982422    1.673819
------------------------------------------------------------------------------

. predict y_hat5, xb                                                     7

. drop _S*                                                               8

. mkspline _Smap = map, nknots(3) cubic                                  9
```

```
. regress log_los _S*                                                    10
                                                             Output omitted
. predict y_hat3, xb                                                     11

. drop _S*

. mkspline _Smap = map, nknots(4) cubic

. regress log_los _S*
                                                             Output omitted

. predict y_hat4, xb

. drop _S*

. mkspline _Smap = map, nknots(6) cubic

. regress log_los _S*
                                                             Output omitted
. predict y_hat6, xb

. drop _S*

. mkspline _Smap = map, nknots(7) cubic displayknots

             |     knot1      knot2      knot3      knot4      knot5      knot6      knot7
-------------+-----------------------------------------------------------------------------
          r1 |        41         60         69         78   101.3251        113    138.075

. regress log_los _S*
                                                             Output omitted

. predict y_hat7, xb

. scatter log_los map, color(gray)                                       12
>     || line y_hat7 y_hat6 y_hat5 y_hat4 y_hat3 map                     13
>     , xlabel(25 (25) 175) xmtick(20 (5) 180)
>       ylabel(1.39 "4" 1.79 "6" 2.08 "8" 2.3 "10" 3 "20"
>           3.69 "40" 4.09 "60" 4.38 "80" 4.61 "100" 5.3 "200")
>       ymtick(1.1 1.39 1.61 1.79 1.95 2.08 2.2 3.4 3.91 4.25 4.5)
>       ytitle(Length of Stay (days))
>       legend(ring(1) position(3) cols(1)                               14
>           subtitle("Number" "of Knots")                                15
>           order( 6 "3" 5 "4" 4 "5" 3 "6" 2 "7"))                       16
. *
. * Plot expected LOS for 7 knot model together with 95%
```

```
. *  confidence bands.  Use the default knot locations.
. *
. predict se, stdp                                                      17

. generate lb = y_hat7 - invttail(_N-7, 0.025)*se                       18

. generate ub = y_hat7 + invttail(_N-7, 0.025)*se

. twoway rarea lb ub map , bcolor(gs14)                                 19
>      || scatter log_los map, color(gray)
>      || line y_hat7 map, lpattern(solid)
>      || line lb ub map , lwidth(vvthin vvthin)                        20
>           lpattern(solid solid)
>      , xlabel(25 (25) 175) xmtick(20 (5) 180)
>        ylabel(1.39 "4" 1.79 "6" 2.08 "8" 2.3 "10" 3 "20"
>           3.69 "40" 4.09 "60" 4.38 "80" 4.61 "100" 5.3 "200")
>        ymtick(1.1 1.39 1.61 1.79 1.95 2.08 2.2 3.4 3.91 4.25 4.5)
>        xline(41 60 69 78 101.3 113 138.1)                             21
>        ytitle(Length of Stay (days))
>        subtitle("Default" "Knot" "Values"                             22
>           , ring(0) position(10)) legend(off)  xsize(4)

. *
. *  Replot 7 knot model with evenly spaced knots.
. *
. drop _S* se lb ub

. mkspline _Smap = map, knots(39 56 73 90 107 124 141)                  23
>    cubic displayknots
```

| | knot1 | knot2 | knot3 | knot4 | knot5 | knot6 | knot7 |
|---|---|---|---|---|---|---|---|
| r1 | 39 | 56 | 73 | 90 | 107 | 124 | 141 |

```
. regress log_los _S*
                                                          Output omitted
. predict y_hat, xb

. predict se, stdp

. generate lb = y_hat - invttail(_N-7, 0.025)*se

. generate ub = y_hat + invttail(_N-7, 0.025)*se
```

```
. twoway rarea lb ub map , bcolor(gs14)                                    24
>      || scatter log_los map, color(gray)
>      || line y_hat map, lpattern(solid)
>      || line lb ub map , lwidth(vvthin vvthin)
>             lpattern(solid solid)
>      , xlabel(25 (25) 175) xmtick(20 (5) 180)
>        xline(39(17)141)
>        ylabel(1.39 "4" 1.79 "6" 2.08 "8" 2.3 "10" 3 "20"
>            3.69 "40" 4.09 "60" 4.38 "80" 4.61 "100" 5.3 "200")
>        ymtick(1.1 1.39 1.61 1.79 1.95 2.08 2.2 3.4 3.91 4.25 4.5)
>        subtitle("Evenly" "Spaced" "Knots", ring(0) position(10))
>        ytitle(Length of Stay (days)) legend(off) xsize(4)
>

. *
. *  Regenerate seven-knot model with default knot values.
. *
. drop _S* y_hat se lb ub

. mkspline _Smap = map, nknots(7)  cubic

. regress log_los _S*

      Source |       SS       df       MS              Number of obs =     996
-------------+------------------------------           F(  6,   989) =   16.92
       Model |  62.5237582     6  10.4206264           Prob > F      =  0.0000   25
    Residual |   609.25106   989  .616027361           R-squared     =  0.0931
-------------+------------------------------           Adj R-squared =  0.0876
       Total |  671.774818   995  .675150571           Root MSE      =  .78487

------------------------------------------------------------------------------
     log_los |      Coef.   Std. Err.      t    P>|t|     [95% Conf. Interval]
-------------+----------------------------------------------------------------
       _Smap1 |   .0389453   .0092924     4.19   0.000     .0207101    .0571804
       _Smap2 |  -.3778786     .12678    -2.98   0.003    -.6266673    -.12909
       _Smap3 |   .9316267   .8933099     1.04   0.297    -.8213739    2.684627
       _Smap4 |   .1269005    1.58931     0.08   0.936    -2.991907    3.245708
       _Smap5 |  -.7282771   1.034745    -0.70   0.482    -2.758824     1.30227
       _Smap6 |  -.3479716   .4841835    -0.72   0.473    -1.298117    .6021733
        _cons |   .6461153   .4496715     1.44   0.151    -.2363046    1.528535
------------------------------------------------------------------------------
```

```
. *
. *  Test for a non-linear association
. *
. test _Smap2  _Smap3 _Smap4  _Smap5  _Smap6                                26

 ( 1)  _Smap2 = 0
 ( 2)  _Smap3 = 0
 ( 3)  _Smap4 = 0
 ( 4)  _Smap5 = 0
 ( 5)  _Smap6 = 0

       F(  5,   989) =   18.59
            Prob > F =    0.0000

. predict rstudent, rstudent                                                27

. generate big = abs(rstudent)>2

. tabulate big

        big |      Freq.     Percent        Cum.
------------+-----------------------------------
          0 |        949       95.28       95.28
          1 |         47        4.72      100.00                            28
------------+-----------------------------------
      Total |        996      100.00

. *
. *  Draw a scatter plot of the studentized residuals against MAP
. *  Overlay the associated lowess regression curve on this graph.
. *
. twoway scatter rstudent map, color(gray)                                  29
>      || lowess rstudent map, lwidth(thick)
>      ,  ytitle(Studentized Residual) yline(-2 0 2) legend(off)

. *
. *  Plot expected LOS against MAP on a linear scale.
. *  Truncate LOS > 70.
. *
. predict y_hat, xb

. predict se, stdp

. generate lb = y_hat - invttail(_N-7, 0.025)*se
```

```
. generate ub = y_hat + invttail(_N-7, 0.025)*se

. generate e_los = exp(y_hat)                                          30

. generate lb_los = exp(lb)

. generate ub_los = exp(ub)

. generate truncated_los = los

. replace truncated_los = 80 if los > 70                               31
(29 real changes made)

. twoway rarea lb_los ub_los map , color(gs14)                         32
>     || scatter truncated_los map ,color(gray)
>     || line e_los map, xlabel(25 (25) 175) xmtick(30 (5) 170)
>     || line lb_los ub_los map , lwidth(vvthin vvthin)
>        ylabel(0 (10) 70) ytitle(Length of Stay)
>        legend(order(3 "Expected MAP"
>            1 "95% Confidence Interval") rows(1)) scale(.8)           33

. log close
```

**Comments**

1 This data set contains a sample of 996 patients from the SUPPORT Study (Knaus et al. 1995) who were admitted to hospital for at least three days (see Section 3.25). The mean arterial blood pressure on day 3 is recorded on each subject together with their length-of-stay and mortal status at discharge. These variables are named *map*, *los*, and *fate*, respectively. The data file is sorted by *map*. Note that the non-linear lines plotted in the subsequent graph commands all require the data to be sorted by this variable.

2 This scatter plot of *los* versus *map* generates the left-hand panel of Figure 3.11.

3 This command generates the right-hand panel of Figure 3.11. The *yscale(log)* option causes the *y*-axis to be plotted on a logarithmic scale. This greatly reduces the degree to which these data are skewed. In the point-and-click version of this command, a logarithmic scale for the *y*-axis is selected from the *Y-axis* tab of the *Overlay twoway graphs* dialog box. This done in the same way as was illustrated in Comment 6 on page 77 for the *x*-axis. The left and right panels of Figure 3.11 were combined using a graphics editor.

4 The *mkspline* command generates either linear or restricted cubic spline covariates. The *cubic* option specifies that restricted cubic spline covariates are to be created. This command generates these covariates for the variable *map*. By default, it defines covariates for a five-knot model with the knot values chosen according to Table 3.3. When the *displayknots* option is given the values of these knots are listed. The number of spline covariates is always one fewer than the number of knots. In this example they are named *_Smap1*, *_Smap2*, *_Smap3*, and *_Smap4*. Stata refers to the label preceding the equal sign (i.e. *_Smap*) as a stubname. The *mkspline* program always names the cubic spline covariates by concatenating the stubname with the integers 1 through $q - 1$. In this text I have adopted the convention of creating the stubname by concatenating the characters *_S* with the name of the original variable. However, any valid variable name may be used as a stubname.

The point-and-click command for generating these cubic spline covariates is Data ▶ Create or change variables ▶ Other variable creation commands ▶ Linear and cubic spline construction [Main] Make spline of variable: *map* ┌ Create spline by specifying — ⦿ New variable stub for restricted cubic spline: *_S* ┘ [Options] [✓] Display the values of the knots used in creating the spline [Submit]

5 This command summarizes the newly created spline covariates. *_Smap1* is identical to *map* and ranges from 20 to 180.

6 In Stata, variables can be specified using a wild-card notation. It interprets *_S** as referring to all variables whose names start with the characters *_S*. The only variables in memory that begin with these characters are our spline covariates. Hence, this command regresses *log_los* against the spline covariates that we have just defined. The command

```
regress log_los _Smap1 _Smap2 _Smap3 _Smap4
```

would have performed exactly the same regression analysis as the one given here. I use the prefix *_S* exclusively for defining spline covariates to reduce the likelihood that some other variable would be incorrectly included as regression covariates in commands such as this one. (Recall that Stata variable names are case-sensitive. Hence, *_Smap* and *_smap* would refer to two distinct variables.)

7 This post-estimation command defines *y_hat5* to be the estimated expected value of *log_los* under the preceding model. See also Comment 11 on page 61 and Comment 12 on page 118.

8 We next want to run other RCS models with different numbers of knots. In order to redefine the spline covariates associated with *map* we first drop the covariates from our five-knot model.

9 The *nknots(3)* option of the *mkspline* command specifies that two spline covariates for a three-knot model will be defined. The default values of the three knots will be chosen according to Table 3.3. In the equivalent point-and-click command the *Options* tab of the *mkspline* dialogue box should be ⌋ Options ⌊ ⌈ Knot specification for restricted cubic spline — ⊙ *3* Number of knots to use ⌋.

10 Regress *log_los* against the covariates for the three-knot model defined above.

11 Define *y_hat3* to be the estimated expected value of *log_los* under the three-knot model.

12 The preceding commands have defined *y_hat3*, *y_hat4*, . . . , *y_hat7* as estimates of the expected value of *log_los* under models with three through seven knots, respectively. We next plot these estimates against *map* overlayed on top of a scatter plot of *log_los* against *map*. The resulting graph is given in Figure 3.12.

13 This *line* command draws five line plots of *y_hat7*, *y_hat6*, *y_hat5*, *y_hat4*, and *y_hat3* against *map*. In this graph, the first plot is the scatter plot and plots two through six are for the line plots of *y_hat7*, *y_hat6*, *y_hat5*, *y_hat4*, and *y_hat3*, respectively. Hence, the default colors and patterns for these lines are those defined for plots two through six of the scheme that is in effect when the command is executed (see Section 1.3.6 and Comment 18 on page 63). The schemes that are used in this text specify black lines. The first two plots have solid lines while plots three through six have dashed lines whose dash-lengths diminish with increasing plot number. I have listed these plots in decreasing knot order to make the dash-lengths increase with the number of knots used to generate each curve. The resulting line patterns are illustrated in Figure 3.12.

Line patterns may also be defined explicitly using the *lpattern* option. For example, the command

```
. line y1 x,          lpattern(shortdash)
>      || line y2 x, lpattern(dash)
>      || line y3 x, lpattern(longdash)
```

would overlay plots of *y1*, *y2*, and *y3* against *x* using lines with short, medium, and long dashes, respectively.

14 The legend suboptions *ring(1) position(3)* place the legend just outside of the *x*- and *y*-axes at the three o'clock position (see Figure 3.12).

15 The *subtitle* suboption gives the legend a title using letters of moderate size. This title is given as two quoted strings: "Number" and "of Knots". Stata places each quoted string on a separate line as shown in Figure 3.12.

16 In this graph we are overlaying five line plots on top of a scatter plot. Stata numbers these plots in the order that they are specified: the scatter plot followed by the line plots. Hence, plot 2 is from the seven-knot model, plot 3 is from the six-knot model, etcetera. This *order* suboption specifies that plots 6, 5, 4, 3, and 2 are to have entries in the legend listed in descending order. The legend keys are given in quotation marks following each plot number. Thus, this suboption will place the number of knots associated with each line plot in the graph legend (see Figure 3.12). Note that *ring, position, cols, subtitle,* and *order* are all suboptions of the *legend* option and must be included within the parentheses following the word *legend.*

The point-and-click version of this entire graph command is Graphics ▶ Twoway graph (scatter plot, line etc) ⌡Plots⌊ [Create] ⌡Plot⌊ ┌ Plot type: (scatter plot) — Y variable: *log_los*, X variable: *map* [Marker properties] ⌡Main⌊ ┌ Marker properties — Color: *Gray* ┘ [Accept] ┘ [Accept] [Create] ⌡Plot⌊ ┌ Choose a plot category and type — Basic plots: (select type) *Line* ┘ ┌ Plot type: (line plot) — Y variable: *y_hat7 y_hat6 y_hat5 y_hat4 y_hat3*, X variable: *map* ┘ [Accept] ⌡Y axis⌊ Title: *Length of Stay (days)* [Major tick/label properties] ⌡Rule⌊ ┌ Axis rule — ⦿ Custom , Custom rule: *1.39 "4" 1.79 "6" 2.08 "8" 2.3 "10" 3 "20" 3.69 "40" 4.09 "60" 4.38 "80" 4.61 "100" 5.3 "200"* ┘ [Accept] [Minor tick/label properties] ⌡Rule⌊ ┌ Axis rule — ⦿ Custom , Custom rule: *1.1 1.39 1.61 1.79 1.95 2.08 2.2 3.4 3.91 4.25 4.5* ┘ [Accept] ⌡X axis⌊ [Major tick/label properties] ⌡Rule⌊ ┌ Axis rule — ⦿ Range/Delta , *25* Minimum value , *175* Maximum value , *25* Delta ┘ [Accept] [Minor tick/label properties] ⌡Rule⌊ ┌ Axis rule — ⦿ Range/Delta , *20* Minimum value , *180* Maximum value , *5* Delta ┘ [Accept] ⌡Legend⌊ ┌ [✓] Override default keys — Specify order of keys and optionally change labels: *6 "3" 5 "4" 4 "5" 3 "6" 2 "7"* ⌋ [Organization / Appearance] ⌡Organization⌊ ⌈ Organization — Rows/Columns: *Columns* ⌋ ⌡Titles⌊ Subtitle: *"Number" "of Knots"* [Accept] [Placement] ⌈ Position: *3 o'clock* [✓] Place legend in an area spanning the entire width ...of the graph, ... [Accept] [Submit].

17 This *predict* command defines *se* to be the standard error of *y_hat7*.

18 We use Equation (3.12) to define *lb* and *ub* as the lower and upper bounds of the 95% confidence interval for *y_hat7*.

19 This command draws the lower panel of Figure 3.13.

20 The density of the scatter plot makes the shaded region of the 95% confidence band hard to see in the center of the graph. The command

*line lb ub map*

draws lines on the boundaries of this confidence band to enhance its visibility. The option *lwidth(vvthin vvthin)* specifies that the line widths of these curves are to be very thin. Had we used the option *lwidth(thin thick)* then the plots of *lb* vs. *map* and *ub* vs. *map* would have used thin and thick lines, respectively.

21 This *xline* option marks the location of the model's knots (see Comment 3 on page 59).

22 This option gives the graph a subtitle using letters of moderate size. Titles and subtitles are positioned in the same way as legends. Placing each word of the subtitle in separate quotes causes these words to be placed on separate lines (see Figure 3.13).

In the point-and-click version of this command the subtitle is specified on the *Titles* tab of the *twoway – Twoway graphs* dialog box as ⌡Titles⌊ Subtitle *"Default" "Knot" "Values"* [Properties] ⌡Text⌊ ⌈ Placement — Position: *11 o'clock*, [✓] Place text inside plot region ⌋ [Accept].

23 The *knots* option of the *mkspline* command explicitly chooses the knot values. In the equivalent point-and-click command the *Options* tab of the *mkspline* dialogue box should be ⌡Options⌊ [✓] Display the values of the knots used in creating the spline ⌈ Knot specification for restricted cubic spline — ⦿ Location of knots *39 56 73 90 107 124 141* ⌋ .

24 This command generates the top panel of Figure 3.13.

25 The *F* statistic for testing whether *log_los* varies with *map* is of overwhelming statistical significance.

26 This *test* command tests the null hypothesis that the parameters associated with the spline covariates *_Smap2*, *_Smap3*, *_Smap4*, *_Smap5*, and *_Smap6* are all simultaneously zero. This is equivalent to testing the null hypothesis that there is a linear relationship between the expected *log_los* and *map* (see Section 3.24). The *F* statistic for this test is also of overwhelming statistical significance.

27 The variable *rstudent* is the studentized residual for this model (see Comment 1 on page 132).

28 There are 4.72% of the studentized residuals with an absolute value greater than two.

29 This command generates Figure 3.14.

30 The variable *e_los* is our estimate of the expected length-of-stay; *lb_los* and *ub_los* estimate the 95% confidence band for this estimate.

31 In order to generate Figure 3.15 we define *truncated_los* to equal *los* for stays <70 days and 80 for stays ≥70.

32 This graph is similar to Figure 3.15. I have used a graphics editor to break the *y*-axis above 70 and add the label ">70" to annotate the 29 patients who were in hospital for more than 70 days.

33 This *rows(1)* suboption arranges the figure legend in a single row. It is printed in its default location at the bottom of the graph.

## 3.26. Additional reading

Armitage et al. (2002) and

Pagano and Gauvreau (2000) provide good introductions to multiple linear regression.

Hamilton (1992) and

Cook and Weisberg (1999) are more advanced texts that emphasize a graphical approach to multiple linear regression. Hamilton (1992) provides a brief introduction to non-linear regression.

Draper and Smith (1998) is a classic reference on multiple linear regression.

Harrell (2001) is a more advanced text on regression modeling strategies. It includes a discussion of restricted cubic splines.

Cook (1977) is the original reference on Cook's distance.

Stone and Koo (1985) and

Devlin and Weeks (1986) are the original references on restricted cubic splines.

Harrell et al. (1988) and

Durrleman and Simon (1989) are early peer-reviewed references on restricted cubic splines that are more accessible than Stone and Koo (1985).

Levy (1999) reviews the findings of the Framingham Heart Study. Knaus et al. (1995) is the original reference on the SUPPORT Study.

## 3.27. Exercises

1 Linear regression was applied to a large data set having age and weight as covariates. The estimated coefficients for these two variables and their standard errors are as follows:

| Covariate | Estimated coefficient | Estimated standard error |
|---|---|---|
| Age | 1.43 | 0.46 |
| Weight | 25.9 | 31.0 |

Can we reject the null hypothesis that the associated parameter equals zero for either of these variables? Can we infer anything about the biologic significance of these variables from the magnitudes of the estimated coefficients? Justify your answers.

The following questions concern the study by Gross et al. (1999) about the relationship between funding by the National Institutes of Health and the burden of 29 diseases. The data from Table 1 of this study are given in a Stata data file called *3.ex.Funding.dta* on the `biostat.mc.vanderbilt.edu/dupontwd/wddtext/` web page. The variable names and definitions in this file are

*disease* = condition or disease,
*id* = a numeric disease identification number,
*dollars* = thousands of dollars of NIH research funds per year,
*incid* = disease incidence rate per 1000,
*preval* = disease prevalence rate per 1000,
*hospdays* = thousands of hospital-days,
*mort* = disease mortality rate per 1000,
*yrslost* = thousands of life-years lost,
*disabil* = thousands of disability-adjusted life-years lost.

2 Explore the relationship between *dollars* and the other covariates listed above. Fit a model that you feel best captures this relationship.

3 Perform a forward stepwise linear regression of log[*dollars*] against the following potential covariates: log[*incid*], log[*preval*], log[*hospdays*], log[*mort*], log[*yrslost*], and log[*disabil*]. Use thresholds for entry and

removal of covariates into or from the model of 0.1 and 0.2, respectively. Which covariates are selected by this procedure?

4 Repeat Question 3 only now using a backward stepwise model selection procedure. Use the same thresholds for entry and removal. Do you get the same model as in Question 3?

5 Regress log[*dollars*] against the same covariates chosen by the stepwise procedure in Question 4. Do you get the same parameter estimates? If not, why not?

6 Regress log[*dollars*] against log[*hospdays*], log[*mort*], log[*yrslost*], and log[*disabil*]. Calculate the expected log[*dollars*] and studentized residuals for this regression. What bounds should contain 95% of the studentized residuals under this model? Draw a scatter plot of these residuals against expected log[*dollars*]. On the graph draw the lowess regression curve of the residuals against the expected values. Draw horizontal lines at zero and the 95% bounds for the studentized residuals. What does this graph tell you about the quality of the fit of this model to these data?

7 In the model from Question 6, calculate the $\Delta\hat{\beta}$ influence statistic for log[*mort*]. List the values of this statistic together with the disease name, studentized residual, and leverage for all diseases for which the absolute value of this $\Delta\hat{\beta}$ statistic is greater than 0.5. Which disease has the largest influence on the log[*mort*] parameter estimate? How many standard errors does this data point shift the log[*mort*] parameter estimate? How big is its studentized residual?

8 Draw scatter plots of log[dollars] against the other covariates in the model from Question 6. Identify the disease in these plots that had the most influence on log[*mort*] in Question 7. Does it appear to be particularly influential in any of these scatter plots?

9 Repeat the regression from Question 6 excluding the observation on perinatal conditions. Compare your coefficient estimates with those from Question 6. What is the change in the estimate of the coefficient for log[*mort*] that results from deleting this disease? Express this difference as a percentage change and as a difference in standard errors.

10 Perform influence analyses on the other covariates in the model from Question 6. Are there any observations that you feel should be dropped from the analysis? Do you think that a simpler model might be more appropriate for these data?

11 Regress log[*dollars*] against log[*disabil*] and log[*hospdays*]. What is the estimated expected amount of research funds budgeted for a disease that causes a million hospital-days a year and the loss of a million disability-adjusted life-years? Calculate a 95% confidence interval for this expected

value. Calculate a 95% prediction interval for the funding that would be provided for a new disease that causes a million hospital-days a year and the loss of a million disability-adjusted life-years.

12 In Question 11, suppose that we increase the number of disability-adjusted life-years lost by two million while keeping the number of hospital-days constant. What will happen to the estimated expected number of research funds spent on this disease under this model?

13 Perform an influence analysis on the model from Question 11. Is this analysis more reassuring than the one that you performed in Question 10? Justify your answer.

14 Drop AIDS from your data set. Define restricted cubic spline covariates for *disabil* using three knots at their default locations. Regress *disease* against these covariates. Is there a significant relationship between NIH funding and disability-adjusted life-years lost under this model? Can you reject the hypothesis that this relationship is linear? Estimate the expected value of *dollars* under this model together with a 95% confidence interval for this estimate. Plot the expected value of *dollars* under this model as a function of *disabil* together with its associated 95% confidence band. Overlay a scatter plot of *dollars* vs. *disabil* on this graph.

15 Calculate the studentized residuals from your model from Question 14. Draw a scatter plot of these residuals against disability-adjusted life-years lost. On your scatter plot, overlay the lowess regression line of these residuals vs. life-years lost. How well does this model fit these data?

16 Compare the graph that you drew in Question 14 with the bottom panel of Figure 2.14. What are the strengths and weaknesses of the models used to generate these graphs?

# 4

# Simple logistic regression

In simple linear regression we fit a straight line to a scatter plot of two continuous variables that are measured on study subjects. Often, however, the response variable of interest has dichotomous outcomes such as survival or death. We wish to be able to predict the probability of a patient's death given the value of an explanatory variable for the patient. Using linear regression to estimate the probability of death is usually unsatisfactory since it can result in probability estimates that are either greater than one (certainty) or less than zero (impossibility). Logistic regression provides a simple and plausible way to estimate such probabilities.

## 4.1. Example: APACHE score and mortality in patients with sepsis

Figure 4.1 shows 30-day mortality in a sample of septic patients as a function of their baseline APACHE scores (see Section 1.2.1). Patients are coded as 1 or 0 depending on whether they are dead or alive at 30 days, respectively. We wish to predict death from baseline APACHE score in these patients. Note that all patients with an APACHE score of less than 17 survived, while all but one patient with a score greater than 27 died. Mortal outcome varied for patients with scores between 17 and 27.

## 4.2. Sigmoidal family of logistic regression curves

Let $\pi[x]$ be the probability that a patient with score $x$ will die. In logistic regression we fit probability functions of the form

$$\pi[x] = \exp[\alpha + \beta x]/(1 + \exp[\alpha + \beta x]), \tag{4.1}$$

where $\alpha$ and $\beta$ are unknown parameters that we will estimate from the data. Equation (4.1) is the **logistic probability function**. This equation describes a family of sigmoidal curves, four examples of which are given in Figure 4.2. For now, assume that $\beta > 0$. If $x$ is negative and the absolute value of $x$ is sufficiently large, then $\alpha + \beta x$ will also be a negative number with a large

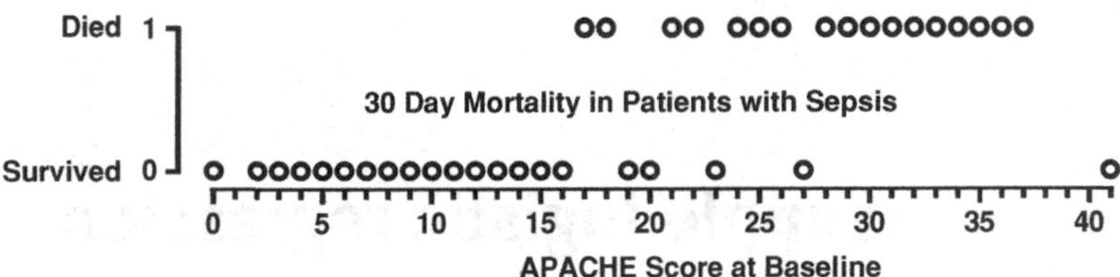


Figure 4.1 Scatter plot showing mortal outcome by baseline APACHE Score for 38 patients admitted to an intensive care unit with sepsis.

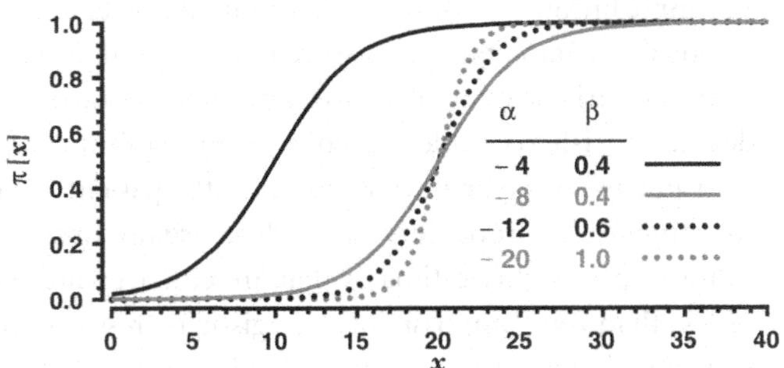


Figure 4.2 Four examples of logistic regression curves given by Equation (4.1). The two solid curves have the same value of the $\beta$ parameter, which gives identical slopes. The different values of the $\alpha$ parameter shifts the gray curve 10 units to the right. The slopes of these curves increase as $\beta$ gets larger.

absolute value (recall that we are assuming that $\beta$ is positive). In this case $\exp[\alpha + \beta x]$ will be very close to zero. Hence, if we choose $x$ sufficiently far to the left in Figure 4.2, then $\pi[x]$ will approach $0/(1 + 0) = 0$. Note that for all of the curves plotted in Figure 4.2 the values of $\alpha$ are negative. For this reason $\pi[x]$ is close to zero for small positive values of $x$. However, regardless of the value of $\alpha$ we can make $\pi[x]$ as close to zero as we want by choosing a sufficiently large value of $-x$. For positive values of $x$, $\exp[\alpha + \beta x]$ is very large when $x$ is big and hence $\pi[x] = a\_big\_number/(1 + a\_big\_number)$ approaches 1 as $x$ gets large. The magnitude of $\beta$ controls how quickly $\pi[x]$ rises from 0 to 1. When $x = -\alpha/\beta$, $\alpha + \beta x = 0$, $e^0 = 1$, and hence $\pi[x] = 1/(1 + 1) = 0.5$. Thus, for given $\beta$, $\alpha$ controls where the 50% survival point is located. In Figure 4.2, the solid black curve reaches $\pi[x] = 0.5$ when $x = -\alpha/\beta = 4/0.4 = 10$. The solid gray curve has the same slope as the black curve but is shifted 10 units to the right. The solid gray curve and the dotted curves all reach their midpoint at $x = -\alpha/\beta = 20$. The slopes of the dotted curves are greater than that of the solid gray curve because of their larger value of $\beta$. It can be shown that the slope of a logistic regression curve when $\pi[x] = 0.5$ equals $\beta/4$.

We wish to choose the best curve to fit data such as that shown in Figure 4.1. Suppose that there is a sharp survival threshold with deaths occurring only in those patients whose $x$ value is above this threshold. Then we would want to fit a regression curve with a large value of $\beta$ that will give a rapid transition between estimated probabilities of death of 0 and 1. On the other hand, if the observed mortality increases gradually with increasing $x$ then we would want a curve with a much smaller value of $\beta$ that will predict a more gradual rise in the probability of death.

## 4.3. The log odds of death given a logistic probability function

Equation (4.1) gives that the probability of death under a logistic probability function is $\pi[x] = \exp[\alpha + \beta x]/(1 + \exp[\alpha + \beta x])$. Hence, the probability of survival is

$$1 - \pi[x] = \frac{1 + \exp[\alpha + \beta x] - \exp[\alpha + \beta x]}{1 + \exp[\alpha + \beta x]} = \frac{1}{1 + \exp[\alpha + \beta x]}.$$

The **odds** of death is

$$\pi[x]/(1 - \pi[x]) = \exp[\alpha + \beta x], \tag{4.2}$$

and the **log odds** of death equals

$$\log\left[\frac{\pi[x]}{1 - \pi[x]}\right] = \alpha + \beta x. \tag{4.3}$$

For any number $\pi$ between 0 and 1 the **logit function** is defined by

$$\text{logit}[\pi] = \log[\pi/(1 - \pi)].$$

In the sepsis example let

$$d_i = \begin{cases} 1: & \text{if the } i^{\text{th}} \text{ patient dies} \\ 0: & \text{if the } i^{\text{th}} \text{ patient lives, and} \end{cases}$$

$x_i$ equal the APACHE score of the $i^{\text{th}}$ patient.

Then we can rewrite Equation (4.3) as

$$\text{logit}[\pi[x_i]] = \alpha + \beta x_i. \tag{4.4}$$

In simple linear regression we modeled a continuous response variable as a linear function of a covariate (see Equation 2.4). In simple logistic regression we will model the logit of the probability of survival as a linear function of a covariate.

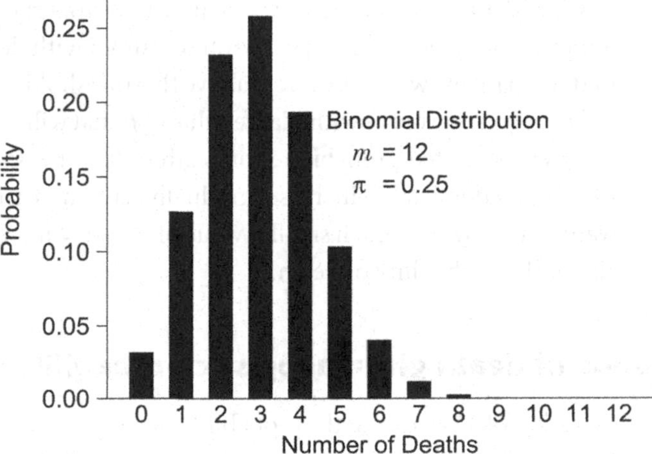


Figure 4.3 Binomial probability distribution resulting from observing 12 patients with an individual probability of death of 0.25.

## 4.4. The binomial distribution

Suppose that $m$ people are at risk of death during some interval and that $d$ of these people die. Let each patient have probability $\pi$ of dying during the interval, and let the fate of each patient be independent of the fates of all the others. Then $d$ has a **binomial distribution** with parameters $m$ and $\pi$. The mean of this distribution is $m\pi$, and its standard deviation is $\sqrt{m\pi(1-\pi)}$. The probability of observing $d$ deaths among these $m$ patients is

$$\Pr[d \text{ deaths}] = \frac{m!}{(m-d)!d!}\pi^d(1-\pi)^{(m-d)} \quad : d = 0, 1, \ldots, m. \qquad (4.5)$$

Equation (4.5) is an example of a **probability distribution** for a discrete random variable, which gives the probability of each possible outcome.

The mean of any random variable $x$ is also equal to its expected value and is written $\mathrm{E}[x]$. Also, if $x$ is a random variable and $k$ is a constant then $\mathrm{E}[kx] = k\mathrm{E}[x]$. Hence

$\mathrm{E}[d] = \pi m$ and $\mathrm{E}[d/m] = \pi$.

For example, if we have $m = 100$ patients whose individual probability of death is $\pi = 1/2$ then the expected number of deaths is $\mathrm{E}[d] = 0.5 \times 100 = 50$. That is, we would expect that one half of the patients will die. Of course, the actual number of deaths may vary considerably from 50 although the probability of observing a number of deaths that is greatly different from this value is small. Figure 4.3 shows the probability distribution for the number of deaths observed in $m = 12$ patients with an individual probability of death of $\pi = 0.25$. In this example the expected number of deaths is three. The probability of observing three deaths is 0.258, which is higher than the probability of any other outcome. The probability of observing nine or more deaths is very small.

A special case of the binomial distribution occurs when we have a single patient who either does, or does not, die. In this case $m = 1$, and we observe either $d = 0$ or $d = 1$ deaths with probability $1 - \pi$ and $\pi$, respectively. The expected value of $d$ is $\mathrm{E}[d] = m\pi = \pi$. The random variable $d$ is said to have a **Bernoulli distribution** when $m = 1$.

## 4.5. Simple logistic regression model

Suppose we have an unbiased sample of $n$ patients from a target population. Let

$$d_i = \begin{cases} 1\text{: if the } i^{\text{th}} \text{ patient suffers some event of interest} \\ 0\text{: otherwise, and} \end{cases}$$

$x_i$ be a continuous covariate observed on the $i^{\text{th}}$ patient.

The **simple logistic regression model** assumes that $d_i$ has a Bernoulli distribution with

$$\mathrm{E}[d_i \mid x_i] = \pi[x_i] = \exp[\alpha + \beta x_i]/(1 + \exp[\alpha + \beta x_i]), \qquad (4.6)$$

where $\alpha$ and $\beta$ are unknown parameters associated with the target population. Equivalently, we can rewrite the logistic regression model using Equation (4.4) as

$$\mathrm{logit}[\mathrm{E}[d_i \mid x_i]] = \alpha + \beta x_i. \qquad (4.7)$$

## 4.6. Generalized linear model

Logistic regression is an example of a **generalized linear model**. These models are defined by three attributes: the distribution of the model's random component, its linear predictor, and its link function. For logistic regression these are defined as follows.

1 The **random component** of the model is $d_i$, the patient's fate. In simple logistic regression, $d_i$ has a Bernoulli distribution with expected value $\mathrm{E}[d_i \mid x_i]$. (In Section 4.14 we will generalize this definition to allow $d_i$ to have any binomial distribution.)

2 The **linear predictor** of the model is $\alpha + \beta x_i$.

3 The **link function** describes a functional relationship between the expected value of the random component and the linear predictor. Logistic regression uses the logit link function
$\text{logit}[\text{E}[d_i \mid x_i]] = \alpha + \beta x_i$.

## 4.7. Contrast between logistic and linear regression

Not surprisingly, linear regression is another example of a generalized linear model. In linear regression, the expected value of $y_i$ given $x_i$ is

$\text{E}[y_i \mid x_i] = \alpha + \beta x_i$ for $i = 1, 2, \ldots, n$.

The random component of the model, $y_i$, has a normal distribution with mean $\alpha + \beta x_i$ and standard deviation $\sigma$. The linear predictor is $\alpha + \beta x_i$, and the link function is the identity function $\text{I}[x] = x$. That is, $\text{I}[\text{E}[y_i \mid x_i]] = \text{E}[y_i \mid x_i] = \alpha + \beta x_i$. The generalized linear model is useful in that it provides a common approach to fitting several important models.

## 4.8. Maximum likelihood estimation

We have yet to discuss how to choose the best logistic regression model to fit a specific data set. In linear regression we used the method of least squares to estimate regression coefficients. That is, we chose those estimates of $\alpha$ and $\beta$ that minimized the sum of the squared residuals. This approach does not work well in logistic regression, or for the entire family of generalized linear models. Instead we use another approach called **maximum likelihood estimation**. The easiest way to explain this approach is through a simple example.

Suppose that we observe an unbiased sample of 50 AIDS patients, and that five of these patients die in one year. We wish to estimate $\pi$, the annual probability of death for these patients. We assume that the number of observed deaths has a binomial distribution obtained from $m = 50$ patients with probability of death $\pi$ for each patient. Let $\text{L}[\pi \mid d = 5] = (50!/45! \times 5!)\pi^5(1 - \pi)^{45}$ be the probability of the observed outcome (five deaths) given different values of $\pi$. $\text{L}[\pi \mid d = 5]$ is called a **likelihood function** and is plotted in Figure 4.4.

The **maximum likelihood estimate** of $\pi$ is the value of $\pi$ that assigns the greatest probability to the observed outcome. In this example the maximum likelihood estimate, denoted $\hat{\pi}$, equals $d/m = 0.1$. This is a plausible estimate in that, if the observed mortality rate is 10%, our best guess of the true mortality rate is also 10%. Note that if $\pi = \hat{\pi} = 0.1$ then

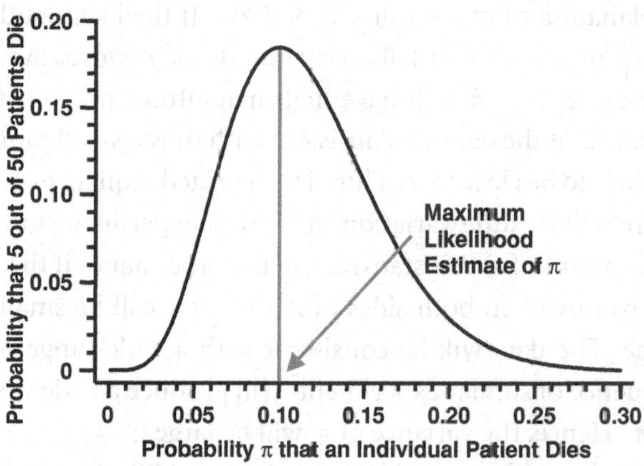


Figure 4.4 Suppose that five of 50 AIDS patients die in a year and that these deaths have a binomial distribution. Let $\pi$ be the probability that an individual patient dies in a given year. Then the likelihood function $L[\pi \mid d = 5]$ for this observation gives the probability of the observed outcome ($d = 5$ deaths) under different hypothesized values of $\pi$.

$E[d] = 50\pi = 5 = d$. Thus, in this example, the maximum likelihood estimate of $\pi$ is also the value that sets the expected number of deaths equal to the observed number of deaths.

In general, maximum likelihood estimates do not have simple closed solutions, but must be solved iteratively using numerical methods. This, however, is not a serious drawback given ubiquitous and powerful desktop computers.

A likelihood function looks deceptively like a probability density function. It is important to realize that they are quite different. A probability density function uses fixed values of the model parameters and indicates the probability of different outcomes under this model. A likelihood function holds the observed outcome fixed and shows the probability of this outcome for the different possible values of the parameters.

### 4.8.1. Variance of maximum likelihood parameter estimates

It can be shown that when a maximum likelihood estimate is based on a large number of patients, its variance is approximately equal to $-1/C$, where $C$ is the curvature of the logarithm of the likelihood function at $\hat{\pi}$. (In mathematical jargon, the curvature of a function is its second derivative. A function that bends downward has a negative curvature. The more sharply it bends the greater the absolute value of its curvature.) An intuitive explanation of this result is as follows. If the likelihood function reaches a sharp peak at $\hat{\pi}$ that falls away rapidly as $\pi$ moves away from $\hat{\pi}$, then the curvature $C$ at $\hat{\pi}$ will have high magnitude and $-1/C$ will be low. This means that the data are consistent with only a small range of $\pi$ and hence $\hat{\pi}$ is likely to be close to $\pi$. Thus, in a repeated sequence of similar experiments there will be little variation in $\hat{\pi}$ from experiment to experiment giving a low variance for this statistic. On the other hand, if the likelihood function drops slowly on both sides of $\hat{\pi}$ then $|C|$ will be small and $-1/C$ will be large. The data will be consistent with a wide range of $\pi$ and a repeated sequence of similar experiments will produce a wide variation in the values of $\hat{\pi}$. Hence, the variance of $\hat{\pi}$ will be large.

In the AIDS example from Section 4.8, $C$ can be shown to equal $-m/(\hat{\pi}(1-\hat{\pi}))$. Hence, the approximate variance of $\hat{\pi}$ is

$$\text{var}[\hat{\pi}] = -1/C = \hat{\pi}(1-\hat{\pi})/m. \tag{4.8}$$

The true variance of $\hat{\pi}$ is $\pi(1-\pi)/m$, and Equation (4.8) converges to this true value as $m$ becomes large. Substituting $\hat{\pi} = 0.1$ and $m = 50$ into Equation (4.8) gives that the variance of $\hat{\pi}$ is approximately $0.1 \times 0.9/50 = 0.0018$. The corresponding standard error is $\text{se}[\hat{\pi}] = \sqrt{0.0018} = 0.0424$.

## 4.9. Statistical tests and confidence intervals

In this section we briefly introduce three fundamental types of statistical tests, which we will use in this and later chapters: likelihood ratio tests, score tests and Wald tests. Each of these tests involves a statistic whose distribution is approximately normal or chi-squared. The accuracy of these approximations increases with increasing study sample size. We will illustrate these tests using the AIDS example from Section 4.8.

### 4.9.1. Likelihood ratio tests

Suppose that we wish to test the null hypothesis that $\pi = \pi_0$. Let $L[\pi]$ denote the likelihood function for $\pi$ given the observed data. We look at the **likelihood ratio** $L[\pi_0]/L[\hat{\pi}]$. If this ratio is small then we would be much more likely to have observed the data that was actually obtained if the true value of $\pi$ was $\hat{\pi}$ rather than $\pi_0$. Hence, small values of $L[\pi_0]/L[\hat{\pi}]$ provide evidence that $\pi \neq \pi_0$. Moreover, it can be shown that if the null hypothesis is true, then

$$\chi^2 = -2\log[L[\pi_0]/L[\hat{\pi}]] \tag{4.9}$$

has an approximately chi-squared distribution with one degree of freedom. Equation (4.9) is an example of a **likelihood ratio test**. The $P$-value associated with this test is the probability that a chi-squared distribution with one degree of freedom exceeds the value of this test statistic.

In our AIDS example, the likelihood ratio is

$$L[\pi_0]/L[\hat{\pi}] = \left(\pi_0^5(1-\pi_0)^{45}\right)/(\hat{\pi}^5(1-\hat{\pi})^{45}).$$

Suppose that we wished to test the null hypothesis that $\pi_0 = 0.2$. Now since $\hat{\pi} = 0.1$, Equation (4.9) gives us that

$$\chi^2 = -2\log[(0.2^5 \times 0.8^{45})/(0.1^5 \times 0.9^{45})] = 3.67.$$

The probability that a chi-squared distribution with one degree of freedom exceeds 3.67 is $P = 0.055$.

### 4.9.2. Quadratic approximations to the log likelihood ratio function

Consider quadratic equations of the form $f[x] = -a(x-b)^2$, where $a \geq 0$. Note that all equations of this form achieve a maximum value of 0 at $x = b$. Suppose that $g[x]$ is any smooth function that has negative curvature at $x_0$. Then it can be shown that there is a unique equation of the form $f[x] = -a(x-b)^2$ such that $f$ and $g$ have the same slope and curvature at $x_0$. Let

$$q[\pi] = \log[L[\pi]/L[\hat{\pi}]] \tag{4.10}$$

equal the logarithm of the likelihood ratio at $\pi$ relative to $\hat{\pi}$. Suppose that we wish to test the null hypothesis that $\pi = \pi_0$. Then the likelihood ratio test is given by $-2q[\pi_0]$ (see Equation (4.9)). In many practical situations, Equation (4.10) is difficult to calculate. For this reason $q[\pi]$ is often approximated by a quadratic equation. The maximum value of $q[\pi]$ is $q[\hat{\pi}] = \log[L[\hat{\pi}]/L[\hat{\pi}]] = 0$. We will consider approximating $q[\pi]$ by a quadratic equation that also has a maximum value of 0. Let

$f_s[\pi]$ be the quadratic equation that has the same slope and curvature as $q[\pi]$ at $\pi_0$ and achieves a maximum value of 0,

$f_w[\pi]$ be the quadratic equation that has the same slope and curvature as $q[\pi]$ at $\hat{\pi}$ and achieves a maximum value of 0.

Tests that approximate $q[\pi]$ by $f_s[\pi]$ are called **score tests**. Tests that approximate $q[\pi]$ by $f_w[\pi]$ are called **Wald tests**. We will introduce these two types of tests in the next two sections.

### 4.9.3. Score tests

Suppose we again wish to test the null hypothesis that $\pi = \pi_0$. If the null hypothesis is true then it can be shown that

$$\chi^2 = -2\, f_s[\pi_0] \tag{4.11}$$

has an approximately chi-squared distribution with one degree of freedom. Equation (4.11) is an example of a **score test**. Score tests are identical to likelihood ratio tests except that a likelihood ratio test is based on the true log likelihood ratio function $q[\pi]$ while a score test approximates $q[\pi]$ by $f_s[\pi]$.

In the AIDS example,

$$\hat{\pi} = 0.1 \text{ and } q[\pi] = \log((\pi/0.1)^5((1-\pi)/0.9)^{45}).$$

It can be shown that

$$q[\pi] \text{ has slope } \frac{5}{\pi} - \frac{45}{1-\pi} \text{ and curvature } -\frac{5}{\pi^2} - \frac{45}{(1-\pi)^2}.$$

We wish to test the null hypothesis that $\pi_0 = 0.2$. The slope and curvature of $q[\pi]$ at $\pi = 0.2$ are $-31.25$ and $-195.3125$, respectively. It can be shown that $f_s[\pi] = -97.656\,25(\pi - 0.04)^2$ also has this slope and curvature at $\pi = 0.2$. Therefore, if the true value of $\pi = 0.2$ then $-2\, f_s[0.2] = 2 \times 97.656\,25(0.2 - 0.04)^2 = 5$ has an approximately chi-squared distribution with one degree of freedom. The *P*-value associated with this score statistic is $P = 0.025$, which is lower than the corresponding likelihood ratio test.

### 4.9.4. Wald tests and confidence intervals

If the null hypothesis that $\pi = \pi_0$ is true, then

$$\chi^2 = -2 f_w[\pi_0] \tag{4.12}$$

also has an approximately chi-squared distribution with one degree of freedom. Equation (4.12) is an example of a **Wald test**. It is identical to the likelihood ratio test except that a likelihood ratio test is based on the true log likelihood ratio function $q[\pi]$, while a Wald test approximates $q[\pi]$ by $f_w[\pi]$. In Section 4.8.1 we said that the variance of a maximum likelihood estimate can be approximated by $\text{var}[\hat{\pi}] = -1/C$. It can be shown that

$$-2 f_w[\pi_0] = (\pi_0 - \hat{\pi})^2/\text{var}[\hat{\pi}]. \tag{4.13}$$

The standard error of $\hat{\pi}$ is approximated by $\text{se}[\hat{\pi}] = \sqrt{-1/C}$. Recall that a chi-squared statistic with one degree of freedom equals the square of a standard normal random variable. Hence, an equivalent way of performing a Wald test is to calculate

$$z = (\hat{\pi} - \pi_0)/\text{se}[\hat{\pi}], \tag{4.14}$$

which has an approximately standard normal distribution. An approximate 95% confidence interval for $\pi$ is given by

$$\hat{\pi} \pm 1.96\ \text{se}[\hat{\pi}]. \tag{4.15}$$

Equations (4.15) is known as a **Wald confidence interval**.

In the AIDS example, $\hat{\pi} = 0.1$ and $\text{se}[\hat{\pi}] = 0.0424$. Consider the null hypothesis that $\pi_0 = 0.2$. Equation (4.14) gives that $z = (0.1 - 0.2)/0.0424 = -2.36$. The probability that a $z$ statistic is less than $-2.36$ or greater than 2.36 is $P = 0.018$. The 95% confidence interval for $\pi$ is $0.1 \pm 1.96 \times 0.0424 = (0.017, 0.183)$.

### 4.9.5. Which test should you use?

The three tests outlined above all generalize to more complicated situations. Given a sufficiently large sample size all of these methods are equivalent. However, likelihood ratio tests and score tests are more accurate than Wald tests for most problems that are encountered in practice. For this reason, you should use a likelihood ratio or score test whenever they are available. The likelihood ratio test has the property that it is unaffected by transformations of the parameter of interest and is preferred over the score test for this reason. The Wald test is much easier to calculate than the other two, which are often not given by statistical software packages. It is common practice to use Wald tests when they are the only ones that can be easily calculated.

Wide divergence between these three tests can result when the log likelihood function is poorly approximated by a quadratic curve. In this case it is desirable to transform the parameter in such a way as to give the log likelihood function a more quadratic shape.

In this text, the most important example of a score test is the log-rank test, which is discussed in Chapter 6. In Chapters 5, 7, and 9 we will look at changes in model deviance as a means of selecting the best model for our data. Tests based on these changes in deviance are important examples of likelihood ratio tests. All of the confidence intervals in this text that are derived from logistic regression, survival, or Poisson regression models

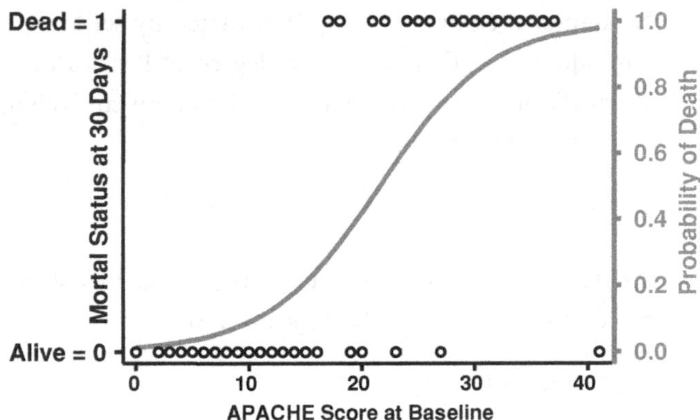


Figure 4.5 The gray curve in this figure shows the estimated probability of death within 30 days for septic patients with the indicated APACHE score at baseline. This curve is obtained by applying a logistic regression model to the observed mortal outcomes of 38 septic patients.

are Wald intervals. Tests of statistical significance in these models that are derived directly from the parameter estimates are Wald tests.

## 4.10. Sepsis example

Let us use logistic regression to model the relationship between mortal risk and APACHE score in the example from Section 4.1. Let $d_i = 1$ if the $i^{\text{th}}$ patient dies within 30 days, and let $d_i = 0$ otherwise. Let $x_i$ be the $i^{\text{th}}$ patient's APACHE score at baseline. Applying the logistic regression Model (4.7) to these data we obtain maximum likelihood parameter estimates of $\hat{\alpha} = -4.3478$ and $\hat{\beta} = 0.201\,24$. Inserting these estimates into Equation (4.6) gives the estimated probability of death associated with each APACHE score. For example, the estimated probability of death associated with an APACHE score of 16 is

$$\begin{aligned}\hat{\pi}[16] &= \exp[\hat{\alpha} + \hat{\beta} \times 16]/(1 + \exp[\hat{\alpha} + \hat{\beta} \times 16]) \\ &= \frac{\exp[-4.348 + 0.2012 \times 16]}{1 + \exp[-4.348 + 0.2012 \times 16]} \\ &= 0.2445.\end{aligned}$$

Figure 4.5 shows a plot of this probability of death as a function of baseline APACHE score.

## 4.11. Logistic regression with Stata

The following log file and comments illustrate how to fit a logistic regression model to the sepsis data set given in Figure 4.1.

```
. *  4.11.Sepsis.log
. *
. *  Simple logistic regression of mortal status at 30 days (fate)
. *  against baseline APACHE II score (apache) in a random sample
. *  of septic patients.
. *
. use C:\WDDtext\4.11.Sepsis.dta, clear

. summarize fate apache                                                1

    Variable |       Obs        Mean    Std. Dev.       Min        Max
-------------+--------------------------------------------------------
        fate |        38    .4473684    .5038966          0          1
      apache |        38    19.55263    11.30343          0         41

. glm fate apache, family(binomial) link(logit)                        2
                                                          Output omitted
Variance function: V(u) = u*(1-u)                 [Bernoulli]
Link function    : g(u) = ln(u/(1-u))             [Logit]
                                                  AIC             =   .8924255
Log likelihood   = -14.95608531                   BIC             = -101.0409

------------------------------------------------------------------------------
             |                 OIM
        fate |      Coef.   Std. Err.      z    P>|z|     [95% Conf. Interval]
-------------+----------------------------------------------------------------
      apache |   .2012365   .0609004     3.30   0.001      .081874     .320599   3
       _cons |  -4.347806   1.371623    -3.17   0.002    -7.036138   -1.659474
------------------------------------------------------------------------------

. predict logodds, xb                                                  4

. generate prob = exp(logodds)/(1 + exp(logodds))                      5

. list apache fate logodds prob in 1/3
```

| | apache | fate | logodds | prob | |
|---|---|---|---|---|---|
| 1. | 16 | Alive | -1.128022 | .2445263 | 6 |
| 2. | 25 | Dead | .6831065 | .6644317 | |
| 3. | 19 | Alive | -.5243126 | .3718444 | |

```
. sort apache
. label variable prob "Probability of Death"
. scatter fate apache || line prob apache, yaxis(2)                7
>     , ylabel(0 1, valuelabel)                                    8
>       yscale(titlegap(-8)) xlabel(0(10)40)                       9
. log close
```

**Comments**

1 This data set contains 38 observations. The variable *fate* equals 1 for patients who die within 30 days; *fate* equals 0 otherwise. Baseline APACHE scores range from 0 to 41.

2 This *glm* command regresses *fate* against *apache* using a generalized linear model. The *family* and *link* options specify that the random component of the model is binomial and the link function is logit. In other words, a logistic model is to be used. The equivalent point-and-click command is Statistics ▶ Generalized linear models (GLM) ▶ Generalized linear model (GLM) Model Dependent variable: *fate* , Independent variables: *apache* , Family and link choices: {Logit ⊙ Binomial} Submit. In the GLM dialog box the Family and link choices are chosen from an array whose columns are random components and whose rows are link functions. By {Logit ⊙ Binomial} I mean that you should click the radio button in the *Logit* row and the *Binomial* column of this array.

Stata has three commands that can perform logistic regression: *glm*, which can analyze any generalized linear model, and the *logistic* and *logit* commands, which can only be used for logistic regression. We will introduce the *logistic* command in Section 4.13.1.

3 The maximum likelihood parameter estimates are $\hat{\alpha} = -4.3478$ and $\hat{\beta} = 0.201\,24$.

4 The *xb* option of this *predict* command specifies that the linear predictor will be estimated for each patient and stored in a variable named

*logodds*. Recall that *predict* is a post-estimation command whose meaning is determined by the latest estimation command, which in this example is *glm*. The equivalent point-and-click command is Statistics ▶ Postestimation ▶ Predictions, residuals, etc ⌋ Main ⌊ New variable name: *logodds* ┌ Produce: — ⦿ Linear prediction (xb) ⌋ Submit . Note that many of the options on the *predict* dialog box following a *glm* command are different from the *predict* options that are available after a *regress* command.

5 This command defines *prob* to equal the estimated probability that a patient will die. It is calculated using Equation (4.6).

Note that from Equation (4.6) this probability is also the expected value of the model's random component. We could have calculated *prob* directly without first calculating *logodds* with the post estimation command

```
predict prob, mu
```

Following a *glm* command, this *predict* command with the *mu* option sets *prob* equal to the estimated expected value of the model's random component.

6 The first patient has an APACHE score of 16. Hence, the estimated linear predictor for this patient is $logodds = \hat{\alpha} + \hat{\beta}x_i = \_cons + apache \times 16 = -4.3478 + 0.201\,24 \times 16 = -1.128$. The second patient has APACHE $= 25$ giving logodds $= -4.3478 + 0.201\,24 \times 25 = 0.683$. For the first patient, $prob = \exp[logodds]/(1 + \exp[logodds]) = 0.2445$, which agrees with our calculation from Section 4.10.

In the *4.11.Sepsis.dta* data file the values of *fate* are coded 0 and 1 for patients who are alive or dead after 30 days, respectively. These values are assigned the labels *Alive* and *Dead* respectively in the data file. These value labels are used in tables, as shown here, and may also be used in graphs. The variable's numeric values are used by regression commands such as the *glm* command illustrated below. We will explain how to define value labels in Section 4.21.

7 This graph command produces a graph that is similar to Figure 4.5. The *yaxis(2)* option draws the *y*-axis for *prob* on the right-hand side of the graph.

8 This *ylabel(0 1, valuelabel)* option causes the *y*-axis to be labeled with the value labels of *fate* rather than this variable's numeric values. Hence, the left axis of Figure 4.5 is labeled *Alive* and *Dead* rather than 0 and 1.

9 By default, the title of the *y*-axis is written outside of the axis labels. This *yscale(titlegap(-8))* option decreases the gap between the title and the *y*-axis. The value 8 indicates that the distance the title is to be moved

is 8% of the minimum dimension of the graph. The equivalent point-and-click command is Graphics ▶ Twoway graph (scatter plot, line etc) ⌡Plots⌊ [Create] ⌡Plot⌊ ⌜ Plot type: (scatter plot) — Y variable: *fate* , X variable: *apache* ⌋ [Accept] [Create] ⌡Plot⌊ ⌜ Choose a plot category and type — Basic plots: (select type) *Line* ⌋ ⌜ Plot type: (line plot) — Y variable: *prob* , X variable: *apache* , [✓] Add a second axis on right ⌋ [Accept] ⌡Y axis⌊ [Properties] ⌡Text⌊ ⌜ Placement — Margin: *Custom* [..] ⌜ Top: *0* , Left: *0* , Right: *-8* , Bottom: *0* [Accept] ⌋ [Accept] [Major tick/label properties] ⌡Rule⌊ ⌜ Axis rule — ⦿ Custom , Custom rule: *0 1* ⌋ ⌡Labels⌊ ⌜ Labels — Angle: *Zero* , [✓] Use value labels ⌋ [Accept] [Edit second y axis] [Major tick/label properties] ⌡Labels⌊ ⌜ Labels — Angle: *Zero* ⌋ [Accept] [Accept] ⌡X axis⌊ [Major tick/label properties] ⌡Rule⌊ ⌜ Axis rule — ⦿ Range/Delta , *0* Minimum value , *40* Maximum value , *10* Delta ⌋ [Accept] ⌡Legend⌊ ⌜ Legend behavior — ⦿ Hide legend ⌋ [Submit].

## 4.12. Odds ratios and the logistic regression model

The log odds of death for patients with APACHE scores of $x$ and $x + 1$ are

$$\text{logit}[\pi[x]] = \alpha + \beta x \tag{4.16}$$

and

$$\text{logit}[\pi[x+1]] = \alpha + \beta(x+1) = \alpha + \beta x + \beta \tag{4.17}$$

respectively. Subtracting Equation (4.16) from Equation (4.17) gives

$$\begin{aligned}\beta &= \text{logit}[\pi[x+1]] - \text{logit}[\pi[x]]\\ &= \log\left[\frac{\pi[x+1]}{1-\pi[x+1]}\right] - \log\left[\frac{\pi[x]}{1-\pi[x]}\right]\\ &= \log\left[\frac{\pi[x+1]/[1-\pi[x+1]]}{\pi[x]/[1-\pi[x]]}\right].\end{aligned}$$

Hence $\exp[\beta]$ is the odds ratio for death associated with a unit increase in $x$. A property of logistic regression is that this ratio remains constant for all values of $x$.

## 4.13. 95% confidence interval for the odds ratio associated with a unit increase in $x$

Let $s_{\hat{\beta}}$ denote the estimated standard error of $\hat{\beta}$ from the logistic regression model. Now $\hat{\beta}$ has an approximately normal distribution. Therefore, a 95% confidence interval for $\beta$ is estimated by $\hat{\beta} \pm 1.96 s_{\hat{\beta}}$, and a 95% confidence interval for the odds ratio associated with a unit increase in $x$ is

$$(\exp[\hat{\beta} - 1.96 s_{\hat{\beta}}], \exp[\hat{\beta} + 1.96 s_{\hat{\beta}}]). \tag{4.18}$$

In the sepsis example in Section 4.10, the parameter estimate for *apache* (that is, $\beta$) was 0.201 24 with a standard error of $s_{\hat{\beta}} = 0.060\,90$. Hence, the 95% confidence interval for $\beta$ is $0.201\,24 \pm z_{0.025} \times 0.060\,90 = 0.201\,24 \pm 1.96 \times 0.060\,90 = (0.0819, 0.3206)$. The odds ratio for death associated with a unit rise in APACHE score is $\exp[0.2012] = 1.223$ with a 95% confidence interval of $(\exp[0.0819], \exp[0.3206]) = (1.085, 1.378)$.

### 4.13.1. Calculating this odds ratio with Stata

Stata can perform these calculations automatically. The following log file and comments illustrates how to do this using the *logistic* command:

```
. *  4.13.1.Sepsis.log
. *
. *  Calculate the odds ratio associated with a unit rise in
. *  APACHE score.
. *
. use C:\WDDtext\4.11.Sepsis.dta, clear
. logistic fate apache                                                    1
Logistic regression                         Number of obs    =        38
                                            LR chi2(1)       =     22.35
                                            Prob > chi2      =    0.0000
Log likelihood = -14.956085                 Pseudo R2        =    0.4276

----------------------------------------------------------------------------
        fate | Odds Ratio   Std. Err.      z    P>|z|    [95% Conf. Interval]
-------------+--------------------------------------------------------------
      apache |   1.222914   .0744759    3.30   0.001     1.085319    1.377953   2
----------------------------------------------------------------------------

. log close
```

**Comments**

1 Regress *fate* against *apache* using logistic regression. This command performs the same calculations as the *glm* command given in Section 4.11. However, the output is somewhat different. Also, there are some useful post-estimation commands that are available after running *logistic* that are not available after running *glm*. The equivalent point-and-click command is Statistics ▶ Binary outcomes ▶ Logistic regression (reporting odds ratios) Model Dependent variable: *fate* , Independent variables: *apache* Submit.

2 The number under the *Odds Ratio* heading is the exponentiated coefficient estimate for *apache*. As indicated above, this is the odds ratio associated with a unit rise in APACHE score. The 95% confidence interval for this odds ratio is identical to that calculated above.

## 4.14. Logistic regression with grouped response data

The number of patients under study often exceeds the number of distinct covariates. For example, in the Ibuprofen in Sepsis Study there were 38 distinct baseline APACHE scores observed on 454 patients (Bernard et al., 1997). Suppose that $\{x_i : i = 1, \ldots, n\}$ denote the distinct values of a covariate, and there are $m_i$ patients who have the identical covariate value $x_i$. Let $d_i$ be the number of deaths in these $m_i$ patients and let $\pi[x_i]$ be the probability that any one of them will die. Then $d_i$ has a binomial distribution with mean $m_i\pi[x_i]$, and hence $\mathrm{E}[d_i \mid x_i]/m_i = \pi[x_i]$. Thus, the logistic model becomes

$$\mathrm{logit}[\mathrm{E}[d_i \mid x_i]/m_i] = \alpha + \beta x_i, \qquad (4.19)$$

or equivalently

$$\mathrm{E}[d_i/m_i \mid x_i] = \pi[x_i] = \exp[\alpha + \beta x_i]/(1 + \exp[\alpha + \beta x_i]). \qquad (4.20)$$

In Equation (4.19) $d_i$ is the random component of the model, which has a binomial distribution. If $i$ indexes patients rather than distinct values of the covariate then $m_i = 1$ for all $i$ and Equation (4.19) reduces to Equation (4.7).

## 4.15. 95% confidence interval for $\pi[x]$

Let $\sigma^2_{\hat\alpha}$ and $\sigma^2_{\hat\beta}$ denote the variances of $\hat\alpha$ and $\hat\beta$, and let $\sigma_{\hat\alpha\hat\beta}$ denote the covariance between $\hat\alpha$ and $\hat\beta$. Then it can be shown that the standard error of $\hat{\alpha} + \hat{\beta}x$ is

$$\text{se}[\hat{\alpha} + \hat{\beta}x] = \sqrt{\sigma^2_{\hat{\alpha}} + 2x\sigma_{\hat{\alpha}\hat{\beta}} + x^2\sigma^2_{\hat{\beta}}}. \tag{4.21}$$

Any logistic regression software that calculates the maximum likelihood estimates of $\alpha$ and $\beta$ can also provide estimates of $\sigma^2_{\hat{\alpha}}$, $\sigma^2_{\hat{\beta}}$, and $\sigma_{\hat{\alpha}\hat{\beta}}$. We substitute these estimates into Equation (4.21) to obtain an estimate of the standard error of $\hat{\alpha} + \hat{\beta}x$. This allows us to estimate the 95% confidence interval for $\alpha + \beta x$ to be $\hat{\alpha} + \hat{\beta}x \pm 1.96 \times \text{se}[\hat{\alpha} + \hat{\beta}x]$. Hence, a 95% confidence interval for $\pi[x]$ is $(\hat{\pi}_{\text{L}}[x], \hat{\pi}_{\text{U}}[x])$, where

$$\hat{\pi}_{\text{L}}[x] = \frac{\exp[\hat{\alpha} + \hat{\beta}x - 1.96 \times \text{se}[\hat{\alpha} + \hat{\beta}x]]}{1 + \exp[\hat{\alpha} + \hat{\beta}x - 1.96 \times \text{se}[\hat{\alpha} + \hat{\beta}x]]} \tag{4.22}$$

and

$$\hat{\pi}_{\text{U}}[x] = \frac{\exp[\hat{\alpha} + \hat{\beta}x + 1.96 \times \text{se}[\hat{\alpha} + \hat{\beta}x]]}{1 + \exp[\hat{\alpha} + \hat{\beta}x + 1.96 \times \text{se}[\hat{\alpha} + \hat{\beta}x]]}. \tag{4.23}$$

## 4.16. Exact 100(1 − α)% confidence intervals for proportions

Let $D$ be the number of deaths among $m$ independent patients with the probability that any individual patient dies being $\pi$. We observe $D = d$ deaths. Let $p = d/m$ be the observed proportion of deaths. We seek probabilities $p_l$ and $p_u$ that give a $100(1 - \alpha)\%$ confidence interval for $\pi$ given $p$. Let $\Pr[a \le D \le b|\pi]$ denote the probability that $D$ lies between $a$ and $b$. For any null hypothesis $\pi = \pi_u > p$ the one-sided critical region associated with alternative hypotheses that $\pi < \pi_u$ is $0 \le D \le d$. We choose $p_u$ such that under the null hypothesis $\pi = p_u$ the one-sided $P$-value associated with smaller values of $\pi$ is $\alpha/2$. That is, we seek $p_u$ such that

$$\Pr[0 \le D \le d|\pi = p_u] = \alpha/2.$$

Similarly, we choose $p_l$ such that under the null hypothesis $\pi = p_l$ the one-sided $P$-value associated with larger values of $\pi$ is $\alpha/2$. That is, we seek $p_l$ such that

$$\Pr[d \le D \le m|\pi = p_l] = \alpha/2.$$

Then $(p_l, p_u)$ is the **exact 100(1 − α)% confidence interval** for $\pi$. This interval has the property that a two-sided test of any probability within this interval cannot be rejected with significance level $\alpha$.

Let $\text{bin}[m, d, \pi] = \Pr[0 \le D \le d|\pi]$ be the binomial cumulative distribution function and let $\text{bin}^{-1}[m, d, \gamma]$ be the inverse of this function such that if $\text{bin}[m, d, \pi] = \gamma$ then $\text{bin}^{-1}[m, d, \gamma] = \pi$. Then it follows from the elementary laws of probability that

$$p_u = \text{bin}^{-1}[m, d, \alpha/2] \tag{4.24}$$

and

$$p_l = 1 - \text{bin}^{-1}[m, m - d, \alpha/2]. \tag{4.25}$$

We will use Equations (4.22) and (4.23) to construct exact confidence intervals for proportions. When $d = 0$ or $m$ these equations reduce to $(0,\ p_u)$ and $(p_l,\ 1)$, respectively. Other formulas for confidence intervals based on normal approximations to the binomial distributions have been proposed (Fleiss et al., 2003). However, these intervals either perform badly when $d$ is near 0 or $m$ or are themselves rather complicated.

## 4.17. Example: the Ibuprofen in Sepsis Study

The Ibuprofen in Sepsis Study contained 454 patients with known baseline APACHE scores. The 30-day mortality data for these patients are summarized in Table 4.1. Let $x_i$ denote the distinct APACHE scores observed in this study. Let $m_i$ be the number of patients with baseline score $x_i$ and let $d_i$ be the number of patients with this score who died within 30 days. Applying the logistic regression model (4.19) to these data yields parameter estimates $\hat{\alpha} = -2.290\,327$ and $\hat{\beta} = 0.115\,627$. The estimated variances of $\hat{\alpha}$ and $\hat{\beta}$ are $s_{\hat{\alpha}}^2 = 0.076\,468$ and $s_{\hat{\beta}}^2 = 0.000\,256$, respectively. The estimated covariance between $\hat{\alpha}$ and $\hat{\beta}$ is $s_{\hat{\alpha}\hat{\beta}} = -0.004\,103$. Substituting these values into Equations (4.20) through (4.25) provides estimates of the probability of death given a baseline score of $x$, 95% confidence intervals for these estimates, and 95% confidence intervals for the observed proportion of deaths at any given score. For example, patients with a baseline score of 20 will have a linear predictor of $\hat{\alpha} + \hat{\beta} \times 20 = 0.0222$. Substituting this value into Equation (4.20) gives $\hat{\pi}[20] = \exp[0.0222]/(1 + \exp[0.0222]) = 0.506$. Equation (4.21) gives us that

$$\begin{aligned}
&\text{se}[\hat{\alpha} + \hat{\beta} \times 20] \\
&\quad = \sqrt{0.076\,468 - 2 \times 20 \times 0.004\,103 + 20^2 \times 0.000\,256} \\
&\quad = 0.1214.
\end{aligned}$$

Substituting into Equations (4.22) and (4.23) gives

$$\hat{\pi}_{\text{L}}[20] = \frac{\exp[0.0222 - 1.96 \times 0.1214]}{1 + \exp[0.0222 - 1.96 \times 0.1214]} = 0.446$$

**Table 4.1.** Survival data from the Ibuprofen in Sepsis Study. The number of patients enrolled with the indicated baseline APACHE score is given together with the number of subjects who died within 30 days of entry into the study (Bernard et al., 1997)

| Baseline APACHE score | Number of patients | Number of deaths | Baseline APACHE score | Number of patients | Number of deaths |
|---|---|---|---|---|---|
| 0 | 1 | 0 | 20 | 13 | 6 |
| 2 | 1 | 0 | 21 | 17 | 9 |
| 3 | 4 | 1 | 22 | 14 | 12 |
| 4 | 11 | 0 | 23 | 13 | 7 |
| 5 | 9 | 3 | 24 | 11 | 8 |
| 6 | 14 | 3 | 25 | 12 | 8 |
| 7 | 12 | 4 | 26 | 6 | 2 |
| 8 | 22 | 5 | 27 | 7 | 5 |
| 9 | 33 | 3 | 28 | 3 | 1 |
| 10 | 19 | 6 | 29 | 7 | 4 |
| 11 | 31 | 5 | 30 | 5 | 4 |
| 12 | 17 | 5 | 31 | 3 | 3 |
| 13 | 32 | 13 | 32 | 3 | 3 |
| 14 | 25 | 7 | 33 | 1 | 1 |
| 15 | 18 | 7 | 34 | 1 | 1 |
| 16 | 24 | 8 | 35 | 1 | 1 |
| 17 | 27 | 8 | 36 | 1 | 1 |
| 18 | 19 | 13 | 37 | 1 | 1 |
| 19 | 15 | 7 | 41 | 1 | 0 |

and

$$\hat{\pi}_{\mathrm{U}}[20] = \frac{\exp[0.0222 + 1.96 \times 0.1214]}{1 + \exp[0.0222 + 1.96 \times 0.1214]} = 0.565.$$

Hence a 95% confidence interval for $\pi(20)$ is (0.446, 0.565).

There are $m = 13$ patients with an APACHE score of 20; $d = 6$ of these subjects died. Hence the observed proportion of patients dying with this score $p = 6/13 = 0.462$. Substituting these values into Equations (4.24) and (4.25) gives $p_u = \mathrm{bin}^{-1}[13, 6, 0.025] = 0.749$ and $p_l = 1 - \mathrm{bin}^{-1}[13, 7, 0.025] = 0.192$ as the bounds of the 95% confidence interval for the true proportion of deaths among people with an APACHE score of 20. Note that the difference between $(\hat{\pi}_{\mathrm{L}}(20), \hat{\pi}_{\mathrm{U}}(20))$ and $(p_l, p_u)$ is that the former is based on all 454 patients and the logistic regression

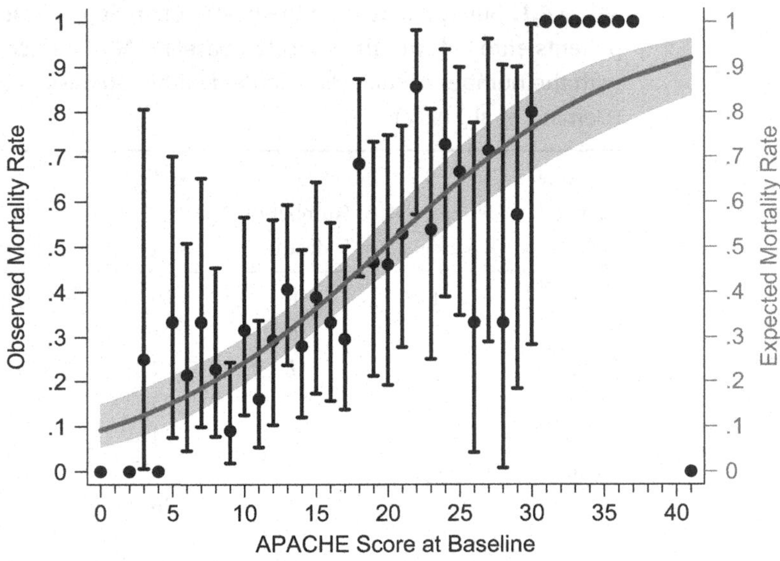


Figure 4.6 **Observed and expected 30-day mortality by APACHE score in patients from the Ibuprofen in Sepsis Study (Bernard et al., 1997). The gray line gives the expected mortality based on a logistic regression model. The shaded region gives the 95% confidence band for this regression line. The black dots give the observed mortality for each APACHE score. The error bars give 95% confidence intervals for the observed mortality at each score.**

model while the latter is based solely on the 13 patients with APACHE scores of 20.

We can perform calculations similar to those given above to generate Figure 4.6. The black dots in this figure give the observed mortality for each APACHE score. The error bars give 95% confidence intervals for the observed mortality at each score using Equations (4.24) and (4.25). Confidence intervals for scores associated with 100% survival or 100% mortality are not given because the numbers of patients with these scores are small and the resulting confidence intervals are very wide. The gray line gives the logistic regression curve using Equation (4.20). This curve depicts the expected 30-day mortality as a function of the baseline APACHE score. The shaded region gives the 95% confidence intervals for the regression curve using Equations (4.22) and (4.23). These intervals are analogous to the confidence intervals for the linear regression line described in Section 2.10. Note that the expected mortality curve lies within all of the 95% confidence intervals for the observed proportion of deaths at each score. This indicates

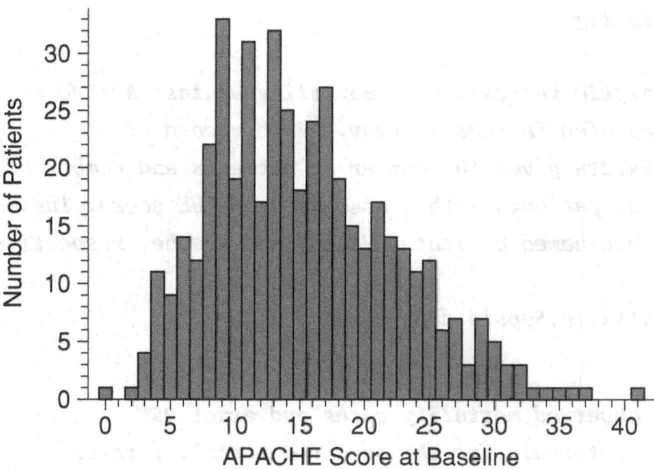


Figure 4.7 Histogram of baseline APACHE scores for patients from the Ibuprofen in Sepsis Study. This distribution is skewed to the right, with few patients having scores greater than 30. The estimate of the expected mortality rate in Figure 4.6 is most accurate over the range of scores that were most common in this study.

that the logistic regression model fits the data quite well. The width of the 95% confidence intervals for the regression curve depends on the number of patients studied, on the distance along the $x$-axis from the central mass of observations and on the proximity of the regression curve to either zero or one. Figure 4.7 shows a histogram of the number of study subjects by baseline APACHE score. This figure shows that the distribution of scores is skewed. The interquartile range is 10–20. Note that the width of the confidence interval at a score of 30 in Figure 4.6 is considerably greater than it is at a score of 15. This reflects the fact that 30 is further from the central mass of observations than is 15, and that as a consequence the accuracy of our estimate of $\pi[30]$ is less than that of $\pi[15]$. For very large values of the $x$ variable, however, we know that $\pi[x]$ converges to one. Hence, $\hat{\pi}_L[x]$ and $\hat{\pi}_U[x]$ must also converge to one. In Figure 4.6 the confidence intervals have started to narrow for this reason for scores of 40 or more. We can think of the 95% confidence intervals for the regression line as defining the region that most likely contains the true regression line given that the logistic regression model is, in fact, correct.

## 4.18. Logistic regression with grouped data using Stata

The following log file and comments illustrates how to use Stata to perform the calculations from the preceding section.

```
. *  4.18.Sepsis.log
. *
. *  Simple logistic regression of mortality against APACHE score
. *  in the Ibuprofen in Sepsis Study.  Each record of
. *  4.18.Sepsis.dta gives the number of patients and number of
. *  deaths among patients with a specified APACHE score. These
. *  variables are named patients, deaths and apache, respectively.
. *
. use C:\WDDtext\4.18.Sepsis.dta, clear

. *
. *  Calculate observed mortality rates and exact 95%
. *  confidence intervals for the observed mortality rates.
. *
. generate p = deaths/patients

. generate ci95ub = invbinomial(patients, deaths, 0.025)                    1
(7 missing values generated)

. generate ci95lb = 1 - invbinomial(patients, patients-deaths,0.025)        2
(4 missing values generated)

. *
. *  Regress deaths against apache
. *
. glm deaths apache, family(binomial patients) link(logit)                 3
                                                                Output omitted
Variance function: V(u) = u*(1-u/patients)        [Binomial]
Link function    : g(u) = ln(u/(patients-u))      [Logit]
Log likelihood   = -60.93390578                   BIC             = -176.2525
```

| deaths | Coef. | OIM Std. Err. | z | P>\|z\| | [95% Conf. | Interval] | |
|---|---|---|---|---|---|---|---|
| apache | .1156272 | .0159997 | 7.23 | 0.000 | .0842684 | .1469861 | 4 |
| _cons | -2.290327 | .2765286 | -8.28 | 0.000 | -2.832314 | -1.748341 | |

```
. estat vce                                                              5

Covariance matrix of coefficients of glm model

             |      deaths
        e(V) |     apache        _cons
-------------+--------------------------
deaths       |
      apache |  .00025599
       _cons | -.00410256    .07646805

. predict logodds, xb                                                    6
. generate e_prob = invlogit(logodds)                                    7
. label variable e_prob "Expected Mortality Rate"
. *
. *  Calculate 95% confidence region for e_prob
. *
. predict stderr, stdp                                                   8
. generate lodds_lb = logodds - 1.96*stderr
. generate lodds_ub = logodds + 1.96*stderr
. generate prob_lb = invlogit(lodds_lb)                                  9
. generate prob_ub = invlogit(lodds_ub)
. list p e_prob prob_lb prob_ub ci95lb ci95ub apache                    10
> if apache == 20
```

| | p | e_prob | prob_lb | prob_ub | ci95lb | ci95ub | apache |
|---|---|---|---|---|---|---|---|
| 20. | .4615385 | .505554 | .4462291 | .564723 | .1922324 | .7486545 | 20 |

```
. twoway rarea prob_ub prob_lb apache, color(gs14)                      11
>   || scatter p apache, symbol(circle)                                 12
>   || rcap ci95ub ci95lb apache                                        13
>   || line e_prob apache, yaxis(2) lwidth(thick) color(gray)           14
```

```
>      , xlabel(0(5)40) xmtick(0(1)41) ylabel(0(.1)1)
>      ytitle(Observed Mortality Rate)                                15
>      ylabel(0(.1)1, axis(2) labcolor(gray) tlcolor(gray))           16
>      ytitle(,axis(2) color(gray)) legend(off)                       17
. histogram apache [freq=patients]                                    18
>      , discrete frequency ytitle(Number of Patients)                19
>      xlabel(0(5)40) xmtick(1(1)41) ylabel(0(5)30) ymtick(1(1)33)
(start=0, width=1)
. log close
```

**Comments**

1 Calculate the upper bound for an exact 95% confidence interval for the observed proportion of deaths using Equation (4.24). The *invbinomial* function calculates the inverse of the cumulative binomial distribution $\text{bin}^{-1}$[*patients, deaths,* 0.025]. The *invbinomial* function returns a missing value when *deaths* = 0 or *deaths* = *patients.*

2 Calculate the corresponding lower bound using Equation (4.25). It should be noted that the *ci* command can also calculate exact confidence intervals for proportions. However, this command requires either that the data be organized as one record per patient or as two records for each APACHE score: one for patients who died and one for those who lived. Since this data set has only one record per APACHE score it is less trouble to calculate these intervals using the *invbinomial* function than to reformat the data.

3 The *family* and *link* option of this *glm* command specify a binomial random component and a logit link function. The *family*(*binomial patients*) option indicates that each observation describes the outcomes of multiple patients with the same value of *apache*; *patients* records the number of subjects with each *apache* value; *deaths* records the number of deaths observed among these subjects. In other words, we are fitting a logistic regression model using Equation (4.20) with $d_i$ = *deaths*, $m_i$ = *patients*, and $x_i$ = *apache*. The equivalent point-and-click command is Statistics ▶ Generalized linear models ▶ Generalized linear model (GLM) Model Dependent variable: *deaths* , Independent variables: *apache* , Family and link choices: {Logit ⊙ Binomial} ⊙ *patients* Variable Submit.

4 The estimated regression coefficients for *apache* and the constant term *_cons* are $\hat{\beta} = 0.115\,627$ and $\hat{\alpha} = -2.290\,327$, respectively.

5 The *estat vce* command prints the variance–covariance matrix for the estimated regression coefficients. This is a triangular array of numbers that gives estimates of the variance of each coefficient estimate and the covariance of each pair of coefficient estimates. In this example there are only two coefficients. The estimated variances of the *apache* and *_cons* coefficient estimates are $s^2_{\hat\beta} = 0.000\,256$ and $s^2_{\hat\alpha} = 0.076\,468$, respectively. The covariance between these estimates is $s_{\hat\alpha\hat\beta} = -0.004\,103$. Note that the square roots of $s^2_{\hat\beta}$ and $s^2_{\hat\alpha}$ equal 0.1600 and 0.2765, which are the standard errors of $\hat\beta$ and $\hat\alpha$ given in the output from the *glm* command. The equivalent point-and-click command is Statistics ▶ Postestimation ▶ Reports and statistics ⌜ Reports and Statistics: *Covariance matrix estimates (vce)* [Submit].

We do not usually need to output the variance–covariance matrix in Stata because the *predict* and *lincom* post estimation commands can usually derive all the statistics of interest. We output these terms here to corroborate the hand calculations performed in Section 4.17. We will introduce the *lincom* command in Section 5.20. The variance–covariance matrix is further discussed in Section 5.17.

6 This command sets *logodds* equal to the linear predictor $\hat\alpha + \hat\beta \times apache$. The equivalent point-and-click command is given on page 172.

7 The *invlogit* function calculates the inverse of the logit function. That is, $invlogit(x) = e^x/(1 + e^x)$. Using this function is slightly simpler than calculating this result directly. The variable *e_prob* equals $\hat\pi[apache]$, the estimated probability of death for patients with the indicated APACHE score.

8 The *stdp* option of this *predict* command sets *stderr* equal to the standard error of the linear predictor. The point-and-click version of this command is Statistics ▶ Postestimation ▶ Predictions, residuals, etc ⌋ Main ⌊ New variable name: *stderr* ⌈ Produce: — ⦿ Standard error of the linear pred. ⌋ [Submit].

9 This generate command defines *prob_lb* to equal $\hat\pi_L[x]$ as defined by Equation (4.22). The next command sets *prob_ub* to equal $\hat\pi_U[x]$.

10 This *list* command outputs the values of variables calculated above for the record with an APACHE score of 20. Note that these values agree with the estimates that we calculated by hand in Section 4.17.

11 The graph produced by this command is similar to Figure 4.6; *rarea* produces the 95% confidence band for the expected mortality rate *e_prob* $= \hat\pi[apache]$.

12 This *scatter* command overlays the observed mortality rates on the graph. The *symbol(circle)* option plots these rates as solid circles.

13 This *rcap* command plots vertical error bars connecting *ci95lb* and *ci95ub* for each value of *apache*.
14 This *line* command plots *e_prob* against *apache*. The *yaxis(2)* option creates a second *y*-axis on the right for this graph for this plot; *lwidth* and *color* control the width and color of this plotted line.
15 This *ytitle* option gives a title to the main *y*-axis (i.e. the axis on the left). Since we have multiple overlayed plots against this axis we need to give it an explicit title.
16 The *axis(2)* suboption of this *ylabel* option indicates that these labels are to be applied to the second *y*-axis on the right. The *labcolor(gray)* and *tlcolor(gray)* suboptions color these labels and tick marks gray.
17 In this graph the only plot that uses the second *y*-axis is the line plot of *e_prob* versus *apache*. For this reason, the default title for this axis is the variable label that we assigned to *e_prob*. This *ytitle* option colors this default title gray. Note that the comma is needed to interpret *axis(2)* and *color(gray)* as suboptions that affect the second axis on the right rather than as a new title for the left *y*-axis.

The point-and-click command for generating Figure 4.6 is Graphics ▶ Twoway graph (scatter plot, line etc) ⌋ Plots ⌊ [Create] ⌋ Plot ⌊ ⌈ Choose a plot category and type — ⦿ Range plots , Range plots: (select type) *Range area* ⌋ ⌈ Plot type: (range plot with area shading) — Y1 variable: *prob_ub* , Y2 variable: *prob_lb* , X variable: *apache* [Area properties] Fill color: *Gray 14* , Outline color *Gray 14* [Accept] ⌋ [Accept] [Create] ⌋ Plot ⌊ ⌈ Plot type: (scatter plot) — Y variable: *p* , X variable: *apache* [Marker properties] ⌋ Main ⌊ ⌈ Marker properties — Symbol: *Circle* ⌋ [Accept] ⌋ [Accept] [Create] ⌋ Plot ⌊ ⌈ Choose a plot category and type — ⦿ Range plots , Range plots: (select type) *Range spike w/cap* ⌋ ⌈ Plot type: (range plot with capped spikes) — Y1 variable: *ci95ub* , Y2 variable: *ci95lb* , X variable: *apache* ⌋ [Accept] [Create] ⌋ Plot ⌊ ⌈ Choose a plot category and type — Basic plots: (select type) *Line* ⌋ ⌈ Plot type: (line plot) — Y variable: *e_prob* , X variable: *apache* , [✓] Add a second y axis on right [Line properties] Color: *Gray* , Width: *Thick* [Accept] ⌋ [Accept] ⌋ Y axis ⌊ Title: *Observed Mortality Rate* [Major tick/label properties] ⌋ Rule ⌊ ⌈ Axis rule — ⦿ Range/Delta , *0* Minimum value , *1* Maximum value , *.1* Delta ⌋ [Accept] [Edit second y axis] [Properties] ⌋ Text ⌊ ⌈ Text properties — Color: *Gray* ⌟ [Accept] [Major tick/label properties] ⌟Rule⌞ ⌜ Axis rule — ⦿ Range/Delta , *0* Minimum value , *1* Maximum value , *.1* Delta ⌟ ⌟Labels⌞ ⌜ Labels — Color: *Gray* ⌟ ⌟Ticks⌞ ⌜ Ticks — Color: *Gray* ⌟ [Accept] [Accept] ⌟X axis⌞ [Major tick/label properties] ⌟Rule⌞ ⌜ Axis rule — ⦿ Range/Delta , *0* Minimum value , *40* Maximum value , *5* Delta ⌟ [Accept] [Minor tick/label properties] ⌟Rule⌞ ⌜ Axis rule — ⦿ Range/Delta , *0* Minimum value , *41* Maximum value , *1* Delta ⌟ [Accept] ⌟Legend⌞ ⌜ Legend behavior — ⦿ Hide legend ⌟ [Submit].

18 This histogram is similar to Figure 4.7. The *[freq = patients]* command qualifier indicates that *patients* describes the number of observations of each record. If we had omitted this qualifier, each data record would have been treated as a single observation.

19 The *discrete* option indicates that a separate bar is to be drawn for each distinct value of *apache*; *frequency* indicates that the *y*-axis will be the number of subjects. A point-and-click command that produces a similar graph is Graphics ▶ Histogram ⌟Main⌞ ⌜ Data — Variable: *apache* , ⦿ Data is discrete ⌟ ⌟Weights⌞ ⦿ Frequency weights , Frequency weight: *patients* ⌟Y axis⌞ Title: *Number of Patients* [Submit].

## 4.19. Simple 2×2 case-control studies

### 4.19.1. Example: the Ille-et-Vilaine study of esophageal cancer and alcohol

Tuyns et al. (1977) conducted a case-control study of alcohol, tobacco, and esophageal cancer in men from the Ille-et-Vilaine district of Brittany. Breslow and Day (1980) subsequently published these data. The cases in this study were 200 esophageal cancer patients who had been diagnosed at a district hospital between January 1972 and April 1974. The controls were 775 men who were drawn from local electoral lists. Study subjects were interviewed concerning their consumption of alcohol and tobacco as well as other dietary risk factors. Table 4.2 shows these subjects divided by whether they were moderate or heavy drinkers.

**Table 4.2.** Cases and controls from the Ille-et-Vilaine study of esophageal cancer, grouped by level of daily alcohol consumption. Subjects were considered heavy drinkers if their daily consumption was ≥80 grams (Breslow and Day, 1980)

| | Daily alcohol consumption | | |
|---|---|---|---|
| Esophageal cancer | ≥80 g | <80 g | Total |
| Yes (cases) | $d_1 = 96$ | $c_1 = 104$ | $m_1 = 200$ |
| No (controls) | $d_0 = 109$ | $c_0 = 666$ | $m_0 = 775$ |
| Total | $n_1 = 205$ | $n_0 = 770$ | $N = 975$ |

### 4.19.2. Review of classical case-control theory

Let $\pi_0$ and $\pi_1$ denote the prevalence of heavy drinking among controls and cases in the Ille-et-Vilaine case-control study, respectively. That is, $\pi_i$ is the probability that a control ($i = 0$) or a case ($i = 1$) is a heavy drinker. Then the **odds** that a control patient is a heavy drinker is $\pi_0/(1 - \pi_0)$, and the odds that a case is a heavy drinker is $\pi_1/(1 - \pi_1)$. The **odds ratio** for heavy drinking among cases relative to controls is

$$\psi = (\pi_1/(1 - \pi_1))/(\pi_0/(1 - \pi_0)). \tag{4.26}$$

Let $m_0$ and $m_1$ denote the number of controls and cases, respectively. Let $d_0$ and $d_1$ denote the number of controls and cases who are heavy drinkers. Let $c_0$ and $c_1$ denote the number of controls and cases who are moderate or non-drinkers. (Note that $m_i = c_i + d_i$ for $i = 0$ or 1.) Then the observed prevalence of heavy drinkers is $d_0/m_0 = 109/775$ for controls and $d_1/m_1 = 96/200$ for cases. The observed prevalence of moderate or non-drinkers is $c_0/m_0 = 666/775$ for controls and $c_1/m_1 = 104/200$ for cases. **The observed odds** that a case or control will be a heavy drinker is

$$(d_i/m_i)/(c_i/m_i) = d_i/c_i$$

$= 109/666$ and $96/104$ for controls and cases, respectively. The **observed odds ratio** for heavy drinking in cases relative to controls is

$$\hat{\psi} = \frac{d_1/c_1}{d_0/c_0} = \frac{96/104}{109/666} = 5.64.$$

If the cases and controls are representative samples from their respective underlying populations then:

1 $\hat{\psi}$ is an appropriate estimate of the true odds ratio $\psi$ for heavy drinking in cases relative to controls in the underlying population.
2 This true odds ratio also equals the true odds ratio for esophageal cancer in heavy drinkers relative to moderate drinkers.
3 If, in addition, the disease under study is rare (as is the case for esophageal cancer) then $\hat{\psi}$ also estimates the relative risk of esophageal cancer in heavy drinkers relative to moderate drinkers.

It is the second of the three facts listed above that makes case-control studies worth doing. We really are not particularly interested in the odds ratio for heavy drinking among cases relative to controls. However, we are very interested in the relative risk of esophageal cancer in heavy drinkers compared with moderate drinkers. It is, perhaps, somewhat surprising that we can estimate this relative risk from the prevalence of heavy drinking among cases and controls. Note that we are unable to estimate the incidence of cancer in either heavy drinkers or moderate drinkers. See Hennekens and Buring (1987) for an introduction to case-control studies. A more mathematical explanation of this relationship is given in Breslow and Day (1980).

### 4.19.3. 95% confidence interval for the odds ratio: Woolf's method

An estimate of the standard error of the log odds ratio is

$$\mathrm{se}_{\log(\hat{\psi})} = \sqrt{\frac{1}{d_0} + \frac{1}{c_0} + \frac{1}{d_1} + \frac{1}{c_1}}, \tag{4.27}$$

and the distribution of $\log(\hat{\psi})$ is approximately normal. Hence, if we let

$$\hat{\psi}_{\mathrm{L}} = \hat{\psi} \exp\left[-1.96\ \mathrm{se}_{\log(\hat{\psi})}\right] \tag{4.28}$$

and

$$\hat{\psi}_{\mathrm{U}} = \hat{\psi} \exp\left[1.96\ \mathrm{se}_{\log(\hat{\psi})}\right], \tag{4.29}$$

then $(\hat{\psi}_{\mathrm{L}}, \hat{\psi}_{\mathrm{U}})$ is a 95% confidence interval for $\psi$ (Woolf, 1955). In the esophageal cancer and alcohol analysis

$$\mathrm{se}_{\log(\hat{\psi})} = \sqrt{\frac{1}{109} + \frac{1}{666} + \frac{1}{96} + \frac{1}{104}} = 0.1752.$$

Therefore, Woolf's estimate of the 95% confidence interval for the odds ratio is $(\hat{\psi}_{\mathrm{L}}, \hat{\psi}_{\mathrm{U}}) = (5.64 \exp[-1.96 \times 0.1752], 5.64 \exp[+1.96 \times 0.1752]) = (4.00, 7.95)$.

### 4.19.4. Test of the null hypothesis that the odds ratio equals one

If there is no association between exposure and disease then the odds ratio $\psi$ will equal one. Let $n_j$ be the number of study subjects who are $(j = 1)$ or are not $(j = 0)$ heavy drinkers and let $N = n_0 + n_1 = m_0 + m_1$ be the total number of cases and controls. Under the null hypothesis that $\psi = 1$, the expected value and variance of $d_1$ are

$$\mathrm{E}[d_1 \mid \psi = 1] = n_1 m_1 / N \text{ and}$$
$$\mathrm{var}[d_1 \mid \psi = 1] = m_0 m_1 n_0 n_1 / N^3.$$

Hence,

$$\chi_1^2 = (|d_1 - \mathrm{E}[d_{1j} \mid \psi = 1]| - 0.5)^2 / \mathrm{var}[d_1 \mid \psi = 1] \tag{4.30}$$

has a $\chi^2$ distribution with one degree of freedom. In the Ille-et-Vilaine study

$$\mathrm{E}[d_1 \mid \psi = 1] = 205 \times 200/975 = 42.051 \text{ and}$$
$$\mathrm{var}[d_1 \mid \psi = 1] = 775 \times 200 \times 770 \times 205/975^3 = 26.397.$$

Therefore, $\chi_1^2 = (|96 - 42.051| - 0.5)^2/(26.397) = 108.22$. The $P$-value associated with this statistic is $<10^{-24}$, providing overwhelming evidence that the observed association between heavy drinking and esophageal cancer is not due to chance.

In Equation (4.30) the constant 0.5 that is subtracted from the numerator is known as Yates' continuity correction (Yates, 1934). It adjusts for the fact that we are approximating a discrete distribution with a continuous normal distribution. There is an ancient controversy among statisticians on whether such corrections are appropriate (Dupont and Plummer, 1999). Mantel and Greenhouse (1968), Fleiss (2003), Breslow and Day (1980), and many others use this correction in calculating this statistic. However, Grizzle (1967) and others, including the statisticians at StataCorp, do not. This leads to a minor discrepancy between output from Stata and other statistical software. Without the continuity correction the $\chi^2$ statistic equals 110.26.

### 4.19.5. Test of the null hypothesis that two proportions are equal

We also need to be able to test the null hypothesis that two proportions are equal. For example, we might wish to test the hypothesis that the proportion of heavy drinkers among cases and controls is the same. It is important to realize that this hypothesis, $H_0 : \pi_0 = \pi_1$, is true if and only if $\psi = 1$. Hence Equation (4.30) may also be used to test this null hypothesis.

## 4.20. Logistic regression models for 2 × 2 contingency tables

Consider the logistic regression model

$$\text{logit}[\text{E}[d_i \mid x_i]/m_i] = \alpha + \beta x_i : i = 0, 1, \tag{4.31}$$

where $x_0 = 0$, $x_1 = 1$, and $\text{E}[d_i \mid x_i]/m_i = \pi_i$ is the probability of being a heavy drinker for controls ($i = 0$) or cases ($i = 1$). Then (4.31) can be rewritten as

$$\text{logit}[\pi_i] = \log[\pi_i/(1 - \pi_i)] = \alpha + \beta x_i. \tag{4.32}$$

Hence,

$$\log[\pi_1/(1 - \pi_1)] = \alpha + \beta x_1 = \alpha + \beta \text{ and} \tag{4.33}$$

$$\log[\pi_0/(1 - \pi_0)] = \alpha + \beta x_0 = \alpha.$$

Subtracting these two equations from each other gives

$$\log[\pi_1/(1 - \pi_1)] - \log[\pi_0/(1 - \pi_0)] = \beta, \text{ and hence}$$

$$\log\left[\frac{\pi_1/(1 - \pi_1)}{\pi_0/(1 - \pi_0)}\right] = \log(\psi) = \beta. \tag{4.34}$$

Thus, the true odds ratio $\psi$ equals $e^{\beta}$. We will use logistic regression to derive an estimate $\hat{\beta}$ of $\beta$. We then can estimate the odds ratio by $\hat{\psi} = e^{\hat{\beta}}$.

In the esophageal cancer and alcohol study $\hat{\beta} = 1.730$ and $\hat{\psi} = e^{1.730} = 5.64$. This is identical to the classical odds ratio estimate obtained in Section 4.19.2. The reader may wonder why we would go to the trouble of calculating $\hat{\psi}$ with logistic regression when the simple classical estimate gives the same answer. The answer is that we will be able to generalize logistic regression to adjust for multiple covariates; classical methods are much more limited in their ability to adjust for confounding variables or effect modifiers.

### 4.20.1. Nuisance parameters

In Equation (4.31) $\alpha$ is called a **nuisance parameter**. This is one that is required by the model but is not used to calculate interesting statistics.

### 4.20.2. 95% confidence interval for the odds ratio: logistic regression

Logistic regression also provides an estimate of the standard error of $\hat{\beta}$. We use this estimate to approximate the 95% confidence interval for the odds ratio in exactly the same way as for Woolf's confidence interval. That is,

$$(\hat{\psi}_L, \hat{\psi}_U) = (\exp[\hat{\beta} - 1.96 s_{\hat{\beta}}],\ \exp[\hat{\beta} + 1.96 s_{\hat{\beta}}]). \tag{4.35}$$

## 4.21. Creating a Stata data file

Up until now we have used previously created data sets in our Stata examples. We next wish to analyze the data in Table 4.2. As this is a very small table, it provides a good opportunity to explain how to create a new Stata data set. We do this in the following example.

```
. *   4.21.EsophagealCa.log
. *
. *   Create a Stata data set from the Ille-et-Vilaine data on esophageal
. *   cancer and alcohol given in Table 4.2.
. *
. edit                                                              1

. list                                                              2

     +------------------------+
     |  var1   var2   var3    |
     |------------------------|
  1. |     0      0    666    |
  2. |     1      0    104    |
  3. |     0      1    109    |
  4. |     1      1     96    |
     +------------------------+

. rename var1 cancer                                                3

. rename var2 alcohol

. rename var3 patients

. label define yesno 0 "No" 1 "Yes"                                 4

. label values cancer yesno                                         5

. label define dose 0 "< 80 g" 1 ">= 80 g"

. label values alcohol dose

. list                                                              6
```

```
     +-----------------------------+
     | cancer   alcohol   patients |
     |-----------------------------|
  1. |     No    < 80 g        666 |
  2. |    Yes    < 80 g        104 |
  3. |     No   >= 80 g        109 |
  4. |    Yes   >= 80 g         96 |
     +-----------------------------+
```

```
. save c:\wddtext\4.21.EsophagealCa.dta, replace
```
7

```
file c:\wddtext\4.21.EsophagealCa.dta saved

. log close
```

## Comments

1 Open the Data Editor window. Enter three columns of values as shown in Figure 4.8. Then, exit the edit window by clicking the "×" in the upper right-hand corner of the window. This creates three variables with the default names *var1*, *var2*, and *var3*. There are four observations corresponding to the four cells in Table 4.2. The variable *var1* classifies the study subjects as either controls (*var1* = 0) or cases (*var1* = 1). Similarly, *var2* classifies subjects as either moderate (*var2* = 0) or heavy (*var2* = 1)

Data Editor

Preserve | Restore | Sort | << | >> | Hide | Delete...

var3[5] =

| | var1 | var2 | var3 |
|---|---|---|---|
| 1 | 0 | 0 | 666 |
| 2 | 1 | 0 | 104 |
| 3 | 0 | 1 | 109 |
| 4 | 1 | 1 | 96 |

Figure 4.8 This figure shows the Data Editor window after the data from Table 4.2 have been entered by hand.

drinkers. The variable *var3* gives the number of subjects in each of the four possible disease–exposure groups.

If you double-click on any of the column headings *var1*, *var2*, or *var3* a dialog box will open that will permit you to redefine the variable's name, variable label, or value labels. This can also be done by typing commands in the Command window or by point-and-click commands as is illustrated below.

2 This *list* command shows the values that we have just entered. Without arguments, this command shows all observations on all variables.

3 This *rename* command changes the name of the first variable from *var1* to *cancer*. The equivalent point-and-click command is Data ▶ Variable utilities ▶ Rename variable ⌜ Existing variable name: *var1* , New variable name: *cancer* Submit.

4 The *cancer* variable takes the values 0 for controls and 1 for cases. It is often useful to associate labels with the numeric values of such classification variables. To do this we first define a value label called *yesno* that links 0 with "No" and 1 with "Yes". To create this value label with the pull-down menus, open the Define value labels dialogue box by clicking Data ▶ Labels ▶ Label values ▶ Define or modify value labels. Click Define... to open the Define new label dialogue box. Enter *yesno* in the Label name field and click OK. The Add value dialogue box will appear. Add *0* and *No* to the Value and Text fields, respectively. Click OK. Assign *1* the label *Yes* in the same way. Click the × in the upper right corner of the Add value dialogue box and then click Close on the Define value labels box.

5 We then use the *label values* command to link the variable *cancer* with the values label *yesno*. Multiple variables can be assigned to the same values label. The equivalent point-and-click command is Data ▶ Labels ▶ Label values ▶ Assign value labels to variable ⌜ Variable: *cancer* , Value label: *yesno* Submit.

6 The *list* command now gives the value labels of the *cancer* and *alcohol* variables instead of their numeric values. The numeric values are still available for use in analysis commands.

7 This save command saves the data set that we have created in the *C:\WDDtext* folder with the name *4.21.EsophagealCa.dta.* If a file with the same name already exists in this folder, the *replace* option will replace the old file with the new version. A standard icon for saving data files is also available on the icon bar of the main Stata window that may be used for saving your data file.

## 4.22. Analyzing case–control data with Stata

The Ille-et-Vilaine data set introduced in Section 4.19 may be analyzed as follows.

```
. * 4.22.EsophagealCa.log
. *
. * Logistic regression analysis of 2x2 case-control data from
. * the Ille-et-Vilaine study of esophageal cancer and alcohol.
. *
. use C:\WDDtext\4.21.EsophagealCa.dta, clear

. cc cancer alcohol [freq=patients], woolf                              1

                 |   alcohol                |             Proportion
                 |   Exposed   Unexposed    |      Total     Exposed
-----------------+--------------------------+----------------------
           Cases |        96         104    |        200      0.4800
        Controls |       109         666    |        775      0.1406
-----------------+--------------------------+----------------------
           Total |       205         770    |        975      0.2103
                 |                          |
                 |      Point estimate      |    [95% Conf. Interval]
                 |--------------------------+----------------------
      Odds ratio |         5.640085         |   4.000589    7.951467  (Woolf)     2
 Attr. frac. ex. |         .8226977         |   .7500368    .8742371  (Woolf)
 Attr. frac. pop |         .3948949         |
                 +-------------------------------------------------
                               chi2(1) =   110.26  Pr>chi2 = 0.0000               3

. logistic alcohol cancer [freq=patients]                                         4

Logistic regression                          Number of obs    =        975
                                             LR chi2(1)       =      96.43
                                             Prob > chi2      =     0.0000
Log likelihood =  -453.2224                  Pseudo R2        =     0.0962

------------------------------------------------------------------------------
     alcohol | Odds Ratio   Std. Err.      z    P>|z|     [95% Conf. Interval]
-------------+----------------------------------------------------------------
      cancer |   5.640085   .9883491    9.87   0.000     4.000589    7.951467      5
------------------------------------------------------------------------------

. log close
```

**Comments**

1 This *cc* command performs a classical case-control analysis of the data in the $2 \times 2$ table defined by *cancer* and *alcohol*. The command qualifier [*freq* = *patients*] gives the number of patients who have the specified values of *cancer* and *alcohol*. The *woolf* option specifies that the 95% confidence interval for the odds ratio is to be calculated using Woolf's method. The equivalent point-and-click command is Statistics ▶ Epidemiology and related ▶ Tables for epidemiologists ▶ Case-control odds ratio [Main] Case variable: *cancer* , Exposed variable: *alcohol* [Weights] ⦿ Frequency weights , Frequency weight: *patients* [Options] ⦿ Woolf approximation [Submit].

An alternative way of performing the same analysis would have been to create a data set with one record per patient. This would have given

666 records with *cancer* = 0 and *alcohol* = 0,
104 records with *cancer* = 1 and *alcohol* = 0,
109 records with *cancer* = 0 and *alcohol* = 1, and
096 records with *cancer* = 1 and *alcohol* = 1.

Then the command

```
cc cancer alcohol, woolf
```

would have given exactly the same results as those shown above.

2 The estimated odds ratio is $\hat{\psi} = 5.64$. Woolf's 95% confidence interval for $\hat{\psi}$ is (4.00, 7.95). These statistics agree with our hand calculations in Sections 4.19.2 and 4.19.3.

3 The test of the null hypothesis that $\psi = 1$ gives an uncorrected $\chi^2$ statistic of 110.26. The *P*-value associated with this statistic is (much) less than 0.000 05.

4 Regress *alcohol* against *cancer* using logistic regression. This command fits Equation (4.31) to the data. We would also have got the same result if we had regressed *cancer* against *alcohol*. The point-and-click version of this command is similar to that given on page 176 except that *patients* is defined as a frequency weight in the same way as in the first comment given above.

5 The estimate of the odds ratio and its 95% confidence interval are identical to those obtained from the classical analysis. Recall that the logistic command outputs $\hat{\psi} = \exp[\hat{\beta}]$ rather than the parameter estimate $\hat{\beta}$ itself.

## 4.23. Regressing disease against exposure

The simplest explanation of simple logistic regression is the one given above. Unfortunately, it does not generalize to multiple logistic regression where we are considering several risk factors at once. To make the next chapter easier to understand, let us return to simple logistic regression one more time.

Suppose we have a population who either are or are not exposed to some risk factor. Let $\pi'_j$ denote the true probability of disease in exposed ($j = 1$) and unexposed ($j = 0$) people. We conduct a case–control study in which we select a representative sample of diseased (case) and healthy (control) subjects from the target population. That is, the selection is done in such a way that the probability that an individual is selected is unaffected by her exposure status. Let

$n_j$ be the number of study subjects who are ($j = 1$) or are not ($j = 0$) exposed,
$d_j$ be the number of cases who are ($j = 1$) or are not ($j = 0$) exposed,
$x_j = j$ denote exposure status, and
$\pi_j$ be the probability that a study subject is a case given that she is ($j = 1$) or is not ($j = 0$) exposed.

Consider the logistic regression model

$$\text{logit}[\text{E}[d_j \mid x_j]/n_j] = \alpha + \beta x_j \quad : j = 0, 1. \tag{4.36}$$

This is a legitimate logistic regression model with $\text{E}[d_j \mid x_j]/n_j = \pi_j$. It can be shown, however, that Equation (4.36) can be rewritten as

$$\text{logit}[\pi'_j] = \alpha' + \beta x_j \quad : j = 0, 1, \tag{4.37}$$

where $\alpha'$ is a different constant. But, by exactly the same argument that we used to derived Equation (4.34) from Equation (4.31), we can deduce from Equation (4.37) that

$$\log\left[\frac{\pi'_1/(1-\pi'_1)}{\pi'_0/(1-\pi'_0)}\right] = \log(\psi) = \beta. \tag{4.38}$$

Hence, $\beta$ also equals the log odds ratio for disease in exposed vs. unexposed members of the target population, and $\hat{\beta}$ from Equation (4.36) estimates this log odds ratio. Thus, in building logistic regression models it makes sense to regress disease against exposure even though we have no estimate of the probability of disease in the underlying population.

In the next chapter we will not always distinguish between terms like $\pi_j$ and $\pi'_j$. It is less awkward to talk about the probability of developing cancer given a set of covariates than to talk about the probability that a study subject with given covariates is also a case. This lack of precision is harmless as long as you remember that in a case–control study we cannot estimate the probability of disease given a patient's exposure status. Moreover, when estimates of $\pi_j$ are used in formulas for odds ratios, they provide valid odds ratio estimates for the underlying population.

## 4.24. Additional reading

McCullagh and Nelder (1989) is a standard, if rather mathematical, reference on Generalized Linear Models.

Breslow and Day (1980) is somewhat easier to read, although it is targeted at an audience with a solid statistical background. They provide an informative contrast between classical methods for case–control studies and logistic regression. This text also has an excellent and extensive discussion of the Ille-et-Vilaine data set that may be read in conjunction with the discussion in this and the next chapter. They provide the complete Ille-et-Vilaine data set in an appendix.

Dobson (2001) is a more recent text on this topic. It is an intermediate level text that is intended for students of statistics.

Fleiss et al. (2003) provides a useful discussion of the analysis of rates and proportions.

Katz (2006) and

Hennekens and Buring (1987) provide good introductions to case–control studies.

Rothman and Greenland (1998) is a more advanced epidemiology text with a worthwhile discussion of case–control studies. This text also has a good discussion of likelihood ratio tests, score tests, and Wald tests.

Clayton and Hills (1993) provide an excellent discussion of the difference between likelihood ratio, score, and Wald tests that includes some helpful graphs.

Wald (1943) is the original reference on Wald tests and confidence intervals.

Yates (1934) is the original reference on the continuity correction for the chi-squared statistic for 2 × 2 tables.

Dupont and Plummer (1999) provide a brief review of the controversy surrounding continuity corrections in the statistical literature. They also provide a Stata program that calculates Yates' corrected chi-squared statistic for 2 × 2 tables.

Tuyns et al. (1977) studied the effect of alcohol and tobacco on the risk of esophageal cancer among men from the Ille-et-Vilaine district of France. We used their data to illustrate classical methods of analyzing case–control studies as well as logistic regression.

## 4.25. Exercises

The following questions relate to the *4.ex.Sepsis.dta* data set from my web site, which you should download onto your computer. This data set contains information on patients from the Ibuprofen in Sepsis Study. Variables in this file include:

$$
\begin{aligned}
&id &&= \text{patient identification number,}\\
&apache &&= \text{baseline APACHE score,}\\
&treat &&= \begin{cases} 0\text{: if patient received placebo} \\ 1\text{: if patient received ibuprofen} \end{cases}\\
&death30d &&= \begin{cases} 0\text{: if patient was alive 30 days after entry into the study} \\ 1\text{: if patient was dead 30 days after entry,} \end{cases}\\
&race &&= \begin{cases} 0\text{: if patient is white} \\ 1\text{: if patient is black.} \end{cases}
\end{aligned}
$$

1 Use logistic regression to estimate the probability of death in treated black patients as a function of baseline APACHE score. Do a similar regression for black patients on placebo. Plot these two curves on a single graph. How would you interpret these curves?

2 What is the odds ratio associated with a unit rise in APACHE score in untreated black patients? Give a 95% confidence interval for this odds ratio.

3 What is the estimated expected mortality for a black control patient with a baseline APACHE score of 10? Give the 95% confidence interval for this expected mortality. How many black control patients had a baseline APACHE score of 15 or less? What proportion of these patients died? Give a 95% confidence interval for this proportion.

4 Have you had an introductory course in probability? If so, prove that Equations (4.24) and (4.25) define an exact confidence interval for a proportion.

## 4.25. Exercises

5

# Multiple logistic regression

Simple logistic regression generalizes to multiple logistic regression in the same way that simple linear regression generalizes to multiple linear regression. We regress a dichotomous response variable, such as survival, against several covariates. This allows us to either adjust for confounding variables or account for covariates that have a synergistic effect on the response variable. We can add interaction terms to our model in exactly the same way as in linear regression.

Before discussing multiple logistic regression we will first describe a traditional method for adjusting an odds ratio estimate for a confounding variable.

## 5.1. Mantel–Haenszel estimate of an age-adjusted odds ratio

In Section 4.19.1 we introduced the Ille-et-Vilaine study of esophageal cancer and alcohol (Breslow and Day, 1980). Table 5.1 shows these data stratified by ten-year age groups. It is clear from this table that the incidence of esophageal cancer increases dramatically with age. There is also some evidence that the prevalence of heavy drinking also increases with age; the prevalence of heavy drinking among controls increases from 7.8% for men aged 25–30 to 17.3% for men aged 45–54. Thus, age may confound the alcohol–cancer relationship, and it makes sense to calculate an age-adjusted odds ratio for the effect of heavy drinking on esophageal cancer. Mantel and Haenszel (1959) proposed the following method for adjusting an odds ratio in the presence of a confounding variable.

Suppose that study subjects are subdivided into a number of strata by a confounding variable. Let

$c_{ij}$ = the number of controls in the $j^{\text{th}}$ stratum who are ($i = 1$) or are not ($i = 0$) exposed (i.e. who are, or are not, heavy drinkers),

$d_{ij}$ = the number of cases in the $j^{\text{th}}$ stratum who are ($i = 1$), or are not ($i = 0$), exposed,

$m_{0j} = c_{0j} + c_{1j}$ = the number of controls in the $j^{\text{th}}$ stratum,

**Table 5.1.** Ille-et-Vilaine data on alcohol consumption and esophageal cancer stratified by age (Breslow and Day, 1980)

| | | Daily alcohol consumption | | | | Odds ratio |
|---|---|---|---|---|---|---|
| Age | Cancer | ≥80 g | <80 g | Total | % ≥80 g | $\hat{\psi}_j$ |
| 25–34 | Yes | 1 | 0 | 1 | 100 | |
| | No | 9 | 106 | 115 | 7.83 | |
| | Total | 10 | 106 | 116 | 8.62 | |
| 35–44 | Yes | 4 | 5 | 9 | 44.4 | 5.05 |
| | No | 26 | 164 | 190 | 13.7 | |
| | Total | 30 | 169 | 199 | 15.1 | |
| 45–54 | Yes | 25 | 21 | 46 | 54.4 | 5.67 |
| | No | 29 | 138 | 167 | 17.4 | |
| | Total | 54 | 159 | 213 | 25.4 | |
| 55–64 | Yes | 42 | 34 | 76 | 55.3 | 6.36 |
| | No | 27 | 139 | 166 | 16.3 | |
| | Total | 69 | 173 | 242 | 28.5 | |
| 65–74 | Yes | 19 | 36 | 55 | 34.6 | 2.58 |
| | No | 18 | 88 | 106 | 17.0 | |
| | Total | 37 | 124 | 161 | 23.0 | |
| ≥75 | Yes | 5 | 8 | 13 | 38.5 | . |
| | No | 0 | 31 | 31 | 0.00 | |
| | Total | 5 | 39 | 44 | 11.4 | |
| All ages | Yes | 96 | 104 | 200 | 48.0 | 5.64 |
| | No | 109 | 666 | 775 | 14.1 | |
| | Total | 205 | 770 | 975 | 21.0 | |

$m_{1j} = d_{0j} + d_{1j}$ = the number of cases in the $j^{\text{th}}$ stratum,
$n_{ij} = d_{ij} + c_{ij}$ = the number of subjects in the $j^{\text{th}}$ stratum who are ($i = 1$) or are not ($i = 0$) exposed,
$N_j = n_{0j} + n_{1j} = m_{0j} + m_{1j}$ = the number of subjects in the $j^{\text{th}}$ stratum,
$\hat{\psi}_j$ = the estimated odds ratio for members of the $j^{\text{th}}$ stratum,
$w_j = d_{0j}c_{1j}/N_j$, and
$W = \sum w_j$.

Then the Mantel–Haenszel estimate of the common odds ratio within these strata is

$$\hat{\psi}_{\text{mh}} = \sum \left(d_{1j}c_{0j}/N_j\right) / W. \tag{5.1}$$

If $\hat{\psi}_j$ is estimable for all strata, then Equation (5.1) can be rewritten

$$\hat{\psi}_{\mathrm{mh}} = \sum \hat{\psi}_j w_j / W. \tag{5.2}$$

This implies that $\hat{\psi}_{\mathrm{mh}}$ is a weighted average of the odds-ratio estimates within each stratum. The weight $w_j$ is approximately equal to the inverse of the variance of $\hat{\psi}_j$ when $\psi$ is near one. Thus, Equation (5.2) gives the greatest weight to those odds-ratio estimates that are estimated with the greatest precision.

In the Ille-et-Vilaine data given in Table 5.1 there are six age strata. We apply Equation (5.1) to these data to calculate the age-adjusted odds ratio for esophageal cancer in heavy drinkers compared with moderate drinkers. For example, in Stratum 2 we have $w_2 = d_{02}c_{12}/N_2 = 5 \times 26/199 = 0.653$ and $d_{12}c_{02}/N_2 = 4 \times 164/199 = 3.296$. Performing similar calculations for the other strata and summing gives the $W = 11.331$ and $\hat{\psi}_{\mathrm{mh}} = 5.158$. The unadjusted odds ratio for this table is 5.640 (see Section 4.19.2). Thus there is a suggestion that age may have a mild confounding effect on this odds ratio.

## 5.2. Mantel–Haenszel $\chi^2$ statistic for multiple 2 × 2 tables

Under the null hypothesis that the common odds ratio $\psi = 1$, the expected value of $d_{1j}$ is

$$\mathrm{E}[d_{1j} \mid \psi = 1] = n_{1j} m_{1j} / N_j \tag{5.3}$$

and the variance of $d_{1j}$ is

$$\mathrm{var}[d_{1j} \mid \psi = 1] = \frac{m_{0j} m_{1j} n_{0j} n_{1j}}{N_j^2 (N_j - 1)}. \tag{5.4}$$

The Mantel–Haenszel test statistic for this null hypothesis is

$$\chi_1^2 = \left( \left| \sum d_{1j} - \sum \mathrm{E}[d_{1j} \mid \psi = 1] \right| - 0.5 \right)^2 \Big/ \sum \mathrm{var}[d_{1j} \mid \psi = 1], \tag{5.5}$$

which has a $\chi^2$ distribution with one degree of freedom (Mantel and Haenszel, 1959). In the Ille-et-Vilaine study $\sum d_{1j} = 96$, $\sum \mathrm{E}[d_{1j} \mid \psi = 1] = 48.891$ and $\sum \mathrm{var}[d_{1j} \mid \psi = 1] = 26.106$. Therefore $\chi_1^2 = (|96 - 48.891| - 0.5)^2/(26.106) = 83.21$. The $P$-value associated with this statistic is $<10^{19}$, providing overwhelming evidence that the observed association between heavy drinking and esophageal cancer is not due to chance.

In Equation (5.5), the constant 0.5 that is subtracted from the numerator is a continuity correction that adjusts for the fact that we are approximating a discrete distribution with a continuous normal distribution (see Section 4.19.4). Without the continuity correction the $\chi^2$ statistic equals 85.01.

## 5.3. 95% confidence interval for the age-adjusted odds ratio

$$\begin{aligned}\text{Let}\quad P_j &= (d_{1j} + c_{0j})/N_j,\\ Q_j &= (c_{1j} + d_{0j})/N_j,\\ R_j &= d_{1j}c_{0j}/N_j, \text{ and}\\ S_j &= c_{1j}d_{0j}/N_j.\end{aligned}$$

Then Robins et al. (1986) estimated the standard error of the log of $\hat{\psi}_{\text{mh}}$ to be

$$\text{se}[\log \hat{\psi}_{\text{mh}}] = \sqrt{\frac{\sum P_j R_j}{2(\sum R_j)^2} + \frac{\sum (P_j S_j + Q_j R_j)}{2\sum R_j \sum S_j} + \frac{\sum Q_j S_j}{2(\sum S_j)^2}}. \tag{5.6}$$

Hence, a 95% confidence interval for the common within-stratum odds ratio $\psi$ is

$$(\hat{\psi}_{\text{mh}} \exp[-1.96\, \text{se}[\log \hat{\psi}_{\text{mh}}]],\ \hat{\psi}_{\text{mh}} \exp[1.96\, \text{se}[\log \hat{\psi}_{\text{mh}}]]). \tag{5.7}$$

In the Ille-et-Vilaine study,

$$\sum R_j = 58.439, \sum S_j = 11.331, \sum P_j R_j = 43.848,$$

$$\sum (P_j S_j + Q_j R_j) = 22.843, \sum Q_j S_j = 3.079, \text{ and } \hat{\psi}_{\text{mh}} = 5.158.$$

Therefore,

$$\begin{aligned}\text{se}(\log \hat{\psi}_{\text{mh}}) &= \sqrt{\frac{43.848}{2\,(58.439)^2} + \frac{22.843}{2 \times 58.439 \times 11.331} + \frac{3.079}{2\,(11.331)^2}}\\ &= 0.189,\end{aligned}$$

and a 95% confidence interval for the age-adjusted odds ratio $\psi$ is $(5.158 \exp[-1.96 \times 0.189], 5.158 \exp[1.96 \times 0.189]) = (3.56, 7.47)$.

## 5.4. Breslow–Day–Tarone test for homogeneity

The derivation of the Mantel–Haenszel odds ratio assumes that there is a single true odds ratio for subjects from each stratum. Breslow and Day

**Table 5.2.** Observed and fitted values for the fifth stratum of the Ille-et-Vilaine data set. The fitted values are chosen so that the resulting odds ratio equals $\hat{\psi}_{mh} = 5.158$, and the total numbers of cases and controls and heavy and moderate drinkers equal the observed totals for this stratum. These calculations are needed for the Breslow–Day–Tarone test for homogeneity of the common odds ratio (Breslow and Day, 1980)

| Esophageal cancer | Daily alcohol consumption ≥80 g | Daily alcohol consumption <80 g | Total |
|---|---|---|---|
| *Observed values* | | | |
| Yes | $d_{15} = 19$ | $d_{05} = 36$ | $m_{15} = 55$ |
| No | $c_{15} = 18$ | $c_{05} = 88$ | $m_{05} = 106$ |
| Total | $n_{15} = 37$ | $n_{05} = 124$ | $N_5 = 161$ |
| *Fitted values* | | | |
| Yes | $d_{15}[\hat{\psi}_{mh}] = 23.557$ | $d_{05}[\hat{\psi}_{mh}] = 31.443$ | $m_{15} = 55$ |
| No | $c_{15}[\hat{\psi}_{mh}] = 13.443$ | $c_{05}[\hat{\psi}_{mh}] = 92.557$ | $m_{05} = 106$ |
| Total | $n_{15} = 37$ | $n_{05} = 124$ | $N_5 = 161$ |

(1980) proposed the following test of this assumption. First, we find fitted values $c_{ij}[\hat{\psi}_{mh}]$ and $d_{ij}[\hat{\psi}_{mh}]$ for the $j^{\text{th}}$ stratum that give $\hat{\psi}_{mh}$ as the within-stratum odds ratio and which add up to the actual number of cases and controls and exposed and unexposed subjects for this stratum. For example, the top and bottom halves of Table 5.2 show the actual and fitted values for the fifth age stratum from the Ille-et-Vilaine study. Note that the fitted values have been chosen so that $(d_{15}[\hat{\psi}_{mh}]/d_{05}[\hat{\psi}_{mh}])/(c_{15}[\hat{\psi}_{mh}]/c_{05}[\hat{\psi}_{mh}]) = (23.557/31.443)/(13.443/92.557) = \hat{\psi}_{mh} = 5.158$ and the column and row totals for the fitted and observed values are identical. The fitted value $d_{1j}[\hat{\psi}_{mh}]$ is obtained by solving for $x$ in the equation

$$\hat{\psi}_{mh} = \frac{(x/(m_{1j} - x))}{(n_{1j} - x)/(n_{0j} - m_{1j} + x)}. \tag{5.8}$$

We then set

$$c_{1j}[\hat{\psi}_{mh}] = n_{1j} - x,\ d_{0j}[\hat{\psi}_{mh}] = m_{1j} - x, \text{ and } c_{0j}[\hat{\psi}_{mh}] = n_{0j} - m_{1j} + x.$$

There is a unique solution to Equation (5.8) for which $c_{ij}[\hat{\psi}_{mh}]$ and $d_{ij}[\hat{\psi}_{mh}]$ are non-negative.

The variance of $d_{1j}$ given $\psi = \hat{\psi}_{\text{mh}}$ is

$$\text{var}[d_{1j} \mid \hat{\psi}_{\text{mh}}] = \left( \frac{1}{c_{0j}[\hat{\psi}_{\text{mh}}]} + \frac{1}{d_{0j}[\hat{\psi}_{\text{mh}}]} + \frac{1}{c_{1j}[\hat{\psi}_{\text{mh}}]} + \frac{1}{d_{1j}[\hat{\psi}_{\text{mh}}]} \right)^{-1}. \tag{5.9}$$

For example, in the fifth stratum

$$\begin{aligned}\text{var}[d_{15} \mid \hat{\psi}_{\text{mh}} = 5.158] &= \left( \frac{1}{92.557} + \frac{1}{31.443} + \frac{1}{13.443} + \frac{1}{23.557} \right)^{-1} \\ &= 6.272.\end{aligned}$$

Let $J$ be the number of strata. Then if the null hypothesis that $\psi_j = \psi$ for all strata is true, and the total study size is large relative to the number of strata,

$$\chi^2_{\text{BD}} = \sum_j \frac{(d_{1j} - d_{1j}[\hat{\psi}_{\text{mh}}])^2}{\text{var}[d_{1j} \mid \hat{\psi}_{\text{mh}}]}$$

has an approximately $\chi^2$ distribution with $J - 1$ degrees of freedom. This equation is the Breslow and Day $\chi^2$ test of homogeneity. Tarone (1985) showed that the asymptotic properties of this test could be improved by subtracting a correction factor giving

$$\chi^2_{J-1} = \chi^2_{\text{BD}} - \frac{(\sum_j d_{1j} - \sum_j d_{1j}[\hat{\psi}_{\text{mh}}])^2}{\sum_j \text{var}[d_{1j} \mid \hat{\psi}_{\text{mh}}]}. \tag{5.10}$$

This sum is performed over all strata. We reject the null hypothesis when $\chi^2_{J-1}$ is too large. For example, in the Ille-et-Vilaine study $\chi^2_{\text{BD}} = 9.32$. Subtracting the correction factor in Equation (5.10) gives $\chi^2_5 = 9.30$. As there are six strata, $J = 5$. The probability that a $\chi^2$ statistic with five degrees of freedom exceeds 9.3 is $P = 0.098$. Hence, although we cannot reject the null hypothesis of equal odds ratios across these strata, there is some evidence to suggest that the odds ratio may vary with age. In Table 5.1 these odds ratios are fairly similar for all strata except for age 65–74, where the odds ratio drops to 2.6. This may be due to chance, or perhaps, to a hardy survivor effect. You must use your judgment in deciding whether it is reasonable to report a single-age adjusted odds ratio in your own work.

## 5.5. Calculating the Mantel–Haenszel odds ratio using Stata

The *5.5.EsophagealCa.dta* data file contains the complete Ille-et-Vilaine data set published by Breslow and Day (1980). The following log file and comments illustrate how to use Stata to perform the calculations given above.

```
. *  5.5.EsophagealCa.log
. *
. *  Calculate the Mantel-Haenszel age-adjusted odds ratio from
. *  the Ille-et-Vilaine study of esophageal cancer and alcohol.
. *
. use C:\WDDtext\5.5.EsophagealCa.dta, clear

. table  cancer heavy [freq=patients]                                    1

-------------------------------
           |   Heavy Alcohol
Esophagea  |    Consumption
l Cancer   |   < 80 g   >= 80 g
-----------+-------------------
        No |     666       109
       Yes |     104        96
-------------------------------

. table  cancer heavy [freq=patients], by(age)                           2

-------------------------------
Age        |
(years)    |
and        |   Heavy Alcohol
Esophagea  |    Consumption
l Cancer   |   < 80 g   >= 80 g
-----------+-------------------
25-34      |
        No |     106         9
       Yes |                 1
-----------+-------------------
35-44      |
        No |     164        26
       Yes |       5         4
-----------+-------------------
45-54      |
        No |     138        29
       Yes |      21        25
-----------+-------------------
55-64      |
        No |     139        27
       Yes |      34        42
```

```
           |
-----------+-----------------
65-74      |
        No |        88     18
       Yes |        36     19
-----------+-----------------
>= 75      |
        No |        31
       Yes |         8      5
-----------------------------

. cc heavy cancer [freq=patients], by(age)                                  3

   Age (years) |       OR      [95% Conf. Interval]   M-H Weight
---------------+---------------------------------------------------
         25-34 |         .            0          .           0 (exact)
         35-44 |  5.046154     .9268668   24.86537    .6532663 (exact)
         45-54 |  5.665025     2.632894   12.16535    2.859155 (exact)
         55-64 |  6.359477     3.299319   12.28473    3.793388 (exact)
         65-74 |  2.580247     1.131489   5.857258    4.024845 (exact)
         >= 75 |         .     4.388738          .           0 (exact)
---------------+---------------------------------------------------
         Crude |  5.640085     3.937435   8.061794                 (exact)  4
  M-H combined |  5.157623     3.562131   7.467743                          5
---------------+---------------------------------------------------
Test of homogeneity (Tarone)   chi2(5) =     9.30  Pr>chi2 = 0.0977         6

                    Test that combined OR = 1:
                                 Mantel-Haenszel chi2(1) =     85.01        7
                                                 Pr>chi2 =    0.0000

. log close
```

**Comments**

1 This *table* command gives a cross tabulation of values of *heavy* by values of *cancer*. The *5.5.EsophagealCa.dta* data set contains one record (row) for each unique combination of the covariate values. The *patients* variable indicates the number of subjects in the study with these values. The [*freq* = *patients*] command qualifier tells Stata the number of subjects represented by each record. The variable *heavy* takes the numeric values 0 and 1, which denote daily alcohol consumption of <80 g and ≥80 g, respectively. The table shows the value labels that have been assigned to this variable rather than its underlying numeric values. Similarly, *cancer*

takes the numeric values 0 and 1, which have been assigned the value labels *No* and *Yes*, respectively. The equivalent point-and-click command is Statistics ▶ Summaries, tables, & tests ▶ Tables ▶ Table of summary statistics (table) ⌋ Main ⌊ Row variable: *cancer* ⌜ [✓] Column variable: — *heavy* ⌋ ⌋ Weights ⌊ ⦿ Frequency weights , Frequency weight: *patients* [Submit].

2 The *by*(*age*) option of the *table* command produces a separate table of *cancer* by *heavy* for each distinct value of *age*. The *age* variable takes a different value for each stratum in the study, producing six subtables. The point-and-click command is the same as that given above except that on the *Main* tab we also enter [✓] Superrow variables: *age*.

3 The *by*(*age*) option of the *cc* command causes odds ratios to be calculated for each age stratum. No estimate is given for the youngest stratum because there were no moderate drinking cases. This results in division by zero when calculating the odds ratio. Similarly, no estimate is given for the oldest stratum because there were no heavy drinking controls. The equivalent point-and-click command is Statistics ▶ Epidemiology and related ▶ Tables for epidemiologists ▶ Case-control odds ratio ⌋ Main ⌊ Case variable: *cancer*, Exposed variable: *heavy* ⌋ Weights ⌊ ⦿ Frequency weights , Frequency weight: *patients* ⌋ Options ⌊ [✓] Stratify on variable: *age* [Submit].

4 The crude odds ratio is 5.640, which we derived in the last chapter. This odds ratio is obtained by ignoring the age strata. The exact 95% confidence interval consists of all values of the odds ratio that cannot be rejected at the $\alpha = 0.05$ level of statistical significance (see Section 1.4.7). The derivation of this interval uses a rather complex iterative formula (Dupont and Plummer, 1999).

5 The Mantel–Haenszel estimate of the common odds ratio within all age strata is 5.158. This is slightly lower than the crude estimate, and is consistent with a mild confounding of age and drinking habits on the risk of esophageal cancer (see Section 5.1). Stata uses the method of Robins et al. (1986) to estimate the 95% confidence interval for this common odds ratio, which is (3.56, 7.47).

6 Tarone's test of homogeneity equals 9.30. This $\chi^2$ statistic has five degrees of freedom giving a $P$-value of 0.098.

7 We test the null hypothesis that the age-adjusted odds ratio equals 1. The Mantel–Haenszel test of this hypothesis equals 85.01. Stata calculates this statistic without the continuity correction. The associated $P$-value is less than 0.000 05.

## 5.6. Multiple logistic regression model

The Mantel–Haenszel method works well when we have a single confounding variable that can be used to create fairly large strata. For a more general approach to modeling dichotomous response data we will need to use logistic regression.

Suppose that we observe an unbiased sample of $n$ patients from some target population. Let

$$d_i = \begin{cases} 1: \text{if the } i^{\text{th}} \text{ patient suffers event of interest} \\ 0: \text{otherwise,} \end{cases}$$

and $x_{i1}, x_{i2}, \ldots, x_{iq}$ be $q$ covariates that are measured on the $i^{\text{th}}$ patient. Let $\mathbf{x}_i = (x_{i1}, x_{i2}, \ldots, x_{iq})$ denote the values of all of the covariates for the $i^{\text{th}}$ patient. Then the multiple logistic regression model assumes that $d_i$ has a Bernoulli distribution, and

$$\text{logit}[\text{E}\,[d_i \mid \mathbf{x}_i]] = \alpha + \beta_1 x_{i1} + \beta_2 x_{i2} + \cdots + \beta_q x_{iq}, \tag{5.11}$$

where $\alpha$, $\beta_1$, $\beta_2$, ... , and $\beta_q$ are unknown parameters.

The probability that $d_i = 1$ given the covariates $\mathbf{x}_i$ is denoted $\pi[x_{i1}, x_{i2}, \ldots, x_{iq}] = \pi[\mathbf{x}_i]$ and equals $\text{E}[d_i \mid \mathbf{x}_i]$. The only difference between simple and multiple logistic regression is that the linear predictor is now $\alpha + \beta_1 x_{i1} + \beta_2 x_{i2} + \cdots + \beta_q x_{iq}$. As in simple logistic regression, the model has a logit link function and a Bernoulli random component.

The data may also be organized as one record per unique combination of covariate values. Suppose that there are $n_j$ patients with identical covariate values $x_{j1}, x_{j2}, \ldots, x_{jq}$ and that $d_j$ of these patients suffer the event of interest. Then the logistic regression Model (5.11) can be rewritten

$$\text{logit}[\text{E}[d_j \mid \mathbf{x}_j]/n_j] = \alpha + \beta_1 x_{j1} + \beta_2 x_{j2} + \cdots + \beta_q x_{jq}. \tag{5.12}$$

(In Equation (5.12) there is a different value of $j$ for each distinct observed pattern of covariates while in Equation (5.11) there is a separate value of $i$ for each patient.) The statistic $d_j$ is assumed to have a binomial distribution obtained from $n_j$ independent dichotomous experiments with probability of success $\pi[x_{j1}, x_{j2}, \ldots, x_{jq}]$ on each experiment. Equation (5.12) implies that

$$\pi[x_{j1}, x_{j2}, \ldots, x_{jq}] = \frac{\exp[\alpha + \beta_1 x_{j1} + \beta_2 x_{j2} + \cdots + \beta_q x_{jq}]}{1 + \exp[\alpha + \beta_1 x_{j1} + \beta_2 x_{j2} + \cdots + \beta_q x_{jq}]}. \tag{5.13}$$

Choose any integer $k$ between 1 and $q$. Suppose that we hold all of the covariates constant except $x_{jk}$, which we allow to vary. Then $\alpha' = \alpha + \beta_1 x_{j1} + \cdots + \beta_{k-1} x_{j,k-1} + \beta_{k+1} x_{j,k+1} + \cdots + \beta_q x_{jq}$ is a constant and Equation (5.13) can be rewritten

$$\pi[x_{jk}] = \frac{\exp[\alpha' + \beta_k x_{jk}]}{1 + \exp[\alpha' + \beta_k x_{jk}]}, \qquad (5.14)$$

which is the equation for a simple logistic regression model. This implies that $\beta_k$ is the log odds ratio associated with a unit rise in $x_{jk}$ while holding the values of all the other covariates constant (see Section 4.12). Thus, the $\beta$ parameters in a multiple logistic regression model have an interpretation that is analogous to that for multiple linear regression. Each parameter equals the log odds ratio associated with a unit rise of its associated covariate adjusted for all of the other covariates in the model.

### 5.6.1. Likelihood ratio test of the influence of the covariates on the response variable

If the model covariates have no effect on the response variable then all of the $\beta$ parameters associated with the covariates will equal zero. Let $\hat{\beta}_1, \hat{\beta}_2, \ldots, \hat{\beta}_q$ denote the maximum likelihood estimates of $\beta_1, \beta_2, \ldots, \beta_q$, respectively. Let $\mathrm{L}[\hat{\boldsymbol{\beta}}]$ denote the maximum value of the likelihood function at $\hat{\beta}_1, \hat{\beta}_2, \ldots, \hat{\beta}_q$ and let $\mathrm{L}[\mathbf{0}]$ denote the value of the likelihood function at $\beta_1 = \beta_2 = \cdots = \beta_q = 0$. Then under the null hypothesis that $\beta_1 = \beta_2 = \cdots = \beta_q = 0$ the likelihood ratio statistic

$$\chi_q^2 = -2\log[\mathrm{L}[\mathbf{0}]/\mathrm{L}[\hat{\boldsymbol{\beta}}]] \qquad (5.15)$$

will have an approximately $\chi^2$ distribution with $q$ degrees of freedom. We will use this statistic to test whether the joint effects of the model covariates have any effect on the outcome of interest.

## 5.7. 95% confidence interval for an adjusted odds ratio

Logistic regression provides maximum likelihood estimates of the model parameters in Equation (5.11) or (5.12) together with estimates of their standard errors. Let $\hat{\beta}_k$ and $\mathrm{se}[\hat{\beta}_k]$ denote the maximum likelihood estimate of $\beta_k$ and its standard error, respectively. Then a 95% confidence interval for the odds ratio associated with a unit rise in $x_{ik}$ adjusted for the other covariates in the model is

$$(\exp[\hat{\beta}_k - 1.96\,\mathrm{se}[\hat{\beta}_k]], \exp[\hat{\beta}_k + 1.96\,\mathrm{se}[\hat{\beta}_k]]). \qquad (5.16)$$

## 5.8. Logistic regression for multiple 2 × 2 contingency tables

We will first consider a model that gives results that are similar to those of the Mantel–Haenszel method. Let us return to the Ille-et-Vilaine data from Section 5.1. Let $d_{ij}$ and $n_{ij}$ be defined as in Section 5.1 and let

$$
\begin{aligned}
J &= \text{the number of strata,}\\
i &= \begin{cases} 1\text{: for subjects who are heavy drinkers} \\ 0\text{: for those who are not,} \end{cases}\\
\pi_{ij} &= \text{the probability that a study subject from the } j^{\text{th}} \text{ age stratum has cancer given that he is } (i = 1) \text{ or is not } (i = 0) \text{ a heavy drinker, and}
\end{aligned}
$$

$\alpha$, $\beta$, and $\alpha_j$ be model parameters.

Consider the logistic model

$$
\text{logit}[\text{E}[d_{ij} \mid ij]/n_{ij}] = \begin{cases} \alpha + \beta \times i & : j = 1 \\ \alpha + \alpha_j + \beta \times i : & j = 2, 3, \ldots, J, \end{cases} \tag{5.17}
$$

where $d_{ij}$ has a binomial distribution obtained from $n_{ij}$ independent trials with success probability $\pi_{ij}$ on each trial. For any age stratum $j$ and drinking habit $i$,

$\text{E}[d_{ij} \mid ij]/n_{ij} = \pi_{ij}$. For any $j > 1$,

$$
\text{logit}[\text{E}[d_{0j} \mid i = 0,\ j]/n_{ij}] = \text{logit}[\pi_{0j}] = \log[\pi_{0j}/(1 - \pi_{0j})] = \alpha + \alpha_j \tag{5.18}
$$

is the log odds that a study subject from the $j^{\text{th}}$ stratum who is a moderate drinker will have cancer. Similarly,

$$
\begin{aligned}
\text{logit}[\text{E}[d_{1j} \mid i = 1,\ j]/n_{ij}] = \text{logit}[\pi_{1j}] &= \log[\pi_{1j}/(1 - \pi_{1j})] \\
&= \alpha + \alpha_j + \beta
\end{aligned} \tag{5.19}
$$

is the log odds that a study subject from the $j^{\text{th}}$ stratum who is a heavy drinker will have cancer. Subtracting Equation (5.18) from Equation (5.19) gives us

$$
\log[\pi_{j1}/(1 - \pi_{j1})] - \log[\pi_{j0}/(1 - \pi_{j0})] = \beta,
$$

or

$$
\log\left[\frac{\pi_{j1}/(1 - \pi_{j1})}{\pi_{j0}/(1 - \pi_{j0})}\right] = \log \psi = \beta. \tag{5.20}
$$

A similar argument shows that Equation (5.20) also holds when $j = 1$. Hence, this model implies that the odds ratio for esophageal cancer among heavy drinkers compared with moderate drinkers is the same in all strata and equals $\psi = \exp[\beta]$. Moreover, as explained in Section 4.23, $\psi$ also equals this odds ratio for members of the target population.

In practice we fit Model (5.17) by defining indicator covariates

$$age_j = \begin{cases} 1: & \text{if subjects are from the } j^{\text{th}} \text{ age stratum} \\ 0: & \text{otherwise.} \end{cases}$$

Then (5.17) becomes

$$\text{logit}[\text{E}[d_{ij} \mid ij]/n_{ij}] = \alpha + \alpha_2 \times age_2 + \alpha_3 \times age_3 + \alpha_4 \times age_4 + \alpha_5 \times age_5 + \alpha_6 \times age_6 + \beta \times i. \quad (5.21)$$

Note that this model places no restraints of the effect of age on the odds of cancer and only requires that the within-strata odds ratio be constant. For example, consider two study subjects from the first and $j^{\text{th}}$ age strata who have similar drinking habits ($i$ is the same for both men). Then the man from the $j^{\text{th}}$ stratum has log odds

$$\text{logit}[E(d_{ij} \mid ij)/n_{ij}] = \alpha + \alpha_j + \beta \times i, \quad (5.22)$$

while the man from the first age stratum has log odds

$$\text{logit}[\text{E}[d_{i1} \mid i, j = 1]/n_{i1}] = \alpha + \beta \times i. \quad (5.23)$$

Subtracting Equation (5.23) from Equation (5.22) gives that the log odds ratio for men with similar drinking habits from stratum $j$ versus stratum 1 is $\alpha_j$. Hence, each of strata 2 through 6 has a separate parameter that determines the odds ratio for men in that stratum relative to men with the same drinking habits from stratum 1.

An alternative model that we could have used is

$$\text{logit}[\text{E}[d_{ij} \mid ij]/n_{ij}] = \alpha \times j + \beta \times i. \quad (5.24)$$

However, this model imposes a linear relationship between age and the log odds for cancer. That is, the log odds ratio

for age stratum 2 vs. stratum 1 is $2\alpha - \alpha = \alpha$,
for age stratum 3 vs. stratum 1 is $3\alpha - \alpha = 2\alpha$, and
for age stratum 6 vs. stratum 1 is $6\alpha - \alpha = 5\alpha$.

As this linear relationship may not be valid, we are often better off using the more general model given by Equation (5.21).

Performing the logistic regression defined by Equation (5.21) gives $\hat{\beta} = 1.670$ with a standard error of $\text{se}[\hat{\beta}] = 0.1896$. Therefore, the age-adjusted estimate of the odds ratio for esophageal cancer in heavy drinkers compared with moderate drinkers is $\hat{\psi} = \exp[\hat{\beta}] = e^{1.670} = 5.31$. From Equation (5.16) we have that the 95% confidence interval for $\psi$ is $(\exp[1.670 - 1.96 \times 0.1896], \exp[1.670 + 1.96 \times 0.1896]) = (3.66, 7.70)$. The results of this logistic regression are similar to those obtained from the Mantel–Haenszel analysis. The age-adjusted odds ratio from this latter test was $\hat{\psi} = 5.16$ as compared with 5.31 from this logistic regression model.

## 5.9. Analyzing multiple 2×2 tables with Stata

The following log file and comments illustrate how to fit the logistic regression Model (5.21) to the Ille-et-Vilaine data set.

```
. *   5.9.EsophagealCa.log
. *
. *   Calculate age-adjusted odds ratio from the Ille-et-Vilaine study
. *   of esophageal cancer and alcohol using logistic regression.
. *
. use C:\WDDtext\5.5.EsophagealCa.dta, clear
. *
. *   First, define indicator variables for age strata 2 through 6
. *
. generate age2 = 0
. replace age2 = 1 if age == 2                                          1
(32 real changes made)
. generate age3 = 0
. replace age3 = 1 if age == 3
(32 real changes made)
. generate age4 = 0
. replace age4 = 1 if age == 4
(32 real changes made)
. generate age5 = 0
. replace age5 = 1 if age == 5
(32 real changes made)
. generate age6 = 0
. replace age6 = 1 if age == 6
(32 real changes made)
. logistic cancer age2 age3 age4 age5 age6 heavy [freq=patients]      2
```

```
Logistic regression                               Number of obs   =        975
                                                  LR chi2(6)      =     200.57    3
                                                  Prob > chi2     =     0.0000
Log likelihood = -394.46094                       Pseudo R2       =     0.2027

------------------------------------------------------------------------------
      cancer | Odds Ratio   Std. Err.      z    P>|z|     [95% Conf. Interval]
-------------+----------------------------------------------------------------
        age2 |   4.675303   4.983382     1.45   0.148      .5787862   37.76602   4
        age3 |   24.50217   25.06914     3.13   0.002      3.298423   182.0131
        age4 |   40.99664   41.75634     3.65   0.000       5.56895   301.8028
        age5 |   52.81958   54.03823     3.88   0.000      7.111389   392.3155
        age6 |   52.57232   55.99081     3.72   0.000      6.519386   423.9432
       heavy |   5.311584   1.007086     8.81   0.000      3.662981   7.702174   5
------------------------------------------------------------------------------

. log close
```

### Comments

1 The numeric values of *age* are 1 through 6 and denote the age strata 25–34, 35–44, 45–54, 55–64, 65–74 and ≥75, respectively. We define *age2* = 1 for subjects from the second stratum and 0 otherwise; *age3* through *age6* are similarly defined for the other strata.

This is the most straightforward but by no means the quickest way of defining indicator variables in Stata. We will illustrate faster ways of doing this in subsequent examples.

2 Regress *cancer* against *age2, age3, age4, age5, age6,* and *heavy* using logistic regression. This command analyzes the model specified by Equation (5.21). (See also Comment 1 from Section 5.5.) The point-and-click command is the same as that given in Comment 1 on page 176 except that all of the independent variables, *age2, age3, age4, age5, age6,* and *heavy,* are entered in the *Independent variables* field.

3 The likelihood ratio $\chi^2$ statistic to test whether the model covariates affect cancer risk is given by Equation (5.15) and equals 220.57. Our model has six covariates (five for age and one for heavy drinking). Hence, this statistic has six degrees of freedom and is of overwhelming statistical significance. (The probability that such a statistic will exceed 220 under this null hypothesis is less than $10^{-39}$.)

4 The estimated cancer odds ratio for men from the second age stratum relative to men from the first with the same drinking habits is 4.68. This odds ratio equals $\exp[\hat{\alpha}_2]$. Note that the odds ratio rises steeply with increasing age until the fourth age stratum and then levels off. Hence, the

model specified by Equation (5.24) would do a poor job of modeling age for these data.

5 The age-adjusted estimated odds ratio for cancer in heavy drinkers relative to moderate drinkers is $\hat{\psi} = \exp[\hat{\beta}] = 5.312$. Hence, $\hat{\beta} = \log[5.312] = 1.670$. The logistic command does not give the value of se$[\hat{\beta}]$. However, the 95% confidence interval for $\hat{\psi}$ is (3.66, 7.70), which agrees with our hand calculations.

## 5.10. Handling categorical variables in Stata

In Section 5.9 *age* is a categorical variable taking six values that are recoded as five separate indicator variables. It is very common to recode categorical variables in this way to avoid forcing a linear relationship on the effect of a variable on the response outcome. In the preceding example we did the recoding by hand. It can also be done much faster using the *xi:* command prefix. We illustrate this by repeating the preceding analysis of the model specified by Equation (5.21).

```
. *  5.10.EsophagealCa.log
. *
. *  Repeat the analysis in 5.9.EsophagealCa.log using
. *  automatic recoding of the age classification variable
. *
. use C:\WDDtext\5.5.EsophagealCa.dta, clear
. xi: logistic cancer i.age heavy [freq=patients]                              1
i.age              _Iage_1-6          (naturally coded; _Iage_1 omitted)

Logistic regression                            Number of obs   =        975
                                               LR chi2(6)      =     200.57
                                               Prob > chi2     =     0.0000
Log likelihood = -394.46094                    Pseudo R2       =     0.2027

------------------------------------------------------------------------------
      cancer | Odds Ratio   Std. Err.      z    P>|z|     [95% Conf. Interval]
-------------+----------------------------------------------------------------
     _Iage_2 |   4.675303   4.983382    1.45   0.148     .5787862    37.76602    2
     _Iage_3 |   24.50217   25.06914    3.13   0.002     3.298423    182.0131
     _Iage_4 |   40.99664   41.75634    3.65   0.000      5.56895    301.8028
     _Iage_5 |   52.81958   54.03823    3.88   0.000     7.111389    392.3155
     _Iage_6 |   52.57232   55.99081    3.72   0.000     6.519386    423.9432
       heavy |   5.311584   1.007086    8.81   0.000     3.662981    7.702174
------------------------------------------------------------------------------

. log close
```

**Comments**

1 The *xi:* prefix before an estimation command (like *logistic*) tells Stata that indicator variables will be created and used in the model; *i.age* indicates that a separate indicator variable is to be created for each distinct value of *age*. These variables are named *_Iage_1*, *_Iage_2*, *_Iage_3*, *_Iage_4*, *_Iage_5*, and *_Iage_6*. Note that these variable names start with "*_I*". When specifying these variables they must be capitalized in exactly the same way they were defined. The variables *_Iage_2* through *_Iage_6* are identical to the variables *age2* through *age6* in Section 5.9. By default, the new variable associated with the smallest value of *age* (that is, *_Iage_1*) is deleted from the model. As a consequence, the model analyzed is that specified by Equation (5.21). The equivalent point-and-click command is Statistics ▶ Binary outcomes ▶ Logistic regression (reporting odds ratios) Model Dependent variable: *cancer*, Independent variables: *i.age heavy* Weights ⦿ Frequency weights , Frequency weight: *patients* Submit .

2 Note that the output of this logistic regression analysis is identical to that in Section 5.9. The only difference is the names of the indicator variables that define the age strata.

## 5.11. Effect of dose of alcohol on esophageal cancer risk

The Ille-et-Vilaine data set provides four different levels of daily alcohol consumption: 0–39 g, 40–79 g, 80–119 g, and ≥120 g. To investigate the joint effects of dose of alcohol on esophageal cancer risk we analyze the model

$$\text{logit}[\text{E}[d_{ij} \mid ij]/n_{ij}] = \alpha + \sum_{h=2}^{6} \alpha_h \times age_h + \sum_{h=2}^{4} \beta_h \times alcohol_{ih}, \tag{5.25}$$

where the terms are analogous to those in Equation (5.21), only now

$i$ denotes the drinking levels 1 through 4,
$j$ denotes age strata 1 through 6, and

$$alcohol_{ih} = \begin{cases} 1: \text{if } i = h \\ 0: \text{otherwise.} \end{cases}$$

Deriving the age-adjusted cancer odds ratio for dose level $k$ relative to dose level 1 is done using an argument similar to that given in Section 5.8. From Equation (5.25) we have that the cancer log odds for a man at the first dose

**Table 5.3.** Effect of dose of alcohol and tobacco on the odds ratio for esophageal cancer in the Ille-et-Vilaine study. These odds ratios associated with alcohol are adjusted for age using the logistic regression Model (5.25). A similar model is used for tobacco. The risk of esophageal cancer increases dramatically with increasing dose of both alcohol and tobacco

| Risk factor | Dose level $i$ | Daily dose | Log odds ratio $\hat{\beta}_i$ | Odds ratio $\hat{\psi}_i$ | 95% confidence interval for $\psi_i$ | *P*-value[†] |
|---|---|---|---|---|---|---|
| *Alcohol* | | | | | | |
| | 1 | 0–39 g | | 1* | | |
| | 2 | 40–79 g | 1.4343 | 4.20 | 2.6–6.8 | <0.0005 |
| | 3 | 80–119 g | 2.0071 | 7.44 | 4.3–13.0 | <0.0005 |
| | 4 | ≥120 g | 3.6800 | 39.6 | 0.19–83.0 | <0.0005 |
| *Tobacco* | | | | | | |
| | 1 | 0–9 g | | 1* | | |
| | 2 | 10–19 g | 0.6073 | 1.84 | 1.2–2.7 | 0.0030 |
| | 3 | 20–29 g | 0.6653 | 1.95 | 1.2–3.2 | 0.0080 |
| | 4 | ≥30 g | 1.7415 | 5.71 | 3.2–10.0 | <0.0005 |

*Denominator (reference group) of following odds ratios

[†]Associated with the two-sided test of the null hypothesis that $\psi_i = 1$

level is

$$\text{logit}[\text{E}[d_{1j} \mid i = 1, j]/n_{1j}] = \log\left[\frac{\pi_{1j}}{1 - \pi_{1j}}\right] = \alpha + \sum_{h=2}^{6} \alpha_h \times age_h$$

$$= \alpha + \alpha_j. \tag{5.26}$$

For a man from the same age stratum at the $i^{\text{th}}$ dose level, the log odds are

$$\log\left[\frac{\pi_{ij}}{1 - \pi_{ij}}\right] = \alpha + \sum_{h=2}^{6} \alpha_h \times age_h + \sum_{h=2}^{4} \beta_h \times alcohol_{ih}$$

$$= \alpha + \alpha_j + \beta_i. \tag{5.27}$$

Subtracting Equation (5.26) from Equation (5.27) gives that the age-adjusted log odds ratio for a man at the $i^{\text{th}}$ dose level relative to the first is

$$\log\left[\frac{\pi_{ij}/(1 - \pi_{ij})}{\pi_{1j}/(1 - \pi_{1j})}\right] = \log\left[\frac{\pi_{ij}}{1 - \pi_{ij}}\right] - \log\left[\frac{\pi_{1j}}{1 - \pi_{1j}}\right] = \beta_i. \tag{5.28}$$

Hence, the age-adjusted odds ratio for dose level $i$ versus dose level 1 is $\exp[\beta_i]$. This model was used to estimate the odds ratios given in the top half of Table 5.3. For example, the odds ratio for the second dose level compared with the first is $\exp[\hat{\beta}_2] = 4.20$. Clearly, the risk of esophageal cancer increases precipitously with increasing dose of alcohol.

### 5.11.1. Analyzing Model (5.25) with Stata

The following log file and comments explain how to analyze Model (5.25) with Stata.

```
. *   5.11.1.EsophagealCa.log
. *
. *   Estimate age-adjusted risk of esophageal cancer due to
. *   dose of alcohol.
. *
. use C:\WDDtext\5.5.EsophagealCa.dta, clear

. *
. *   Show frequency tables of effect of dose of alcohol on
. *   esophageal cancer.
. *
. tabulate cancer alcohol [freq=patients] , column                          1
```

```
+-------------------+
| Key               |
|-------------------|
|     frequency     |
| column percentage |
+-------------------+
```

| Esophageal Cancer | Alcohol (g/day) 0-39 | 40-79 | 80-119 | >= 120 | Total |
|---|---|---|---|---|---|
| No | 386<br>93.01 | 280<br>78.87 | 87<br>63.04 | 22<br>32.84 | 775<br>79.49 |
| Yes | 29<br>6.99 | 75<br>21.13 | 51<br>36.96 | 45<br>67.16 | 200<br>20.51 |
| Total | 415<br>100.00 | 355<br>100.00 | 138<br>100.00 | 67<br>100.00 | 975<br>100.00 |

```
. *
. *  Analyze the Ille-et-Vilaine data using logistic regression
. *  model (5.24).
. *
. xi: logistic cancer i.age i.alcohol [freq=patients]
```

```
i.age             _Iage_1-6         (naturally coded; _Iage_1 omitted)
i.alcohol         _Ialcohol_1-4     (naturally coded; _Ialcohol_1 omitted)

Logistic regression                           Number of obs   =        975
                                              LR chi2(8)      =     262.07
                                              Prob > chi2     =     0.0000
Log likelihood = -363.70808                   Pseudo R2       =     0.2649
```

| cancer | Odds Ratio | Std. Err. | z | P>\|z\| | [95% Conf. | Interval] |
|---|---|---|---|---|---|---|
| _Iage_2 | 5.109602 | 5.518316 | 1.51 | 0.131 | .6153163 | 42.43026 |
| _Iage_3 | 30.74859 | 31.9451 | 3.30 | 0.001 | 4.013298 | 235.5858 |
| _Iage_4 | 51.59663 | 53.38175 | 3.81 | 0.000 | 6.791573 | 391.9876 |
| _Iage_5 | 78.00528 | 81.22778 | 4.18 | 0.000 | 10.13347 | 600.4678 |
| _Iage_6 | 83.44844 | 91.07367 | 4.05 | 0.000 | 9.827359 | 708.5975 |
| _Ialcohol_2 | 4.196747 | 1.027304 | 5.86 | 0.000 | 2.597472 | 6.780704 |
| _Ialcohol_3 | 7.441782 | 2.065952 | 7.23 | 0.000 | 4.318873 | 12.82282 |
| _Ialcohol_4 | 39.64689 | 14.92059 | 9.78 | 0.000 | 18.9614 | 82.8987 |

2

```
. log close
```

**Comments**

1 The *tabulate* command produces one- and two-way frequency tables. The variable *alcohol* gives the dose level. The numeric values of this variable are 1, 2, 3, and 4. The *column* option expresses the number of observations in each cell as a percentage of the total number of observations in the associated column. If we had added a *row* option, row percentages would also have been given. The equivalent point-and-click command is Statistics ► Summaries, tables, & tests ► Tables ► Two-way tables with measures of association [Main] Row variable: *cancer*, Column variable: *alcohol* [Weights] ⦿ Frequency weights , Frequency weight: *patients* [Submit].

It is always a good idea to produce such tables as a cross-check of the results of our regression analyses. Note that the proportion of cancer cases increases dramatically with increasing dose.

2 The indicator variables *_Ialcohol_2*, *_Ialcohol_3* and *_Ialcohol_4* are the covariates $alcohol_{i2}$, $alcohol_{i3}$ and $alcohol_{i4}$ in Model (5.25). The shaded odds ratios and confidence intervals that are associated with these covariates are also given in Table 5.3.

## 5.12. Effect of dose of tobacco on esophageal cancer risk

The Ille-et-Vilaine data set also provides four different levels of daily tobacco consumption: 0–9 g, 10–19 g, 20–29 g, and ≥30 g. This risk factor is modeled in exactly the same way as alcohol. The log file named *5.12.EsophagealCa.log* on my web site illustrates how to perform this analysis in Stata. The bottom panel of Table 5.3 shows the effect of increasing tobacco dose on esophageal cancer risk. This risk increases significantly with increasing dose. Note, however, that the odds ratios associated with 10–19 g and 20–29 g are very similar. For this reason, it makes sense to combine subjects with these two levels of tobacco consumption into a single group. In subsequent models, we will recode tobacco dosage to permit tobacco to be modeled with two parameters rather than three. In general, it is a good idea to avoid having unnecessary parameters in our models as this reduces their statistical power.

## 5.13. Deriving odds ratios from multiple parameters

Model (5.25) also permits us to calculate the age-adjusted odds ratio for, say, alcohol dose level 4 relative to dose level 3. From Equation (5.27) we have that the log odds of cancer for two men from the $j^{\text{th}}$ age stratum who are at dose levels 3 and 4 are

$$\log\left[\frac{\pi_{3j}}{1-\pi_{3j}}\right] = \alpha + \alpha_j + \beta_3$$

and

$$\log\left[\frac{\pi_{4j}}{1-\pi_{4j}}\right] = \alpha + \alpha_j + \beta_4.$$

Subtracting the first of these log odds from the second gives that the cancer log odds ratio for men at dose level 4 relative to dose level 3 is

$$\log\left[\frac{\pi_{4j}/(1-\pi_{4j})}{\pi_{3j}/(1-\pi_{3j})}\right] = \log\left[\frac{\pi_{4j}}{1-\pi_{4j}}\right] - \log\left[\frac{\pi_{3j}}{1-\pi_{3j}}\right] = \beta_4 - \beta_3,$$

and the corresponding odds ratio is $\exp[\beta_4 - \beta_3]$.

In more complex multiple logistic regression models we often need to make inferences about odds ratios that are estimated from multiple parameters. The preceding is a simple example of such an odds ratio. To derive confidence intervals and perform hypothesis tests on these odds ratios we need to compute the standard errors of weighted sums of parameter estimates.

## 5.14. The standard error of a weighted sum of regression coefficients

Suppose that we have a model with $q$ parameters $\beta_1, \beta_2, \ldots, \beta_q$. Let

$\hat{\beta}_1, \hat{\beta}_2, \ldots, \hat{\beta}_q$ be estimates of these parameters,
$c_1, c_2, \ldots, c_q$ be a set of known weights,
$f = \sum c_j \beta_j$ be the weighted sum of the coefficients that equals some log odds ratio of interest, and

$$\hat{f} = \sum c_j \hat{\beta}_j \quad \text{be an estimate of } f. \tag{5.29}$$

For example, in Model (5.25) there is the constant parameter $\alpha$, the five age parameters $\alpha_2, \alpha_3, \ldots, \alpha_6$, and the three alcohol parameters $\beta_2$, $\beta_3$, and $\beta_4$, giving a total of $q = 9$ parameters. Let us reassign $\alpha, \alpha_2, \alpha_3, \alpha_4, \alpha_5$, and $\alpha_6$ with the names $\beta_1, \beta_5, \beta_6, \beta_7, \beta_8$, and $\beta_9$. Let $c_4 = 1$, $c_3 = -1$, and $c_1 = c_2 = c_5 = c_6 = c_7 = c_8 = c_9 = 0$. Then $\hat{f} = \hat{\beta}_4 - \hat{\beta}_3$. From Table 5.3 we have that $\hat{\beta}_4 = 3.6800$ and $\hat{\beta}_3 = 2.0071$. Therefore, $\hat{f} = 3.6800 - 2.0071 = 1.6729$ and $\exp[\hat{f}] = \exp[1.6729] = 5.33$ is the estimated odds ratio of level 4 drinkers relative to level 3 drinkers. Let

$s_{jj}$ be the estimated variance of $\hat{\beta}_j$ for $j = 1, \ldots, q$, and
$s_{ij}$ be the estimated covariance of $\hat{\beta}_i$ and $\hat{\beta}_j$ for any $i \neq j$.

Then it can be shown that the variance of $\hat{f}$ may be estimated by

$$s_f^2 = \sum_{i=1}^{q} \sum_{j=1}^{q} c_i c_j s_{ij}. \tag{5.30}$$

## 5.15. Confidence intervals for weighted sums of coefficients

The estimated standard error of $\hat{f}$ is $s_f$. For large studies the 95% confidence interval for $f$ is approximated by

$$\hat{f} \pm 1.96 s_f. \tag{5.31}$$

A 95% confidence interval for the odds ratio $\exp[f]$ is given by

$$(\exp[\hat{f} - 1.96 s_f], \ \exp[\hat{f} + 1.96 s_f]). \tag{5.32}$$

Equation (5.32) is an example of a Wald confidence interval (see Section 4.9.4).

In our example comparing level 4 drinkers with level 3 drinkers, our logistic regression program estimates $s_{33} = 0.077\,07$, $s_{34} = s_{43} = 0.042\,24$, and

$s_{44} = 0.141\,63$. Hence, $s_f^2 = (-1)^2 s_{33} + (-1) \times 1 \times s_{34} + 1 \times (-1) s_{43} + 1^2 s_{44} = 0.077\,07 - 2 \times 0.042\,24 + 0.141\,63 = 0.134\,22$, which gives $s_f = 0.3664$. This is the standard error of the log odds ratio for level 4 drinking compared with level 3. Equation (5.32) gives the 95% confidence interval for this odds ratio to be $(\exp[1.6729 - 1.96 \times 0.3664], \exp[1.6729 + 1.96 \times 0.3664]) = (2.60, 10.9)$. Fortunately, Stata has a powerful post-estimation command called *lincom*, which rarely makes it necessary for us to calculate Equations (5.30) or (5.32) explicitly.

## 5.16. Hypothesis tests for weighted sums of coefficients

For large studies

$$z = \hat{f}/s_f \tag{5.33}$$

has an approximately standard normal distribution. Equation (5.33) is an example of a Wald test (see Section 4.9.4). We use this statistic to test the null hypothesis that $f = \sum c_j \beta_j = 0$, or, equivalently, that $\exp[f] = 1$. For example, to test the null hypothesis that $\beta_4 - \beta_3 = 0$ we calculate $z = (1.6729/0.3664) = 4.57$. The $P$-value associated with a two-sided test of this null hypothesis is $P = 0.000\,005$. Note that this null hypothesis is equivalent to the hypothesis that $\exp[\beta_4 - \beta_3] = 1$ (i.e., that the odds ratio for level 4 drinkers relative to level 3 equals 1). Hence, we can reject the hypothesis that these two consumption levels are associated with equivalent cancer risks with overwhelming statistical significance.

## 5.17. The estimated variance–covariance matrix

The estimates of $s_{ij}$ can be written in a square array

$$\begin{bmatrix} s_{11} & s_{12} & \cdots & s_{1q} \\ s_{21} & s_{22} & \cdots & s_{2q} \\ \vdots & \vdots & \ddots & \vdots \\ s_{q1} & s_{q2} & \cdots & s_{qq} \end{bmatrix},$$

which is called the estimated variance–covariance matrix. For any two variables $x$ and $y$ the covariance of $x$ with $y$ equals the covariance of $y$ with $x$. Hence, $s_{ij} = s_{ji}$ for any $i$ and $j$ between 1 and $q$, and the variance–covariance matrix is symmetric about the main diagonal that runs from

$s_{11}$ to $s_{qq}$. For this reason it is common to display this matrix in the lower triangular form

$$\begin{bmatrix} s_{11} & & & \\ s_{21} & s_{22} & & \\ \vdots & \vdots & \ddots & \\ s_{q1} & s_{q2} & \cdots & s_{qq} \end{bmatrix}.$$

The Stata *estat vce* post-estimation command introduced in Section 4.18 uses this format to display the variance–covariance matrix. We use this command whenever we wish to print the variance and covariance estimates for the parameters from our regression models.

## 5.18. Multiplicative models of two risk factors

Suppose that subjects either were or were not exposed to alcohol and tobacco and we do not adjust for age. Consider the model

$$\text{logit}[\text{E}[d_{ij} \mid ij]/n_{ij}] = \text{logit}[\pi_{ij}] = \alpha + \beta_1 \times i + \beta_2 \times j, \tag{5.34}$$

$$\text{where } i = \begin{cases} 1: & \text{if subject drank} \\ 0: & \text{otherwise,} \end{cases}$$

$$j = \begin{cases} 1: & \text{if subject smoked} \\ 0: & \text{otherwise,} \end{cases}$$

$n_{ij}$ = the number of subjects with drinking status $i$ and smoking status $j$,
$d_{ij}$ = the number of cancer cases with drinking status $i$ and smoking status $j$,
$\pi_{ij}$ = the probability that someone with drinking status $i$ and smoking status $j$ develops cancer,

and $\alpha$, $\beta_1$, and $\beta_2$ are model parameters.
Then the cancer log odds of a drinker with smoking status $j$ is

$$\text{logit}[\text{E}[d_{1j} \mid i = 1, j]/n_{1j}] = \text{logit}[\pi_{1j}] = \alpha + \beta_1 + \beta_2 \times j. \tag{5.35}$$

The log odds of a non-drinker with smoking status $j$ is

$$\text{logit}[\text{E}[d_{0j} \mid i = 0, j]/n_{0j}] = \text{logit}[\pi_{0j}] = \alpha + \beta_2 \times j. \tag{5.36}$$

Subtracting Equation (5.36) from (5.35) gives

$$\log\left[\frac{\pi_{1j}/(1-\pi_{1j})}{\pi_{0j}/(1-\pi_{0j})}\right] = \beta_1.$$

In other words, $\exp[\beta_1]$ is the cancer odds ratio in drinkers compared with non-drinkers adjusted for smoking. Note that this implies that the relative risk of drinking is the same in smokers and non-smokers. By an identical argument, $\exp[\beta_2]$ is the odds ratio for cancer in smokers compared with non-smokers adjusted for drinking.

For people who both drink and smoke the model is

$$\text{logit}[\text{E}[d_{11} \mid i = 1, j = 1]/n_{11}] = \text{logit}[\pi_{11}] = \alpha + \beta_1 + \beta_2, \tag{5.37}$$

while for people who neither drink nor smoke it is

$$\text{logit}[\text{E}[d_{00} \mid i = 0, j = 0]/n_{00}] = \text{logit}[\pi_{00}] = \alpha. \tag{5.38}$$

Subtracting Equation (5.38) from (5.37) gives that the log odds ratio for people who both smoke and drink relative to those who do neither is $\beta_1 + \beta_2$. The corresponding odds ratio is $\exp[\beta_1 + \beta_2] = \exp[\beta_1] \times \exp[\beta_2]$. Thus, our model implies that the odds ratio of having both risk factors equals the product of the individual odds ratios for drinking and smoking. It is for this reason that this is called a **multiplicative model**.

## 5.19. Multiplicative model of smoking, alcohol, and esophageal cancer

The multiplicative assumption is a very strong one that is often not justified. Let us see how it works with the Ille-et-Vilaine data set. The model that we will use is

$$\text{logit}[\text{E}[d_{ijk} \mid ijk]/n_{ijk}] = \alpha + \sum_{h=2}^{6} \alpha_h \times age_h + \sum_{h=2}^{4} \beta_h \times alcohol_{ih} + \sum_{h=2}^{3} \gamma_h \times smoke_{kh}, \tag{5.39}$$

where

- $i$ is one of four dose levels of alcohol,
- $k$ is one of three dose levels of tobacco,
- $n_{ijk}$ is the number of subjects from the $j^{\text{th}}$ age stratum who are at the $i^{\text{th}}$ dose level of alcohol and the $k^{\text{th}}$ dose level of tobacco,
- $d_{ijk}$ is the number of cancer cases from the $j^{\text{th}}$ age stratum who are at the $i^{\text{th}}$ dose level of alcohol and the $k^{\text{th}}$ dose level of tobacco,

**Table 5.4.** Effect of alcohol and tobacco on the risk of esophageal cancer in the Ille-et-Vilaine study. These estimates are based on the multiplicative Model (5.39). This model requires that the odds ratio associated with the joint effects of alcohol and tobacco equal the product of the odds ratios for the individual effects of these risk factors

| | Daily tobacco consumption | | | | | |
|---|---|---|---|---|---|---|
| | 0–9 g | | 10–29 g | | ≥30 g | |
| Daily alcohol consumption | Odds ratio | 95% confidence interval | Odds ratio | 95% confidence interval | Odds ratio | 95% confidence interval |
| 0–39 g | 1.0* | | 1.59 | (1.1–2.4) | 5.16 | (2.6–10) |
| 40–79 g | 4.21 | (2.6–6.9) | 6.71 | (3.6–12) | 21.7 | (9.2–51) |
| 80–119 g | 7.22 | (4.1–13) | 11.5 | (5.9–22) | 37.3 | (15–91) |
| ≥120 g | 36.8 | (17–78) | 58.6 | (25–140) | 190 | (67–540) |

*Denominator of odds ratios

$\gamma_h$ is a parameter associated with the $h^{\text{th}}$ dose level of tobacco,

$$smoke_{kh} = \begin{cases} 1: \text{if } k = h \\ 0: \text{otherwise,} \end{cases}$$

and $\alpha$, $\alpha_h$, $age_h$, $\beta_h$, and $alcohol_{ih}$ are as defined in Equation (5.25).

In Table 5.3 we found that the middle two levels of tobacco consumption were associated with similar risks of esophageal cancer. In this model we combine these levels into one; dose levels $k = 1$, 2, and 3 correspond to daily consumption levels 0–9 g, 10–29 g, and ≥30 g, respectively.

Let $\psi_{ik}$ be the odds ratio for men at alcohol dose level $i$ and tobacco dose level $k$ relative to men at level 1 for both drugs. Then for $i > 1$ and $j > 1$ we have by the same argument used in Section 5.18 that

$$\psi_{i1} = \exp[\beta_i],$$

$$\psi_{1k} = \exp[\gamma_k], \text{ and}$$

$$\psi_{ik} = \exp[\beta_i] \times \exp[\gamma_k].$$

Solving Model (5.39) yields maximum likelihood parameter estimates $\hat{\beta}_i$ and $\hat{\gamma}_k$, which can be used to generate Table 5.4 using the preceding formulas. For example, $\hat{\beta}_4 = 3.6053$ and $\hat{\gamma}_3 = 1.6408$. Therefore, $\hat{\psi}_{41} = \exp[3.6053] = 36.79$, $\hat{\psi}_{13} = \exp[1.6408] = 5.16$, and $\hat{\psi}_{43} =$

$36.79 \times 5.16 = 189.8$. The confidence intervals in this table are derived using Equation (5.32).

If Model (5.39) is to be believed, then the risk of esophageal cancer associated with the highest levels of alcohol and tobacco consumption are extraordinary. There is no biologic reason, however, why the odds ratio associated with the combined effects of two risk factors should equal the product of the odds ratios for the individual risk factors. Indeed, the joint risk is usually less than the product of the individual risks. To investigate whether this is the case here we will need to analyze a more general model. We will do this in Section 5.22.

## 5.20. Fitting a multiplicative model with Stata

In the following Stata log file we first combine subjects at smoking levels 2 and 3 into a single group. We then fit the age-adjusted multiplicative Model (5.39) to estimate the effect of dose of alcohol and tobacco on the risk of esophageal cancer.

```
. *  5.20.EsophagealCa.log
. *
. *  Regress esophageal cancers against age and dose of alcohol
. *  and tobacco using a multiplicative model.
. *
. use C:\WDDtext\5.5.EsophagealCa.dta, clear

. *
. *  Combine tobacco levels 2 and 3 in a new variable called smoke
. *
. generate smoke = tobacco
. recode smoke 3=2 4=3                                              1

(smoke: 96 changes made)

. label variable smoke "Smoking (g/day)"

. label define  smoke 1 "0-9" 2 "10-29" 3 ">= 30"

. label values smoke smoke

. table smoke tobacco [freq=patients], row col                      2
```

| Smoking (g/day) | Tobacco (g/day) 0-9 | 10-19 | 20-29 | >= 30 | Total |
|---|---|---|---|---|---|
| 0-9 | 525 | | | | 525 |
| 10-29 | | 236 | 132 | | 368 |
| >= 30 | | | | 82 | 82 |
| Total | 525 | 236 | 132 | 82 | 975 |

```
. *
. *   Regress cancer against age, alcohol and smoke
. *   using a multiplicative model.
. *
. xi: logistic cancer i.age i.alcohol i.smoke [freq=patients]          3

i.age            _Iage_1-6          (naturally coded; _Iage_1 omitted)
i.alcohol        _Ialcohol_1-4      (naturally coded; _Ialcohol_1 omitted)
i.smoke          _Ismoke_1-3        (naturally coded; _Ismoke_1 omitted)

Logistic regression                          Number of obs   =      975
                                             LR chi2(10)     =   285.55
                                             Prob > chi2     =   0.0000
Log likelihood = -351.96823                  Pseudo R2       =   0.2886   4
```

| cancer | Odds Ratio | Std. Err. | z | P>\|z\| | [95% Conf. | Interval] |
|---|---|---|---|---|---|---|
| _Iage_2 | 7.262526 | 8.017364 | 1.80 | 0.072 | .8344795 | 63.2062 |
| _Iage_3 | 43.65627 | 46.6239 | 3.54 | 0.000 | 5.382485 | 354.0873 |
| _Iage_4 | 76.3655 | 81.32909 | 4.07 | 0.000 | 9.470422 | 615.7792 |
| _Iage_5 | 133.7632 | 143.9718 | 4.55 | 0.000 | 16.22455 | 1102.81 |
| _Iage_6 | 124.4262 | 139.5027 | 4.30 | 0.000 | 13.82203 | 1120.088 |
| _Ialcohol_2 | 4.213304 | 1.05191 | 5.76 | 0.000 | 2.582905 | 6.872853 5 |
| _Ialcohol_3 | 7.222005 | 2.053956 | 6.95 | 0.000 | 4.135937 | 12.61077 |
| _Ialcohol_4 | 36.7912 | 14.1701 | 9.36 | 0.000 | 17.29435 | 78.26787 |
| _Ismoke_2 | 1.592701 | .3200883 | 2.32 | 0.021 | 1.074154 | 2.361576 |
| _Ismoke_3 | 5.159309 | 1.775205 | 4.77 | 0.000 | 2.628523 | 10.12678 |

```
. lincom _Ialcohol_2 + _Ismoke_2, or
```

See comment 6 below

```
( 1)  _Ialcohol_2 + _Ismoke_2 = 0
```

| cancer | Odds Ratio | Std. Err. | z | P>\|z\| | [95% Conf. | Interval] |
|---|---|---|---|---|---|---|
| (1) | 6.710535 | 2.110331 | 6.05 | 0.000 | 3.623022 | 12.4292 |

```
. lincom _Ialcohol_3 + _Ismoke_2, or

( 1)  _Ialcohol_3 + _Ismoke_2 = 0
```

| cancer | Odds Ratio | Std. Err. | z | P>\|z\| | [95% Conf. | Interval] |
|---|---|---|---|---|---|---|
| (1) | 11.5025 | 3.877641 | 7.25 | 0.000 | 5.940747 | 22.27118 |

```
. lincom _Ialcohol_4 + _Ismoke_2, or

( 1)  _Ialcohol_4 + _Ismoke_2 = 0
```

| cancer | Odds Ratio | Std. Err. | z | P>\|z\| | [95% Conf. | Interval] |
|---|---|---|---|---|---|---|
| (1) | 58.59739 | 25.19568 | 9.47 | 0.000 | 25.22777 | 136.1061 |

```
. lincom _Ialcohol_2 + _Ismoke_3, or

( 1)  _Ialcohol_2 + _Ismoke_3 = 0
```

| cancer | Odds Ratio | Std. Err. | z | P>\|z\| | [95% Conf. | Interval] |
|---|---|---|---|---|---|---|
| (1) | 21.73774 | 9.508636 | 7.04 | 0.000 | 9.223106 | 51.23319 |

```
. lincom _Ialcohol_3 + _Ismoke_3, or

( 1)  _Ialcohol_3 + _Ismoke_3 = 0
```

```
------------------------------------------------------------------------------
      cancer | Odds Ratio   Std. Err.      z    P>|z|     [95% Conf. Interval]
-------------+----------------------------------------------------------------
         (1) |   37.26056   17.06685     7.90   0.000     15.18324    91.43957
------------------------------------------------------------------------------

. lincom _Ialcohol_4 + _Ismoke_3, or
```
6

```
( 1)  _Ialcohol_4 + _Ismoke_3 = 0

------------------------------------------------------------------------------
      cancer | Odds Ratio   Std. Err.      z    P>|z|     [95% Conf. Interval]
-------------+----------------------------------------------------------------
         (1) |   189.8171   100.9788     9.86   0.000     66.91353    538.4643
------------------------------------------------------------------------------
```

## Comments

1 We want to combine the 2nd and 3rd levels of tobacco exposure. We do this by defining a new variable called *smoke* that is identical to *tobacco* and then using the *recode* statement, which, in this example, changes values of *smoke* = 3 to *smoke* = 2, and values of *smoke* = 4 to *smoke* = 3. The equivalent point-and-click command is Data ▶ Create or change variables ▶ Other variable transformation commands ▶ Recode categorical variable ⌋Main⌊ Variables: *smoke*, Required: *3=2*, Optional: *4=3* [Submit].

2 This *table* statement gives a cross-tabulation of values of *smoke* by values of *tobacco*. The *row* and *col* options specify that row and column totals are to be given. The resulting table shows that the previous *recode* statement had the desired effect. The equivalent point-and-click command is Statistics ▶ Summaries, tables, & tests ▶ Tables ▶ Table of summary statistics (table) ⌋Main⌊ Row variable: *smoke* ┌ [✓] Column variable — *tobacco* ┘ ⌋Weights⌊ ⦿ Frequency weights , Frequency weight: *patients* ⌋Options⌊ [✓] Add row totals [✓] Add column totals [Submit].

3 This statement performs the logistic regression specified by Model (5.39). The point-and-click command is the same as that given in Comment 1 on page 217 except that the variables *i.age i.alcohol* and *i.smoke* are entered in the *Independent variables* field of the *Model* tab.

4 The maximum value of the log likelihood function is −351.968 23. We will discuss this statistic in Section 5.24.

5 The highlighted odds ratios and confidence intervals are also given in Table 5.4. For example, *_IalcohoL4* and *_Ismoke_3* are the covariates $alcohol_{i4}$ and $smoke_{k3}$, respectively, in Model (5.39). The associated parameter estimates are $\hat{\beta}_4$ and $\hat{\gamma}_3$, which give odds ratio estimates $\hat{\psi}_{41} = \exp[\hat{\beta}_4] = 36.7912$ and $\hat{\psi}_{13} = \exp[\hat{\gamma}_3] = 5.159\,309$. Hence $\hat{\beta}_4 = \log[36.7912] = 3.6053$, and $\hat{\gamma}_3 = \log[5.159\,309] = 1.6408$. The 95% confidence intervals for these odds ratios are calculated using Equation (5.16).

6 The *lincom* post-estimation command calculates any linear combination of parameter estimates, tests the null hypothesis that the true value of this combination equals zero, and gives a 95% confidence interval for this estimate. In this example, the parameters associated with *_IalcohoL4* and *_Ismoke_3* are $\hat{\beta}_4$ and $\hat{\gamma}_3$, respectively, and the linear combination is $\hat{\beta}_4 + \hat{\gamma}_3$. When the *or* option is specified, *lincom* exponentiates this sum in its output, giving the odds ratio $\hat{\psi}_{43} = \exp[\hat{\beta}_4 + \hat{\gamma}_3] = \exp[3.6053 + 1.6408] = 189.8$. The 95% confidence interval for $\hat{\psi}_{43}$ is 66.9 – 538. This interval is calculated using Equation (5.32). The weights in Equation (5.29) are 1 for $\hat{\beta}_4$ and $\hat{\gamma}_3$, and 0 for the other parameters in the model. Thus, the cancer odds ratio for men who consume more than 119 g of alcohol and 29 g of tobacco a day is 189.8 relative to men whose daily consumption is less than 40 g of alcohol and 10 g of tobacco. The test of the null hypothesis that this odds ratio equals 1 is done using the $z$ statistic given in Equation (5.33). This hypothesis is rejected with overwhelming statistical significance. The equivalent point-and-click command is Statistics ▶ Postestimation ▶ Linear combinations of estimates ⌜ Linear expression: *_IalcohoL4* + *_IalcohoL3* ⌜ ☑ Exponentiate coefficients — ⦿ Odds ratio ⌟ Submit.

The results of this *lincom* command together with the other *lincom* commands given above are used to complete Table 5.4.

## 5.21. Model of two risk factors with interaction

Let us first return to the simple model of Section 5.18 where people either do or do not drink or smoke and where we do not adjust for age. Our multiplicative model was

$$\text{logit}[\text{E}[d_{ij} \mid ij]/n_{ij}] = \log\left[\frac{\pi_{ij}}{1-\pi_{ij}}\right] = \alpha + \beta_1 \times i + \beta_2 \times j,$$

where

$i$ = 1 or 0 for people who do or do not drink,
$j$ = 1 or 0 for people who do or do not smoke, and
$\pi_{ij}$ = the probability that someone with drinking status $i$ and smoking status $j$ develops cancer.

We next allow alcohol and tobacco to have a synergistic effect on cancer odds by including a fourth parameter as follows:

$$\text{logit}[\text{E}[d_{ij} \mid ij]/n_{ij}] = \alpha + \beta_1 \times i + \beta_2 \times j + \beta_3 \times i \times j. \qquad (5.40)$$

Note that $\beta_3$ only enters the model for people who both smoke and drink since for everyone else $i \times j = 0$. Under this model, subjects can be divided into four categories determined by whether they do or do not drink and whether they do or do not smoke. We can derive the cancer odds ratio associated with any one of these categories relative to any other by the type of argument that we have used in the preceding sections. Specifically, we write down the log odds for people in the numerator of the odds ratio, write down the log odds for people in the denominator of the odds ratio, and then subtract the denominator log odds from the numerator log odds. This gives us the desired log odds ratio. You should be able to show that

$\beta_1$ is the log odds ratio for cancer associated with alcohol among non-smokers,
$\beta_2$ is the log odds ratio for cancer associated with smoking among non-drinkers,
$\beta_1 + \beta_3$ is the log odds ratio for cancer associated with alcohol among smokers,
$\beta_2 + \beta_3$ is the log odds ratio for cancer associated with smoking among drinkers, and
$\beta_1 + \beta_2 + \beta_3$ is the log odds ratio for cancer associated with people who both smoke and drink compared with those who do neither.

Let $\psi_{ij}$ be the odds ratio associated with someone with drinking status $i$ and smoking status $j$ relative to people who neither smoke nor drink. Then $\psi_{10} = \exp[\beta_1]$, $\psi_{01} = \exp[\beta_2]$, and $\psi_{11} = \exp[\beta_1 + \beta_2 + \beta_3] = \psi_{10}\psi_{01}\exp[\beta_3]$. Hence, if $\beta_3 = 0$, then the multiplicative model holds. We can test the validity of the multiplicative model by testing the null hypothesis that $\beta_3 = 0$. If $\beta_3 > 0$, then the risk of both smoking and drinking will be greater than the product of the risk of smoking but not drinking and that of drinking but not smoking. If $\beta_3 < 0$, then the risk of both habits will be less than that of this product.

## 5.22. Model of alcohol, tobacco, and esophageal cancer with interaction terms

In order to weaken the multiplicative assumption implied by Model (5.39) we add interaction terms to the model. Specifically, we use the model

$$\text{logit}[\text{E}[d_{ijk} \mid ijk]/n_{ijk}] = \alpha + \sum_{h=2}^{6} \alpha_h \times age_h + \sum_{h=2}^{4} \beta_h \times alcohol_{ih}$$
$$+ \sum_{h=2}^{3} \gamma_h \times smoke_{kh} + \sum_{g=2}^{4}\sum_{h=2}^{3} \delta_{gh} \times alcohol_{ig} \times smoke_{kh}, \qquad (5.41)$$

where $i$, $j$, $k$, $d_{ijk}$, $n_{ijk}$, $\alpha$, $\alpha_h$, $age_h$, $\beta_h$, $alcohol_{ih}$, $\gamma_h$, and $smoke_{kh}$ are as defined in Model (5.39), and $\delta_{gh}$ is one of six new parameters that we have added to the model. This parameter is an interaction term that only appears in the model when both $i = g$ and $k = h$. For any $i > 1$ and $k > 1$, the log odds of cancer for a man from the $j^{\text{th}}$ age stratum who consumes alcohol level $i$ and tobacco level $k$ is

$$\log\left[\frac{\pi_{ijk}}{1 - \pi_{ijk}}\right] = \alpha + \alpha_j + \beta_i + \gamma_k + \delta_{ik}, \qquad (5.42)$$

where $\pi_{ijk}$ is his probability of having cancer. The log odds of cancer for a man from this age stratum who consumes both alcohol and tobacco at the first level is

$$\log\left[\frac{\pi_{1j1}}{1 - \pi_{1j1}}\right] = \alpha + \alpha_j. \qquad (5.43)$$

Subtracting Equation (5.43) from Equation (5.42) gives that the age-adjusted log odds ratio for men at the $i^{\text{th}}$ and $k^{\text{th}}$ levels of alcohol and tobacco exposure relative to men at the lowest levels of these drugs is

$$\log\left[\frac{\pi_{ijk}/(1 - \pi_{ijk})}{\pi_{1j1}/(1 - \pi_{1j1})}\right] = \beta_i + \gamma_k + \delta_{ik}. \qquad (5.44)$$

It is the presence of the $\delta_{ik}$ term in Equation (5.44) that permits this log odds ratio to be unaffected by the size of the other log odds ratios that can be estimated by the model. By the usual argument, $\beta_i$ is the log odds ratio for alcohol level $i$ versus level 1 among men at tobacco level 1, and $\gamma_k$ is the log odds ratio for tobacco level $k$ versus level 1 among men at alcohol level 1.

**Table 5.5.** Effect of alcohol and tobacco on the risk of esophageal cancer in the Ille-et-Vilaine study. These estimates are based on Model (5.41). This model contains interaction terms that permit the joint effects of alcohol and tobacco to vary from those dictated by the multiplicative model. Compare these results with those of Table 5.4

| | Daily tobacco consumption | | | | | |
|---|---|---|---|---|---|---|
| | 0–9 g | | 10–29 g | | ≥30 g | |
| Daily alcohol consumption | Odds ratio | 95% confidence interval | Odds ratio | 95% confidence interval | Odds ratio | 95% confidence interval |
| 10–39 g | 1.0* | | 3.80 | (1.6–9.2) | 8.65 | (2.4–31) |
| 40–79 g | 7.55 | (3.4–17) | 9.34 | (4.2–21) | 32.9 | (10–110) |
| 80–119 g | 12.7 | (5.2–31) | 16.1 | (6.8–38) | 72.3 | (15–350) |
| ≥120 g | 65.1 | (20–210) | 92.3 | (29–290) | 196 | (30–1300) |

*Denominator of odds ratios

Table 5.5 contains the age-adjusted odds ratios obtained by fitting Model (5.41) to the Ille-et-Vilaine data set and then applying Equation (5.44). The odds ratios in this table should be compared with those in Table 5.4. Note that among men who smoke less than 10 g a day the odds ratios increase more rapidly with increasing dose of alcohol in Table 5.5 than in Table 5.4. For example, $\hat{\psi}_{41}$ equals 65.1 in Table 5.5 but only 36.8 in Table 5.4. A similar comparison can be made among men at the lowest level of alcohol consumption with regard to rising exposure to tobacco. In Table 5.5 the odds ratios associated with the combined effects of different levels of alcohol and tobacco consumption are uniformly less than the product of the corresponding odds ratios for alcohol and tobacco alone. Note, however, that both models indicate a dramatic increase in cancer risk with increasing dose of alcohol and tobacco. The confidence intervals are wider in Table 5.5 than in Table 5.4 because they are derived from a model with more parameters and because some of the interaction parameter estimates have large standard errors due to the small number of subjects with the corresponding combined levels of alcohol and tobacco consumption.

## 5.23. Fitting a model with interaction using Stata

We next fit Model (5.41) to the Ille-et-Vilaine data set. The *5.20.EsophagealCa.log* log file that was started in Section 5.20 continues as follows.

```
. *
. * Regress cancer against age, alcohol and smoke.
. * Include alcohol-smoke interaction terms.
. *
. xi: logistic cancer i.age i.alcohol*i.smoke [freq=patients]            1

i.age              _Iage_1-6          (naturally coded; _Iage_1 omitted)
i.alcohol          _Ialcohol_1-4      (naturally coded; _Ialcohol_1 omitted)
i.smoke            _Ismoke_1-3        (naturally coded; _Ismoke_1 omitted)
i.alc~l*i.smoke    _IalcXsmo_#_#      (coded as above)

Logistic regression                               Number of obs   =       975
                                                  LR chi2(16)     =    290.90
                                                  Prob > chi2     =    0.0000
Log likelihood = -349.29335                       Pseudo R2       =    0.2940

------------------------------------------------------------------------------
      cancer | Odds Ratio   Std. Err.      z    P>|z|     [95% Conf. Interval]
-------------+----------------------------------------------------------------
     _Iage_2 |   6.697614   7.410168     1.72   0.086     .7658787    58.57068
     _Iage_3 |    40.1626   42.67237     3.48   0.001      5.00528    322.2665
     _Iage_4 |   69.55115   73.73317     4.00   0.000     8.708053    555.5044
     _Iage_5 |   123.0645   131.6687     4.50   0.000     15.11535    1001.953
     _Iage_6 |   118.8368   133.2476     4.26   0.000     13.19858    1069.977
  _Ialcohol_2 |   7.554406   3.043768     5.02   0.000     3.429574    16.64027     2
  _Ialcohol_3 |   12.71358   5.825001     5.55   0.000     5.179307    31.20787
  _Ialcohol_4 |   65.07188   39.54144     6.87   0.000     19.77671    214.1079
    _Ismoke_2 |   3.800862   1.703912     2.98   0.003     1.578671    9.151083     3
    _Ismoke_3 |   8.651205   5.569299     3.35   0.001     2.449668    30.55245
_IalcXsm~2_2 |   .3251915   .1746668    -2.09   0.036     .1134859    .9318291     4
_IalcXsm~2_3 |   .5033299   .4154535    -0.83   0.406     .0998303    2.537716
_IalcXsm~3_2 |   .3341452   .2008274    -1.82   0.068     .1028839    1.085233
_IalcXsm~3_3 |    .657279   .6598906    -0.42   0.676     .0918684     4.70255
_IalcXsm~4_2 |   .3731549   .3018038    -1.22   0.223     .0764621    1.821093
_IalcXsm~4_3 |   .3489097   .4210271    -0.87   0.383     .0327773    3.714089
------------------------------------------------------------------------------

. lincom _Ialcohol_2 + _Ismoke_2 + _IalcXsmo_2_2, or                      5

 ( 1)  _Ialcohol_2 + _Ismoke_2 + _IalcXsmo_2_2 = 0

------------------------------------------------------------------------------
      cancer | Odds Ratio   Std. Err.      z    P>|z|     [95% Conf. Interval]
-------------+----------------------------------------------------------------
```

| | | | | | | |
|---|---|---|---|---|---|---|
| (1) | 9.337306 | 3.826162 | 5.45 | 0.000 | 4.182379 | 20.84586 |

```
. lincom _Ialcohol_2 + _Ismoke_3 + _IalcXsmo_2_3, or
( 1)  _Ialcohol_2 + _Ismoke_3 + _IalcXsmo_2_3 = 0
```

| cancer | Odds Ratio | Std. Err. | z | P>\|z\| | [95% Conf. | Interval] |
|---|---|---|---|---|---|---|
| (1) | 32.89498 | 19.73769 | 5.82 | 0.000 | 10.14824 | 106.6274 |

```
. lincom _Ialcohol_3 + _Ismoke_2 + _IalcXsmo_3_2, or
( 1)  _Ialcohol_3 + _Ismoke_2 + _IalcXsmo_3_2 = 0
```

| cancer | Odds Ratio | Std. Err. | z | P>\|z\| | [95% Conf. | Interval] |
|---|---|---|---|---|---|---|
| (1) | 16.14675 | 7.152595 | 6.28 | 0.000 | 6.776802 | 38.47207 |

```
. lincom _Ialcohol_3 + _Ismoke_3 + _IalcXsmo_3_3, or
( 1)  _Ialcohol_3 + _Ismoke_3 + _IalcXsmo_3_3 = 0
```

| cancer | Odds Ratio | Std. Err. | z | P>\|z\| | [95% Conf. | Interval] |
|---|---|---|---|---|---|---|
| (1) | 72.29267 | 57.80896 | 5.35 | 0.000 | 15.08098 | 346.5446 |

```
. lincom _Ialcohol_4 + _Ismoke_2 + _IalcXsmo_4_2, or
( 1)  _Ialcohol_4 + _Ismoke_2 + _IalcXsmo_4_2 = 0
```

| cancer | Odds Ratio | Std. Err. | z | P>\|z\| | [95% Conf. | Interval] |
|---|---|---|---|---|---|---|
| (1) | 92.29212 | 53.97508 | 7.74 | 0.000 | 29.33307 | 290.3833 |

```
. lincom _Ialcohol_4 + _Ismoke_3 + _IalcXsmo_4_3, or
( 1)  _Ialcohol_4 + _Ismoke_3 + _IalcXsmo_4_3 = 0
```

| cancer | Odds Ratio | Std. Err. | z | P>\|z\| | [95% Conf. | Interval] |
|---|---|---|---|---|---|---|
| (1) | 196.4188 | 189.1684 | 5.48 | 0.000 | 29.74417 | 1297.072 |

**Comments**

1 This command performs the logistic regression specified by Model (5.41). The Stata variable *age* equals $j$ in this model, *alcohol* $= i$, and *smoke* $= k$. The syntax *i.alcohol**i.smoke* defines the following categorical variables that are included in the model:

$$\_IalcohoL2 = alcohol_{i2} = \begin{cases} 1\text{: if } alcohol = 2 \\ 0\text{: otherwise,} \end{cases}$$

$$\_IalcohoL3 = alcohol_{i3} = \begin{cases} 1\text{: if } alcohol = 3 \\ 0\text{: otherwise,} \end{cases}$$

$$\_IalcohoL4 = alcohol_{i4} = \begin{cases} 1\text{: if } alcohol = 4 \\ 0\text{: otherwise,} \end{cases}$$

$$\_Ismoke\_2 = smoke_{k2} = \begin{cases} 1\text{: if } smoke = 2 \\ 0\text{: otherwise,} \end{cases}$$

$$\_Ismoke\_3 = smoke_{k3} = \begin{cases} 1\text{: if } smoke = 3 \\ 0\text{: otherwise,} \end{cases}$$

$$\_IalcXsmo\_2\_2 = alcohol_{i2} \times smoke_{k2} = \_IalcohoL2 \times \_Ismoke\_2,$$
$$\_IalcXsmo\_2\_3 = alcohol_{i2} \times smoke_{k3} = \_IalcohoL2 \times \_Ismoke\_3,$$
$$\_IalcXsmo\_3\_2 = alcohol_{i3} \times smoke_{k2} = \_IalcohoL3 \times \_Ismoke\_2,$$
$$\_IalcXsmo\_3\_3 = alcohol_{i3} \times smoke_{k3} = \_IalcohoL3 \times \_Ismoke\_3,$$
$$\_IalcXsmo\_4\_2 = alcohol_{i4} \times smoke_{k2} = \_IalcohoL4 \times \_Ismoke\_2,$$

and

$$\_IalcXsmo\_4\_3 = alcohol_{i4} \times smoke_{k3} = \_IalcohoL4 \times \_Ismoke\_3.$$

A separate parameter is fitted for each of these variables. In addition, the model specifies five parameters for the five age indicator variables and a constant parameter.

The point-and-click command is the same as that given in Comment 1 on page 217 except that the variables *i.age* and *i.alcohol**i.smoke* are entered in the *Independent variables* field of the *Model* tab.

2 The parameter associated with the covariate *_IalcohoL2* $= alcohol_{i2}$ is $\beta_2$; $\hat{\psi}_{21} = \exp[\hat{\beta}_2] = 7.5544$ is the estimated age-adjusted odds ratio for men at alcohol level 2 and tobacco level 1 relative to men at alcohol level 1 and tobacco level 1. The odds ratios and confidence intervals highlighted in this output were used to produce Table 5.5.

3 The parameter associated with the covariate *_Ismoke_2* $= smoke_{k2}$ is $\gamma_2$; $\hat{\psi}_{12} = \exp[\hat{\gamma}_2] = 3.8009$ is the estimated age-adjusted odds ratio for men at alcohol level 1 and tobacco level 2 relative to men at alcohol level 1 and tobacco level 1.

4 The parameter associated with the covariate *_IalcXsmo_2_2* = $alcohol_{i2} \times smoke_{k2}$ is $\delta_{22}$. Note that due to lack of room, Stata abbreviates this covariate in the left-hand column as *_IalcXsmo~2_2*. This interaction parameter does not equal any specific odds ratio. Nevertheless, Stata outputs $\exp[\hat{\delta}_{22}] = 0.3252$ in the odds ratio column.
5 This statement uses Equation (5.44) to calculate $\hat{\psi}_{22} = \exp[\hat{\beta}_2 + \hat{\gamma}_2 + \hat{\delta}_{22}] = 9.3373$. This is the age-adjusted odds ratio for men at the second level of alcohol and tobacco consumption relative to men at the first level of both of these variables.

Stata also has the ability to efficiently execute repetitive commands. The six *lincom* commands given here could also have been executed with the following syntax:

```
forvalues i = 2/4 {
  forvalues j = 2/3 {
    lincom _Ialcohol_`i' + _Ismoke_`j' + _IalcXsmo_`i'_`j'
  }
}
```

Users who have had some previous experience with programming languages that permit iterative looping may wish to consider the *forvalues* command. It can save time in situations that call for a tedious repetition of combinations of Stata commands. See the Stata Programming Manual for additional details.

## 5.24. Model fitting: nested models and model deviance

A model $\hat{y}$ is said to be **nested** within a second model if the first model is a special case of the second. For example, the multiplicative Model (5.35) was

$$\text{logit}[\text{E}[d_{ij} \mid ij]/n_{ij}] = \alpha + \beta_1 \times i + \beta_2 \times j,$$

while Model (5.40), which contained an interaction term, was

$$\text{logit}[\text{E}[d_{ij} \mid ij]/n_{ij}] = \alpha + \beta_1 \times i + \beta_2 \times j + \beta_3 \times i \times j.$$

Model (5.35) is nested within Model (5.40) since Model (5.35) is a special case of Model (5.40) with $\beta_3 = 0$.

The model **deviance** $D$ is a statistic derived from the likelihood function that measures goodness of fit of the data to the model. Suppose that a model has parameters $\beta_1, \beta_2, \ldots, \beta_q$. Let $L[\beta_1, \beta_2, \ldots, \beta_q]$ denote the likelihood function for this model and let $\hat{L} = L[\hat{\beta}_1, \hat{\beta}_2, \ldots, \hat{\beta}_q]$ denote the maximum value of the likelihood function over all possible values of the parameters. Then the model deviance is

$$D = K - 2\log[\hat{L}], \tag{5.45}$$

where $K$ is a constant. The value of $K$ is always the same for any two models that are nested. $D$ is always non-negative. Large values of $D$ indicate poor model fit; a perfect fit has $D = 0$.

Suppose that $D_1$ and $D_2$ are the deviances from two models and that model 1 is nested within model 2. Let $\hat{L}_1$ and $\hat{L}_2$ denote the maximum values of the likelihood functions for these models. Then it can be shown that if model 1 is true,

$$\Delta D = D_1 - D_2 = 2(\log[\hat{L}_2] - \log[\hat{L}_1]) = -2\log[\hat{L}_1/\hat{L}_2] \tag{5.46}$$

has an approximately $\chi^2$ distribution with the number of degrees of freedom equal to the difference in the number of parameters between the two models. We use this reduction in deviance as a guide to building reasonable models for our data. Equation (5.46) is an example of a likelihood ratio test (see Section 4.9.1).

To illustrate the use of this test consider the Ille-et-Vilaine data. The multiplicative Model (5.39) of alcohol and tobacco levels is nested within Model (5.41). The log file given in Sections 5.20 and 5.23 show that the maximum log likelihoods for Models (5.39) and (5.41) are

$\log[\hat{L}_1] = -351.968$ and $\log[\hat{L}_2] = -349.293$, respectively.

Therefore, the reduction in deviance is

$$\Delta D = 2(\log[\hat{L}_2] - \log[\hat{L}_1]) = 2(-349.293 + 351.968) = 5.35.$$

Since there are six more parameters in the interactive model than the multiplicative model, $\Delta D$ has a $\chi^2$ distribution with six degrees of freedom if the multiplicative model is true. The probability that this $\chi^2$ statistic exceeds 5.35 is $P = 0.50$. Thus, there is no statistical evidence to suggest that the multiplicative model is false, or that any meaningful improvement in the model fit can be obtained by adding interaction terms to the model.

There are no hard and fast guidelines to model building other than that it is best not to include uninteresting variables in the model that have a trivial effect on the model deviance. In general, I am guided by deviance reduction statistics when deciding whether to include variables that may, or may not, be true confounders, but that are not intrinsically of interest. It is important to bear in mind, however, that failure to reject the null hypothesis that the nested model is true does not prove the validity of this model. We will discuss this further in the next section.

## 5.25. Effect modifiers and confounding variables

An **effect modifier** is a variable that influences the effect of a risk factor on the outcome variable. In the preceding example, smoking is a powerful effect modifier of alcohol and vice versa. The key difference between confounding variables and effect modifiers is that confounding variables are not of primary interest in our study while effect modifiers are. A variable is an important effect modifier if there is a meaningful interaction between it and the exposure of interest on the risk of the event under study. Clearly, any variable that requires an interaction term in a regression model is an effect modifier. It is common practice to be fairly tolerant of the multiplicative model assumption for confounding variables but less tolerant of this assumption when we are considering variables of primary interest. For example, Model (5.41) assumes that age and either of the other two variables have a multiplicative effect on the cancer odds ratio. Although this assumption may not be precisely true, including age in the model in this way does adjust to a considerable extent for the confounding effects of age on the relationship between alcohol, smoking, and esophageal cancer. Similarly, if you only wanted to present the effects of alcohol on esophageal cancer adjusted for age and smoking, or the effects of smoking on esophageal cancer adjusted for age and alcohol, then the multiplicative Model (5.39) would do just fine. The lack of significance of the deviance reduction statistic between Models (5.39) and (5.41) provides ample justification for using Model (5.39) to adjust for the confounding effects of age and smoking on the cancer risk associated with alcohol consumption. On the other hand, when we present a table such as Table 5.5, we need to be careful to neither overestimate nor underestimate the joint effects of two risk factors on the outcome of interest. For this reason, I recommend that you include an interaction term when presenting the joint effects of two variables unless there is strong evidence that the multiplicative assumption is true. Hence, my personal preference is for Table 5.5 over Table 5.4 even though we are unable to reject Model (5.39) in favor of Model (5.41) with statistical significance.

## 5.26. Goodness-of-fit tests

We need to be able to determine whether our model gives a good fit to our data, and to detect outliers that have an undue effect on our inferences. Many of the concepts that we introduced for linear regression have counterparts in logistic regression.

### 5.26.1. The Pearson $\chi^2$ goodness-of-fit statistic

Let us return to the general multiple logistic regression Model (5.12). Suppose that there are $J$ distinct covariate patterns and that $d_j$ events occur among $n_j$ patients with the covariate pattern $x_{j1}, x_{j2}, \ldots, x_{jq}$. Let $\pi_j = \pi[x_{j1}, x_{j2}, \ldots, x_{jq}]$ denote the probability that a patient with the $j^{\text{th}}$ pattern of covariate values suffers an event, which is given by Equation (5.13). Then $d_j$ has a binomial distribution with expected value $n_j\pi_j$ and standard error $\sqrt{n_j\pi_j(1-\pi_j)}$. Hence

$$(d_j - n_j\pi_j)\Big/\sqrt{n_j\pi_j(1-\pi_j)} \tag{5.47}$$

will have a mean of 0 and a standard error of 1. Let

$$\hat{\pi}_j = \frac{\exp[\alpha + \hat{\beta}_1 x_{j_1} + \hat{\beta}_2 x_{j2} + \cdots + \hat{\beta}_q x_{jq}]}{1 + \exp[\hat{\alpha} + \hat{\beta}_1 x_{j_1} + \hat{\beta}_2 x_{j2} + \cdots + \hat{\beta}_q x_{jq}]} \tag{5.48}$$

be the estimate of $\pi_j$ obtained by substituting the maximum likelihood parameter estimates into Equation (5.13). Then the **residual** for the $j^{\text{th}}$ covariate pattern is $d_j - n_j\hat{\pi}_j$. Substituting $\hat{\pi}_j$ for $\pi_j$ in the Equation (5.47) gives the **Pearson residual**, which is

$$r_j = (d_j - n_j\hat{\pi}_j)\Big/\sqrt{n_j\hat{\pi}_j(1-\hat{\pi}_j)}. \tag{5.49}$$

If Model (5.12) is correct and $n_j$ is sufficiently large, then

$$\chi^2 = \sum r_j^2 \tag{5.50}$$

will have a chi-squared distribution with $J - (q+1)$ degrees of freedom. Equation (5.50) is the **Pearson chi-squared goodness-of-fit statistic**. It can be used as a goodness-of-fit test of Model (5.12) as long as $J$, the number of distinct covariate patterns, is small in comparison with the number of study subjects. A conservative rule of thumb is that the estimated expected number of events $n_j\hat{\pi}_j$ should be at least 5 and not greater than $n_j - 5$ for each distinct pattern of covariates. In this case, we can reject Model (5.12) if the *P*-value associated with this chi-squared statistic is less than 0.05.

It should be noted that the meaning of $\hat{\pi}_j$ depends on whether we are analyzing data from a prospective or case–control study. In an unbiased prospective study, $\hat{\pi}_j$ estimates the probability that someone from the underlying population with the $j^{\text{th}}$ covariate pattern will suffer the event of interest. In a case–control study we are unable to estimate this probability (see Sections 4.19.2 and 4.23). Nevertheless, we can still perform valid goodness-of-fit tests and residual analyses even though the value of $\hat{\pi}_j$ is greatly affected by our study design and is not directly related to the probability of disease in the underlying population.

## 5.27. Hosmer–Lemeshow goodness-of-fit test

When some of the covariates are continuous we may have a unique covariate pattern for each patient, and it is likely that the number of covariate patterns will increase with increasing sample size. In this situation, Equation (5.50) will not provide a valid goodness-of-fit test. Hosmer and Lemeshow (1980, 2000) proposed the following test for this situation. First, sort the covariate patterns by increasing values of $\hat{\pi}_j$. Then, divide the patients into $g$ groups containing approximately equal numbers of subjects in such a way that subjects with the lowest values of $\hat{\pi}_j$ are in group 1, subjects with the next lowest values of $\hat{\pi}_j$ are in group 2, and so on – the last group consisting of subjects with the largest values of $\hat{\pi}_j$. Summing within each group, let $m_k = \sum n_j$ and $o_k = \sum d_j$ be the total number of subjects and events in the $k^{\text{th}}$ group, respectively. Let $\bar{\pi}_k = \sum n_j \hat{\pi}_j / m_k$ be a weighted average of the values of $\hat{\pi}_j$ in the $k^{\text{th}}$ group. Then the **Hosmer–Lemeshow goodness-of-fit statistic** is

$$\hat{C} = \sum_{k=1}^{g} \frac{(o_k - m_k\bar{\pi}_k)^2}{m_k\bar{\pi}_k(1 - \bar{\pi}_k)}. \tag{5.51}$$

If Model (5.12) is true, then $\hat{C}$ has an approximately chi-squared distribution with $g - 2$ degrees of freedom. We reject this model if $\hat{C}$ exceeds the critical value associated with the 0.05 significance level of a chi-squared statistic with $g - 2$ degrees of freedom. A value of $g = 10$ is often used in this test.

### 5.27.1. An example: the Ille-et-Vilaine cancer data set

In Section 5.22 we fitted Model (5.41) to the Ille-et-Vilaine esophageal cancer data set. Under this model there are 68 distinct covariate patterns in the data. The number of patients associated with these patterns varies considerably from pattern to pattern. For example, there is only one subject age 25–34 who drank 80–119 grams of alcohol and smoked 10–29 grams of tobacco each day, while there were 34 subjects age 65–74 who drank 40–79 grams of alcohol and smoked 0–9 grams of tobacco a day. Let's designate this latter group as having the $j^{\text{th}}$ covariate pattern. Then in this group there were $d_j = 17$ esophageal cancer cases among $n_j = 34$ subjects. Under Model (5.41), the estimated probability that a subject in this group was a case is $\hat{\pi}_j = 0.393\,38$. Hence, the expected number of esophageal cancers is $n_j\hat{\pi}_j = 34 \times 0.393\,38 = 13.375$ and the residual for this pattern is

$$d_j - n_j\hat{\pi}_j = 17 - 13.375 = 3.625.$$

The Pearson residual is

$$r_j = (d_j - n_j\hat{\pi}_j)\Big/\sqrt{n_j\hat{\pi}_j(1-\hat{\pi}_j)}$$
$$= \frac{3.625}{\sqrt{34 \times 0.393\,38 \times (1 - 0.393\,38)}} = 1.2727.$$

Performing similar calculations for all of the other covariate patterns and summing the squares of these residuals gives

$$\chi^2 = \sum_{j=1}^{68} r_j^2 = 55.85.$$

As there are $q = 16$ covariates in Model (5.41) this Pearson goodness-of-fit statistic will have $68 - 16 - 1 = 51$ degrees of freedom. The probability that such a statistic exceeds 55.85 equals 0.30.

In this example there are 27 covariate patterns in which the expected number of cancers is less than one and there are 51 patterns in which the expected number of cancers is less than five. This raises serious doubts as to whether we can assume that the Pearson goodness-of-fit statistic has a chi-squared distribution under the null hypothesis that Model (5.41) is true. For this reason, the Hosmer–Lemeshow goodness-of-fit test is a better statistic for this model. Sorting the covariate patterns by the values of $\hat{\pi}_j$ gives probabilities that range from $\hat{\pi}_1 = 0.000\,697$ to $\hat{\pi}_{68} = 0.944\,011$. To calculate this test with $g = 10$ we first divide the covariate patterns into ten groups with approximately equal numbers of patients in each group. There are 975 patients in the study so we would prefer to have 97 or 98 patients in each group. We may be forced to deviate from this target in order to keep all patients with the same pattern in the same group. For example, the three lowest cancer probabilities associated with distinct covariate patterns are $\hat{\pi}_1 = 0.000\,697$, $\hat{\pi}_2 = 0.002\,644\,2$, and $\hat{\pi}_3 = 0.004\,65$. The numbers of patients with these patterns are $n_1 = 40$, $n_2 = 16$, and $n_3 = 60$. Now $n_1 + n_2 + n_3 = 116$ is closer to 97.5 than $n_1 + n_2 = 56$. Hence, we choose the first of the ten groups to consist of the 116 patients with the three lowest estimated cancer probabilities. The remaining nine groups are chosen similarly. Among patients with the three covariate patterns associated with the smallest cancer probabilities, there were no cancer cases giving $d_1 = d_2 = d_3 = 0$. Hence, for the first group

$$m_1 = n_1 + n_2 + n_3 = 116,\ o_1 = d_1 + d_2 + d_3 = 0,$$
$$\bar{\pi}_1 = (n_1\hat{\pi}_1 + n_2\hat{\pi}_2 + n_3\hat{\pi}_3)/m_1 = (40 \times 0.000\,697 + 16 \times 0.002\,644 + 60 \times 0.004\,65)/116 = 0.003\,01,$$

and

$$\frac{(o_1 - m_1\bar{\pi}_1)^2}{m_1\bar{\pi}_1(1-\bar{\pi}_1)} = (0 - 116 \times 0.003\,01)^2/(116 \times 0.003\,01 \times (1 - 0.003\,01)) = 0.350.$$

Performing the analogous computations for the other nine groups and summing the standardized squared residuals gives

$$\hat{C} = \sum_{k=1}^{10} \frac{(o_k - m_k\bar{\pi}_k)^2}{m_k\bar{\pi}_k(1-\bar{\pi}_k)} = 4.728.$$

This Hosmer–Lemeshow test statistic has eight degrees of freedom. The probability that a chi-squared statistic with eight degrees of freedom exceeds 4.728 is $P = 0.7862$. Hence, this test provides no evidence to reject Model (5.41).

## 5.28. Residual and influence analysis

Of course, the failure to reject a model by a goodness-of-fit test does not prove that the model is true or fits the data well. For this reason, residual analyses are always advisable for any results that are to be published. A residual analysis for a logistic regression model is analogous to one for linear regression. Although the standard error of $d_j$ is $\text{se}[d_j] = \sqrt{n_j\pi_j(1-\pi_j)}$, the standard error of the residual $d_j - n_j\hat{\pi}_j$ is less than $\text{se}[d_j]$ due to the fact that the maximum likelihood values of the parameter estimates tend to shift $n_j\hat{\pi}_j$ in the direction of $d_j$. The ability of an individual covariate pattern to reduce the standard deviation of its associated residual is measured by the **leverage** $h_j$ (Pregibon, 1981). The formula for $h_j$ is complex and not terribly edifying. For our purposes, we can define $h_j$ by the formula

$$\text{var}[d_j - n_j\hat{\pi}_j] = n_j\hat{\pi}_j(1-\hat{\pi}_j)(1-h_j) \cong \text{var}[d_j - n_j\pi_j](1-h_j). \tag{5.52}$$

In other words, $100(1 - h_j)$ is the percent reduction in the variance of the $j^{\text{th}}$ residual due to the fact that the estimate of $n_j\hat{\pi}_j$ is pulled towards $d_j$. The value of $h_j$ lies between 0 and 1. When $h_j$ is very small, $d_j$ has almost no effect on its estimated expected value $n_j\hat{\pi}_j$. When $h_j$ is close to one, then $d_j \cong n_j\hat{\pi}_j$. This implies that both the residual $d_j - n_j\hat{\pi}_j$ and its variance will be close to zero. This definition of leverage is highly analogous to that given for linear regression. See, in particular, Equation (2.26).

### 5.28.1. Standardized Pearson residual

The **standardized Pearson residual** for the $j^{\text{th}}$ covariate pattern is the residual divided by its standard error. That is,

$$r_{sj} = \frac{d_j - n_j\pi_j}{\sqrt{n_j\hat{\pi}_j(1 - \hat{\pi}_j)(1 - h_j)}} = \frac{r_j}{\sqrt{1 - h_j}}. \tag{5.53}$$

This residual is analogous to the standardized residual for linear regression (see Equation 2.27). The key difference between Equation (2.27) and Equation (5.53) is that the standardized residual has a known $t$ distribution under the linear model. Although $r_{sj}$ has mean zero and standard error one it does not have a normally shaped distribution when $n_j$ is small. The square of the standardized Pearson residual is denoted by

$$\Delta X_j^2 = r_{sj}^2 = r_j^2/(1 - h_j). \tag{5.54}$$

We will use the critical value $(z_{0.025})^2 = 1.96^2 = 3.84$ as a very rough guide to identifying large values of $\Delta X_j^2$. Approximately 95% of these squared residuals should be less than 3.84 if the logistic regression model is correct.

### 5.28.2. $\Delta\hat{\beta}_j$ influence statistic

Covariate patterns that are associated with both high leverage and large residuals can have a substantial influence on the parameter estimates of the model. The $\Delta\hat{\beta}_j$ **influence statistic** is a measure of the influence of the $j^{\text{th}}$ covariate pattern on all of the parameter estimates taken together (Pregibon, 1981), and equals

$$\Delta\hat{\beta}_j = r_{sj}^2 h_j/(1 - h_j). \tag{5.55}$$

Note that $\Delta\hat{\beta}_j$ increases with both the magnitude of the standardized residual and the size of the leverage. It is analogous to Cook's distance for linear

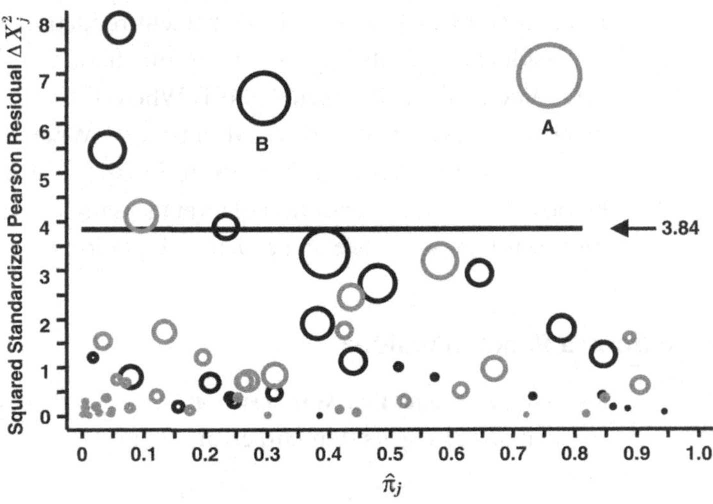


Figure 5.1 Squared residual plot of $\Delta X_j^2$ against $\hat{\pi}_j$ for the esophageal cancer data analyzed with model (5.41). A separate circle is plotted for each distinct covariate pattern. The area of each circle is proportional to the influence statistic $\Delta\hat{\beta}_j$. $\Delta X_j^2$ is the squared standardized Pearson residual for the $j^{\text{th}}$ covariate pattern; $\hat{\pi}_j$ is the estimated probability that a study subject with this pattern is one of the case patients. Black and gray circles indicate positive and negative residuals, respectively. Two circles associated with covariate patterns having large influence and big squared residuals are labeled A and B (see text).

regression (see Section 3.21.2). Covariate patterns associated with large values of $\Delta X_j^2$ and $\Delta\hat{\beta}_j$ merit special attention.

### 5.28.3. Residual plots of the Ille-et-Vilaine data on esophageal cancer

Figure 5.1 shows a plot of the squared residuals $\Delta X_j^2$ against the estimated cancer probability for Model (5.41). Each circle represents the squared residual associated with a unique covariate pattern. The area of each circle is proportional to $\Delta\hat{\beta}_j$. Black circles are used to indicate positive residuals while gray circles indicate negative residuals. Hosmer and Lemeshow (2000) first suggested this form of residual plot. They recommend that the area of the plotted circles be 1.5 times the magnitude of $\Delta\hat{\beta}_j$. Figure 5.1 does not reveal any obvious relationship between the magnitude of the residuals and the values of $\hat{\pi}_j$. There are 68 unique covariate patterns in this data set. Five percent of 68 equals 3.4. Hence, if Model (5.41) is correct we would expect three or four squared residuals to be greater than 3.84. There are six such

**Table 5.6.** Effects on odds ratios from Model (5.41) due to deleting patients with covariates A and B identified in Figure 5.1 (see text)

| Daily drug consumption | | Complete data | | Deleted covariate pattern | | | |
|---|---|---|---|---|---|---|---|
| | | | | A† | | B‡ | |
| Tobacco | Alcohol | Odds ratio | 95% confidence interval | Odds ratio | Percent change from complete data | Odds ratio | Percent change from complete data |
| 0–9 g | 0–39 g | 1.0* | | 1.0* | | 1.0* | |
| 0–9 g | 40–79 g | 7.55 | (3.4–17) | 7.53 | −0.26 | 7.70 | 2.0 |
| 0–9 g | 80–119 g | 12.7 | (5.2–31) | 12.6 | −0.79 | 13.0 | 2.4 |
| 0–9 g | ≥120 g | 65.1 | (20–210) | 274 | 321 | 66.8 | 2.6 |
| 10–29 g | 0–39 g | 3.80 | (1.6–9.2) | 3.77 | −0.79 | 3.86 | 1.6 |
| 10–29 g | 40–79 g | 9.34 | (4.2–21) | 9.30 | −0.43 | 9.53 | 2.0 |
| 10–29 g | 80–119 g | 16.1 | (6.8–38) | 16.0 | −0.62 | 16.6 | 3.1 |
| 10–29 g | ≥120 g | 92.3 | (29–290) | 95.4 | −3.4 | 94.0 | 1.8 |
| ≥30 g | 0–39 g | 8.65 | (2.4–31) | 8.66 | −0.12 | 1.88 | −78 |
| ≥30 g | 40–79 g | 32.9 | (10–110) | 33.7 | −2.4 | 33.5 | 1.8 |
| ≥30 g | 80–119 g | 72.3 | (15–350) | 73.0 | −0.97 | 74.2 | 2.6 |
| ≥30 g | ≥120 g | 196 | (30–1300) | 198 | −1.02 | 203 | 3.6 |

* Denominator of odds ratios

† Patients age 55–64 who drink at least 120 g a day and smoke 0–9 g a day deleted

‡ Patients age 55–64 who drink 0–39 g a day and smoke at least 30 g a day deleted

residuals with two of them being close to 3.84. Thus, the magnitude of the residuals is reasonably consistent with Model (5.41).

There are two large squared residuals in Figure 5.1 that have high influence. These squared residuals are labeled A and B in this figure. Residual A is associated with patients who are age 55–64 and consume, on a daily basis, at least 120 g of alcohol and 0–9 g of tobacco. Residual B is associated with patients who are age 55–64 and consume, on a daily basis, 0–39 g of alcohol and at least 30 g of tobacco. The $\Delta\hat{\beta}_j$ influence statistics associated with residuals A and B are 6.16 and 4.15, respectively. Table 5.6 shows the effects of deleting patients with these covariate patterns from the analysis. Column 3 of this table repeats the odds ratio given in Table 5.5. Columns 5 and 7 show the odds ratios that result when patients with covariate patterns A and B are deleted from Model (5.41). Deleting patients with pattern A increases the odds ratio for men who smoke 0–9 g and drink ≥120 g from

65.1 to 274. This is a 321% increase that places this odds ratio outside of its 95% confidence interval based on the complete data. The other odds ratios in Table 5.5 are not greatly changed by deleting these patients. Deleting the patients associated with covariate pattern B causes a 78% reduction in the odds ratio for men who smoke at least 30 g and drink 0–39 g a day. Their deletion does not greatly affect the other odds ratios in this table.

How should these analyses guide the way in which we present these results? Here, reasonable investigators may disagree on the best way to proceed. My own inclination would be to publish Table 5.5. This table provides compelling evidence that tobacco and alcohol are strong independent risk factors for esophageal cancer and indicates an impressive synergy between these two risk factors. Deleting patients with covariate patterns A and B does not greatly alter this conclusion, although it does profoundly alter the size of two of these odds ratios. On the other hand, the size of some of the $\Delta\hat{\beta}_j$ influence statistics in Figure 5.1 and the width of the confidence intervals in Table 5.5 provide a clear warning that Model (5.41) is approaching the upper limit of complexity that is reasonable for this data set. A more conservative approach would be not to report the combined effects of alcohol and smoking, or to use just two levels of consumption for each drug rather than three or four. Model (5.39) could be used to report the odds ratios associated with different levels of alcohol consumption adjusted for tobacco usage. This model could also be used to estimate odds ratios associated with different tobacco levels adjusted for alcohol.

Residual analyses in logistic regression are in many ways similar to those for linear regression. There is, however, one important difference. In linear regression, an influential observation is made on a single patient and there is always the possibility that this result is invalid and should be discarded from the analysis. In logistic regression, an influential observation usually is due to the response from multiple patients with the same covariate pattern. Hence, deleting these observations is not an option. Nevertheless, residual analyses are worthwhile in that they help us evaluate how well the model fits the data and can indicate instabilities that can arise from excessively complicated models.

## 5.29. Using Stata for goodness-of-fit tests and residual analyses

We next perform the analyses discussed in the preceding sections. The *5.20.EsophagealCa.log* that was discussed in Sections 5.20 and 5.23 continues as follows:

```
. *
. *   Perform Pearson chi-squared and Hosmer-Lemeshow tests of
. *   goodness of fit.
. *
. estat gof                                                    1

Logistic model for cancer, goodness-of-fit test

        number of observations =         975
  number of covariate patterns =          68
             Pearson chi2(51)  =        55.85
                  Prob > chi2  =        0.2977

. estat gof, group(10) table                                   2

Logistic model for cancer, goodness-of-fit test

  (Table collapsed on quantiles of estimated probabilities)
```

| Group | Prob | Obs_1 | Exp_1 | Obs_0 | Exp_0 | Total |
|---|---|---|---|---|---|---|
| 1 | 0.0046 | 0 | 0.3 | 116 | 115.7 | 116 |
| 2 | 0.0273 | 2 | 2.0 | 118 | 118.0 | 120 |
| 3 | 0.0418 | 4 | 3.1 | 76 | 76.9 | 80 |
| 4 | 0.0765 | 4 | 5.1 | 87 | 85.9 | 91 |
| 5 | 0.1332 | 5 | 7.8 | 81 | 78.2 | 86 |
| 6 | 0.2073 | 21 | 20.2 | 91 | 91.8 | 112 |
| 7 | 0.2682 | 22 | 22.5 | 65 | 64.5 | 87 |
| 8 | 0.3833 | 32 | 28.5 | 56 | 59.5 | 88 |
| 9 | 0.5131 | 46 | 41.6 | 52 | 56.4 | 98 |
| 10 | 0.9440 | 64 | 68.9 | 33 | 28.1 | 97 |

```
        number of observations =         975
              number of groups =          10
     Hosmer-Lemeshow chi2(8)   =         4.73
                  Prob > chi2  =        0.7862

. *
. *  Perform residual analysis
. *
```

```
. predict p, p                                                                3

. label variable p "Estimate of pi for the jth Covariate Pattern"

. predict dx2, dx2                                                            4

(57 missing values generated)

. predict rstandard, rstandard                                                5

(57 missing values generated)

. generate dx2_pos = dx2 if rstandard >= 0                                    6

(137 missing values generated)

. generate dx2_neg = dx2 if rstandard <  0

(112 missing values generated)

. predict dbeta, dbeta                                                        7

(57 missing values generated)

. scatter dx2_pos p [weight=dbeta], symbol(oh) mlwidth(thick)                 8
>     || scatter dx2_neg p [weight=dbeta]                                     9
>          , symbol(oh) mlwidth(thick) color(gray)
>     , ylabel(0(1)8) ytick(0(.5)8) yline(3.84)
>       xlabel(0(.1)1) xtick(0(.05)1) legend(off)
>       ytitle("Squared Standardized Pearson Residual")
                                                                 Output omitted

. save temporary, replace                                                    10

file temporary.dta saved

. drop if patients == 0                                                      11
(57 observations deleted)

. generate ca_no = cancer*patients

. collapse (sum) n = patients ca = ca_no                                     12
>    , by(age alcohol smoke dbeta dx2 p)

. *
. *  Identify covariate patterns associated with
. *  large squared residuals.
```

```
. *
. list n ca age alcohol smoke dbeta dx2 p if dx2 > 3.84                    13
```

| | n | ca | age | alcohol | smoke | dbeta | dx2 | p |
|---|---|---|---|---|---|---|---|---|
| 11. | 2 | 1 | 25-34 | >= 120 | 10-29 | 1.335425 | 7.942312 | .060482 |
| 17. | 37 | 4 | 35-44 | 40-79 | 10-29 | 1.890465 | 5.466789 | .041798 |
| 22. | 3 | 2 | 35-44 | >= 120 | 0-9 | .9170162 | 3.896309 | .2331274 |
| 25. | 28 | 0 | 45-54 | 0-39 | 10-29 | 1.564479 | 4.114906 | .0962316 |
| 38. | 6 | 4 | 55-64 | 0-39 | >= 30 | 4.159096 | 6.503713 | .2956251 |
| 45. | 10 | 5 | 55-64 | >= 120 | 0-9 | 6.159449 | 6.949361 | .7594333 |

```
. *
. *  Rerun analysis without the covariate pattern A
. *
. use temporary, clear                                                      14
. drop if age == 4 & alcohol == 4 & smoke == 1                              15
(2 observations deleted)
. xi: logistic cancer i.age i.alcohol*i.smoke [freq=patients]               16
```

Output omitted

| cancer | Odds Ratio | Std. Err. | z | P>\|z\| | [95% Conf. | Interval] |
|---|---|---|---|---|---|---|
| Output omitted | | | | | | |
| _Ialcohol_2 | 7.525681 | 3.032792 | 5.01 | 0.000 | 3.416001 | 16.57958 |
| _Ialcohol_3 | 12.62548 | 5.790079 | 5.53 | 0.000 | 5.139068 | 31.01781 |
| _Ialcohol_4 | 273.8578 | 248.0885 | 6.20 | 0.000 | 46.38949 | 1616.705 |
| _Ismoke_2 | 3.76567 | 1.6883 | 2.96 | 0.003 | 1.563921 | 9.067132 |
| _Ismoke_3 | 8.65512 | 5.583627 | 3.35 | 0.001 | 2.444232 | 30.64811 |
| Output omitted | | | | | | |

```
. lincom _Ialcohol_2 + _Ismoke_2 + _IalcXsmo_2_2, or
```

Output omitted

| cancer | Odds Ratio | Std. Err. | z | P>\|z\| | [95% Conf. Interval] | |
|---|---|---|---|---|---|---|
| (1) | 9.298176 | 3.811849 | 5.44 | 0.000 | 4.163342 | 20.76603 |

```
. lincom _Ialcohol_2 + _Ismoke_3 + _IalcXsmo_2_3, or
( 1) _Ialcohol_2 + _Ismoke_3 + _IalcXsmo_2_3 = 0
```

| cancer | Odds Ratio | Std. Err. | z | P>\|z\| | [95% Conf. Interval] | |
|---|---|---|---|---|---|---|
| (1) | 33.6871 | 20.40138 | 5.81 | 0.000 | 10.27932 | 110.3985 |

```
. lincom _Ialcohol_3 + _Ismoke_2 + _IalcXsmo_3_2, or
( 1) _Ialcohol_3 + _Ismoke_2 + _IalcXsmo_3_2 = 0
```

| cancer | Odds Ratio | Std. Err. | z | P>\|z\| | [95% Conf. Interval] | |
|---|---|---|---|---|---|---|
| (1) | 16.01118 | 7.097924 | 6.26 | 0.000 | 6.715472 | 38.1742 |

```
. lincom _Ialcohol_3 + _Ismoke_3 + _IalcXsmo_3_3, or
( 1) _Ialcohol_3 + _Ismoke_3 + _IalcXsmo_3_3 = 0
```

| cancer | Odds Ratio | Std. Err. | z | P>\|z\| | [95% Conf. Interval] | |
|---|---|---|---|---|---|---|
| (1) | 73.00683 | 58.92606 | 5.32 | 0.000 | 15.00833 | 355.1358 |

```
. lincom _Ialcohol_4 + _Ismoke_2 + _IalcXsmo_4_2, or
( 1) _Ialcohol_4 + _Ismoke_2 + _IalcXsmo_4_2 = 0
```

| cancer | Odds Ratio | Std. Err. | z | P>\|z\| | [95% Conf. Interval] | |
|---|---|---|---|---|---|---|
| (1) | 95.43948 | 56.55247 | 7.69 | 0.000 | 29.87792 | 304.8638 |

```
. lincom _Ialcohol_4 + _Ismoke_3 + _IalcXsmo_4_3, or
```

```
( 1)  _Ialcohol_4 + _Ismoke_3 + _IalcXsmo_4_3 = 0
```

| cancer | Odds Ratio | Std. Err. | z | P>\|z\| | [95% Conf. | Interval] |
|---|---|---|---|---|---|---|
| (1) | 197.7124 | 192.6564 | 5.43 | 0.000 | 29.28192 | 1334.96 |

```
. *
. *  Rerun analysis without the covariate pattern B
. *
. use temporary, clear
```
17

```
. drop if age == 4 & alcohol == 1 & smoke == 3
```
18

```
(2 observations deleted)

. xi: logistic cancer i.age i.alcohol*i.smoke [freq=patients]
```
19

Output omitted

| cancer | Odds Ratio | Std. Err. | z | P>\|z\| | [95% Conf. | Interval] |
|---|---|---|---|---|---|---|
| Output omitted | | | | | | |
| _Ialcohol_2 | 7.695185 | 3.109016 | 5.05 | 0.000 | 3.485907 | 16.98722 |
| _Ialcohol_3 | 13.04068 | 5.992019 | 5.59 | 0.000 | 5.298882 | 32.09342 |
| _Ialcohol_4 | 66.83578 | 40.63582 | 6.91 | 0.000 | 20.29938 | 220.057 |
| _Ismoke_2 | 3.864114 | 1.735157 | 3.01 | 0.003 | 1.602592 | 9.317017 |
| _Ismoke_3 | 1.875407 | 2.107209 | 0.56 | 0.576 | .2073406 | 16.96315 |
| Output omitted | | | | | | |

```
. lincom _Ialcohol_2 + _Ismoke_2 + _IalcXsmo_2_2, or

( 1)  _Ialcohol_2 + _Ismoke_2 + _IalcXsmo_2_2 = 0
```

| cancer | Odds Ratio | Std. Err. | z | P>\|z\| | [95% Conf. | Interval] |
|---|---|---|---|---|---|---|
| (1) | 9.526812 | 3.914527 | 5.49 | 0.000 | 4.25787 | 21.31586 |

```
. lincom _Ialcohol_2 + _Ismoke_3 + _IalcXsmo_2_3, or

( 1)  _Ialcohol_2 + _Ismoke_3 + _IalcXsmo_2_3 = 0
```

| cancer | Odds Ratio | Std. Err. | z | P>\|z\| | [95% Conf. Interval] | |
|---|---|---|---|---|---|---|
| (1) | 33.48594 | 20.08865 | 5.85 | 0.000 | 10.33274 | 108.5199 |

**. lincom _Ialcohol_3 + _Ismoke_2 + _IalcXsmo_3_2, or**

```
( 1)  _Ialcohol_3 + _Ismoke_2 + _IalcXsmo_3_2 = 0
```

| cancer | Odds Ratio | Std. Err. | z | P>\|z\| | [95% Conf. Interval] | |
|---|---|---|---|---|---|---|
| (1) | 16.58352 | 7.369457 | 6.32 | 0.000 | 6.940903 | 39.62209 |

**. lincom _Ialcohol_3 + _Ismoke_3 + _IalcXsmo_3_3, or**

```
( 1)  _Ialcohol_3 + _Ismoke_3 + _IalcXsmo_3_3 = 0
```

| cancer | Odds Ratio | Std. Err. | z | P>\|z\| | [95% Conf. Interval] | |
|---|---|---|---|---|---|---|
| (1) | 74.22997 | 59.24187 | 5.40 | 0.000 | 15.53272 | 354.7406 |

**. lincom _Ialcohol_4 + _Ismoke_2 + _IalcXsmo_4_2, or**

```
( 1)  _Ialcohol_4 + _Ismoke_2 + _IalcXsmo_4_2 = 0
```

| cancer | Odds Ratio | Std. Err. | z | P>\|z\| | [95% Conf. Interval] | |
|---|---|---|---|---|---|---|
| (1) | 94.0049 | 54.92414 | 7.78 | 0.000 | 29.91024 | 295.448 |

**. lincom _Ialcohol_4 + _Ismoke_3 + _IalcXsmo_4_3, or**

```
( 1)  _Ialcohol_4 + _Ismoke_3 + _IalcXsmo_4_3 = 0
```

| cancer | Odds Ratio | Std. Err. | z | P>\|z\| | [95% Conf. Interval] | |
|---|---|---|---|---|---|---|
| (1) | 202.6374 | 194.6184 | 5.53 | 0.000 | 30.84628 | 1331.179 |

**. log close**

**Comments**

1 The *estat gof* command is a post-estimation command that can be used with logistic regression. Without options it calculates the Pearson chi-squared goodness-of-fit test for the preceding logistic regression analysis. In this example, the preceding logistic command analyzed Model (5.41) (see Section 5.23). As indicated in Section 5.27.1, this statistic equals 55.85 and has 51 degrees of freedom. The associated *P*-value is 0.30. The equivalent point-and-click command is Statistics ▶ Postestimation ▶ Reports and statistics ⌋Main⌊ Reports and statistics: (subcommand) *Pearson or Hosmer-Lemeshow goodness-of-fit test (gof)* Submit.

2 The *group(10)* option causes *estat gof* to calculate the Hosmer–Lemeshow goodness-of-fit test with the study subjects subdivided into $g = 10$ groups. The *table* option displays information about these groups. The columns in the subsequent table are defined as follows: *Group* $= k$ is the group number, *Prob* is the maximum value of $\hat{\pi}_j$ in the $k^{\text{th}}$ group, *Obs_1* $= o_k$ is the observed number of events in the $k^{\text{th}}$ group, *Exp_1* $= \sum n_j \hat{\pi}_j$ is the expected number of events in the $k^{\text{th}}$ group, *Obs_0* $= m_k - o_k =$ the number of subjects who did not have events in the $k^{\text{th}}$ group, *Exp_0* $= m_k - \sum n_j \hat{\pi}_j$ is the expected number of subjects who did not have events in the $k^{\text{th}}$ group, and *Total* $= m_k$ is the total number of subjects in the $k^{\text{th}}$ group. The Hosmer–Lemeshow goodness-of-fit statistic equals 4.73 with eight degrees of freedom. The *P*-value associated with this test is 0.79. The point-and-click command is Statistics ▶ Postestimation ▶ Reports and statistics ⌋Main⌊ Reports and statistics: (subcommand) *Pearson or Hosmer-Lemeshow goodness-of-fit test (gof)* ⌜Test — ⊙ Hosmer-Lemeshow goodness-of-fit ⌟ ☑ Display table of groups used for test Submit.

3 The *p* option in this *predict* command defines the variable *p* to equal $\hat{\pi}_j$. In this and the next two *predict* commands the name of the newly defined variable is the same as the command option. The equivalent point-and-click command is Statistics ▶ Postestimation ▶ Predictions, residuals, etc ⌋Main⌊ New variable name: *p* Submit.

4 Define the variable *dx2* to equal $\Delta X_j^2$. All records with the same covariate pattern are given the same value of *dx2*. The point-and-click command is the same as in Comment 3 except that we click the *Delta chi-squared influence statistic* radio button in the *Produce* rectangle.

5 Define *rstandard* to equal the standardized Pearson residual $r_{sj}$. In the equivalent point-and-click command we click on the radio button labeled *Standardized Pearson residual (adusted for # sharing covariate pattern).*

6 We are going to draw a scatter plot of $\Delta X_j^2$ against $\hat{\pi}_j$. We would like to color code the plotting symbols to indicate whether the residual is positive or negative. This command defines *dx2_pos* to equal $\Delta X_j^2$ if and only if $r_{sj}$ is non-negative. The next command defines *dx2_neg* to equal $\Delta X_j^2$ if $r_{sj}$ is negative. See Comment 8 below.

7 Define the variable *dbeta* to equal $\Delta\hat{\beta}_j$. The values of *dx2*, *dbeta*, and *rstandard* are affected by the number of subjects with a given covariate pattern, and the number of events that occur to these subjects. They are not affected by the number of records used to record this information. Hence, it makes no difference whether there is one record per patient or just two records specifying the number of subjects with the specified covariate pattern who did, or did not, suffer the event of interest. In the equivalent point-and-click command we click the *Delta-Beta influence statistic* radio button on the *Predict* dialogue box.

8 This graph produces a scatter plot of $\Delta X_j^2$ against $\hat{\pi}_j$ that is similar to Figure 5.1. The *[weight = dbeta]* command modifier causes the plotting symbols to be circles whose areas are proportional to the variable *dbeta*; *mlwidth(thick)* chooses a thick width for these circles. (Hosmer and Lemeshow (1989) recommend a symbol area for these plots that is 1.5 × $\Delta\hat{\beta}_j$. However, Stata determines the relative size of these symbols, which is beyond the control of the user.)

The point-and-click commands do not allow scatter plots with symbol sizes that are proportional to some variable. One can, of course, generate all other aspects of this plot by point-and-click, recall the resulting graph command from the Review window and then edit this command by adding *[weight = dbeta]* as command qualifiers to the two scatter plots.

9 We plot both *dx2_pos* and *dx2_neg* against *p* in order to be able to assign different pen colors to values of $\Delta X_j^2$ that are associated with positive or negative residuals.

10 We need to identify and delete patients with covariate patterns A and B in Figure 5.1. Before doing this we save the current data file so that we can restore it to its current form when needed. This *save* command saves the data in a file called *temporary*, which is located in the Stata default file folder.

11 Delete covariate patterns that do not pertain to any patients in the study.

12 The *collapse* (*sum*) command reduces the data to one record for each unique combination of values for the variables listed in the *by* option. This command defines *n* and *ca* to be the sum of *patients* and *ca_no*, respectively over all records with identical values of *age, alcohol, smoke, dbeta, dx2*, and *p*. In other words, for each specific pattern of these covariates, *n* is the number of patients and *ca* is the number of cancer cases with this pattern. All other covariates that are not included in the *by* option are deleted from memory. The covariates *age, alcohol*, and *smoke* uniquely define the covariate pattern. The variables *dbeta, dx2*, and *p* are the same for all patients with the same covariate pattern. However, we include them in this *by* statement in order to be able to list them in the following command.

The equivalent point-and-click command is Data ▶ Create or change variables ▶ Other variable transformation commands ▶ Make data set of means, medians, etc. ⌋ Main ⌊ ⌈ Statistics to collapse — 1: Statistic *Sum*, Variables *n* = *patients*, [✓] 2: Statistic *Sum*, Variables *ca* = *ca_no* ⌋ ⌋ Options ⌊ Grouping variables: *age alcohol smoke dbeta dx2 p* [Submit].

13 List the covariate values and other variables for all covariate patterns for which $\Delta X_j^2 > 3.84$. The two largest values of $\Delta\beta_j$ are highlighted. The record with $\Delta\beta_j = 6.16$ corresponds to squared residual A in Figure 5.1. Patients with the covariate pattern associated with this residual are age 55–64, drink at least 120 g of alcohol and smoke less than 10 g of tobacco a day. Squared residual B has $\Delta\beta_j = 4.16$. The associated residual pattern is for patients aged 55–64 who drink 0–39 g alcohol and smoke ≥30 g tobacco a day.

14 Restore the complete data file that we saved earlier.

15 Delete records with covariate pattern A. That is, the record is deleted if *age* = 4 and *alcohol* = 4 and *smoke* = 1. These coded values correspond to age 55–64, ≥120 g alcohol, and 0–9 g tobacco, respectively.

16 Analyze the data with covariate pattern A deleted using Model (5.41). The highlighted odds ratios in the subsequent output are also given in column 5 of Table 5.6.

17 Restore complete database.

18 Delete records with covariate pattern B.

19 Analyze the data with covariate pattern B deleted using Model (5.41). The highlighted odds ratios in the subsequent output are also given in column 7 of Table 5.6.

## 5.30. Frequency matched case–control studies

We often have access to many more potential control patients than case patients for case–control studies. If the distribution of some important confounding variable, such as age, differs markedly between cases and controls, we may wish to adjust for this variable when designing the study. One way to do this is through **frequency matching**. The cases and potential controls are stratified into a number of groups based on, say, age. We then randomly select from each stratum the same number of controls as there are cases in the stratum. The data can then be analyzed by logistic regression with a classification variable to indicate these strata.

It is important, however, to keep the strata fairly large if logistic regression is to be used for the analysis. Otherwise the estimates of the parameters of real interest may be seriously biased. Breslow and Day (1980) recommend that the strata be large enough so that each stratum contains at least ten cases and ten controls when the true odds ratio is between one and two. They show that even larger strata are needed to avoid appreciable bias when the true odds ratio is greater than 2.

## 5.31. Conditional logistic regression

Sometimes there is more than one important confounder that we would like to adjust for in the design of our study. In this case we typically match each case patient to one or more controls with the same values of the confounding variables. This approach is often quite reasonable. However, it usually leads to strata (matched pairs or sets of patients) that are too small to be analyzed accurately with logistic regression. In this case, an alternative technique called **conditional logistic regression** should be used. This technique is discussed in Breslow and Day (1980). In Stata, the *clogit* command may be used to implement these analyses. The syntax of the *clogit* command is similar to that for *logistic*. A mandatory "option" for this command is

**group(*groupvar*)**

where *groupvar* is a variable that links cases to their matched controls. That is, each case and her matched control share a unique value of *varname*.

## 5.32. Analyzing data with missing values

Frequently, data sets will contain missing values of some covariates. Most regression programs, including those of Stata, deal with missing values by excluding all records with missing values in any of the covariates. This can result in the discarding of substantial amounts of information and a considerable loss of power. Missing data can also induce bias if the response of patients with a missing value of some covariate tends to be different from the response of otherwise similar patients for whom the value of this covariate is known.

### 5.32.1. Imputing data that is missing at random

We classify missing data in one of three ways (Little and Rubin, 2002). The value of a covariate is said to be **missing completely at random** if there is no relationship between whether or not the covariate is missing and the value of any other data that may be available on the patient. It is **missing at random** if there is no relationship between whether or not the covariate is missing and the value of the patient's response variable. This does not preclude the possibility that the values of other covariates may affect the probability that the covariate is missing. Data are **informatively missing** if the value of the response variable is likely to be affected by whether or not the covariate is missing. In this case our inferences may be seriously biased if there is a substantial quantity of missing data. Regardless of the cause of missing data it is always advisable to make every feasible effort to collect all of the data specified by your study design.

Some statisticians recommend using methods of **data imputation** to estimate the values of missing covariates (Little and Rubin, 2002; Harrell, 2001). The basic idea of these methods is as follows. Suppose that $x_{ij}$ represents the $j^{\text{th}}$ covariate value on the $i^{\text{th}}$ patient, and that $x_{kj}$ is missing for the $k^{\text{th}}$ patient. We first identify all patients who have non-missing values of both the $j^{\text{th}}$ covariate and all other covariates that are available on the $k^{\text{th}}$ patient. Using this patient subset, we regress $x_{ij}$ against these other covariates. We use the results of this regression to predict the value of $x_{kj}$ from the other known covariate values of the $k^{\text{th}}$ patient. This predicted value is called the **imputed value** of $x_{kj}$. This process is then repeated for all of the other missing covariates in the data set. The imputed covariate values are then used in the final regression in place of the missing values.

The preceding approach is known as **single imputation**. It provides unbiased estimates of the model's parameters as long as the data is missing at random. The Stata program *impute* is an example of a single imputation program. Even when the data is missing at random, this approach tends to underestimate the standard errors of the parameter estimates. This is because the missing values are estimated by their expected values conditioned on the known covariates while the true missing values will deviate from this expected value due to random error. This results in the imputed values having less dispersion than the true values. For this reason advocates of imputation recommend using **multiple imputation**. These methods simulate the dispersion of the missing values in order to obtain more accurate estimates the standard errors of the model coefficients. As of version 10, StataCorp has yet to provide a multiple imputation program as part of their core set of programs. Royston (2004, 2005) has provided a multiple imputation program to the Stata community that implements the approach of van Buuren et al. (1999). For more information on this program type *search multiple imputation* in the Stata command window.

There is still some controversy as to when to impute missing values in medical research. In my opinion, the most compelling use of imputation occurs when we are doing an observational study to determine the effect of one or two variables on an outcome of interest; there are a number of other variables that are known or suspected to confound the association between the variables of primary interest and the patient outcome. In this case it makes sense to include the confounding variables in our model. However, if missing values are scattered throughout these confounding variables we may lose a substantial amount of power if we restrict the analyses to patients with complete data on all variables. It is also possible that patients with complete data on all covariates may be a biased sample of the target population of interest. Using multiple imputation in this situation to estimate the values of missing confounding variables makes good sense. In general, however, I am hesitant to impute the values of the variables of primary interest.

The hardest part about dealing with missing data is that we rarely know for sure if data are missing at random or if they are informatively missing. When the latter is thought to be true it is prudent to be circumspect about the conclusions that we can draw from our data. In the next section we consider a data set that contains a large quantity of missing data that is almost certainly informatively missing.

### 5.32.2. Cardiac output in the Ibuprofen in Sepsis Study

An important variable for assessing and managing severe pulmonary morbidity is oxygen delivery, which is the rate at which oxygen is delivered to the body by the lungs. Oxygen delivery is a function of cardiac output and several other variables (Marini and Wheeler, 1997). Unfortunately, cardiac output can only be reliably measured by inserting a catheter into the pulmonary artery. This is an invasive procedure that is only performed in the sickest patients. In the Ibuprofen in Sepsis Study, baseline oxygen delivery was measured in 37% of patients. However, we cannot assume that the oxygen delivery was similar in patients who were, or were not, catheterized. Hence, any analysis that assesses the influence of baseline oxygen delivery on 30 day mortality must take into account the fact that this covariate is only known on a biased sample of study subjects.

Let us restrict our analyses to patients who are either black or white. Consider the model

$$\text{logit}[\text{E}[d_i \mid x_i, y_i]] = \alpha + \beta_1 x_i + \beta_2 y_i, \tag{5.56}$$

where

$$d_i = \begin{cases} 1: & \text{if the } i^{\text{th}} \text{ patient dies within 30 days} \\ 0: & \text{otherwise,} \end{cases}$$

$$x_i = \begin{cases} 1: & \text{if the } i^{\text{th}} \text{ patient is black} \\ 0: & \text{otherwise, and} \end{cases}$$

$y_i =$ the rate of oxygen delivery for the $i^{\text{th}}$ patient.

The analysis of Model (5.56) excludes patients with missing oxygen delivery. This, together with the exclusion of patients of other race, restricts this analysis to 161 of the 455 subjects in the study. The results of this analysis are given in the left-hand side of Table 5.7. The mortality odds ratio for black patients of 1.38 is not significantly different from one, and the confidence interval for this odds ratio is wide. As one would expect, survival improves with increasing oxygen delivery ($P = 0.01$).

In this study, oxygen delivery was measured in every patient who received a pulmonary artery catheter. Hence, a missing value for oxygen delivery indicates that the patient was not catheterized. A problem with Model (5.56) is that it excludes 262 patients of known race because they did not have their oxygen delivery measured. A better model is

$$\text{logit}[\text{E}[d_i \mid x_i, y_i', z_i]] = \alpha + \beta_1 x_i + \beta_2 y_i' + \beta_3 z_i, \tag{5.57}$$

where

$d_i$ and $x_i$ and are as in Model (5.56),

$$y_i' = \begin{cases} y_i: & \text{the oxygen delivery for the } i^{\text{th}} \text{ patient if measured} \\ 0: & \text{if oxygen delivery was not measured, and} \end{cases}$$

$$z_i = \begin{cases} 1: & \text{if oxygen delivery was not measured for } i^{\text{th}} \text{ patient} \\ 0: & \text{otherwise.} \end{cases}$$

An analysis of Model (5.57) gives the odds ratio estimates in the right half of Table 5.7. Note that the mortal odds ratio for black patients is higher

**Table 5.7.** Effect of race and baseline oxygen delivery on mortality in the Ibuprofen in Sepsis Study. Oxygen delivery can only be reliably measured in patients with pulmonary artery catheters. In the analysis of Model (5.56) 262 patients were excluded because of missing oxygen delivery. These patients were retained in the analysis of Model (5.57). In this latter model, black patients had a significantly higher mortality than white patients, and uncatheterized patients had a significantly lower mortality than those who were catheterized. In contrast, race did not significantly affect mortality in the analysis of Model (5.56) (see text)

| | Model (5.56) | | | Model (5.57) | | |
|---|---|---|---|---|---|---|
| Risk factor | Odds ratio | 95% confidence interval | *P* value | Odds ratio | 95% confidence interval | *P* value |
| *Race* | | | | | | |
| White | 1.0* | | | 1.0* | | |
| Black | 1.38 | 0.60–3.2 | 0.45 | 1.85 | 1.2–2.9 | 0.006 |
| *Unit increase in oxygen delivery*† | 0.9988 | 0.9979–0.9997 | 0.01 | 0.9988 | 0.9979–0.9997 | 0.01 |
| *Pulmonary artery catheter* | | | | | | |
| Yes | | | | 1.0* | | |
| No | | | | 0.236 | 0.087–0.64 | 0.005 |

*Denominator of odds ratio

†Oxygen delivery is missing in patients who did not have a pulmonary artery catheter

than in Model (5.56) and is significantly different from one. The confidence interval for this odds ratio is substantially smaller than in Model (5.57) due to the fact that it is based on all 423 subjects rather than just the 161 patients who where catheterized. The odds ratio associated with oxygen delivery is the same in both models. This is because $\beta_2$ only enters the likelihood function through the linear predictor, and $y_i'$ is always 0 when oxygen delivery is missing. Hence, in Model (5.57), patients with missing oxygen delivery have no influence on the maximum likelihood estimate of $\beta_2$.

It is particularly noteworthy that the odds ratio associated with $z_i$ is both highly significant and substantially less than one. This means that patients who were not catheterized were far less likely to die than patients who were catheterized. Thus, we need to be very cautious in interpreting the meaning of the significant odds ratio for oxygen consumption. We can only say that increased oxygen delivery was beneficial among those patients in whom it was measured. The effect of oxygen delivery on mortality among other uncatheterized patients may be quite different since this group had a much better prognosis. For example, it is possible that oxygen delivery in the uncatheterized is sufficiently good that variation in the rate of oxygen delivery has little effect on mortality. Using a data imputation method for these data would be highly inappropriate.

This analysis provides evidence that black patients have a higher mortality rate from sepsis than white patients and catheterized patients have higher mortality than uncatheterized patients. It says nothing, however, about why these rates differ. As a group, black patients may differ from white patients with respect to the etiology of their sepsis and the time between onset of illness and admission to hospital. Certainly, critical care physicians do not catheterize patients unless they consider it necessary for their care, and it is plausible that patients who are at the greatest risk of death are most likely to be monitored in this way.

### 5.32.3. Modeling missing values with Stata

The following Stata log file regresses death within 30 days against race and baseline oxygen delivery in the Ibuprofen in Sepsis Study using Models (5.56) and (5.57).

```
. *  5.32.3.Sepsis.log
. *
. *  Regress fate against race and oxygen delivery in black and
. *  white patients from the Ibuprofen in Sepsis Study
. *  (Bernard et al., 1997).
. *
. use C:\WDDtext\1.4.11.Sepsis.dta ,clear

. keep if race < 2                                                    1

(32 observations deleted)

. logistic fate race o2del                                            2

Logistic regression                          Number of obs   =        161
                                             LR chi2(2)      =       7.56
                                             Prob > chi2     =     0.0228
Log likelihood = -105.19119                  Pseudo R2       =     0.0347
```

```
------------------------------------------------------------------------------
        fate | Odds Ratio   Std. Err.      z    P>|z|     [95% Conf. Interval]
-------------+----------------------------------------------------------------
        race |   1.384358   .5933089     0.76   0.448     .5976407    3.206689
       o2del |   .9988218   .0004675    -2.52   0.012     .9979059    .9997385
------------------------------------------------------------------------------

. *
. *  Let o2mis indicate whether o2del is missing.
. *  Set o2del1 = o2del when oxygen delivery is
. *  available and = 0 when it is not.
. *
. generate o2mis = missing(o2del)                                              3
(262 real changes made)

. generate o2del1 = o2del
(262 missing values generated)

. replace o2del1 =  0 if o2mis
(262 real changes made)

. logistic fate race o2del1 o2mis                                              4

Logistic regression                               Number of obs   =        423
                                                  LR chi2(3)      =      14.87
                                                  Prob > chi2     =     0.0019
Log likelihood = -276.33062                       Pseudo R2       =     0.0262

------------------------------------------------------------------------------
        fate | Odds Ratio   Std. Err.      z    P>|z|     [95% Conf. Interval]
-------------+----------------------------------------------------------------
        race |   1.847489   .4110734     2.76   0.006     1.194501    2.857443
      o2del1 |   .9987949   .0004711    -2.56   0.011     .9978721    .9997186
       o2mis |   .2364569   .1205078    -2.83   0.005     .0870855    .6420338
------------------------------------------------------------------------------

. log close
```

**Comments**

1 The values of *race* are 0 and 1 for white and black patients, respectively. This statement excludes patients of other races from our analyses.

2 The variable *o2del* denotes baseline oxygen delivery. We regress *fate* against *race* and *o2del* using Model (5.56).
3 This *missing* function returns the value *true* (i.e. 1) if *o2del* is missing and *false* (i.e. 0) otherwise.
4 We regress *fate* against *race*, *o2del1* and *o2mis* using Model (5.57).

## 5.33. Logistic regression using restricted cubic splines

Restricted cubic splines (RCSs) can be used in logistic regression in much the same way as linear regression. Suppose that we wished to model the relationship between a dichotomous outcome variable $d_i$ and a continuous covariate $x_i$. We define spline covariates $f_1[x_i]$, $f_2[x_i]$, $\cdots$, $f_{q-1}[x_i]$ for $x_i$ in exactly the same way as in Section 3.24. Then we can rewrite Equation (5.11) as

$$\text{logit}[\text{E}[d_i \mid x_i]] = \alpha + \beta_1 f_1[x_i] + \beta_2 f_2[x_i] + \cdots + \beta_{q-1} f_{q-1}[x_i], \tag{5.58}$$

which defines an RCS logistic regression model with $q$ knots. In other words, this model assumes that the log odds of the expected value of $d_i$ given $x_i$ is an RCS function that looks like Figure 3.10. The only difference between using this technique in linear versus logistic regression is that in the former, the $y$-axis of Figure 3.10 represents the expected value of $y_i$ while in the latter it represents the logit of the expected value of $d_i$.

Let $\pi\,[x_i] = \text{E}\,[d_i|x_i]$ be the probability that a patient with covariate $x_i$ suffers the event of interest ($d_i = 1$). Equation (5.58) defines both the linear predictor for this model and the log odds of this event (see Section 4.6). Let

$$\text{lp}[x] = \hat{\alpha} + \hat{\beta}_1 f_1[x] + \hat{\beta}_2 f_2[x] + \cdots + \hat{\beta}_{q-1} f_{q-1}[x] \tag{5.59}$$

be the estimate of the linear predictor at $x$ obtained by substituting the model's parameter estimates into Equation (5.58). Then the analysis of this model is analogous to that for simple logistic regression given in Chapter 4. Our estimate of the probability that the $i^{\text{th}}$ patient will suffer the event of interest is

$$\hat{\pi}[x_i] = \exp[\text{lp}[x_i]]/(1 + \exp[\text{lp}[x_i]]). \tag{5.60}$$

The standard error of $\text{lp}[x]$ is a function of $x$, the spline knots, and the variance–covariance matrix of the model's parameter estimates (see Section 5.17). Let $\text{se}[\text{lp}[x]]$ denote the estimate of this standard error. Then a 95%

confidence interval for lp[$x$] may be estimated by

$$\text{lp}[x] \pm 1.96\,\text{se}[\text{lp}[x]]. \tag{5.61}$$

The lower and upper bounds of a 95% confidence interval for $\hat{\pi}[x_i]$ are

$$\hat{\pi}_{\text{L}}[x] = \frac{\exp[\text{lp}[x_i] - 1.96\,\text{se}[\text{lp}[x_i]]]}{1 + \exp[\text{lp}[x_i] - 1.96\,\text{se}[\text{lp}[x_i]]]} \tag{5.62}$$

and

$$\hat{\pi}_{\text{U}}[x] = \frac{\exp[\text{lp}[x_i] + 1.96\,\text{se}[\text{lp}[x_i]]]}{1 + \exp[\text{lp}[x_i] + 1.96\,\text{se}[\text{lp}[x_i]]]} \tag{5.63}$$

respectively. (See Section 4.15 for an analogous discussion of confidence intervals for $\hat{\pi}[x]$ for simple logistic regression.)

### 5.33.1. Odds ratios from restricted cubic spline models

It is often useful to plot the odds ratio of some event, say death, as a function of the covariate in a RCS logistic regression model. Suppose that we wish the denominator of this odds ratio to be with respect to patients with a covariate value of $x_0$. Then the estimated log odds of death for patients with covariate values $x$ and $x_0$ are

$$\log[\hat{\pi}[x]/(1 - \hat{\pi}[x])] = \text{logit}[\hat{\pi}[x]] = \text{lp}[x] \tag{5.64}$$

and

$$\log[\hat{\pi}[x_0]/(1 - \hat{\pi}[x_0])] = \text{logit}[\hat{\pi}[x_0]] = \text{lp}[x_0] \tag{5.65}$$

respectively. Subtracting Equation (5.65) from Equation (5.64) gives the estimated log odds ratio for patients with covariate $x$ relative to those with covariate $x_0$, which is

$$\log[\hat{\psi}[x]] = \log\left[\frac{\hat{\pi}[x]/(1 - \hat{\pi}[x])}{\hat{\pi}[x_0]/(1 - \hat{\pi}[x_0])}\right] = \text{lp}[x] - \text{lp}[x_0]. \tag{5.66}$$

We calculate Equation (5.66) by substituting Equation (5.59) into (5.66), which gives

$$\log[\hat{\psi}[x]] = \hat{\beta}_1(f_1[x] - f_1[x_0]) + \hat{\beta}_2(f_2[x] - f_2[x_0]) + \cdots \\ + \hat{\beta}_{q-1}\left(f_{q-1}[x] - f_{q-1}[x_0]\right). \tag{5.67}$$

Exponentiating both sides of Equation (5.66) gives the odds ratio for death in patients with covariate $x$ compared with those with covariate $x_0$, which is

$$\hat{\psi}[x] = \exp[\mathrm{lp}[x] - \mathrm{lp}[x_0]]. \tag{5.68}$$

### 5.33.2. 95% confidence intervals for $\hat{\psi}[x]$

Let $\mathrm{se}[\mathrm{lp}[x] - \mathrm{lp}[x_0]]$ denote the estimated standard error of $\mathrm{lp}[x] - \mathrm{lp}[x_0]$. This standard error is a function of $x$, $x_0$, and the variance–covariance matrix of the model's parameter estimates. A 95% confidence interval for this difference in linear predictors is

$$\mathrm{lp}[x] - \mathrm{lp}[x_0] \pm 1.96\,\mathrm{se}[\mathrm{lp}[x] - \mathrm{lp}[x_0]]. \tag{5.69}$$

Hence, the lower and upper bounds of a 95% confidence interval for $\hat{\psi}[x]$ are

$$\hat{\psi}_{\mathrm{L}}[x] = \exp[\mathrm{lp}[x] - \mathrm{lp}[x_0] - 1.96\,\mathrm{se}[\mathrm{lp}[x] - \mathrm{lp}[x_0]]] \tag{5.70}$$

and

$$\hat{\psi}_{\mathrm{U}}[x] = \exp[\mathrm{lp}[x] - \mathrm{lp}[x_0] + 1.96\,\mathrm{se}[\mathrm{lp}[x] - \mathrm{lp}[x_0]]]. \tag{5.71}$$

## 5.34. Modeling hospital mortality in the SUPPORT Study

Figure 5.2 shows overlayed histograms of subjects in the SUPPORT Study categorized by baseline (day 3) mean arterial pressure (MAP) (see Section 3.25). Both the number of study subjects and number of in-hospital deaths are shown for each 5 mm Hg baseline MAP interval. The observed MAP-specific in-hospital mortality rates are also shown. The distributions of both deaths and study subjects are bimodal. By their third day of admission, patients are much more likely to have high or low blood pressure than to be normotensive. The mortality rate is U-shaped with mortal risk increasing with the severity of hypotension or hypertension.

Figure 5.3 shows the estimated probability of death from a simple logistic regression of in-hospital death against MAP. It provides an instructive lesson of how badly misleading results can arise from an inappropriate statistical model. This estimated mortality curve completely misses the rise in mortal risk associated with high blood pressure and badly underestimates the risk of being severely hypotensive. Recall that simple logistic regression always estimates the event probability by a sigmoidal curve that is either strictly increasing or decreasing. It is thus quite inappropriate for data in which the greatest or lowest risk lies in the middle of the range of the independent covariate.

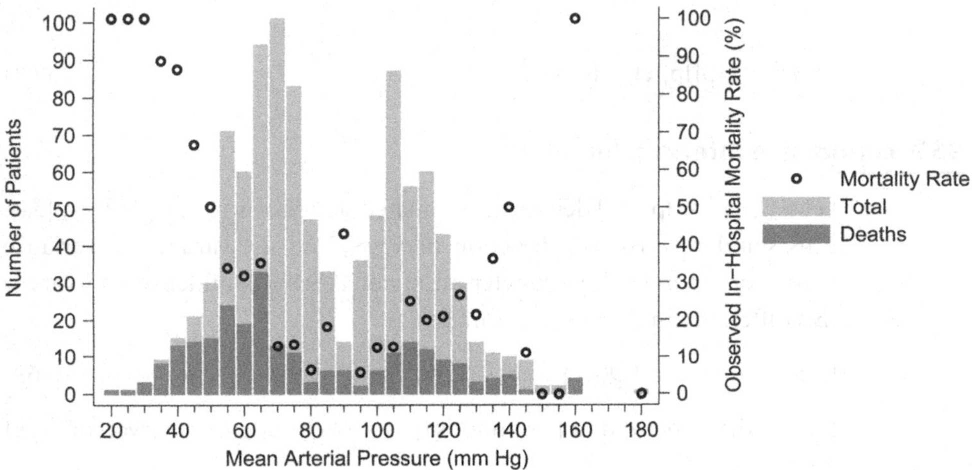


Figure 5.2 Histograms showing the total numbers of subjects and numbers of in-hospital deaths among patients in the SUPPORT data set (see Section 3.25). Patients are stratified by baseline (day 3) mean arterial pressure (MAP). MAP-specific in-hospital mortality rates are also shown. Mortality rates are lowest for patients who were normotensive by the third day of their hospitalization. These rates increase with increasing severity of either hypotension or hypertension.

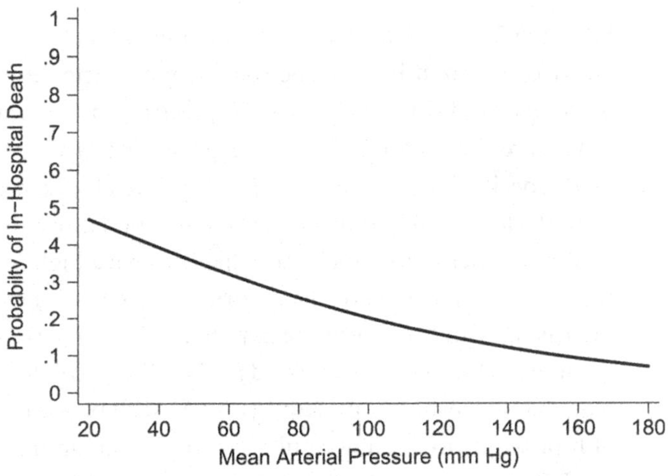


Figure 5.3 Probability of in-hospital death in the SUPPORT Study estimated by simple logistic regression. Compare this figure to Figure 5.2. This model fails to recognize the increasing mortal risk associated with increasing hypertension and badly underestimates the mortal risk associated with being in shock. It illustrates how seriously misleading estimates can be obtained from inappropriate models.

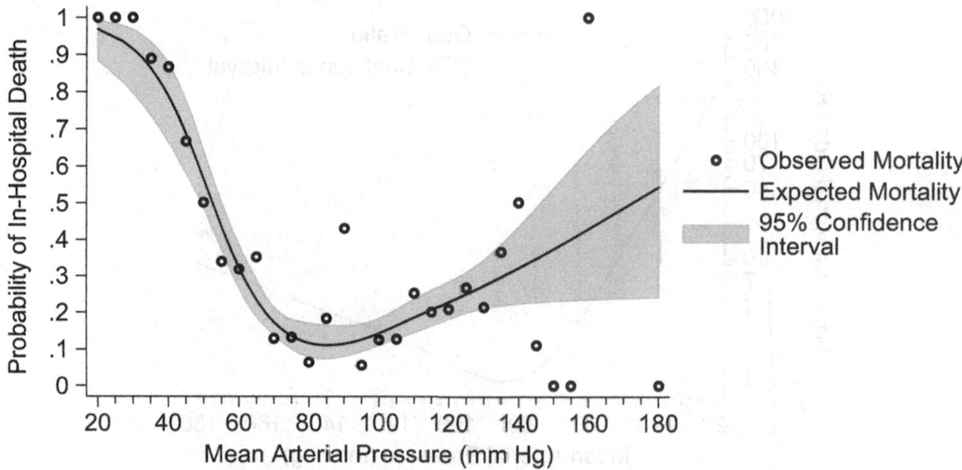


**Figure 5.4** Estimated probability of in-hospital death as a function of the patients' MAP. This curve was derived from a 5-knot RCS logistic regression model using default knot values. A 95% confidence band for this curve is also shown. This mortality curve effectively tracks the observed MAP-specific mortality rates.

Let $map_i$ and $d_i$ denote the $i^{\text{th}}$ patient's baseline MAP and mortal status at discharge, respectively. Then from Equation (5.58) a logistic regression model using RCS covariates with five knots would be

$$\begin{aligned} \text{logit}[\text{E}[d_i \mid map_i]] &= \alpha + \beta_1 f_1[map_i] + \beta_2 f_2[map_i] \\ &\quad + \beta_3 f_3[map_i] + \beta_4 f_4[map_i]. \end{aligned} \tag{5.72}$$

Substituting $map_i$ for $x_i$ in Equations (5.60), (5.62), and (5.63) gives the estimated probability of in-hospital death from this model and the 95% confidence interval for this probability. Figure 5.4 uses these equations to plot $\hat{\pi}[map_i]$ against $map_i$ together with its 95% confidence band. The observed mortality rates are overlayed on this figure. Note that the estimated mortality curve from this model is consistent with the observed mortality rates. The confidence band widens for patients with either very low or very high blood pressure due to the small number of subjects with these pressures. This is particularly true of severely hypertensive patients and reflects our uncertainty of the true mortal risk for these subjects.

Testing the null hypothesis that mortality rates are unaffected by baseline MAP is equivalent to testing the hypothesis that $\beta_1 = \beta_2 = \beta_3 = \beta_4 = 0$. We do this with the likelihood ratio test given by Equation (5.15), which yields a $\chi^2$ statistic of 122.86 with four degrees of freedom and a $P$-value $<10^{-24}$. Recall that $f_1[map_i] = map_i$ (see Section 3.24). Hence, to test the

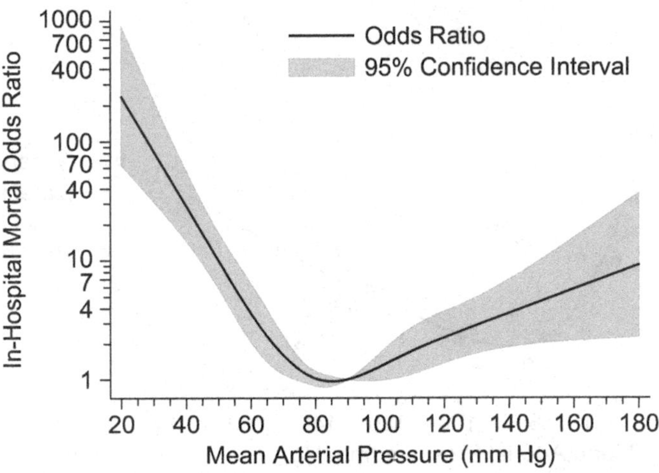


Figure 5.5 **Odds ratio for in-hospital mortality for patients with the indicated MAP in comparison with patients with a MAP of 90 mm Hg. The 95% confidence bands for this odds ratio curve are also given.**

hypothesis that there is a linear relationship between the log odds of death and baseline MAP we test the hypothesis that $\beta_2 = \beta_3 = \beta_4 = 0$. Note that the simple logistic regression model is nested within Model (5.72). Thus, we can test this hypothesis by calculating the change in model deviance between the simple and RCS models. This statistic equals 93.2 and has a $\chi^2$ distribution under this hypothesis with three degrees of freedom. This test is also of overwhelming statistical significance ($P < 10^{-19}$).

Figure 5.4 illustrates the flexibility of using RCS covariates in multiple logistic regression models. The mortality curve depicted in this figure looks nothing like the sigmoidal curves of simple logistic regression. Nevertheless, this curve was obtained from a straightforward application of multiple logistic regression using spline covariates.

Suppose that we wished to calculate odds ratios associated with different MAPs. In normal subjects MAPs usually lie between 70 and 110 mm Hg. Let us choose as a denominator for these odds ratios patients with a MAP of 90. Letting $x$ denote MAP and $x_0 = 90$ in Equation (5.67) gives the log odds ratio for in-hospital mortality associated with patients with a specific MAP in comparison with patients with a MAP of 90. Exponentiating this value gives the corresponding odds ratio in Equation (5.68). The 95% confidence intervals for these odds ratios are given by Equations (5.70) and (5.71). These odds ratios and confidence bands are plotted in Figure 5.5. The odds ratios for patients with very low baseline blood pressures are very high due to the almost 100% mortality among these patients. For this reason, these odds ratios are plotted on a logarithmic scale. Note that the odds ratio for patients with a MAP of 90 is one, since the same patients are used to derive the odds in the numerator and denominator of this odds ratio. This explains why the confidence interval for this odds ratio at 90 has zero width.

In plots like Figure 5.5 it is important to choose the denominator of the odds ratio from results reported in the literature or based on hypotheses specified in advance of data collection. Choosing this denominator after data collection on the basis of the lowest or highest estimated probability of death is likely to lead to odds ratios with spurious statistical significance due to a multiple comparisons artifact.

## 5.35. Using Stata for logistic regression with restricted cubic splines

The following log file and comments illustrate how to fit a RCS logistic regression model to the relationship between in-hospital mortality and baseline MAP.

```
. * 5.35.SUPPORT.log
. *
. *  Regress mortal status at discharge against MAP
. *  in the SUPPORT data set.
. *
. use "C:\WDDtext\3.25.2.SUPPORT.dta"

. *
. *  Calculate the proportion of patients who die in hospital
. *  stratified by MAP.
. *
. generate map_gr = round(map,5)                                    1

. label variable map_gr "Mean Arterial Pressure (mm Hg)"

. sort map_gr

. by map_gr: egen proportion = mean(fate)                           2

. generate rate = 100*proportion

. label variable rate "Observed Hospital Mortality Rate (%)"
. generate deaths = map_gr if fate

(747 missing values generated)
```

```
. *
. *  Draw an exploratory graph showing the number of patients,
. *  the number of deaths, and the mortality rate for each MAP.
. *
. twoway histogram map_gr, discrete frequency color(gs12) gap(20)      3
>     || histogram deaths, discrete frequency color(gray) gap(20)      4
>     || scatter rate map_gr, yaxis(2) symbol(Oh)
>     , xlabel(20 (20) 180) xtitle(Mean Arterial Pressure (mm Hg))
>       ylabel(0(10)100) xmtick(25 (5) 175)
>       ytitle(Number of Patients) ylabel(0 (10) 100, axis(2))
>       legend(ring(1) position(3) order(3 "Mortality Rate"
>          1 "Total" 2 "Deaths" ) cols(1)) xsize(5.25)

. *
. *  Regress in-hospital mortality against MAP using simple
. *  logistic regression.
. *
. logistic fate map                                                    5

Logistic regression                         Number of obs   =        996
                                            LR chi2(1)      =      29.66
                                            Prob > chi2     =     0.0000
Log likelihood = -545.25721                 Pseudo R2       =     0.0265

------------------------------------------------------------------------------
        fate | Odds Ratio   Std. Err.      z    P>|z|     [95% Conf. Interval]
-------------+----------------------------------------------------------------
         map |   .9845924   .0028997    -5.27   0.000     .9789254    .9902922
------------------------------------------------------------------------------

. estimates store simple                                               6

. predict p,p

. label variable p "Probability of In-Hospital Death"

. line p map, ylabel(0(.1)1)                                           7

. drop p

. *
. *  Repeat the preceding model using restricted cubic splines
. *  with 5 knots at their default locations.
```

```
. *
. mkspline _Smap = map, cubic displayknots

             |     knot1      knot2      knot3      knot4      knot5
-------------+-------------------------------------------------------
          r1 |        47         66         78        106        129

. logistic fate _S*                                                    8

Logistic regression                          Number of obs   =        996
                                             LR chi2(4)      =     122.86  9
                                             Prob > chi2     =     0.0000
Log likelihood = -498.65571                  Pseudo R2       =     0.1097

------------------------------------------------------------------------------
        fate | Odds Ratio   Std. Err.      z    P>|z|     [95% Conf. Interval]
-------------+----------------------------------------------------------------
      _Smap1 |   .8998261   .0182859    -5.19   0.000      .8646907    .9363892
      _Smap2 |    1.17328   .2013998     0.93   0.352       .838086    1.642537
      _Smap3 |     1.0781   .7263371     0.11   0.911      .2878645    4.037664
      _Smap4 |   .6236851   .4083056    -0.72   0.471      .1728672    2.250185
------------------------------------------------------------------------------

. *
. *   Test null hypothesis that the logit of the probability of
. *   in-hospital death is a linear function of MAP.
. *
. lrtest simple .                                                      10

Likelihood-ratio test                            LR chi2(3)  =      93.20
(Assumption: simple nested in .)                 Prob > chi2 =     0.0000

. display 2*(545.25721 -498.65571)                                    11

93.203

. *
. *   Plot the estimated probability of death against MAP together
. *   with the 95% confidence interval for this curve.  Overlay
. *   the MAP-specific observed mortality rates.
. *
. predict p,p                                                          12
. predict logodds, xb
```

```
. predict stderr, stdp

. generate lodds_lb = logodds - 1.96*stderr

. generate lodds_ub = logodds + 1.96*stderr

. generate ub_p = exp(lodds_ub)/(1+exp(lodds_ub))                    13

. generate lb_p = exp(lodds_lb)/(1+exp(lodds_lb))

. twoway rarea lb_p ub_p map, color(gs14)                            14
>       || line p map, lwidth(medthick)
>       || scatter proportion map_gr,  symbol(Oh)
>       ,  ylabel(0(.1)1) xlabel(20 (20) 180)
>          xmtick(25(5)175) ytitle(Probability of In-Hospital Death)
>          legend(ring(1) position(3) order(3 "Observed Mortality"
>             2 "Expected Mortality" 1 "95% Confidence" "Interval")
>             cols(1)) xsize(5.25)

. *
. *  Determine the spline covariates at MAP = 90
. *
. list _S* if map == 90                                              15

     +------------------------------------------+
     | _Smap1     _Smap2     _Smap3     _Smap4  |
     |------------------------------------------|
575. |     90   11.82436   2.055919   .2569899  |
                                                          Output omitted
     +------------------------------------------+

. *
. *  Let or1 = _Smap1 minus the value of _Smap1 at 90.
. *  Define or2, or3 and or3 in a similar fashion.
. *
. generate or1 = _Smap1 - 90

. generate or2 = _Smap2 - 11.82436

. generate or3 = _Smap3 -  2.055919

. generate or4 = _Smap4 -   .2569899

. *
```

```
. * Calculate the log odds ratio for in-hospital death
. * relative to patients with MAP = 90.
. *
. predictnl log_or = or1*_b[_Smap1] + or2*_b[_Smap2]                    16
>     + or3*_b[_Smap3] + or4*_b[_Smap4], se(se_or)                       17

. generate lb_log_or = log_or - 1.96*se_or

. generate ub_log_or = log_or + 1.96*se_or

. generate or = exp(log_or)                                              18

. generate lb_or = exp(lb_log_or)                                        19

. generate ub_or = exp(ub_log_or)

. twoway rarea lb_or ub_or map, color(gs14)                              20
>     || line or map, lwidth(medthick)
>     , ylabel(1 (3) 10 40(30)100 400(300)1000)
>     ymtick(2(1)10 20(10)100 200(100)900) yscale(log)
>     xlabel(20 (20) 180) xmtick(25 (5) 175)
>     ytitle(In-Hospital Mortal Odds Ratio)
>     legend(ring(0) position(2) order(2 "Odds Ratio"
>         1 "95% Confidence Interval") cols(1))
. log close
```

**Comments**

1 This *round* command defines *map_gr* to equal the integer nearest to *map* that is evenly divisible by 5. In general, *round(y,x)* is the value closest to *y* that is evenly divisible by *x*.

2 The *egen* command defines a new variable on the basis of the values of other variables in multiple records of the data file. This command defines *proportion* to equal the average value of *fate* over all records with the same value of *map_gr*. Since *fate* is a zero-one indicator variable, *proportion* will be equal to the proportion of patients with the same value of *map_gr* who die (have *fate* = 1). This command requires that the data set be sorted by the *by* variable (*map_gr*). The equivalent point-and-click command is Graphics ▶ Create or change variables ▶ Create new variable (extended) ⌋ Main ⌊ Generate variable: *proportion*, Egen function: *Mean* ⌈ Egen function argument — Expression: *fate* ⌋ ⌋ by/if/in ⌊ ⌈ ☑ Repeat command by groups — Variables that define groups: *map_gr* ⌋ Submit .

3 The command *twoway histogram map_gr* produces a histogram of the variable *map_gr*. The *discrete* option specifies that a bar is to be drawn for each distinct value of *map_gr*; *frequency* specifies that the *y*-axis will be the number of patients at each value of *map_gr*; *color(gs12)* specifies that the bars are to be light gray and *gap(20)* reduces the bar width by 20% to provide separation between adjacent bars.

The point-and-click version of the first line of this command is Graphics ▶ Twoway graph (scatter plot, line etc) ⌡Plots⌊ [Create] ⌡Plot⌊ ┌ Choose a plot category and type — ⦿ Advanced plots , Advanced plots: (select type) *Histogram* ┘ ┌ Plot type: (histogram plot) — X variable: *map_gr* ┌ Type of data — ⦿ Discrete data ┘ [Histogram options] ┌ ┌ Scale — ⦿ Scale to number of observations in each category ┘ [Accept] [Bar properties] ┌ Fill color: *Gray 12*, Outline color: *Gray 12* [Accept] ┘ [Accept] [Submit].

4 This line of this command overlays a histogram of the number of in-hospital deaths on the histogram of the total number of patients. The entire command produces Figure 5.2.

5 This command regresses *fate* against *map* using simple logistic regression.

6 This command stores parameter estimates and other statistics from the most recent regression command. These statistics are stored under the name *simple*. We will use this information later to calculate the change in model deviance. The equivalent point-and-click command is Statistics ▶ Postestimation ▶ Manage estimation results ▶ Store in memory ┌ ┌ Store active estimation results in memory — Name: *simple* ┘ [Submit].

7 This command generated Figure 5.3.

8 Regress *fate* against MAP using a 5-knot RCS logistic regression model.

9 Testing the null hypothesis that mortality is unrelated to MAP under this model is equivalent to testing the null hypothesis that all of the parameters associated with the spline covariates are zero. The likelihood ratio $\chi^2$ statistic to test this hypothesis equals 122.86. It has four degrees of freedom and is highly significant ($P < 0.000\,05$).

10 This *lrtest* command calculates the likelihood ratio test of the null hypothesis that there is a linear relationship between the log odds of in-hospital death and baseline MAP. This is equivalent to testing the null hypothesis that *_Smap2* = *_Smap3* = *_Smap4* = 0. The *lrtest* command calculates the change in model deviance between two nested models

using Equation (5.46). In this command *simple* is the name of the model output saved by the previous *estimates store* command (see Comment 6). The period (.) refers to the estimates from the most recently executed regression command. The user must insure that the two models specified by this command are nested. The change in model deviance equals 93.2. Under the null hypothesis that the simple logistic regression model is correct this statistic will have an approximately $\chi^2$ distribution with three degrees of freedom. The $P$-value associated with this statistic is (much) less than 0.000 05.

The equivalent point-and-click command is Statistics ▶ Postestimation ▶ Tests ▶ Likelihood-ratio test ⌜ First set of models: (leave empty for the most recent) *simple* | Submit |.

11 Here we calculate the change in model deviance by hand from the maximum values of the log likelihood functions of the two models under consideration. Note that this gives the same answer as the preceding *lrtest* command.

12 The variable $p$ is the estimated probability of in-hospital death $\hat{\pi}[map_i]$ from Model (5.72) using Equation (5.60).

13 The variables *lb_p* and *ub_p* are the lower and upper 95% confidence bounds for $\hat{\pi}[map_i]$ calculated with Equations (5.62) and (5.63), respectively.

14 This command produces Figure 5.4.

15 List the values of the spline covariates for the seven patients in the data set with a baseline MAP of 90. Only one of these identical lines of output is shown here.

16 Define *log_or* to be the mortal log odds ratio for the $i^{\text{th}}$ patient in comparison with patients with a MAP of 90. That is, it is the log odds ratio associated with MAP $= map_i$ compared with MAP $= 90$. It is calculated using Equation (5.67). The parameter estimates from the most recent regression command may be used in *generate* commands and are named _b[*varname*]. For example, in this RCS model _b[*_Smap2*] $= \hat{\beta}_2 =$ 1.17328. Note also that *or2* = *_Smap2* − 11.824 36 $= f_2[map_i] - f_2[90]$.

The command *predictnl* may be used to estimate non-linear functions of the parameter estimates. It is also very useful for calculating linear combinations of these estimates as is illustrated here. It may be thought of as a generalization of the *lincom* command, which can calculate any single weighted sum of the parameter estimates. In contrast, this *predictnl* command calculates a new variable that equals a different weighted sum of parameter estimates for each distinct value of MAP.

17 The option *se(se_or)* calculates a new variable called *se_or* which equals the standard error of *log_or*, the log odds ratio.

The point-and-click version of this *predictnl* command is Statistics ▶ Postestimation ▶ Nonlinear predictions ⌋Main⌊ Generate variable: *log_or*, Nonlinear expression *or1*_b[_Smap1] + or2*_b[_Smap2] + or3*_b[_Smap3] + or4*_b[_Smap4]* ⌈ Additionally generate variables containing — [✓] Standard errors: *se_or* ⌋ [Submit].

18 The variable *or* equals the odds ratio $\hat{\psi}[map_i]$ defined by Equation (5.68).

19 The variables *lb_or* and *ub_or* equal the lower and upper bounds of the 95% confidence interval for $\hat{\psi}[map_i]$ defined by Equations (5.70) and (5.71), respectively.

20 This command generates Figure 5.5.

## 5.36. Regression methods with a categorical response variable

Logistic regression generalizes to situations in which the response variable has more than two response values. We wish to model each patient's response in terms of one or more independent covariates. There are two regression methods that are commonly used in this situation. The first approach is called **proportional odds logistic regression** or **ordered logistic regression**. It is often used when there is a natural ordering of the values of the response variable. For example, in a study of breast cancer each patient might be classified as having carcinoma *in situ*, local invasive cancer, or metastatic cancer. In this case the severity of the outcome increases in the order in which they are listed and patients can progress from milder outcomes to more severe ones.

The second method is called **polytomous logistic regression**, or **multinomial logistic regression**. It is used when the response categories are not ordered. For example, in a study of respiratory infections, each patient might be classified as being infected by respiratory syncytial virus, rhinovirus, human metapneumovirus, or some other microbe. See Agresti (2002) for a complete introduction to these two methods.

### 5.36.1. Proportional odds logistic regression

Suppose that $d_i$, the response variable for the $i^{\text{th}}$ patient, can take any integer value between 1 and $K$ and that these responses are ordered in such a way that it is biologically relevant to consider the probability that $d_i \leq k$ for any $k < K$. Let $x_{ij} : j = 1, 2, \ldots, q$ be the values of the covariates for the $i^{\text{th}}$

patient. Let $\mathbf{x}_i = (x_{i1}, x_{i2}, \ldots, x_{iq})$ denote the values of all of the covariates for the $i^{\text{th}}$ patient. Then the proportional odds logistic regression model assumes that

$$\text{logit}[\Pr[d_i \le k|\mathbf{x}_i]] = \alpha_k + \beta_1 x_{i1} + \beta_2 x_{i2} + \cdots + \beta_k x_{iq} \quad (5.73)$$

for $k = 1, 2, \ldots, K-1$.

In the breast cancer example described above $\Pr[d_i \le 1|\mathbf{x}_i]$ would be the probability that the $i^{\text{th}}$ patient had carcinoma *in situ*, while $\Pr[d_i \le 2|\mathbf{x}_i]$ would be the probability that she had either carcinoma *in situ* or invasive disease. Note that Equation (5.73) is a generalization of the multiple logistic regression model. If there are only two response outcomes ($K = 2$) then Equation (5.73) reduces to Equation (5.11) since $\Pr[d_i \le 1|\mathbf{x}_i] = \Pr[d_i = 1|\mathbf{x}_i]$, and $\Pr[d_i = 1|\mathbf{x}_i] = \text{E}[d_i|\mathbf{x}_i]$ if $d_i$ takes the values 0 or 1. Also, the log odds ratio that $d_i \le k$ relative to $d_i \le k'$ equals $\alpha_k - \alpha_{k'}$ regardless of the values of the covariates $x_{i1}, x_{i2}, \ldots, x_{iq}$.

If there is a single covariate $x_i$ then Equation (5.73) reduces to

$$\text{logit}[\Pr[d_i \le k|\mathbf{x}_i]] = \alpha_k + \beta x_i \quad (5.74)$$

for $k = 1, 2, \ldots, K-1$. This model allows a separate value of $\alpha$ for the $K-1$ curves defined by Equation (5.74) but only one parameter $\beta$ to describe the rate at which $\Pr[d_i \le k]$ increases with $x_i$. Regardless of the value of $k$, the log odds ratio that $d_i \le k$ for a patient with covariate $x$ relative to a patient with covariate $x'$ equals $\beta(x - x')$. That is, the size of this log odds ratio is proportional to the difference between $x$ and $x'$. It is this property that gives this model the name "proportional odds logistic regression". Figure 5.6 shows plots of the probabilities that $d_i \le k$ in an example of Model (5.74) in which $K = 4$. Note that all of these curves have the identical sigmoidal shape of a logistic regression curve. If the rate at which $\Pr[d_i \le 3]$ increased with increasing $x_i$ was appreciably greater than the corresponding rate at which, say, $\Pr[d_i \le 1]$ increased then we would need to use the polytomous logistic regression model described in the next section.

In Stata proportional odds logistic regression models are evaluated using the *ologit* command.

### 5.36.2. Polytomous logistic regression

Suppose that $d_i$, $x_{ij}$, and $\mathbf{x}_i$ are defined as in Model (5.73) only now there is no natural ordering of the response outcomes $d_i$. Let $\pi_k[\mathbf{x}_i]$ denote the probability that the $i^{\text{th}}$ subject has the $k^{\text{th}}$ response value given her covariates.

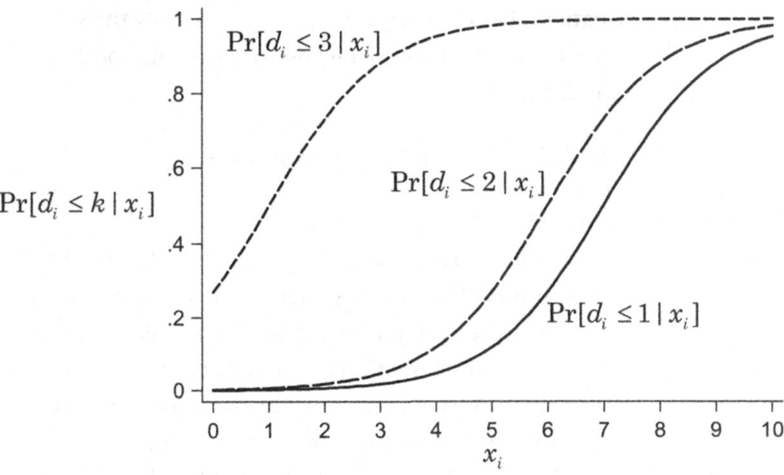


Figure 5.6 Plot of the probabilities that $d_i \leq k$ in a proportional odds logistic regression model with a single covariate $x_i$ and $K = 4$ possible outcomes. In these models a separate $\alpha$ parameter controls the horizontal position of each probability curve. There is only a single $\beta$ parameter controlling the speed at which $\Pr[d_i \leq k|\mathbf{x}_i]$ increases with $x_i$. This causes the shapes of these curves to be identical.

Then the polytomous logistic regression model assumes that

$$\log\left[\frac{\pi_k[\mathbf{x}_i]}{\pi_K[\mathbf{x}_i]}\right] = \alpha_k + \beta_{k1}x_{i1} + \beta_{k2}x_{i2} + \cdots + \beta_{kq}x_{iq} \tag{5.75}$$

for $k = 1, 2, \ldots, K-1$ and that

$$\pi_K[\mathbf{x}_i] = 1 - \sum_{k=1}^{K-1} \pi_k[\mathbf{x}_i]. \tag{5.76}$$

This model requires that each subject has one of the $K$ distinct possible outcomes but is considerably less restrictive than the proportional odds model. Note that when $K = 2$ that $\pi_2[\mathbf{x}_i] = 1 - \pi_1[\mathbf{x}_i]$. Hence,

$$\log\left[\frac{\pi_1[\mathbf{x}_i]}{\pi_2[\mathbf{x}_i]}\right] = \text{logit}\,[\pi_1[\mathbf{x}_i]]$$

and Equation (5.75) reduces to Equation (5.11). In other words, polytomous logistic regression is another generalization of multiple logistic regression to situations where there are more than two response outcomes.

It is important to realize that the reduction in model assumptions in the polytomous model compared with the proportional odds model is bought at the cost of a considerable increase in model parameters. The proportional

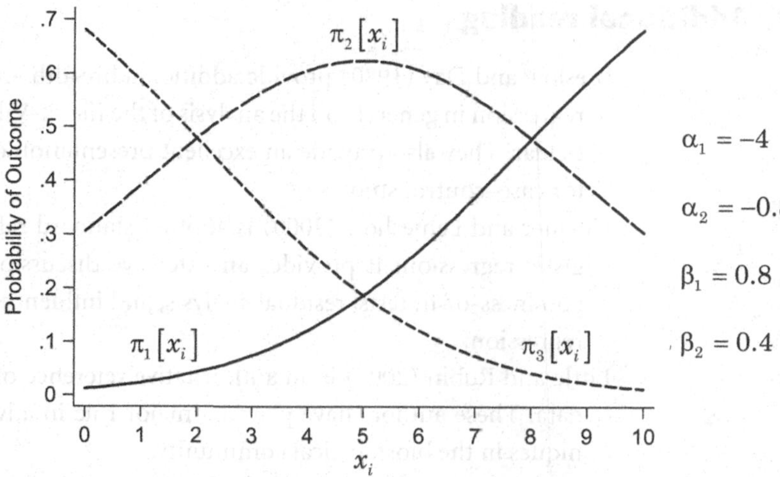


**Figure 5.7** **Plots of the probabilities of each outcome in a polytomous logistic regression model with a single covariate $x_i$ and $K = 3$ possible outcomes. This model requires that $\pi_1[x_i] + \pi_2[x_i] + \pi_3[x_i] = 1$. The relationship between the shapes of these curves and the model parameters is less intuitive than is the case for the other simple regression models that we have considered in this text.**

odds model has $K - 1 + q$ parameters while the polytomous model has $(K - 1)(q + 1)$ parameters. If there are many response outcomes and covariates then the sample sizes needed to avoid overfitting of the polytomous model will be large. For example, if there are five response outcomes and ten covariates then the proportional odds model would have 14 parameters while the polytomous model would have 44.

The interpretation of the coefficients of the polytomous model is more difficult than for the proportional odds model. Figure 5.7 shows plots of $\pi_1[x_i]$, $\pi_2[x_i]$, and $\pi_3[x_i]$ for a polytomous model with a single covariate $x_i$, $K = 3$ response outcomes, $\alpha_1 = -4$, $\alpha_2 = -0.8$, $\beta_1 = 0.8$, and $\beta_2 = 0.4$. Note in particular that $\pi_2[x_i]$ has its maximal value in the middle of the range of $x_i$. Equation (5.76) ensures that $\pi_1[x_i] + \pi_2[x_i] + \pi_3[x_i] = 1$ for all values of $x_i$. This forces $\pi_2[x_i]$ to be high for values of $x_i$ where both $\pi_1[x_i]$ and $\pi_3[x_i]$ are low.

In Stata, polytomous regression models can be fitted using the *mlogit* program. These models should be used cautiously in view of the ease with which they can over-fit the data. For many data sets, the power with which it is possible to distinguish between polytomous models having different shapes for the probability curves of different outcomes will be low.

## 5.37. Additional reading

Breslow and Day (1980) provide additional breadth and depth on logistic regression in general and the analysis of the Ille-et-Vilaine data set in particular. They also provide an excellent presentation of classical methods for case–control studies.

Hosmer and Lemeshow (2000) is another standard reference work on logistic regression. It provides an extensive discussion of model fitting, goodness-of-fit tests, residual analysis, and influence analysis for logistic regression.

Little and Rubin (2002) is an authoritative reference on imputing missing data. These authors have played a major role in advocating these techniques in the biostatistical community.

Harrell (2001) also discusses and advocates the use of multiple imputation methods for missing data.

Agresti (2002) discusses proportional odds logistic regression and polytomous logistic regression.

van Buuren et al. (1999) is the original reference for one of the standard methods used for multiple imputation of missing data.

Royston (2004) discusses and presents software for implementing van Buuren et al.'s (1999) approach in Stata.

Royston (2005) provides an update to his 2004 paper.

Marini and Wheeler (1997) provide a good overview of the biology and treatment of acute pulmonary disease.

Dupont and Plummer (1999) explain how to derive an exact confidence interval for the odds ratio from a $2 \times 2$ case–control study.

Hosmer and Lemeshow (1980) is the original reference for the Hosmer–Lemeshow goodness-of-fit test.

Mantel and Haenszel (1959) is another classic original reference that is discussed by many authors, including Pagano and Gauvreau (2000).

Pregibon (1981) is the original reference for the $\Delta\hat{\beta}_j$ influence statistic.

McCullagh (1980) is the original reference on proportional odds logistic regression.

Tuyns et al. (1977) is the original reference on the Ille-et-Vilaine Study.

Robins et al. (1986) derived the confidence interval for the Mantel–Haenszel odds ratio given in Equation (5.7).

Tarone (1985) is the original reference on Tarone's $\chi^2$ test of homogeneity for $2 \times 2$ tables.

See Section 3.26 for references on restricted cubic splines.

## 5.38. Exercises

1 In Section 5.21 we said that $\beta_1$ is the log odds ratio for cancer associated with alcohol among non-smokers, $\beta_2$ is the log odds ratio for cancer associated with smoking among non-drinkers, $\beta_1 + \beta_3$ is the log odds ratio for cancer associated with alcohol among smokers, $\beta_2 + \beta_3$ is the log odds ratio for cancer associated with smoking among drinkers, and $\beta_1 + \beta_2 + \beta_3$ is the log odds ratio for cancer associated with people who both smoke and drink compared with those who do neither. Write down the log odds for the appropriate numerator and denominator groups for each of these odds ratios. Subtract the denominator log odds from the numerator log odds to show that these statements are all true.

The following exercises are based on a study by Scholer et al. (1997). This was a nested case–control study obtained from a cohort of children age 0 through 4 years in Tennessee between January 1, 1991 and December 31, 1995. Case patients consist of all cohort members who suffered injury deaths. Control patients were frequency matched to case patients by birth year. The data set that you will need for these exercises is posted on my web site and is called *5.ex.InjuryDeath.dta*. The variables in this file are

$$byear = \text{year of birth},$$

$$injflag = \begin{cases} 1: & \text{if subject died of injuries} \\ 0: & \text{otherwise,} \end{cases}$$

$$pnclate = \begin{cases} 1: & \text{if no prenatal care was received in the first four months of pregnancy} \\ 0: & \text{if such care was given, or if information is missing,} \end{cases}$$

$$illegit = \begin{cases} 1: & \text{if born out of wedlock} \\ 0: & \text{otherwise.} \end{cases}$$

2 Calculate the Mantel–Haenszel estimate of the birth-year adjusted odds ratio for injury death among children with unmarried mothers compared with those with married mothers. Test the homogeneity of this odds ratio across birth-year strata. Is it reasonable to estimate a common odds ratio across these strata?

3 Using logistic regression, calculate the odds ratio for injury death of children with unmarried mothers compared with married mothers, adjusted for birth year. What is the 95% confidence interval for this odds ratio?

4 Fit a multiplicative model of the effect of illegitimacy and prenatal care on injury death adjusted for birth year. Complete the following table.

(Recall that for rare events the odds ratio is an excellent estimate of the corresponding relative risk.)

| Numerator of relative risk | Denominator of relative risk | Relative risk | 95% confidence interval |
|---|---|---|---|
| Unmarried mother | Married mother | | |
| Inadequate prenatal care | Adequate prenatal care | | |
| Married mother | Unmarried mother | | |

5 Add an interaction term to your model in Question 4 for the effect of being illegitimate and not having adequate prenatal care. Complete the following table.

| Numerator of relative risk | Denominator of relative risk | Relative risk | 95% confidence interval |
|---|---|---|---|
| Married mother without prenatal care | Married mother with prenatal care | | |
| Unmarried mother with prenatal care | Married mother with prenatal care | | |
| Unmarried mother without prenatal care | Married mother with prenatal care | | |
| Unmarried mother without prenatal care | Unmarried mother with prenatal care | | |
| Unmarried mother without prenatal care | Married mother without prenatal care | | |

6 Are your models in Questions 4 and 5 nested? Derive the difference in deviance between them. Is this difference significant? If you were writing a paper on the effects of illegitimacy and adequate prenatal care on the risk of injury death, which model would you use?

7 Generate a squared residual plot similar to Figure 5.1 only using Model (5.39). What does this plot tell you about the adequacy of this model?

The following questions concern the SUPPORT Study data set *5.35.SUPPORT.dta*.

8 Regress *fate* against *map* using RCS logistic regression models with four, five, and six knots, respectively. Use the default knot values for these models. For each model, plot the estimated probability of in-hospital deaths against MAP. Does the choice of the number of knots have a critical effect on the resulting probability plots?

9 Regress *fate* against *map* using two RCS logistic regression models with five knots. Use the default knot locations for one model and evenly spaced knots between 50 and 150 for the other. Plot the estimated mortality rates from these models against MAP. How important are the precise knot locations in determining the shape of this mortality curve?

10 For Model (5.72) with default knot values, draw a scatter plot of the squared standardized Pearson residual $\Delta X_j^2$ against $\hat{\pi}_j$ for each distinct value of MAP in the data set. Use an open circular plot symbol whose size is proportional to the $\Delta\hat{\beta}_j$ influence statistic. Draw another plot of $\Delta X_j^2$ against the observed MAP values. Which plot do you prefer? What proportion of these residuals are greater than 3.84? Are any of the MAP values particularly influential? How well do you think this model fits these data?

11 For your model from the previous question, calculate the odds ratio for in-hospital mortality for each patient in comparison with patients with a MAP of 50. Plot these odds ratios against MAP together with the associated 95% confidence band. Provide separate plots showing the odds-ratios on linear and logarithmic scales. Compare your plots with Figure 5.5. Are these plots mutually consistent? Why is the width of the confidence intervals at MAP = 50 so different in your plots from that in Figure 5.5?

12 From Figure 5.5 give the approximate range of MAP values associated with a significant elevation in in-hospital mortality compared with patients with a MAP of 90 mm Hg.

The following questions concern the Ibuprofen in Sepsis Study data set *4.18.Sepsis.dta*.

13 Regress 30-day mortality against baseline APACHE score using a three-knot logistic regression model with default knot values. Plot the estimated probability of death from this model against the baseline APACHE score. Show the 95% confidence band for this curve. Overlay a scatter plot of the observed mortality at each APACHE score. Compare your

plot with Figure 4.6. Does your plot increase your confidence in the validity of the simple logistic regression model for these data?

14 In your model from the previous question, test the null hypothesis that baseline APACEI score is unrelated to 30-day mortality. What is the $\chi^2$ statistic for this test? How many degrees of freedom does it have? What is the $P$-value?

15 Test the null hypothesis that Model (4.20) is valid. What is the $P$-value associated with this hypothesis? Is this $P$-value consistent with your graph from Question 13 and Figure 4.6? If your were publishing these data which model would you use?

6

# Introduction to survival analysis

In a **survival analysis** we start with a cohort of patients and then follow them forwards in time to determine some clinical outcome. The covariates in a survival analysis are treatments or attributes of the patient when they are first recruited. Follow-up continues for each patient until some event of interest occurs, the study ends, or further observation becomes impossible. The response variables in a survival analysis consist of the patient's fate and length of follow-up at the end of the study. A critical aspect of survival analysis is that the outcome of interest may not occur to all patients during follow-up. For such patients, we know only that this event did not occur while the patient was being followed. We do not know whether or not it will occur at some later time.

## 6.1. Survival and cumulative mortality functions

Suppose we have a cohort of $n$ patients who we wish to follow. Let

$t_i$ be the time that the $i^{\text{th}}$ person dies,
$m[t]$ be the number of patients for whom $t < t_i$, and
$d[t]$ be the number of patients for whom $t_i \le t$.

Then $m[t]$ is the number of patients who we know survived beyond time $t$ while $d[t]$ is the number who are known to have died by this time. The **survival function** is

$S[t] = \Pr[t_i > t] =$ the probability of surviving beyond time $t$.

The **cumulative mortality function** is

$D[t] = \Pr[t_i \le t] =$ the probability of dying by time $t$.

If $t_i$ is known for all members of the cohort we can estimate $S[t]$ and $D(t)$ by

$\hat{S}[t] = m[t]/n,$ the proportion of subjects who are alive at time $t$, and
$\hat{D}[t] = d[t]/n,$ the proportion of subjects who have died by time $t$.

**Table 6.1.** Survival and mortality in the Ibuprofen in Sepsis Study. In this study, calculating the proportion of patients who have survived a given number of days is facilitated by the fact that all patients were followed until death or 30 days, and no patients were lost to follow-up before death

| Days since entry $t$ | Number of patients alive $m[t]$ | Number of deaths since entry $d[t]$ | Proportion alive $\hat{S}[t] = m[t]/n$ | Proportion dead $\hat{D}[t] = d[t]/n$ |
|---|---|---|---|---|
| 0 | 455 | 0 | 1.00 | 0.00 |
| 1 | 431 | 24 | 0.95 | 0.05 |
| 2 | 416 | 39 | 0.91 | 0.09 |
| . | . | . | . | . |
| . | . | . | . | . |
| . | . | . | . | . |
| 28 | 284 | 171 | 0.62 | 0.38 |
| 29 | 282 | 173 | 0.62 | 0.38 |
| 30 | 279 | 176 | 0.61 | 0.39 |

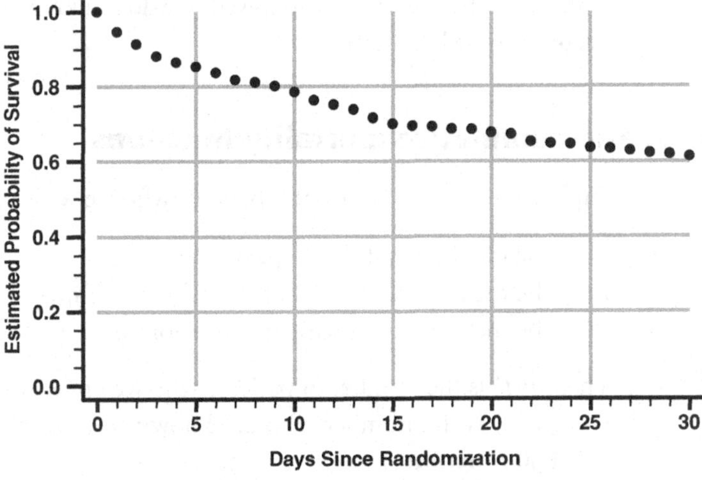


Figure 6.1 Estimated survival function for patients in the Ibuprofen in Sepsis Study. In this study all patients were followed until death or thirty days. Hence, $S[t]$ is estimated by the number of patients alive at time $t$ divided by the total number of study subjects.

For example, Table 6.1 shows the values of $\hat{S}[t]$ and $\hat{D}[t]$ for patients from the Ibuprofen in Sepsis Study. Figure 6.1 shows a plot of the survival function for this study.

Often the outcome of interest is some morbid event rather than death, and $t_i$ is the time that the $i^{\text{th}}$ patient suffers this event. In this case, $S[t]$ is called the **disease-free survival curve** and is the probability of surviving until time $t$ without suffering this event. $D[t]$ is called the **cumulative morbidity curve** and is the probability of suffering the event of interest by time $t$. The equations used to estimate morbidity and mortality curves are the same.

## 6.2. Right censored data

In clinical studies, patients are typically recruited over a recruitment interval and then followed for an additional period of time (see Figure 6.2). Patients are followed forward in time until some event of interest, say death, occurs. For each patient, the follow-up interval runs from recruitment until death or the end of the study. Patients who are alive at the end of follow-up are said to be **right censored**. This means that we know that they survived their follow-up interval but do not know how much longer they lived thereafter (further to the right on the survival graph). In survival studies we are usually concerned with elapsed time since recruitment rather than calendar time. Figure 6.3 shows the same patients as in Figure 6.2 only with the $x$-axis showing time since recruitment. Note that the follow-up time is highly variable, and that some patients are censored before others die. With censored data, the proportion of patients who are known to have died by time $t$ underestimates the true cumulative mortality by this time. This is because some patients may die after their censoring times but before time $t$. In the next section, we will introduce a method of calculating the survival function that provides unbiased estimates from censored survival data. Patients who are censored are also said to be **lost to follow-up**.

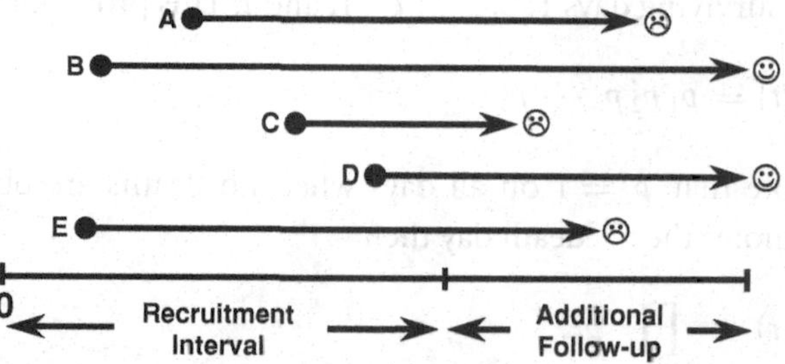


Figure 6.2 Schematic diagram showing the time of recruitment and length of follow-up for five patients in a hypothetical clinical trial. The ☹ and ☺ symbols denote death or survival at the end of follow-up, respectively. The length of follow-up can vary widely in these studies. Note that patient E, who dies, has a longer follow-up time than patient D, who survives.

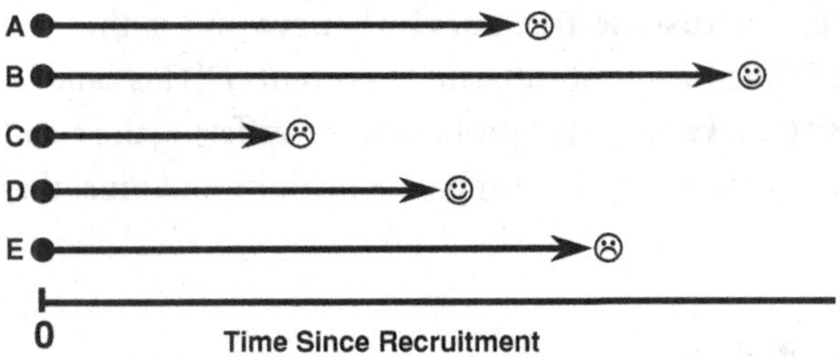


Figure 6.3 Figure 6.2 is redrawn with the $x$-axis denoting time since recruitment. Note that patient D is censored before patients A and E die. Such censoring must be taken into account when estimating the survival function since some censored patients may die after their follow-up ends.

## 6.3. Kaplan–Meier survival curves

Suppose that we have censored survival data on a cohort of patients. We divide the follow-up into short time intervals, say days, that are small enough that few patients die in any one interval. Let

$n_i$ be the number of patients known to be at risk at the beginning of the $i^{\text{th}}$ day, and

$d_i$ be the number of patients who die on day $i$.

Then for the patients alive at the beginning of the $i^{\text{th}}$ day, the estimated probability of surviving the day given that $d_i$ of them die is

$$p_i = \frac{n_i - d_i}{n_i}. \tag{6.1}$$

The probability that a patient survives the first $t$ days is the joint probability of surviving days 1, 2, . . . , $t-1$, and $t$. This probability is estimated by

$$\hat{S}[t] = p_1 p_2 p_3 \cdots p_t.$$

Note that $p_i = 1$ on all days when no deaths are observed. Hence, if $t_k$ denotes the $k^{\text{th}}$ death day then

$$\hat{S}(t) = \prod_{\{k:t_k<t\}} p_k. \tag{6.2}$$

This estimate is the **Kaplan–Meier survival function** (Kaplan and Meier, 1958). It is also sometimes referred to as the **product limit survival function**. The **Kaplan–Meier cumulative mortality function** is

$$\hat{D}[t] = 1 - \hat{S}[t]. \tag{6.3}$$

The Kaplan–Meier survival and mortality functions avoid bias that might be induced by censored patients because patients censored before the $k^{th}$ day are not included in the denominator of Equation (6.1).

Equations (6.2) and (6.3) are also used to estimate disease-free survival and cumulative morbidity curves. The only difference is that $n_i$ is now the number of patients who are known to have not suffered the event by the beginning of the $i^{th}$ day, and $d_i$ is the number of these patients who suffer the event on day $i$.

Tabulated values of $t_j$, $n_j$, $d_j$, and $\hat{S}[t_j]$ are often called **life tables**. These tables are typically given for times $t_i$ at which patients die. This term is slightly old-fashioned but is still used.

## 6.4. An example: genetic risk of recurrent intracerebral hemorrhage

O'Donnell et al. (2000) have studied the effect of the apolipoprotein E gene on the risk of recurrent lobar intracerebral hemorrhage in patients who have survived such a hemorrhage. Follow-up was obtained for 70 patients who had survived a lobar intracerebral hemorrhage and whose genotype was known. There are three common alleles for the apolipoprotein E gene: $\varepsilon 2$, $\varepsilon 3$, and $\varepsilon 4$. The genotype of all 70 patients was composed of these three alleles. Patients were classified either as being homozygous for $\varepsilon 3$ (Group 1), or as having at least one of the other two alleles (Group 2). Table 6.2 shows the follow-up for these patients. There were four recurrent

**Table 6.2.** Length of follow-up and fate for patients in the study by O'Donnell et al. (2000). Patients are divided into two groups defined by their genotype for the apolipoprotein E gene. Follow-up times marked with an asterisk indicate patients who had a recurrent lobar intracerebral hemorrhage at the end of follow-up. All other patients did not suffer this event during follow-up

| Length of follow-up (months) | | | | | | | | | |
|---|---|---|---|---|---|---|---|---|---|
| *Homozygous ε3/ε3 (Group 1)* | | | | | | | | | |
| 0.23* | 1.051 | 1.511 | 3.055* | 8.082 | 12.32* | 14.69 | 16.72 | 18.46 | 18.66 |
| 19.55 | 19.75 | 24.77* | 25.56 | 25.63 | 26.32 | 26.81 | 32.95 | 33.05 | 34.99 |
| 35.06 | 36.24 | 37.03 | 37.75 | 38.97 | 39.16 | 42.22 | 42.41 | 45.24 | 46.29 |
| 47.57 | 53.88 | | | | | | | | |
| *At least one ε2 or ε4 allele (Group 2)* | | | | | | | | | |
| 1.38 | 1.413* | 1.577 | 1.577* | 3.318* | 3.515* | 3.548* | 4.041 | 4.632 | 4.764* |
| 8.444 | 9.528* | 10.61 | 10.68 | 11.86 | 13.27 | 13.60 | 15.57* | 17.84 | 18.04 |
| 18.46 | 18.46 | 19.15* | 20.11 | 20.27 | 20.47 | 24.87* | 28.09* | 30.52 | 33.61* |
| 37.52* | 38.54 | 40.61 | 42.78 | 42.87* | 43.27 | 44.65 | 46.88 | | |

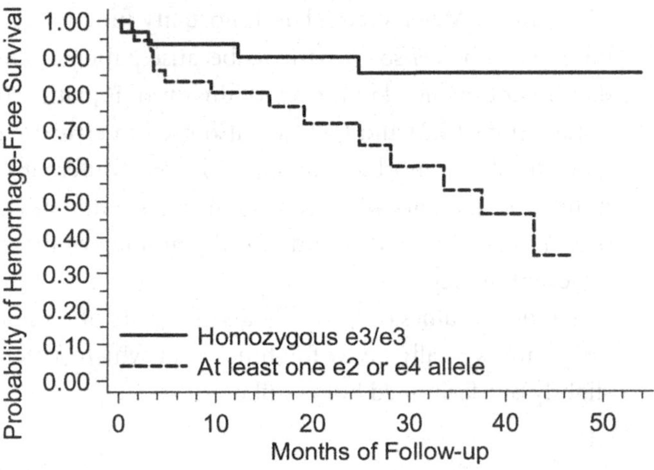


Figure 6.4 Kaplan–Meier estimates of hemorrhage-free survival functions for patients who had previously survived a lobular intracerebral hemorrhage. Patients are subdivided according to their apolipoprotein E genotype. Patients who were homozygous for the $\varepsilon 3$ allele of this gene had a much better prognosis than other patients (O'Donnell et al., 2000).

hemorrhages among the 32 patients in Group 1 and 14 hemorrhages among the 38 patients in Group 2. Figure 6.4 shows the Kaplan–Meier disease-free survival function for these two groups of patients. These curves were derived using Equation (6.2). For example, suppose that we wish to calculate the disease-free survival function at 15 months for the 32 patients in Group 1. Three hemorrhages occurred in this group before 15 months at 0.23, 3.055, and 12.32 months. Therefore,

$$\hat{S}[15] = p_1 p_2 p_3 = \prod_{k=1}^{3} p_k,$$

where $p_k$ is the probability of avoiding a hemorrhage on the $k^{\text{th}}$ day on which hemorrhages occurred. At 12.3 months there are 27 patients at risk; two of the original 32 have already had hemorrhages and three have been censored. Hence, $p_3 = (27 - 1)/27 = 0.9629$. Similarly, $p_1 = (32 - 1)/32 = 0.9688$ and $p_2 = (29 - 1)/29 = 0.9655$. Therefore, $\hat{S}[15] = 0.9688 \times 0.9655 \times 0.9629 = 0.9007$. $\hat{S}[t]$ is constant and equals 0.9007 from $t = 12.32$ until just before the next hemorrhage in Group 1, which occurs at time 24.77.

In Figure 6.4, the estimated disease-free survival functions are constant over days when no hemorrhages are observed and drop abruptly on days when hemorrhages occur. If the time interval is short enough that there is rarely more than one death per interval, then the height of the drop at each death day indicates the size of the cohort remaining on that day. The accuracy of the survival curve gets less as we move towards the right, as it is based on fewer and fewer patients. Large drops in these curves are warnings of decreasing accuracy of our survival estimates due to diminishing numbers of study subjects.

If there is no censoring and there are $q$ death days before time $t$ then

$$\hat{S}(t) = \left(\frac{n_1 - d_1}{n_1}\right)\left(\frac{n_2 - d_2}{n_1 - d_1}\right)\cdots\left(\frac{n_q - d_q}{n_{q1} - d_{q1}}\right)$$

$$= \frac{n_q - d_q}{n_1} = \frac{m(t)}{n}.$$

Hence the Kaplan–Meier survival curve reduces to the proportion of patients alive at time $t$ if there is no censoring.

## 6.5. 95% confidence intervals for survival functions

The variance of $\hat{S}(t)$ is estimated by Greenwood's formula (Kalbfleisch and Prentice, 2002), which is

$$s^2_{\hat{S}(t)} = \hat{S}(t)^2 \sum_{\{k:\ t_k<t\}} \frac{d_k}{n_k(n_k - d_k)}. \tag{6.4}$$

A 95% confidence interval for $S[t]$ could be estimated by $\hat{S}(t) \pm 1.96 s_{\hat{S}(t)}$. However, this interval is unsatisfactory when $\hat{S}(t)$ is near 0 or 1. This is because $\hat{S}(t)$ has a skewed distribution near these extreme values. The true survival curve is never less than zero or greater than one, and we want our confidence intervals to never exceed these bounds. For this reason we calculate the statistic $\log[-\log[\hat{S}(t)]]$, which has variance

$$\hat{\sigma}^2(t) = \frac{\displaystyle\sum_{\{k:\ t_k<t\}} \frac{d_k}{n_k(n_k - d_k)}}{\left[\displaystyle\sum_{\{k:\ t_k<t\}} \log\left[\frac{(n_k - d_k)}{d_k}\right]\right]^2} \tag{6.5}$$

(Kalbfleisch and Prentice, 2002). A 95% confidence interval for this statistic is

$$\log[-\log[\hat{S}(t)]] \pm 1.96\hat{\sigma}(t). \tag{6.6}$$

Exponentiating Equation (6.6) twice gives a 95% confidence interval for $\hat{S}(t)$ of

$$\hat{S}(t)^{\exp(\mp 1.96\hat{\sigma}(t))}. \tag{6.7}$$

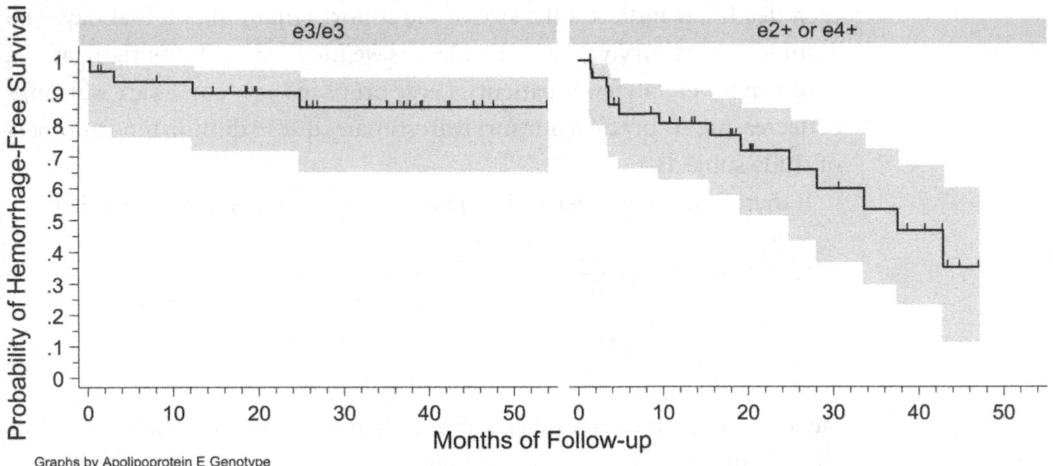


Figure 6.5 Kaplan–Meier survival curves for patients subdivided by whether or not they are homozygous with the $\varepsilon 2$ allele in the study by O'Donnell et al. (2000). The gray shaded areas give 95% confidence intervals for these curves. The hatch marks on the survival curves indicate times when patients were lost to follow-up. Note that the confidence intervals widen with increasing time. This reflects the reduced precision of the estimated survival function due to the reduced numbers of patients with lengthy follow-up.

Equation (6.7) provides reasonable confidence intervals for the entire range of values of $\hat{S}(t)$. If we return to the homozygous $\varepsilon 3$ patients in Section 6.4 and let $t = 15$ then

$$\sum_{\{k:t_k<15\}} \frac{d_k}{n_k(n_k - d_k)} = \frac{1}{32 \times 31} + \frac{1}{29 \times 28} + \frac{1}{27 \times 26} = 0.003\,66$$

and

$$\sum_{\{k:t_k<15\}} \log\left[\frac{(n_k - d_k)}{d_k}\right] = \log\left[\frac{32-1}{32}\right] + \log\left[\frac{29-1}{29}\right] + \log\left[\frac{27-1}{27}\right]$$
$$= -0.104\,58.$$

Therefore, $\hat{\sigma}^2(15) = 0.003\,66/(-0.104\,58)^2 = 0.335$, and a 95% confidence interval for $\hat{S}[15]$ is $0.9007^{\exp(\mp 1.96\times\sqrt{0.335})} = (0.722, 0.967)$. This interval remains constant from the previous Group 1 hemorrhage recurrence at time 12.32 until just before the next at time 24.77.

Figure 6.5 shows confidence intervals calculated using Equation (6.7) plotted for the hemorrhage-free survival curves of patients who either are, or are not, homozygous for the $\varepsilon 2$ allele in O'Donnell et al. (2000).

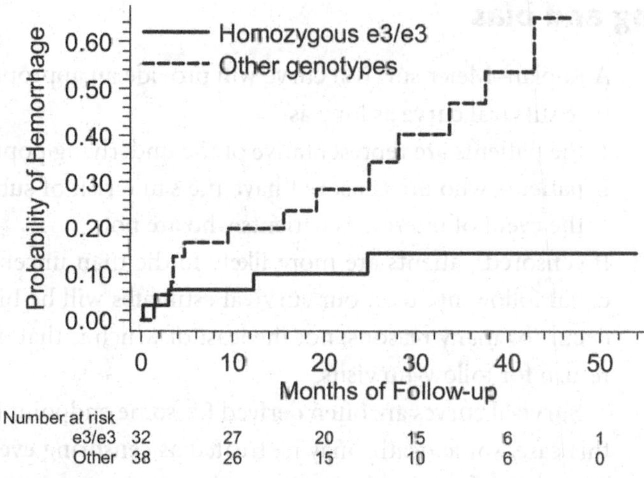


Figure 6.6 Kaplan–Meier cumulative morbidity curves for patients who are, or are not, homozygous $\varepsilon3/\varepsilon3$ from the study of O'Donnell et al. (2000). Below the morbidity plot is a table showing the number of patients still at risk of hemorrhage as follow-up progresses.

## 6.6. Cumulative mortality function

The cumulative mortality function $D[t] = 1 - S[t]$ is estimated by $1 - \hat{S}[t]$. The 95% confidence interval for the cumulative mortality function may also be estimated by

$$1 - \hat{S}(t)^{\exp(\pm 1.96\hat{\sigma}(t))}. \tag{6.8}$$

Figure 6.6 shows the cumulative morbidity function for patients who are or are not homozygous $\varepsilon3/\varepsilon3$ patients from O'Donnell et al. (2000). Plotting cumulative morbidity rather than disease-free survival is a good idea when the total morbidity is low. This is because the $y$-axis can be plotted on a larger scale and need only extend up to the maximum observed morbidity. An alternative to Figure 6.6 would have been to plot the hemorrhage-free survival curve with the $y$-axis ranging from 0.35 to 1.00. Although this would achieve the same magnification of the $y$-axis as Figure 6.6, it tends to exaggerate the extent of the morbidity, particularly if the reader does not notice that the $y$-axis starts at 0.35 rather than zero.

Below the survival curve in Figure 6.6 is a table showing the number of disease free patients in each genotype who are still at risk as follow-up progresses. For example, after 30 months of follow-up there are only 15 $\varepsilon3/\varepsilon3$ patients remaining who are still at risk of hemorrhage. Of the original 32 patients in this group, four have developed hemorrhage and 13 have been lost to follow-up.

## 6.7. Censoring and bias

A Kaplan–Meier survival curve will provide an appropriate estimate of the true survival curve as long as

1 the patients are representative of the underlying population, and
2 patients who are censored have the same risk of subsequently suffering the event of interest as patients who are not.

If censored patients are more likely to die than uncensored patients with equal follow-up, then our survival estimates will be biased. Such bias can occur for many reasons, not the least of which is that dead patients do not return for follow-up visits.

Survival curves are often derived for some endpoint other than death. In this case, some deaths may be treated as censoring events. For example, if the event of interest is developing breast cancer, then we may treat death due to heart disease as a censoring event. This is reasonable as long as there is no relationship between heart disease and breast cancer. That is, when we censor a woman who died of heart disease, we are assuming that she would have had the same subsequent risk of breast cancer as other women if she had lived. If we were studying lung cancer and smoking, however, then treating death from heart disease as a censoring event would bias our results since smoking increases the risk of both lung cancer morbidity and cardiovascular mortality.

## 6.8. Log-rank test

Suppose that two treatments have survival functions $S_1[t]$ and $S_2[t]$. We wish to know whether these functions are equal. One approach that we could take is to test whether $S_1[t_0] = S_2[t_0]$ at some specific time point $t_0$. The problem with doing this is that it is difficult to know how to choose $t_0$. It is tempting to choose the value of $t_0$ where the estimated survival functions are most different. However, this results in underestimating the true $P$-value of the test, and hence, overestimating the statistical significance of the difference in survival curves. A better approach is to test the null hypothesis

$$H_0\colon\ S_1[t] = S_2[t] \text{ for all } t.$$

Suppose that on the $k^{\text{th}}$ death day there are $n_{1k}$ and $n_{2k}$ patients at risk on treatments 1 and 2 and that $d_{1k}$ and $d_{2k}$ deaths occur in these groups on this day. Let $N_k = n_{1k} + n_{2k}$ and $D_k = d_{1k} + d_{2k}$ denote the total number of patients at risk and observed deaths on the $k^{\text{th}}$ death day. Then the observed death rate on the $k^{\text{th}}$ death day is $D_k/N_k$. If the null hypothesis $H_0$ is true, then the expected number of deaths among patients on treatment 1 given

**Table 6.3.** To test the null hypothesis of equal survivorship we form the following $2 \times 2$ table for each day on which a death occurs. This table gives the numbers of patients at risk and the number of deaths for each treatment on that day. We then perform a Mantel–Haenszel chi-squared test on these tables (see text).

| $k^{\text{th}}$ death day | Treatment 1 | Treatment 2 | Total |
|---|---|---|---|
| Died | $d_{1k}$ | $d_{2k}$ | $D_k$ |
| Survived | $n_{1k} - d_{1k}$ | $n_{2k} - d_{2k}$ | $N_k - D_k$ |
| Total at risk at the start of the day | $n_{1k}$ | $n_{2k}$ | $N_k$ |

that $D_k$ deaths occurred in both groups is

$$\mathrm{E}[d_{1k} \mid D_k] = n_{1k}(D_k/N_k). \tag{6.9}$$

The greater the difference between $d_{1k}$ and $\mathrm{E}[d_{1k} \mid D_k]$, the greater the evidence that the null hypothesis is false.

Mantel (1966) proposed the following test of this hypothesis. For each death day, create a $2 \times 2$ table of the number of patients who die or survive on each treatment (see Table 6.3). Then perform a Mantel–Haenszel test on these tables. In other words, apply Equation (5.5) to strata defined by the different death days. This gives

$$\chi_1^2 = \left(\left|\sum d_{1k} - \sum \mathrm{E}[d_{1k} \mid D_k]\right| - 0.5\right)^2 \Big/ \sum \mathrm{var}[d_{1k} \mid D_k], \tag{6.10}$$

which has a chi-squared distribution with one degree of freedom if $H_0$ is true. In Equation (6.10) the estimated variance of $d_{1k}$ given a total of $D_k$ deaths and assuming that $H_0$ is true is

$$\mathrm{var}[d_{1k} \mid D_k] = \frac{n_{1k} n_{2k} D_k (N_k - D_k)}{N_k^2 (N_k - 1)}. \tag{6.11}$$

Equation (6.11) is Equation (5.4) rewritten in the notation of this section.

In the intracerebral hemorrhage study the tenth hemorrhage among both groups occurs at time 12.32 months. Before this time, two patients have hemorrhages and three patients are lost to follow-up in Group 1 (the homozygous patients). In Group 2, seven patients have hemorrhages and eight patients are lost to follow-up before time 12.32. Therefore, just before the tenth hemorrhage there are $n_{1,10} = 32 - 2 - 3 = 27$ patients at risk in Group 1, and $n_{2,10} = 38 - 7 - 8 = 23$ patients at risk in Group 2, giving a total of $N_{10} = 27 + 23 = 50$ patients at risk of hemorrhage. The tenth hemorrhage occurs in Group 1 and there are no hemorrhages in Group 2 at the same time. Therefore $d_{1,10} = 1$, $d_{2,10} = 0$ and $D_{10} = 1 + 0 = 1$. Under the null hypothesis $H_0$ of equal risk in both groups,

$$E[d_{1,10} \mid D_{10}] = n_{1,10}(D_{10}/N_{10}) = 27 \times 1/50 = 0.54$$

and

$$\text{var}[d_{1,10} \mid D_{10}] = \frac{n_{1,10}n_{2,10}D_{10}(N_{10}-D_{10})}{N_{10}^2(N_{10}-1)} = \frac{27 \times 23 \times 1 \times 49}{50^2 \times (50-1)}$$
$$= 0.2484.$$

Performing similar calculations for all of the other recurrence times and summing over recurrence days gives that $\sum E[d_{1k} \mid D_k] = 9.277$ and $\sum \text{var}[d_{1k} \mid D_k] = 4.433$. There are a total of $\sum d_{1k} = 4$ recurrences in Group 1. Therefore, Equation (6.10) gives us $\chi_1^2 = (|4 - 9.277| - 0.5)^2/4.433 = 5.15$. Without the continuity correction this statistic equals 6.28. The probability that a chi-squared statistic with one degree of freedom exceeds 6.28 equals 0.01. Hence, Group 1 patients have significantly fewer recurrent hemorrhages than Group 2 patients.

Equation (6.10) is sometimes called the **Mantel–Haenszel test for survival data**. It was renamed the **log-rank test** by Peto and Peto (1972) who studied its mathematical properties. If the time interval is short enough so that $d_k \leq 1$ for each interval, then the test of $H_0$ depends only on the order in which the deaths occur and not on their time of occurrence. It is in this sense that this statistic is a rank order test. It can also be shown that the log-rank test is a score test (see Section 4.9.3). Currently, the most commonly used name for this statistic is the log-rank test.

It should also be noted that we could perform a simple 2×2 chi-squared test on the total number of recurrences in the two patient groups (see Section 4.19.4). However, differences in survivorship are affected by time to death as well as the number of deaths, and the simple test does not take time into consideration. Consider the hypothetical survival curves shown in Figure 6.7. These curves are quite different, with Group 1 patients dying sooner than Group 2 patients. However, the overall mortality at the end of follow-up is the same in both groups. The 2×2 chi-squared test would not be able to detect this difference in survivorship. For a sufficiently large study, the log-rank test would be significant.

## 6.9. Using Stata to derive survival functions and the log-rank test

The following log file and comments illustrate how to perform the preceding analyses with Stata.

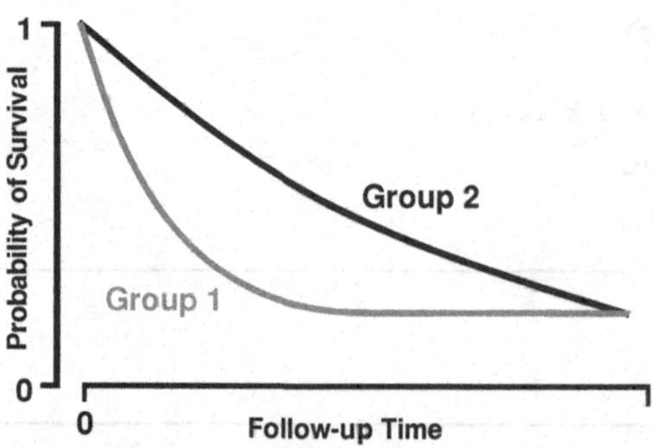


Figure 6.7 In these hypothetical survival curves the total mortality at the end of follow-up is the same in both groups. Mortality, however, tends to happen sooner in Group 1 than in Group 2. This difference in time to death may be detected by the log-rank test but will not be detected by a 2 × 2 chi-squared test of overall mortality in the two groups.

```
. *  6.9.Hemorrhage.log
. *
. *  Plot Kaplan-Meier Survival functions for recurrent
. *  lobar intracerebral hemorrhage in patients who are
. *  or are not homozygous for the epsilon3 allele of
. *  the apolipoprotein E gene (O'Donnell et al. 2000).
. *
. use  C:\WDDtext\6.9.Hemorrhage.dta                                    1

. summarize

    Variable |     Obs        Mean    Std. Dev.        Min        Max
-------------+-------------------------------------------------------
    genotype |      70    .5428571    .5017567          0          1
        time |      71    22.50051    15.21965   .2299795   53.88091
       recur |      71    .2676056    .4458618          0          1

. table genotype recur, col row                                         2

-----------------------------
Apolipopro |
tein E     |    Recurrence
Genotype   |   No   yes  Total
-----------+-----------------
     e3/e3 |   28     4     32
e2+ or e4+ |   24    14     38
           |
     Total |   52    18     70
-----------------------------
```

```
. stset time, failure(recur)                                                    3

     failure event:  recur != 0 & recur < .
obs. time interval:  (0, time]
 exit on or before:  failure

------------------------------------------------------------------------------
       71  total obs.
        0  exclusions
------------------------------------------------------------------------------
       71  obs. remaining, representing
       19  failures in single record/single failure data
 1597.536  total analysis time at risk, at risk from t =         0
                             earliest observed entry t =         0
                                  last observed exit t =  53.88091

. *
. *  Graph survival function by genotype.
. *
. sts graph, by(genotype) plot2opts(lpattern(dash))                             4
>     ylabel(0(.1)1) ymtick(0(.05)1) xlabel(0(10)50)
>     xmtick(0(2)54) xtitle("Months of Follow-up")                              5
>     ytitle("Probability of Hemorrhage-Free Survival")
>     title(" ", size(0)) legend(ring(0) cols(1)                                6
>       position(7) order(1 "Homozygous e3/e3"
>       2 "At least one e2 or e4 allele"))                                      7

         failure _d:  recur
   analysis time _t:  time

. *
. *  List survival statistics.
. *
. sts list, by(genotype)                                                        8

         failure _d:  recur
   analysis time _t:  time

           Beg.          Net            Survivor      Std.
  Time    Total   Fail   Lost           Function     Error     [95% Conf. Int.]
-------------------------------------------------------------------------------
e3/e3
   .23      32      1      0             0.9688    0.0308     0.7982    0.9955
 1.051      31      0      1             0.9688    0.0308     0.7982    0.9955
 1.511      30      0      1             0.9688    0.0308     0.7982    0.9955
```

```
 3.055      29      1      0      0.9353   0.0443   0.7651   0.9835
 8.082      28      0      1      0.9353   0.0443   0.7651   0.9835
 12.32      27      1      0      0.9007   0.0545   0.7224   0.9669
                                                          Output omitted
 47.57       2      0      1      0.8557   0.0679   0.6553   0.9441
 53.88       1      0      1      0.8557   0.0679   0.6553   0.9441
e2+ or e4+
  1.38      38      0      1      1.0000        .        .        .
 1.413      37      1      0      0.9730   0.0267   0.8232   0.9961
 1.577      36      1      1      0.9459   0.0372   0.8007   0.9862
 3.318      34      1      0      0.9181   0.0453   0.7672   0.9728
 3.515      33      1      0      0.8903   0.0518   0.7335   0.9574
 3.548      32      1      0      0.8625   0.0571   0.7005   0.9404
 4.041      31      0      1      0.8625   0.0571   0.7005   0.9404
 4.632      30      0      1      0.8625   0.0571   0.7005   0.9404
                                                          Output omitted
 42.78       5      0      1      0.4641   0.1156   0.2346   0.6659
 42.87       4      1      0      0.3480   0.1327   0.1174   0.5946
 43.27       3      0      1      0.3480   0.1327   0.1174   0.5946
 44.65       2      0      1      0.3480   0.1327   0.1174   0.5946
 46.88       1      0      1      0.3480   0.1327   0.1174   0.5946
--------------------------------------------------------------------

. *
. *  Graph survival functions by genotype with 95% confidence
. *   intervals.  Show loss to follow-up.
. *
. sts graph, by(genotype) ci censored(single) separate                    9
>      ciopts(lcolor(none)) byopts(title(" ", size(0))                    10
>        legend(off)) ylabel(0(.1)1) ymtick(0(.05)1)
>      xtitle("Months of Follow-up") xlabel(0(10)50)
>      xmtick(0(2)54) xsize(5.6) ysize(3.2)
>      ytitle("Probability of Hemorrhage-Free Survival")                  11

         failure _d:  recur
   analysis time _t:  time

. *
. *  Plot cumulative morbidity for homozygous e3 patients
. *  together with 95% confidence intervals for this morbidity.
. *
. sts graph , by(genotype) plot2opts(lpattern(dash))
```

```
>      failure risktable(,order(1 "e3/e3" 2 "Other"))                    12
>      ylabel(0(.1).6) ymtick(0(.02).64)
>      ytitle("Probability of Hemorrhage") xlabel(0(10)50)
>      xmtick(0(2)54) xtitle("Months of Follow-up")
>      title(" ",size(0)) legend(ring(0) cols(1)
>         position(11) order(1 "Homozygous e3/e3"
>         2 "Other genotypes" ))

         failure _d:  recur
   analysis time _t:  time
. *
. * Compare survival functions for the two genotypes using
. * the log-rank test.
. *
. sts test genotype                                                      13

         failure _d:  recur
   analysis time _t:  time

Log-rank test for equality of survivor functions

            |  Events         Events
genotype    |  observed       expected
------------+-------------------------
e3/e3       |         4           9.28
e2+ or e4+  |        14           8.72
------------+-------------------------
Total       |        18          18.00

                 chi2(1) =        6.28
                 Pr>chi2 =      0.0122

.log close
```

**Comments**

1 The hemorrhage data set contains three variables on 71 patients. The variable *time* denotes length of follow-up in months; *recur* records whether the patient had a hemorrhage (*recur* = 1) or was censored (*recur* = 0) at the end of follow-up; *genotype* divides the patients into two groups determined by their genotype. The value of *genotype* is missing on one patient who did not give a blood sample.

2 This command tabulates study subjects by hemorrhage recurrence and genotype. The value labels of these two variables are shown.

3 This *stset* command specifies that the data set contains survival data. Each patient's follow-up time is denoted by *time*; her fate at the end

of follow-up is denoted by *recur*. Stata interprets *recur* = 0 to mean that the patient is censored and *recur* ≠ 0 to mean that she suffered the event of interest at exit. A *stset* command must be specified before other survival commands such as *sts list*, *sts graph*, *sts test* or *sts generate*. The equivalent point-and-click command is Statistics ▶ Survival analysis ▶ Setup utilities ▶ Declare data to be survival-time data ⌋Main⌊ Time variable: *time* , ⌈ Failure event — Failure variable: *recur* ⌋ Submit.

4 The *sts graph* command plots Kaplan–Meier survival curves; *by(genotype)* specifies that separate plots will be generated for each value of *genotype*. The *plot2opts* option specifies the appearance of the second plot on this curve. (This plot is for the second largest value of *genotype*, which is this example is for patients with at least one ε2 or ε4 allele.) The *lpattern(dash)* suboption of the *plot2opts* option specifies that a dashed line is to be used for this survival plot.

5 By default, the *sts graph* command titles the *x*-axis "*analysis time*" and does not title the *y*-axis. These *xtitle* and *ytitle* options provide the titles "*Months of Follow-up*" and "*Probability of Hemorrhage-Free Survival*" for the *x*- and *y*-axes, respectively.

6 By default, *sts graph* commands produce graphs with the title *Kaplan–Meier survival estimate*. This *title* option suppresses this default title.

7 This entire command produces Figure 6.4. A point-and-click command that generates the curves in this figure is Graphics ▶ Survival analysis graphs ▶ Survivor & cumulative hazard functions ⌋Main⌊ ⌈ ✓ Make separate calculations by group — Grouping variables: *genotype* ⌋ ⌋Plot⌊ Select Plot: *Plot 2* Edit Line properties Pattern: *Dash* Accept Accept Submit. This point-and-click command uses the default values of the options specified on the *Y axis*, *X axis*, *Titles* and *Legend* tabs. These tabs on the *sts graph* dialog box are identical to those given on the *Twoway graphs* dialog box.

8 This command lists the values of the survival functions that are plotted by the preceding command. The *by(genotype)* option specifies that a separate survival function is to be calculated for each value of *genotype*. The number of patients at risk before each failure or loss to follow-up is also given, together with the 95% confidence interval for the survival function. The highlighted values agree with the hand calculations in Sections 6.4 and 6.5. The point-and-click version of this command is Statistics ▶ Survival analysis ▶ Summary statistics, tests,

& tables ▶ List survivor & cumulative hazard functions ⌋Main⌊ ⌈ Calculation — ☑ Separate on different groups of specified variables: (by variables) *genotype* ⌋ Submit.

The *sts list* command lists a line of output for every time at which a patient dies or is lost to follow-up. This can produce a very large listing for large studies. The *at* option can restrict this listing to the times that we are really interested in. For example,

```
sts list, by(genotype) at(10 15 20)
```

would restrict the output of the *sts list* command to times 10, 15 and 20 months.

9 Stata also permits 95% confidence bounds for $\hat{S}(t)$ to be included for Kaplan–Meier graphs and to indicate the times at which patients are lost to follow-up. This is done with the *ci* and *censored(single)* options, respectively. In this example, the *separate* option draws a separate plot for each value of *genotype*.

An alternative way to indicate when patients are censored is the *lost* option. This option prints the number of subjects lost to follow-up between consecutive death days just above the survival curve.

10 By default, the *ci* option draws the confidence bounds with a boundary whose color is different from that of the shaded region. This *ciopts(lcolor(none))* option suppresses these boundary lines.

The *title(" "), size(0))* and *legend(off)* suboptions of the *byopts* option suppress the figure title and figure legend, respectively. Surprisingly, when the *by* option is given, *legend* and *title* must be suboptions of the *byopts* option rather than options of the *sts graph* command.

11 The entire command produces Figure 6.5. A similar point-and-click command that uses default titles and labels for the *x*- and *y*-axes is Graphics ▶ Survival analysis graphs ▶ Survivor & cumulative hazard functions ⌋Main⌊ ⌈ ☑ Make separate calculations by group — Grouping variables: *genotype* , ☑ Show plots on separate graphs ⌋ ☑ Show pointwise confidence bands ⌋Options⌊ Plot censorings, entries, etc... Plot the following additional information: *Number lost (number censored minus number who enter)* Accept ⌋CI plot⌊ Area properties Outline color: *None* Accept ⌋Titles⌊ Title: Properties ⌋Text⌊ ⌈ Text properties — Size: *Zero* ⌋ Accept ⌋Legend⌊ ⌈ Legend behavior — ⊙ Hide legend ⌋ Submit.

12 The *failure* option of this *sts graph* command produces cumulative morbidity plots. The *risktable* option creates a table below the graph showing the number of patients still at risk of failure at different follow-up times. The *order* suboption of the *risktable* option labels each row of the risk table in the same way as *order* suboption of the *label* option of most graph commands. The resulting graph is given in Figure 6.6. A point-and-click command that is similar to this one is Graphics ▶ Survival analysis graphs ▶ Survivor & cumulative hazard functions [Main] ┌ Function — ⦿ Graph Kaplan–Meier failure function ┌ [✓] Make separate calculations by group — Grouping variables: *genotype* ┘ [At-risk table] [✓] Show at-risk table beneath graph [At-risk table properties (global)] [Main] Order specification: *1 2* [Accept] [Edit] [Row title] Row title: *e3/e3* [Accept] At-risk table properties: (row specific) *Row2* [Edit] [Row title] Row title: *Other* [Accept] [Plot] Select Plot: *Plot 2* [Edit] [Line properties] Pattern: *Dash* [Accept] [Accept] [Submit].

13 Perform a log-rank test for the equality of survivor functions in patient groups defined by different values of *genotype*. In this example, patients who are homozygous for the $\varepsilon 3$ allele are compared to other patients. The highlighted chi-squared statistic and $P$-value agree with our hand calculations for the uncorrected test. The point-and-click version of this command is Statistics ▶ Survival analysis ▶ Summary statistics, tests, & tables ▶ Test equality of survivor functions [Main] Variables: *genotype* [Submit].

## 6.10. Log-rank test for multiple patient groups

The log-rank test generalizes to allow the comparison of survival in several groups. The test statistic has an asymptotic chi-squared distribution with one degree of freedom fewer than the number of patient groups being compared. In Stata, these groups are defined by the number of distinct levels taken by the variable specified in the *sts test* command. If, in the hemorrhage study, a variable named *geno6* indicated each of the six possible genotypes that can result from three alleles for one gene, then *sts test geno6* would compare the six survival curves for these groups of patients; the test statistic would have five degrees of freedom.

## 6.11. Hazard functions

Our next topic is the estimation of relative risks in survival studies. Before doing this we need to introduce the concept of a hazard function. Suppose that a patient is alive at time $t$ and that her probability of dying in the next short time interval $(t, t + \Delta t)$ is $\lambda[t]\Delta t$. Then $\lambda[t]$ is said to be the **hazard function** for the patient at time $t$. In other words

$$\lambda(t) = \frac{\Pr[\text{patient dies by time } t + \Delta t \mid \text{patient alive at time } t]}{\Delta t}. \qquad (6.12)$$

Of course, both the numerator and the denominator of Equation (6.12) approach zero as $\Delta t$ gets very small. However, the ratio of numerator to denominator approaches $\lambda[t]$ as $\Delta t$ approaches zero. For a very large population,

$$\lambda[t]\Delta t \cong \frac{\text{number of deaths in the interval}(t, t + \Delta t)}{\text{number of people alive at time } t}.$$

The hazard function $\lambda[t]$ is the instantaneous rate per unit time at which people are dying at time $t$; $\lambda[t] = 0$ implies that there is no risk of death and $S[t]$ is flat at time $t$. Large values of $\lambda[t]$ imply a rapid rate of decline in $S[t]$. The hazard function is related to the survival function through the equation $S[t] = \exp[-\int_0^t \lambda[x]dx]$, where $\int_0^t \lambda[x]dx$ is the area under the curve $\lambda[t]$ between 0 and $t$. The simplest hazard function is a constant, which implies that a patient's risk of death does not vary with time. If $\lambda[t] = k$, then the area under the curve between 0 and $t$ is $kt$ and the survival function is $S[t] = e^{-kt}$. Examples of constant hazard functions and the corresponding survival curves are given in Figure 6.8.

## 6.12. Proportional hazards

Suppose that $\lambda_0[t]$ and $\lambda_1[t]$ are the hazard functions for patients on control and experimental treatments, respectively. Then these treatments have **proportional hazards** if

$$\lambda_1[t] = R\lambda_0[t]$$

for some constant $R$. The proportional hazards assumption places no restrictions on the shape of $\lambda_0(t)$ but requires that

$$\lambda_1[t]/\lambda_0[t] = R$$

at all times $t$. Figure 6.9 provides an artificial example that may help to increase your intuitive understanding of hazard functions, survival functions,

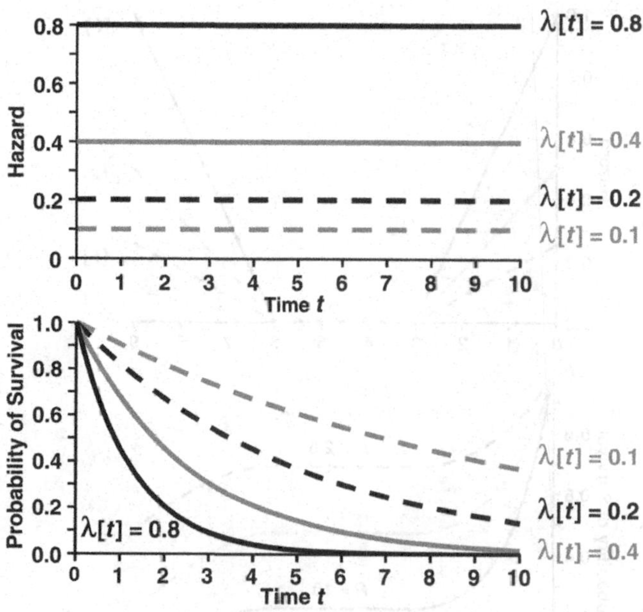


Figure 6.8 The hazard function equals the rate of instantaneous mortality for study subjects. This graph shows the relationship between different constant hazard functions and the associated survival curves. If $\lambda[t] = k$ then $S[t] = \exp[-kt]$. The higher the hazard function the more rapidly the probability of survival drops to zero with increasing time.

and the proportional hazards assumption. In this figure, $\lambda_0[t] = 0.1$ when $t = 0$. It decreases linearly until it reaches 0 at $t = 3$; is constant at 0 from $t = 3$ until $t = 6$ and then increases linearly until it reaches 0.1 at $t = 9$. The hazard functions $\lambda_0[t]$, $\lambda_1[t]$, $\lambda_2[t]$, and $\lambda_3[t]$ meet the proportional hazards assumption in that $\lambda_1[t] = 2.5\lambda_0[t]$, $\lambda_2[t] = 5\lambda_0[t]$, and $\lambda_3[t] = 10\lambda_0[t]$. The associated survival functions are also shown in Figure 6.9. The fact that these hazard functions all equal zero between 3 and 6 implies that no-one may die in this interval. For this reason, the associated survival functions are constant from 3 to 6. Regardless of the shape of the hazard function, the survival curve is always non-increasing, and is always between one and zero. The rate of decrease of the survival curve increases with increasing hazard and with increasing size of the survival function itself.

## 6.13. Relative risks and hazard ratios

Suppose that the risks of death by time $t + \Delta t$ for patients on control and experimental treatments who are alive at time $t$ are $\lambda_0[t]\Delta t$ and $\lambda_1[t]\Delta t$,

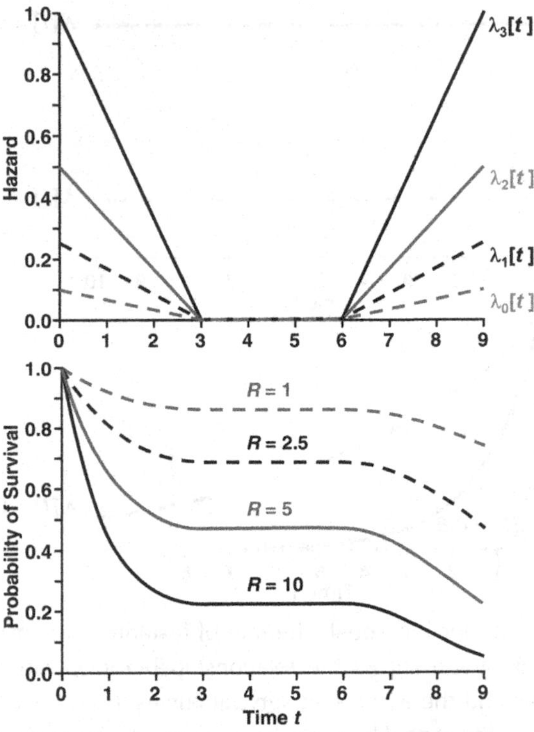


Figure 6.9 Hypothetical example of hazard functions that meet the proportional hazards assumption. Although the hazard functions themselves vary with time the ratio of any two hazard functions is constant. The associated survival functions are shown in the lower panel. The relative risks $R$ of patients with hazards $\lambda_1[t]$, $\lambda_2[t]$, and $\lambda_3[t]$ compared with $\lambda_0[t]$ are given in the lower panel.

respectively. Then the risk of experimental subjects at time $t$ relative to controls is

$$\frac{\lambda_1[t]\Delta t}{\lambda_0[t]\Delta t} = \frac{\lambda_1[t]}{\lambda_0[t]}.$$

If $\lambda_1[t] = R\lambda_0[t]$ at all times, then this relative risk is

$$\frac{\lambda_1[t]}{\lambda_0[t]} = \frac{R\lambda_0[t]}{\lambda_0[t]} = R.$$

Thus, the ratio of two hazard functions can be thought of as an instantaneous relative risk. If the proportional hazards assumption is true, then this hazard ratio remains constant over time and equals the relative risk of experimental subjects compared with controls. In Figure 6.9, the hazard ratios $\lambda_1[t]/\lambda_0[t]$, $\lambda_2[t]/\lambda_0[t]$, and $\lambda_3[t]/\lambda_0[t]$ equal 2.5, 5, and 10, respectively. Therefore, the relative risks of patients with hazard functions $\lambda_1[t]$, $\lambda_2[t]$, and $\lambda_3[t]$ relative to patients with hazard function $\lambda_0[t]$ are 2.5, 5, and 10.

## 6.14. Proportional hazards regression analysis

Suppose that patients are randomized to an experimental or control therapy. Let

$\lambda_0[t]$ be the hazard function for patients on the control therapy,

and

$$x_i = \begin{cases} 1: & \text{if the } i^{\text{th}} \text{ patient receives the experimental therapy} \\ 0: & \text{if she receives the control therapy.} \end{cases}$$

Then the **simple proportional hazards model** assumes that the $i^{\text{th}}$ patient has hazard

$$\lambda_i[t] = \lambda_0[t] \exp[\beta x_i], \tag{6.13}$$

where $\beta$ is an unknown parameter. Note that if the $i^{\text{th}}$ patient is on the control therapy then $\beta x_i = 0$ and $\lambda_i[t] = \lambda_0[t]e^0 = \lambda_0[t]$. If she is on the experimental therapy, then $\beta x_i = \beta$ and $\lambda_i[t] = \lambda_0[t]e^{\beta}$. This model is said to be **semi-nonparametric** in that it makes no assumptions about the shape of the control hazard function $\lambda_0[t]$. Under this model, the relative risk of experimental therapy relative to control therapy is $\lambda_0[t]e^{\beta}/\lambda_0[t] = e^{\beta}$. Hence, $\beta$ is the log relative risk of the experimental therapy relative to the control therapy. Cox (1972) developed a regression method for survival data that uses the proportional hazards model. This method is in many ways similar to logistic regression. It provides an estimate, $\hat{\beta}$, of $\beta$ together with an estimate, $\text{se}[\hat{\beta}]$, of the standard error of $\hat{\beta}$. For large studies $\hat{\beta}$ has an approximately normal distribution. We use these estimates in the same way that we used the analogous estimates from logistic regression. The estimated relative risk of experimental therapy relative to control therapy is

$$\hat{R} = \exp[\hat{\beta}]. \tag{6.14}$$

A 95% confidence interval for this relative risk is

$$\hat{R} \exp[\pm 1.96 \times \text{se}[\hat{\beta}]]. \tag{6.15}$$

The two therapies will be equally efficacious if $R = 1$, or, equivalently, if $\beta = 0$. Hence, testing the null hypothesis that $\beta = 0$ is equivalent to testing the null hypothesis of equal treatment efficacy. Under this null hypothesis

$$z = \hat{\beta}/\text{se}[\hat{\beta}] \tag{6.16}$$

has an approximately standard normal distribution. Equations (6.15) and (6.16) are a Wald confidence interval and Wald test, respectively (see Section 4.9.4).

## 6.15. Hazard regression analysis of the intracerebral hemorrhage data

Let $\lambda_i[t]$ be the hemorrhage hazard function for the $i^{\text{th}}$ patient in the study of O'Donnell et al. (2000). Let $\lambda_0[t]$ be the hazard for patients who are homozygous for the $\varepsilon 3$ allele, and let

$$x_i = \begin{cases} 1: & \text{if the } i^{\text{th}} \text{ patient has an } \varepsilon 2 \text{ or } \varepsilon 4 \text{ allele} \\ 0: & \text{otherwise.} \end{cases}$$

We will assume the proportional hazards model $\lambda_i[t] = \lambda_0[t] \exp[\beta x_i]$. Performing a proportional hazards regression analysis on these data gives an estimate of $\hat{\beta} = 1.3317$ with a standard error of $\text{se}[\hat{\beta}] = 0.5699$. Therefore, the relative risk of recurrence for patients with an $\varepsilon 2$ or $\varepsilon 4$ allele relative to homozygous $\varepsilon 3/\varepsilon 3$ patients is $\exp[1.3317] = 3.79$. A 95% confidence interval for this relative risk is $3.79 \exp[\pm 1.96 \times 0.5699] = (1.2, 12)$. To test the null hypothesis that the two patient groups are at equal risk of recurrence, we calculate $z = 1.3317/0.5699 = 2.34$. The probability that a standard normal random variable is less than $-2.34$ or more than 2.34 is $P = 0.019$. Hence, the hemorrhage recurrence rate is significantly greater in patients with an $\varepsilon 2$ or $\varepsilon 4$ allele compared with homozygous $\varepsilon 3/\varepsilon 3$ patients. This $P$-value is similar to that obtained from the log-rank test, which is testing the same null hypothesis.

## 6.16. Proportional hazards regression analysis with Stata

The following log file and comments illustrate a simple proportional hazards regression analysis that compares two groups of patients.

```
. *  6.16.Hemorrhage.log
. *
. *  Perform a proportional hazards regression analysis of recurrent
. *  lobar intracerebral hemorrhage in patients who are or are not
. *  homozygous for the epsilon3 allele of the apolipoprotein E gene
. *  (O'Donnell et al. 2000).
. *
. use  C:\WDDtext\6.9.Hemorrhage.dta, clear

. stset time, failure(recur)
```

```
                                                          Output omitted
. stcox genotype                                                     1

        failure _d:  recur
  analysis time _t:  time
                                                          Output omitted
Cox regression -- no ties

No. of subjects =           70                Number of obs   =        70
No. of failures =           18
Time at risk    =  1596.320341
                                              LR chi2(1)      =      6.61
Log likelihood  =   -63.370953                Prob > chi2     =    0.0102

------------------------------------------------------------------------------
         _t | Haz. Ratio   Std. Err.      z    P>|z|     [95% Conf. Interval]
------------+-----------------------------------------------------------------
   genotype |   3.787366   2.158422     2.34   0.019     1.239473    11.57278    2
------------------------------------------------------------------------------
. log close
```

**Comments**

1 This command fits the proportional hazards regression model
$\lambda(t, genotype) = \lambda_0(t) \exp(\beta \times genotype)$.

That is, we fit Model (6.13) using *genotype* as the covariate $x_i$. A *stset* command must precede the *stcox* command to define the fate and follow-up variables. The point-and-click version of this command is Statistics ▶ Survival analysis ▶ Regression models ▶ Cox proportional hazards model ⌋ Model ⌊ Independent variables: *genotype* [Submit].

2 The *stcox* command outputs the hazard ratio $\exp[\hat{\beta}] = 3.787$ and the associated 95% confidence interval using Equation (6.15). This hazard ratio is the relative risk of patients with an $\varepsilon 2$ or $\varepsilon 4$ allele compared with homozygous $\varepsilon 3/\varepsilon 3$ patients. The *z* statistic is calculated using Equation (6.16). Note that the highlighted output agrees with our hand calculations given in the preceding section.

## 6.17. Tied failure times

The most straightforward computational approach to the proportional hazards model can produce biased parameter estimates if a large proportion of the failure times are identical. For this reason, it is best to record failure times as precisely as possible to avoid ties in this variable. If there are extensive ties in the data, there are other approaches which are computationally intensive but which can reduce this bias (see StataCorp, 2007). An alternative approach is to use Poisson regression, which will be discussed in Chapters 8 and 9.

## 6.18. Additional reading

Kalbfleisch and Prentice (2002),
Lawless (2002), and
Cox and Oakes (1984) are three standard references on survival analysis. These texts all assume that the reader has a solid grounding in statistics.
Cox (1972) is the original reference on proportional hazards regression.
Greenwood (1926) is the original reference on Greenwood's formula for the variance of the survival function.
O'Donnell et al. (2000) studied the relationship between apolipoprotein E genotype and intracerebral hemorrhage. We used their data to illustrate survival analysis in this chapter.
Kaplan and Meier (1958) is the original reference on the Kaplan–Meier survival curve.
Mantel (1966) is the original reference on the Mantel–Haenszel test for survival data that is also known as the log-rank test.
Peto and Peto (1972) studied the mathematical properties of the Mantel–Haenszel test for survival data, which they renamed the log-rank test.

## 6.19. Exercises

The following exercises are based on a study by Dupont and Page (1985). A cohort of 3303 Nashville women underwent benign breast biopsies between 1950 and 1968. We obtained follow-up information from these women or their next of kin. You will find a data set on my webpage called *6.ex.breast.dta* that contains some of the information from this cohort. The variables in this file are

$$
\begin{aligned}
&id &&= \text{patient identification number},\\
&entage &&= \text{age at entry biopsy},\\
&follow &&= \text{years of follow-up},\\
&pd &&= \text{diagnosis of entry biopsy}\\
& &&= \begin{cases} 0\text{: no proliferative disease (No PD)}\\ 1\text{: proliferative disease without atypia (PDWA)}\\ 2\text{: atypical hyperplasia (AH)},\end{cases}\\
&fate &&= \text{fate at end of follow-up} = \begin{cases} 0\text{: censored}\\ 1\text{: invasive breast cancer},\end{cases}\\
&fh &&= \text{first degree family history of breast cancer} = \begin{cases} 0\text{: no}\\ 1\text{: yes.}\end{cases}
\end{aligned}
$$

1 Plot Kaplan–Meier breast cancer free survival curves for women with entry diagnoses of AH, PDWA, and No PD as a function of years since biopsy. Is this a useful graphic? If not, why not?
2 Plot the cumulative breast cancer morbidity in patient groups defined by entry histology. What is the estimated probability that a woman with PDWA will develop breast cancer within 15 years of her entry biopsy? Give a 95% confidence interval for this probability. Use the *at* option of the *sts list* command to answer this question.
3 Derive the log-rank test to compare the cumulative morbidity curves for women with these three diagnoses. Are these morbidity curves significantly different from each other? Is the cumulative incidence curve for women with AH significantly different from the curve for women with PDWA? Is the curve for women with PDWA significantly different from the curve for women without PD?
4 Calculate the breast cancer risk of women with AH relative to women without PD. Derive a 95% confidence interval for this relative risk. Calculate this relative risk for women with PDWA compared with women without PD.
5 What are the mean ages of entry biopsy for these three diagnoses? Do they differ significantly from each other? Does your answer complicate the interpretation of the preceding results?

7

# Hazard regression analysis

In the last chapter we introduced the concept of proportional hazards regression analysis to estimate the relative risk associated with a single risk factor from survival data. In this chapter we generalize this technique. We will regress survival outcome against multiple covariates. The technique can be used to deal with multiple confounding variables or effect modifiers in precisely the same way as in logistic or linear regression. Indeed, many of the basic principles of multiple regression using the proportional hazards model have already been covered in previous chapters.

## 7.1. Proportional hazards model

We expand the simple proportional hazards model to handle multiple covariates as follows. Suppose we have a cohort of $n$ patients who we follow forward in time as described in Chapter 6. Let

$t_i$ be the time from entry to exit for the $i^{\text{th}}$ patient,

$$f_i = \begin{cases} 1: & \text{if the } i^{\text{th}} \text{ patient dies at exit} \\ 0: & \text{if the } i^{\text{th}} \text{ patient is censored at exit, and} \end{cases}$$

$x_{i1}, x_{i2}, \ldots, x_{iq}$ be the values of $q$ covariates for the $i^{\text{th}}$ patient.

Let $\lambda_0[t]$ be the hazard function for patients with covariates $x_{i1} = x_{i2} = \cdots = x_{iq} = 0$. Then the proportional hazards model assumes that the hazard function for the $i^{\text{th}}$ patient is

$$\lambda_i[t] = \lambda_0[t] \exp[\beta_1 x_{i1} + \beta_2 x_{i2} + \cdots + \beta_q x_{iq}]. \tag{7.1}$$

## 7.2. Relative risks and hazard ratios

Suppose that patients in risk groups 1 and 2 have covariates $x_{11}, x_{12}, \ldots, x_{1q}$ and $x_{21}, x_{22}, \ldots, x_{2q}$, respectively. Then the relative risk of patients in

Group 2 with respect to those in Group 1 in the time interval $(t, t + \Delta t)$ is

$$\frac{\lambda_2[t]\Delta t}{\lambda_1[t]\Delta t} = \frac{\lambda_0[t]\exp[x_{21}\beta_1 + x_{22}\beta_2 + \cdots + x_{2q}\beta_q]}{\lambda_0[t]\exp[x_{11}\beta_1 + x_{12}\beta_2 + \cdots + x_{1q}\beta_q]}$$
$$= \exp[(x_{21} - x_{11})\beta_1 + (x_{22} - x_{12})\beta_2 + \cdots + (x_{2q} - x_{1q})\beta_q]. \tag{7.2}$$

Note that $\lambda_0[t]$ drops out of this equation, and that this instantaneous relative risk remains constant over time. Thus, if the proportional hazards model is reasonable, we can interpret

$$(x_{21} - x_{11})\beta_1 + (x_{22} - x_{12})\beta_2 + \cdots + (x_{2q} - x_{1q})\beta_q \tag{7.3}$$

as being the log relative risk associated with Group 2 patients as compared with Group 1 patients. Proportional hazards regression provides maximum likelihood estimates $\hat{\beta}_1, \hat{\beta}_2, \ldots, \hat{\beta}_q$ of the model parameters $\beta_1, \beta_2, \ldots \beta_q$. We use these estimates in Equation (7.2) to estimate relative risks from the model.

It should be noted that there are strong similarities between logistic regression and proportional hazards regression. Indeed, if $d_i$ denotes the fates of two patients selected from risk groups $i = 1$ and 2, respectively, who followed the multiple logistic model (5.11), then

$$\text{logit}[\text{E}[d_i \mid \mathbf{x}_i]] = \log[\pi_i/(1 - \pi_i)] = \alpha + \beta_1 x_{i1} + \beta_2 x_{i2} + \cdots + \beta_q x_{iq}.$$

Subtracting the log odds for the first patient from the second gives us

$$\log\left[\frac{\pi_2/(1 - \pi_2)}{\pi_1/(1 - \pi_1)}\right] = (x_{21} - x_{11})\,\beta_1 + (x_{22} - x_{12})\,\beta_2 + \cdots$$
$$+ (x_{2q} - x_{1q})\beta_q.$$

Hence, the only difference in the interpretation of logistic and proportional hazards regression models is that in logistic regression Equation (7.3) is interpreted as a log odds ratio while in proportional hazards regression it is interpreted as a log relative risk.

Proportional hazards regression also provides an estimate of the variance–covariance matrix for $\hat{\beta}_1, \hat{\beta}_2, \ldots, \hat{\beta}_q$ (see Section 5.17). The elements of this matrix are $s_{ij}$, the estimated covariance between $\hat{\beta}_i$ and $\hat{\beta}_j$, and $s_{ii}$, the estimated variance of $\hat{\beta}_i$. These variance and covariance terms are used in the same way as in Chapter 5 to calculate confidence intervals and to test hypotheses. Changes in model deviance between nested models are also used in the same way as in Chapter 5 as a guide to model building. I recommend that you read Chapter 5 before this chapter.

## 7.3. 95% confidence intervals and hypothesis tests

Suppose that $f = \Sigma c_j \beta_j$ is a weighted sum of the model coefficients and that $\hat{f} = \Sigma c_j \hat{\beta}_j$ is as in Equation (5.29). Then the variance of $\hat{f}$ is estimated by $s_f^2$ in Equation (5.30). If $\exp[f]$ is a relative risk, then the 95% confidence interval for this risk is given by Equation (5.32). We test the null hypotheses that $\exp[f] = 1$ using the $z$ statistic defined in Equation (5.33).

## 7.4. Nested models and model deviance

We fit appropriate models to the data by comparing the change in model deviance between nested models. The model deviance is defined by Equation (5.45). Suppose that we are considering two models and that model 1 is nested within model 2. Then the change in deviance $\Delta D$ between these models is given by Equation (5.46). Under the null hypothesis that model 1 is true, $\Delta D$ will have an approximately chi-squared distribution whose degrees of freedom equal the difference in the number of parameters in the two models.

## 7.5. An example: the Framingham Heart Study

Let us return to the Framingham didactic data set introduced in Sections 2.19.1 and 3.11. This data set contains long-term follow-up and cardiovascular outcome data on a large cohort of men and women. We will investigate the effects of gender and baseline diastolic blood pressure (DBP) on coronary heart disease (CHD) adjusted for other risk factors. Analyzing a complex real data set involves a considerable degree of judgment, and there is no single correct way to proceed. The following, however, includes the typical components of such an analysis.

### 7.5.1. Kaplan–Meier survival curves for DBP

The first step is to perform a univariate analysis on the effects of DBP on CHD. Figure 7.1 shows a histogram of baseline DBP in this cohort. The range of blood pressures is very wide. Ninety-five per cent of the observations lie between 60 and 110 mm Hg. However, the data set is large enough that there are still 150 subjects with DBP $\leq$60 and 105 patients with pressures greater than 110. We subdivide the study subjects into seven groups based on their DBPs. Group 1 consists of patients with DBP $\leq$60, Group 2 has DBPs between 61 and 70, Group 3 has DBPs between 71 and 80, etcetera. The last

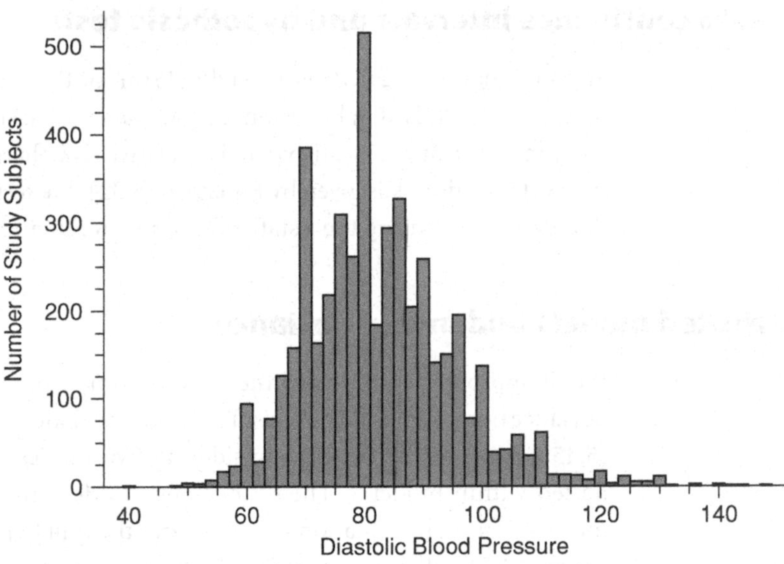


Figure 7.1 Histogram of baseline diastolic blood pressure among subjects from the Framingham Heart Study (Levy et al., 1999). These pressures were collected before the era of effective medical control of hypertension. (The jagged shape of this histogram is due to a digit preference in recording blood pressures. Blood pressures ending in a 0 were recorded most often, followed by even pressures and then pressures ending in a 5. Blood pressures ending in a 1, 3, 7 or 9 were rarely recorded.)

group (Group 7) has DBPs greater than 110. Figure 7.2 shows the Kaplan–Meier CHD free survival curves for these groups. The risk of CHD increases markedly with increasing DBP. The log-rank $\chi^2$ statistic equals 260 with six degrees of freedom ($P < 10^{-52}$). Hence, we can reject the hypothesis that the survival curves for these groups are all equal with overwhelming statistical significance. Moreover, the log-rank tests of each adjacent pair of survival curves are also statistically significant. Hence, the data provide clear evidence that even modest increases in baseline DBP are predictive of increased risk of CHD.

## 7.5.2. Simple hazard regression model for CHD risk and DBP

Suppose that we would like to calculate the relative risk of CHD associated with baseline DBP. Let us choose the denominator for this relative risk to be patients with a baseline DBP of 60 mm Hg. Then a simple model of this

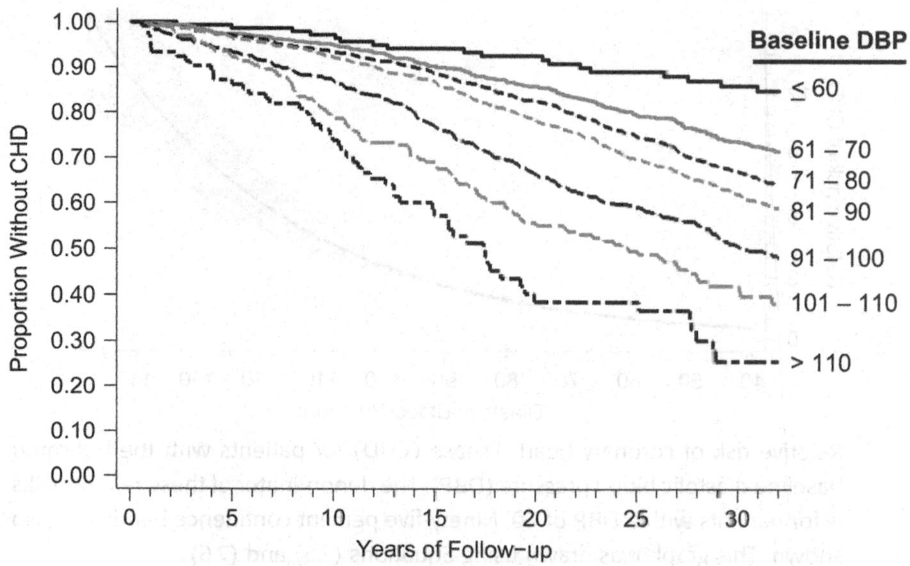


Figure 7.2 Effect of baseline diastolic blood pressure (DBP) on the risk of subsequent coronary heart disease (CHD). The proportion of subjects who subsequently develop CHD increases steadily with increasing DBP. This elevation in risk persists for over 30 years (Framingham Heart Study, 1997).

risk is

$$\lambda_i[t] = \lambda_0[t] \exp\left[\beta\left(dbp_i - 60\right)\right], \tag{7.4}$$

where $dbp_i$ is the baseline DBP for the $i^{\text{th}}$ patient. We calculate the desired relative risk by Equation (7.2). Note that when $dbp_i = 60$ that Equation (7.4) reduces to $\lambda_0[t]$. Hence, dividing a patient's hazard function by the hazard function for some other patient with a baseline DBP of 60 gives the patient's estimated relative risk of CHD to be

$$\exp\left[\hat{\beta}\left(dbp_i - 60\right)\right], \tag{7.5}$$

where $\hat{\beta}$ is the maximum likelihood estimate of $\beta$ under this model. A 95% confidence interval for this relative risk is

$$\exp\left[\hat{\beta}\left(dbp_i - 60\right) \pm 1.96 \times \text{se}[\hat{\beta}]\right], \tag{7.6}$$

Figure 7.3 shows a plot of the relative risk of CHD together with 95% confidence bands using Equations (7.5) and (7.6).

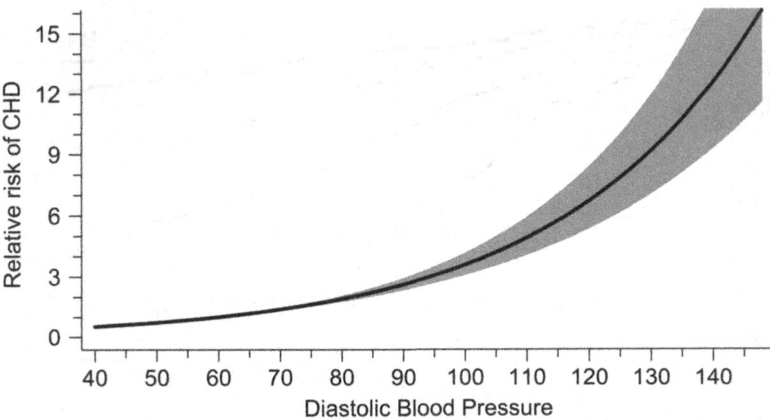


Figure 7.3 Relative risk of coronary heart disease (CHD) for patients with the indicated baseline diastolic blood pressure (DBP). The denominator of these relative risks is for patients with a DBP of 60. Ninety-five percent confidence bands are also shown. This graph was drawn using Equations (7.5) and (7.6).

### 7.5.3. Restricted cubic spline model of CHD risk and DBP

A potential problem with Model (7.5) is that it forces an exponential relationship between CHD relative risk and baseline DBP. This could be quite misleading if this relationship was false, given the wide range of baseline DBPs in the Framingham study. An effective way of weakening this assumption is through fitting a restricted cubic spline (RCS) model (see Section 3.24). Let

$dbp60_i = dbp_i - 60$ and let
$f_1[dbp60_i], f_2[dbp60_i], \ldots, f_{q-1}[dbp60_i]$ be spline covariates associated with $q$ knot values at $dbp60 = u_1, u_2, \ldots, u_q$. Consider the model

$$\lambda_i[t] = \lambda_0[t] \exp\big[\beta_1 f_1[dbp60_i] + \beta_2 f_2[dbp60_i] + \cdots + \beta_{q-1} f_{q-1}[dbp60_i]\big]. \tag{7.7}$$

Now a property of any set of RCS covariates is that $f_1[x] = x$ and $f_2[x] = f_3[x] = \cdots = f_{q-1}[x] = 0$ for all values of $x$ that are less than the first knot. If we calculate the spline covariates for $dbp60_i$ with five knots at their default locations the smallest knot value is 4. For a patient with DBP = 60, $f_1[dbp60_i] = dbp60_i = 0 < 4$ and hence $f_1[dbp60_i] = f_2[dbp60_i] = f_3[dbp60_i] = f_4[dbp60_i] = 0$. Thus, Equation (7.7) reduces to $\lambda_i[t] = \lambda_0[t]$ when $dbp60_i = 0$. It follows from the same argument given in Section 7.5.2 that the risk of CHD associated with a specific DBP relative to a DBP of 60 is

$$\exp[\beta_1 f_1[dbp60_i] + \beta_2 f_2[dbp60_i] + \beta_3 f_3[dbp60_i] + \beta_4 f_4[dbp60_i]]. \tag{7.8}$$

Note that Equation (7.8) is just the exponentiated value of the linear predictor in Model (7.7). This makes calculating relative risks from RCS proportional hazards models particularly easy in languages like Stata.

In general, if $x$ is a continuous covariate and we are interested in calculating relative risks with respect to some baseline value $x_0$ then we set $y = x - x_0$, calculate spline covariates $f_1[y]$, $f_2[y]$, ..., $f_{q-1}[y]$ with knots $u_1, u_2, \ldots, u_q$ and analyze the model

$$\lambda_i[t] = \lambda_0[t] \exp[\beta_1 f_1[y_i] + \beta_2 f_2[y_i] + \cdots + \beta_{q-1} f_{q-1}[y_i]]. \tag{7.9}$$

Then as long as $x_0 < u_1$ the risk associated with having a covariate value $x$ relative to someone with a covariate value $x_0$ is estimated by

$$\exp[\hat{\beta}_1 f_1[y_i] + \hat{\beta}_2 f_2[y_i] + \cdots + \hat{\beta}_{q-1} f_{q-1}[y_i]] \tag{7.10}$$

under this model. If

$$xb = \hat{\beta}_1 f_1[y_i] + \hat{\beta}_2 f_2[y_i] + \cdots + \hat{\beta}_{q-1} f_{q-1}[y_i]$$

is the estimated linear predictor under this model, then a 95% confidence interval for this relative risk is

$$\exp[xb \pm 1.96 \times \mathrm{se}[xb]] \tag{7.11}$$

where se[$xb$] is the estimated standard error of $xb$.

Now Model (7.4) is nested within Model (7.7). Hence, we can use a likelihood ratio test of the validity of Model (7.4) (see Section 5.24). This test is not significant ($P = 0.18$) and indicates that there is no statistical evidence to reject the simple Model (7.4). The next thing we might try is a simpler RCS model. A three-knot model yields a likelihood ratio test with $P = 0.56$ and the resulting relative risk estimates track those of the simple model closely. The default knots for this three-knot model are at 8, 20, and 40. One of the challenging aspects of this data set is that it is highly skewed, with a small proportion of patients having baseline DBPs that range as high as 148. This latter blood pressure translates into a value of *dbp60* of 88. There is no obvious best way of modeling these data. You could use the RSC models describe above as justification for using the simple

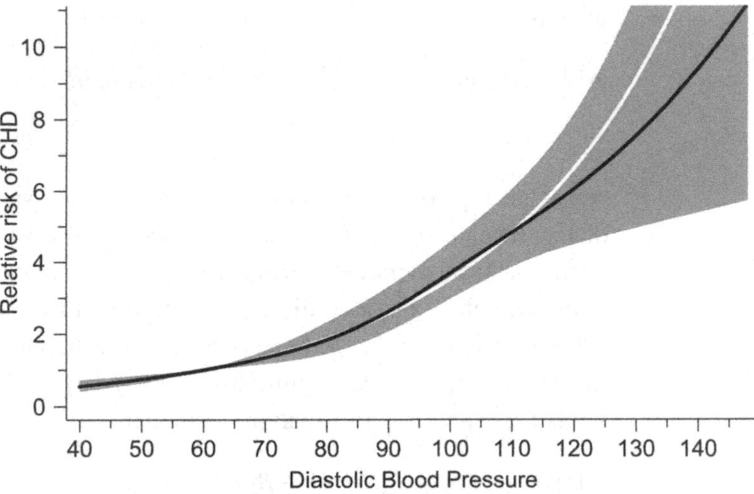


Figure 7.4 This graph is similar to Figure 7.3 but is derived from a four-knot RCS model. The knots in this model correspond to DBPs of 68, 80, 100, and 120 mm Hg. The white curve gives the relative risks from Figure 7.3 for comparison. These analyses are highly consistent for blood pressures below 110 mm Hg. For higher pressures the dearth of data creates great uncertainty about the true relative risks. There is, however, impressive evidence that these risks are very high.

model, or settle on the three-knot model. The three-knot model is reasonable in many ways, but I was concerned about the fact that baseline blood pressures could range as high as 48 units above the largest knot. In this range, the three knot model imposes a linear relationship between the log relative risk and *dbp60*. Since there is no a priori reason why this should be true, I decided to weaken the three-knot model by adding an additional knot at $dbp60 = 60$. Figure 7.4 shows a graph of the relative risk of CHD under this model. In this figure the relative risk curve is plotted using Equation (7.10) with $y$ replaced by *dbp60* and $q = 4$ knots at 8, 20, 40, and 60. The 95% confidence band is derived using Equation (7.11). The relative risk curve from the simple Model (7.5) is also shown in white for comparison. These analyses provide convincing evidence that the relationship between CHD relative risk and baseline DBP is approximately exponential between 40 and 110 mm Hg. The relative risk continues to rise with higher blood pressures but the confidence intervals become very wide due to the small number of patients with blood pressures in this range. There is no statistical evidence to reject the simple exponential model over the entire blood pressure range. However, our four-knot RCS model provides relative risk estimates that are less than those of the exponential model for extremely high values of DBP.

### 7.5.4. Categorical hazard regression model of CHD risk and DBP

A more traditional way of estimating the relative risks associated with a continuous risk factor is to group the observations into a discrete number of categories. The analysis then precedes in exactly the same way as for estimating odds ratios associated with categorical risk factors in logistic regression. For example, let

$$dbp_{ij} = \begin{cases} 1: & \text{if the } i^{\text{th}} \text{ patient is in DBP Group } j \\ 0: & \text{otherwise,} \end{cases}$$

where the blood pressure groups are defined as in Section 7.5.1. Then a simple proportional hazards model for estimating the relative risks associated with these blood pressures is

$$\lambda_i[t] = \lambda_0[t] \exp[\beta_2 \times dbp_{i2} + \beta_3 \times dbp_{i3} + \beta_4 \times dbp_{i4} + \beta_5 \times dbp_{i5} + \beta_6 \times dbp_{i6} + \beta_7 \times dbp_{i7}]. \tag{7.12}$$

For a patient in DBP Group 1, the hazard equals $\lambda_0[t] \exp[\beta_2 \times 0 + \beta_3 \times 0 + \cdots + \beta_7 \times 0] = \lambda_0[t]$. For a patient in Group $j$, the hazard is $\lambda_0[t] \exp[\beta_j \times 1]$ for $2 \le j \le 7$. Dividing $\lambda_0[t] \exp[\beta_j]\Delta t$ by $\lambda_0[t]\Delta t$ gives the relative risk for patients in DBP Group $j$ relative to Group 1, which is $\exp[\beta_j]$. The log relative risk for Group $j$ compared to Group 1 is $\beta_j$. Let $\hat{\beta}_j$ denote the maximum likelihood estimate of $\beta_j$ and let $\text{se}[\hat{\beta}_j] = \sqrt{s_{jj}}$ denote the estimated standard error of $\hat{\beta}_j$. Then the estimated relative risk for subjects in Group $j$ relative to those in Group 1 is $\exp[\hat{\beta}_j]$. The 95% confidence interval for this risk is

$$(\exp[\hat{\beta}_j - 1.96\,\text{se}[\hat{\beta}_j]], \exp[\hat{\beta}_j + 1.96\,\text{se}[\hat{\beta}_j]]). \tag{7.13}$$

Table 7.1 shows the estimates of $\beta_j$ together with the corresponding relative risk estimates and 95% confidence intervals that result from Model (7.12). These estimates are consistent with Figure 7.2 and confirm the importance of DBP as a predictor of subsequent risk of coronary heart disease. It is also instructive to compare Table 7.1 with Figure 7.4. Note that the reference group in Figure 7.4 consist of patients with a DBP of 60, while in Table 7.1 it consists of all patients with a DBP ≤60. This latter group has less risk of CHD than patients with a DBP of exactly 60. It is for this reason that the relative risks in Table 7.1 are higher than those in Figure 7.4.

**Table 7.1.** Effect of baseline diastolic blood pressure on coronary heart disease. The Framingham Heart Study data were analyzed using Model (7.12)

| Baseline diastolic blood pressure | Number of subjects | Cases of coronary heart disease | $\hat{\beta}_j$ | Relative risk | 95% confidence interval |
|---|---|---|---|---|---|
| ≤60 mm Hg | 150 | 18 | | 1.0* | |
| 61 – 70 mm Hg | 774 | 182 | 0.677 | 1.97 | (1.2–3.2) |
| 71 – 80 mm Hg | 1467 | 419 | 0.939 | 2.56 | (1.6–4.1) |
| 81 – 90 mm Hg | 1267 | 404 | 1.117 | 3.06 | (1.9–4.9) |
| 91 –100 mm Hg | 701 | 284 | 1.512 | 4.54 | (2.8–7.3) |
| 101 – 110 mm Hg | 235 | 110 | 1.839 | 6.29 | (3.8–10) |
| >110 mm Hg | 105 | 56 | 2.247 | 9.46 | (5.6–16) |
| Total | 4699 | 1473 | | | |

*Denominator of relative risk

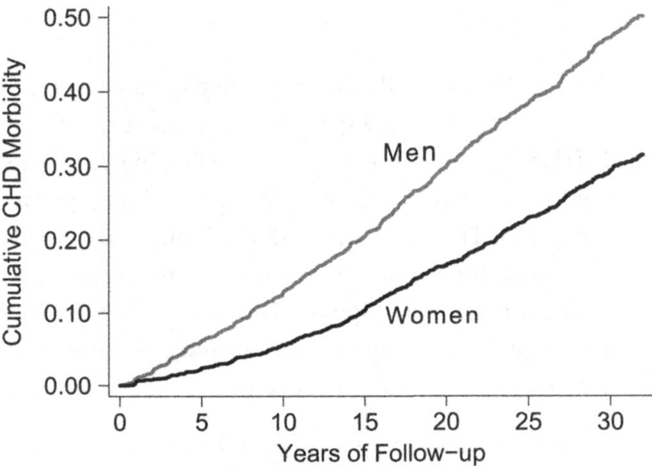


Figure 7.5 Cumulative incidence of coronary heart disease (CHD) in men and women from the Framingham Heart Study (Levy et al., 1999).

## 7.5.5. Simple hazard regression model of CHD risk and gender

Figure 7.5 shows the Kaplan–Meier CHD morbidity curves for men and women from the Framingham Heart Study. The log-rank statistic for comparing these curves has one degree of freedom and equals 155. This statistic is also highly significant ($P < 10^{-34}$). Let

$$male_i = \begin{cases} 1: & \text{if } i^{\text{th}} \text{ subject is a man} \\ 0: & \text{if } i^{\text{th}} \text{ subject is a woman.} \end{cases}$$

Then a simple hazard regression model for estimating the effects of gender on CHD is

$$\lambda_i[t] = \lambda_0[t] \exp[\beta \times male_i]. \tag{7.14}$$

This model gives $\hat{\beta} = 0.642$ with standard error $\text{se}[\hat{\beta}] = 0.0525$. Therefore, the estimated relative risk of CHD in men relative to women is $\exp[0.642] = 1.90$. We calculate the 95% confidence interval for this risk to be (1.71–2.11) using Equation (7.13).

### 7.5.6. Multiplicative model of DBP and gender on risk of CHD

The next step is to fit a multiplicative model of DBP and gender on CHD (see Section 5.18). Consider the model

$$\lambda_i[t] = \lambda_0[t] \exp\left[\sum_{h=2}^{7} \beta_h \times dbp_{ih} + \gamma \times male_i\right]. \tag{7.15}$$

The interpretation of this model is precisely analogous to that for Model (5.39) in Section 5.19. To derive any relative risk under this model, write down the hazards for patients in the numerator and denominator of the desired relative risk. Then, divide the numerator hazard by the denominator hazard. You should be able to convince yourself that

- $\beta_h$ is the log relative risk of women in DBP Group $h$ relative to women in DBP Group 1,
- $\gamma$ is the log relative risk of men in DBP Group 1 relative to women in DBP Group 1, and
- $\beta_h + \gamma$ is the log relative risk of men in DBP Group $h$ relative to women in DBP Group 1.
- If $R_h$ is the relative risk of being in Group $h$ vs. Group 1 among women, and $R_m$ is the relative risk of men vs. women among people in Group 1, then the relative risk of men in Group $h$ relative to women in Group 1 equals $R_h \times R_m$. In other words, the effects of gender and blood pressure in Model (7.15) are multiplicative.

Model (7.15) was used to produce the relative risk estimates in Table 7.2. Note that Model (7.12) is nested within Model (7.15). That is, if $\gamma = 0$ then Model (7.15) reduces to Model (7.12). This allows us to use the change

**Table 7.2.** Effect of gender and baseline diastolic blood pressure on coronary heart disease. The Framingham Heart Study data are analyzed using the multiplicative Model (7.15).

| | Gender | | | |
|---|---|---|---|---|
| | Women | | Men | |
| Baseline diastolic blood pressure | Relative risk | 95% confidence interval | Relative risk | 95% confidence interval |
| ≤60 mm Hg | 1.0* | | 1.83 | (1.7–2.0) |
| 61–70 mm Hg | 1.91 | (1.2–3.1) | 3.51 | (2.1–5.7) |
| 71–80 mm Hg | 2.43 | (1.5–3.9) | 4.46 | (2.8–7.2) |
| 81–90 mm Hg | 2.78 | (1.7–4.5) | 5.09 | (3.2–8.2) |
| 91–100 mm Hg | 4.06 | (2.5–6.5) | 7.45 | (4.6–12) |
| 101–110 mm Hg | 5.96 | (3.6–9.8) | 10.9 | (6.6–18) |
| >110 mm Hg | 9.18 | (5.4–16) | 16.8 | (9.8–29) |

*Denominator of relative risk

in model deviance to test whether adding gender improves the fit of the model to the data. This change in deviance is $\Delta D = 133$, which has an approximately chi-squared distribution with one degree of freedom under the null hypothesis that $\gamma = 0$. Hence, we can reject this null hypothesis with overwhelming statistical significance ($P < 10^{-30}$).

### 7.5.7. Using interaction terms to model the effects of gender and DBP on CHD

We next add interaction terms to weaken the multiplicative assumption in Model (7.15) (see Sections 5.18 and 5.19). Let

$$\lambda_i[t] = \lambda_0[t] \exp\left[\sum_{h=2}^{7} \beta_h \times dbp_{ih} + \gamma \times male_i + \sum_{h=2}^{7} \delta_h \times dbp_{ih} \times male_i\right]. \tag{7.16}$$

This model is analogous to Model (5.41) for esophageal cancer. For men in DBP Group $h$, the hazard is $\lambda_0[t]\exp[\beta_h + \gamma + \delta_h]$. For women in Group 1, the hazard is $\lambda_0[t]$. Hence, the relative risk for men in DBP Group $h$ relative to women in DBP Group 1 is $(\lambda_0[t]\exp[\beta_h + \gamma + \delta_h])/\lambda_0[t] = \exp[\beta_h + \gamma + \delta_h]$. This model was used to generate the relative risks in

**Table 7.3.** Effect of gender and baseline diastolic blood pressure on coronary heart disease. The Framingham Heart Study data are analyzed using Model (7.16), which includes interaction terms for the joint effects of gender and blood pressure

| | Gender | | | |
|---|---|---|---|---|
| | Women | | Men | |
| Baseline diastolic blood pressure | Relative risk | 95% confidence interval | Relative risk | 95% confidence interval |
| ≤60 mm Hg | 1.0* | | 2.37 | (0.94–6.0) |
| 61–70 mm Hg | 1.83 | (0.92–3.6) | 4.59 | (2.3–9.1) |
| 71–80 mm Hg | 2.43 | (1.2–4.7) | 5.55 | (2.9–11) |
| 81–90 mm Hg | 3.52 | (1.8–6.9) | 5.28 | (2.7–10) |
| 91–100 mm Hg | 4.69 | (2.4–9.3) | 8.28 | (4.2–16) |
| 101–110 mm Hg | 7.64 | (3.8–15) | 10.9 | (5.4–22) |
| >110 mm Hg | 13.6 | (6.6–28) | 13.0 | (5.9–29) |

*Denominator of relative risk

Table 7.3. Note the marked differences between the estimates in Table 7.2 and 7.3. Model (7.16) indicates that the effect of gender on the risk of CHD is greatest for people with low or moderate blood pressure and diminishes as blood pressure rises. Gender has no apparent effect on CHD for people with a DBP above 110 mm Hg, although the associated confidence intervals are wide.

Model (7.15) is nested within Model (7.16). Hence, we can use the change in the model deviance to test the null hypothesis that the multiplicative model is correct. This change in deviance is $\Delta D = 21.23$. Model (7.16) has six more parameters than Model (7.15). Therefore, under the null hypothesis $\Delta D$ has an approximately chi-squared distribution with six degrees of freedom. The probability that this statistic exceeds 21.23 is $P = 0.002$. Thus, the evidence of interaction between DBP and gender on CHD risk is statistically significant.

### 7.5.8. Adjusting for confounding variables

So far we have not adjusted our results for other confounding variables. Of particular importance is age at baseline exam. Figure 7.6 shows that this age varied widely among study subjects. As both DBP and risk of CHD increases

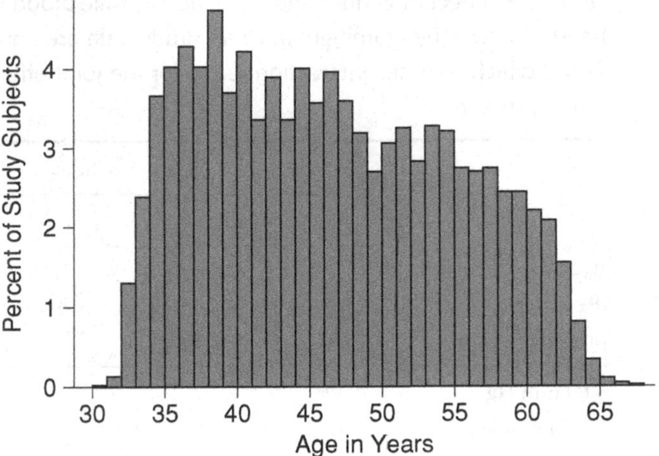


Figure 7.6 Histogram showing the age at baseline exam of subjects in the Framingham Heart Study (Levy et al., 1999).

markedly with age, we would expect age to strongly confound the effect of DBP on CHD. Other potential confounding variables that we may wish to consider include body mass index and serum cholesterol. Let $age_i$, $bmi_i$, and $scl_i$ denote the age, body mass index, and serum cholesterol of the $i^{\text{th}}$ patient. We add these variables one at a time, giving models

$$\lambda_i[t] = \lambda_0[t] \exp\left[\sum_{h=2}^{7} \beta_h \times dbp_{ih} + \gamma \times male_i + \sum_{h=2}^{7} \delta_h \times dbp_{ih} \times male_i + \theta_1 \times age_i\right], \tag{7.17}$$

$$\lambda_i[t] = \lambda_0[t] \exp\left[\sum_{h=2}^{7} \beta_h \times dbp_{ih} + \gamma \times male_i + \sum_{h=2}^{7} \delta_h \times dbp_{ih} \times male_i + \theta_1 \times age_i + \theta_2 \times bmi_i\right], \text{ and} \tag{7.18}$$

$$\lambda_i[t] = \lambda_0[t] \exp\left[\sum_{h=2}^{7} \beta_h \times dbp_{ih} + \gamma \times male_i + \sum_{h=2}^{7} \delta_h \times dbp_{ih} \times male_i + \theta_1 \times age_i + \theta_2 \times bmi_i + \theta_3 \times scl_i\right]. \tag{7.19}$$

Note that Model (7.16) is nested within Model (7.17), Model (7.17) is nested within Model (7.18), and Model (7.18) is nested within Model (7.19). Hence,

**Table 7.4.** Effect of gender and baseline diastolic blood pressure (DBP) on coronary heart disease. The Framingham Heart Study data are analyzed using Model (7.19). This model includes gender–DBP interaction terms and adjusts for age, body mass index, and serum cholesterol

| | Gender | | | |
|---|---|---|---|---|
| | Women | | Men | |
| Baseline diastolic blood pressure | Relative risk† | 95% confidence interval | Relative risk† | 95% confidence interval |
| ≤60 mm Hg | 1.0* | | 1.98 | (0.79–5.0) |
| 61–70 mm Hg | 1.51 | (0.76–3.0) | 3.53 | (1.8–7.0) |
| 71–80 mm Hg | 1.65 | (0.85–3.2) | 3.88 | (2.0–7.6) |
| 81–90 mm Hg | 1.91 | (0.98–3.7) | 3.33 | (1.7–6.5) |
| 91–100 mm Hg | 1.94 | (0.97–3.9) | 4.86 | (2.5–9.5) |
| 101–110 mm Hg | 3.10 | (1.5–6.3) | 6.29 | (3.1–13) |
| >110 mm Hg | 5.27 | (2.5–11) | 6.40 | (2.9–14) |

*Denominator of relative risk

†Adjusted for age, body mass index, and serum cholesterol.

we can derive the change in model deviance with each successive model to test whether each new term significantly improves the model fit. These tests show that age, body mass index, and serum cholesterol all substantially improve the model fit, and that the null hypotheses $\theta_1 = 0$, $\theta_2 = 0$, and $\theta_3 = 0$ may all be rejected with overwhelming statistical significance. These tests also show that these variables are important independent predictors of CHD. Table 7.4 shows the estimated relative risks of CHD associated with DBP and gender that are obtained from Model (7.19).

### 7.5.9. Interpretation

Tables 7.2, 7.3, and 7.4 are all estimating similar relative risks from the same data set. It is therefore sobering to see how different these estimates are. It is very important to understand the implications of the models used to derive these tables. Men in DBP Group 1 have a lower risk in Table 7.2 than in Table 7.3 while the converse is true for men in DBP Group 7. This is because Model (7.15) forces the relative risks in Table 7.2 to obey the multiplicative assumption while Model (7.16) permits the effect of gender on CHD to diminish with increasing DBP.

The relative risks in Table 7.4 are substantially smaller than those in Table 7.3. It is important to realize that the relative risks in Table 7.4 compare people of the same age, body mass index, and serum cholesterol while those of Table 7.3 compare people without regard to these three risk factors. Our analyses show that age, body mass index, and serum cholesterol are risk factors for CHD in their own right. Also, these risk factors are positively correlated with DBP. Hence, it is not surprising that the unadjusted risks of DBP and gender in Table 7.3 are inflated by confounding due to these other variables. In general, the decision as to which variables to include as confounding variables is affected by how the results are to be used and our knowledge of the etiology of the disease being studied. For example, since it is easier to measure blood pressure than serum cholesterol, it might be more clinically useful to know the effect of DBP on CHD without adjustment for serum cholesterol. If we are trying to establish a causal link between a risk factor and a disease, then it is important to avoid adjusting for any condition that may be an intermediate outcome between the initial cause and the final outcome.

### 7.5.10. Alternative models

In Model (7.19) we treat age, body mass index, and serum cholesterol as continuous variables while DBP is recoded into seven dichotomous variables involving six parameters. We could have treated these confounding variables in the same way as DBP. In our analysis of esophageal cancer in Chapter 5 we treated age in precisely this way. In general, it is best to recode those continuous variables that are of primary interest into several dichotomous variables or to use restricted cubic splines to avoid assuming a linear relationship between these risk factors and the log relative risk. It may, however, be reasonable to treat confounding variables as continuous. The advantage of putting a continuous variable directly into the model is that it requires only one parameter. The cost of making the linear assumption may not be too important for a variable that is included in the model only because it is a confounder. It is also important to note that we can build models with restricted cubic splines and interaction terms. For example, a model similar to Model (7.16) but with the $dbp_{ih}$ indicator covariates replaced by spline covariates may be used to estimate relative risk curves that have different shapes for men and women. Therneau and Grambsch (2000) provide a comprehensive discussion of advanced modeling methods for survival data.

## 7.6. Proportional hazards regression analysis using Stata

The following log file and comments illustrate how to perform the analyses from the preceding sections using Stata.

```
. *   7.6.Framingham.log
. *
. *   Proportional hazards regression analysis of the effect of gender
. *   and baseline diastolic blood pressure (DBP) on coronary heart
. *   disease (CHD) adjusted for age, body mass index (BMI), and serum
. *   cholesterol (SCL).
. *
. set memory 2000                                                          1
Current memory allocation

                  current                                    memory usage
    settable        value     description                    (1M = 1024k)
    ---------------------------------------------------------------------
    set maxvar       5000     max. variables allowed             1.909M
    set memory      2000k     max. data space                    1.953M
    set matsize       400     max. RHS vars in models            1.254M
                                                             -----------
                                                                 5.116M

. use C:\WDDtext\2.20.Framingham.dta
. *
. *   Univariate analysis of the effect of DBP on CHD
. *
. histogram dbp, start(39) width(2) frequency ylabel(0(100)500)            2
>     ymtick(0(25)525) xlabel(40(20)140) xmtick(40(5)140)
>     ytitle(Number of Study Subjects)
(bin=55, start=39, width=2)
. generate dbpgr = recode(dbp,60,70,80,90,100,110,111)                      3
. tabulate dbpgr chdfate                                                    4

           |   Coronary Heart
           |      Disease
     dbpgr |  Censored        CHD |     Total
-----------+----------------------+----------
        60 |       132         18 |       150
        70 |       592        182 |       774
```

| | | | |
|---|---|---|---|
| 80 | 1,048 | 419 | 1,467 |
| 90 | 863 | 404 | 1,267 |
| 100 | 417 | 284 | 701 |
| 110 | 125 | 110 | 235 |
| 111 | 49 | 56 | 105 |
| Total | 3,226 | 1,473 | 4,699 |

```
. label define dbp 60 "        DBP <= 60"   70 "60  < DBP <= 70"
>                  80 "70  < DBP <= 80"   90 "80  < DBP <= 90"
>                 100 "90  < DBP <= 100" 110 "100 < DBP <= 110"
>                 111 "110 < DBP"
. label variable dbpgr "DBP level"
. label values dbpgr dbp
. generate time = followup/365.25                                          5
. label variable time "Follow-up in Years"
. stset time, failure(chdfate)

     failure event:  chdfate != 0 & chdfate < .
obs. time interval:  (0, time]
 exit on or before:  failure

------------------------------------------------------------------------------
     4699  total obs.
        0  exclusions
------------------------------------------------------------------------------
     4699  obs. remaining, representing
     1473  failures in single record/single failure data
 103710.1  total analysis time at risk, at risk from t =         0
                             earliest observed entry t =         0
                                  last observed exit t =        32

. sts graph, by(dbpgr) ytitle(Proportion Without CHD)                      6
>    ylabel(0(.1)1) xlabel(0(5)30) xmtick(1(1)32)
>    xtitle(Years of Follow-up) plot2opts(color(gray))                     7
>    plot3opts(color(black) lpattern(dash))
>    plot4opts(color(gray)  lpattern(dash))
>    plot5opts(color(black) lpattern(longdash))
>    plot6opts(color(gray)  lpattern(longdash))                            8
>    plot7opts(color(black) lpattern("_-"))                                9
>    title(" ",size(zero)) legend(ring(0) position(7) col(1))
```

```
>     order(1 "DBP <= 60" 2 "60  < DBP <= 70"
>         3 "70 < DBP <=  80"   4 "80 < DBP <=  90"
>         5 "90  < DBP <= 100"  6 "100 < DBP <= 110" 7 "110 < DBP"))
         failure _d:  chdfate
   analysis time _t:  time
```

```
. sts test dbpgr
```
10

```
         failure _d:  chdfate
   analysis time _t:  time
```

Log-rank test for equality of survivor functions

| dbpgr | Events observed | Events expected |
|---|---|---|
| DBP <= 60 | 18 | 53.63 |
| 60 < DBP <= 70 | 182 | 275.72 |
| 70 < DBP <= 80 | 419 | 489.41 |
| 80 < DBP <= 90 | 404 | 395.62 |
| 90 < DBP <= 100 | 284 | 187.97 |
| 100 < DBP <= 110 | 110 | 52.73 |
| 110 < DBP | 56 | 17.94 |
| Total | 1473 | 1473.00 |

```
                 chi2(6) =      259.71
                 Pr>chi2 =      0.0000
```

```
. sts test dbpgr if dbpgr ==  60 | dbpgr == 70
```
11

```
         failure _d:  chdfate
   analysis time _t:  time
```

Log-rank test for equality of survivor functions

| dbpgr | Events observed | Events expected |
|---|---|---|
| DBP <= 60 | 18 | 32.58 |
| 60 < DBP <= 70 | 182 | 167.42 |
| Total | 200 | 200.00 |

```
            chi2(1) =      7.80
            Pr>chi2 =      0.0052
```

```
. sts test dbpgr if dbpgr ==  70 | dbpgr == 80
```
12

Output omitted

```
            Pr>chi2 =      0.0028
```

```
. sts test dbpgr if dbpgr ==  80 | dbpgr == 90
```

Output omitted

```
                 Pr>chi2 =    0.0090
. sts test dbpgr if dbpgr ==  90 | dbpgr == 100
```

Output omitted

```
                 Pr>chi2 =    0.0000
. sts test dbpgr if dbpgr == 100 | dbpgr == 110
```

Output omitted

```
                 Pr>chi2 =    0.0053
. sts test dbpgr if dbpgr == 110 | dbpgr == 111
```

Output omitted

```
                 Pr>chi2 =    0.0215
. *
. *  Hazard regression analysis with dbp - 60 as a continuous
. *  covariate.
. *
. generate dbp60 = dbp - 60
. stcox dbp60
         failure _d:  chdfate
   analysis time _t:  time
```

Output omitted

```
Cox regression -- Breslow method for ties
No. of subjects =         4699                Number of obs    =      4699
No. of failures =         1473
Time at risk    =  103710.0917
                                              LR chi2(1)       =    242.08
Log likelihood  =   -11713.816                Prob > chi2      =    0.0000
```

| _t | Haz. Ratio | Std. Err. | z | P>\|z\| | [95% Conf. Interval] | |
|---|---|---|---|---|---|---|
| dbp60 | 1.032064 | .0019926 | 16.35 | 0.000 | 1.028166 | 1.035977 |

13

```
. estimates store simple
. predict loghaz, xb                                              14
. predict relhaz1, hr                                             15
. predict se, stdp                                                16
. generate logcil = loghaz - 1.96*se
```

```
. generate logciu = loghaz + 1.96*se
. generate cil = exp(logcil)                                          17
. generate ciu = exp(logciu)
. sort dbp                                                            18
. *
. *  Plot risk of CHD for patients with a given baseline DBP
. *  relative to patients with a basline DBP of 60.  Show
. *  the 95% confidence band for this plot.
. *
. twoway rarea cil ciu dbp, color(gray)                               19
>     || line relhaz1 dbp
>     , legend(off) ytitle(Relative risk of CHD)
>       ymtick(1(1)16) ylabel(0(3)15) xlabel(40(10)140)
>       xmtick(45(5)145)
. *
. *  Restricted cubic spline model of the effect of DBP on CHD
. *  risk.  Use a 5 knot model with default knot values.
. *
. mkspline _Sdbp60 = dbp60, cubic displayknots

             |     knot1      knot2      knot3      knot4      knot5
-------------+-------------------------------------------------------
          r1 |         4         14         20       29.5         45

. stcox _S*, nohr                                                     20

         failure _d:  chdfate
   analysis time _t:  time
                                                          Output omitted
Cox regression -- Breslow method for ties

No. of subjects =         4699                 Number of obs    =      4699
No. of failures =         1473
Time at risk    =  103710.0917
                                                 LR chi2(4)       =    246.93
Log likelihood  =   -11711.393                   Prob > chi2      =    0.0000

------------------------------------------------------------------------------
          _t |      Coef.   Std. Err.      z    P>|z|     [95% Conf. Interval]
-------------+----------------------------------------------------------------
    _Sdbp601 |   .0618603    .016815     3.68   0.000     .0289035     .094817
    _Sdbp602 |  -.2268319    .1120642   -2.02   0.043    -.4464737   -.0071902
```

```
    _Sdbp603 |     .93755   .4547913     2.06   0.039    .0461754    1.828925
    _Sdbp604 |   -.982937   .4821521    -2.04   0.041   -1.927938   -.0379362
------------------------------------------------------------------------------
```

```
. lrtest simple .
Likelihood-ratio test                           LR chi2(3)  =       4.85
(Assumption: simple nested in .)                Prob > chi2 =     0.1835
```

21

```
. *
. *  Let's try a three knot model.
. *
. drop _S*
. mkspline _Sdbp60 = dbp60, cubic nknots(3) displayknots

             |     knot1      knot2      knot3
-------------+---------------------------------
          r1 |         8         20         40

. stcox _S*, nohr

         failure _d:  chdfate
   analysis time _t:  time
```

Output omitted

```
Cox regression -- Breslow method for ties

No. of subjects =         4699             Number of obs   =       4699
No. of failures =         1473
Time at risk    =  103710.0917
                                           LR chi2(2)      =     242.43
Log likelihood  =   -11713.643             Prob > chi2     =     0.0000

------------------------------------------------------------------------------
          _t |      Coef.   Std. Err.      z    P>|z|     [95% Conf. Interval]
-------------+----------------------------------------------------------------
    _Sdbp601 |   .0347213   .0057337     6.06   0.000     .0234835    .0459592
    _Sdbp602 |  -.0041479   .0070762    -0.59   0.558    -.0180169    .0097212
------------------------------------------------------------------------------
```

22

```
. lrtest simple .

Likelihood-ratio test                           LR chi2(1)  =       0.35
(Assumption: simple nested in .)                Prob > chi2 =     0.5560
```

23

```
. *
. *  The range of DBPs above the last knot is 40 mm Hg.
. *  let's add another knot at DBP = 120 to try to avoid
. *  excessive model extrapolation for high DBPs.
. *
```

```
. drop _S*

. mkspline _Sdbp60 = dbp60, cubic knots(8 20 40 60)

. stcox _S*, nohr                                                      24

         failure _d:  chdfate
   analysis time _t:  time
                                                          Output omitted

Cox regression -- Breslow method for ties

No. of subjects =        4699              Number of obs    =      4699
No. of failures =        1473
Time at risk    =  103710.0917
                                            LR chi2(3)       =    243.93
Log likelihood  =    -11712.89              Prob > chi2      =    0.0000

------------------------------------------------------------------------------
          _t |      Coef.   Std. Err.      z    P>|z|     [95% Conf. Interval]
-------------+----------------------------------------------------------------
   _Sdbp601 |    .029958    .0068727     4.36   0.000     .0164878    .0434282
   _Sdbp602 |   .0229262    .0332729     0.69   0.491    -.0422876    .0881399
   _Sdbp603 |  -.0569008    .0676407    -0.84   0.400     -.189474    .0756725
------------------------------------------------------------------------------

. lrtest simple .

Likelihood-ratio test                                 LR chi2(2)  =      1.85
(Assumption: simple nested in .)                      Prob > chi2 =    0.3963

. drop loghaz se logcil logciu cil ciu

. predict relhaz4, hr

. predict loghaz, xb

. predict se, stdp

. generate logcil = loghaz - 1.96*se

. generate logciu = loghaz + 1.96*se

. generate cil = exp(logcil)

. generate ciu = exp(logciu)

. *

. * Plot relative risks of CHD with 95% confidence bands

. * for this model.

. *

. twoway rarea cil ciu dbp, color(gray)                                25
>     || line relhaz1 dbp, color(white)
>     || line relhaz4 dbp, lpattern(solid)
```

```
>      , legend(off) ytitle(Relative risk of CHD)
>        ymtick(1(1)11) ylabel(0(2)10) xlabel(40(10)140)
>        xmtick(45(5)145)
. *
. *  Model effects of DBP on CHD risk using a categorical
. *  variable for DBP.
. *
. xi: stcox  i.dbpgr                                                    26
i.dbpgr           _Idbpgr_60-111      (naturally coded; _Idbpgr_60 omitted)

         failure _d:  chdfate
   analysis time _t:  time
                                                          Output omitted

Cox regression -- Breslow method for ties

No. of subjects =         4699                Number of obs   =       4699
No. of failures =         1473
Time at risk    =  103710.0917
                                              LR chi2(6)      =     221.83
Log likelihood  =   -11723.942                Prob > chi2     =     0.0000

-------------------------------------------------------------------------
          _t | Haz. Ratio  Std. Err.      z   P>|z|   [95% Conf. Interval]   27
-------------+-----------------------------------------------------------
  _Idbpgr_70 |   1.968764   .486453    2.74  0.006    1.213037   3.195312
  _Idbpgr_80 |   2.557839  .6157326    3.90  0.000    1.595764   4.099941
  _Idbpgr_90 |   3.056073  .7362768    4.64  0.000    1.905856   4.900466
 _Idbpgr_100 |    4.53703  1.103093    6.22  0.000    2.817203   7.306767
 _Idbpgr_110 |   6.291702  1.600738    7.23  0.000    3.821246   10.35932
 _Idbpgr_111 |   9.462228  2.566611    8.29  0.000    5.560408   16.10201
-------------------------------------------------------------------------
. *
. *  Store estimates from this model for future likelihood ratio
. *  tests (tests of change in model deviance).
. *
. estimates store _dbpgr
. *
. *  Univariate analysis of the effect of gender on CHD
. *
. sts graph, by(sex) plot1opts(color(gray)) failure ylabel(0(.1).5)      28
>    ytitle(Cumulative CHD Morbidity)  xlabel(0(5)30)
>    xtitle(Years of Follow-up) title(" ", size(zero)) legend(off)
```

```
         failure _d:  chdfate
   analysis time _t:  time
. sts test sex
```
29

```
         failure _d:  chdfate
   analysis time _t:  time

Log-rank test for equality of survivor functions

       |   Events         Events
sex    |  observed       expected
-------+-------------------------
Men    |       823         589.47
Women  |       650         883.53
-------+-------------------------
Total  |      1473        1473.00

             chi2(1) =     154.57
             Pr>chi2 =     0.0000
. generate male = sex == 1 if !missing(sex)
```
30

```
. tabulate male sex

           |          Sex
      male |      Men      Women |     Total
-----------+---------------------+----------
         0 |        0      2,650 |     2,650
         1 |    2,049          0 |     2,049
-----------+---------------------+----------
     Total |    2,049      2,650 |     4,699
. stcox male
```
31

Output omitted

```
----------------------------------------------------------------------------
        _t | Haz. Ratio   Std. Err.      z    P>|z|     [95% Conf. Interval]
-----------+----------------------------------------------------------------
      male |   1.900412   .0998308    12.22   0.000     1.714482    2.106504
----------------------------------------------------------------------------
. *
. *  Fit multiplicative model of DBP and gender on risk of CHD.
. *
. xi: stcox  i.dbpgr male
```
32

```
i.dbpgr           _Idbpgr_60-111       (naturally coded; _Idbpgr_60 omitted)
```

Output omitted

```
Log likelihood  =   -11657.409                 Prob > chi2      =    0.0000

------------------------------------------------------------------------------
          _t | Haz. Ratio  Std. Err.     z    P>|z|     [95% Conf. Interval]
-------------+----------------------------------------------------------------
  _Idbpgr_70 |   1.911621   .4723633   2.62   0.009    1.177793    3.102662
  _Idbpgr_80 |   2.429787    .585021   3.69   0.000    1.515737    3.895044
  _Idbpgr_90 |   2.778377   .6697835   4.24   0.000    1.732176    4.456464
 _Idbpgr_100 |   4.060083   .9879333   5.76   0.000    2.520075    6.541184
 _Idbpgr_110 |   5.960225   1.516627   7.02   0.000    3.619658    9.814262
 _Idbpgr_111 |   9.181868   2.490468   8.17   0.000    5.395767     15.6246
        male |   1.833729   .0968002  11.49   0.000    1.653489    2.033616
------------------------------------------------------------------------------

. lrtest _dbpgr .                                                          33
Likelihood-ratio test                            LR chi2(1)  =     133.07
(Assumption: _dbpgr nested in .)                 Prob > chi2 =     0.0000

. estimates store dbp_male

. lincom _Idbpgr_70 + male , hr                                            34
 ( 1)  _Idbpgr_70 + male = 0

------------------------------------------------------------------------------
          _t | Haz. Ratio   Std. Err.      z    P>|z|     [95% Conf. Interval]
-------------+----------------------------------------------------------------
         (1) |   3.505395   .8837535    4.98   0.000     2.138644      5.7456
------------------------------------------------------------------------------

. lincom _Idbpgr_80 + male , hr
```

Output omitted. See Table 7.2

```
. lincom _Idbpgr_90 + male , hr
```

Output omitted. See Table 7.2

```
. lincom _Idbpgr_100 + male , hr
```

Output omitted. See Table 7.2

```
. lincom _Idbpgr_110 + male , hr
```

Output omitted. See Table 7.2

```
. lincom _Idbpgr_111 + male , hr
```

Output omitted. See Table 7.2

```
. *
. *  Fit model of DBP and gender on risk of CHD using interaction terms.
. *
```

```
. xi: stcox  i.dbpgr*male                                                    35
i.dbpgr           _Idbpgr_60-111        (naturally coded; _Idbpgr_60 omitted)
i.dbpgr*male      _IdbpXmal_#           (coded as above)
```

Output omitted

```
Log likelihood  =   -11646.794                  Prob > chi2       =     0.0000

------------------------------------------------------------------------------
          _t | Haz. Ratio   Std. Err.      z    P>|z|     [95% Conf. Interval]
-------------+----------------------------------------------------------------
  _Idbpgr_70 |    1.82731   .6428651    1.71   0.087      .9169625    3.64144
  _Idbpgr_80 |   2.428115   .8298216    2.60   0.009        1.2427   4.744299
  _Idbpgr_90 |   3.517929   1.201355    3.68   0.000      1.801384   6.870179
 _Idbpgr_100 |   4.693559   1.628053    4.46   0.000      2.378188   9.263141
 _Idbpgr_110 |   7.635131   2.736437    5.67   0.000      3.782205   15.41302
 _Idbpgr_111 |   13.62563   5.067901    7.02   0.000      6.572973   28.24565
        male |   2.372645   1.118489    1.83   0.067      .9418198   5.977199
_IdbpXmal_70 |   1.058632   .5235583    0.12   0.908      .4015814    2.79072
_IdbpXmal_80 |   .9628061   .4637697   -0.08   0.937      .3745652   2.474858
_IdbpXmal_90 |   .6324678   .3047828   -0.95   0.342      .2459512   1.626402
_IdbpXma~100 |   .7437487   .3621623   -0.61   0.543      .2863787   1.931576
_IdbpXma~110 |   .6015939   .3059896   -1.00   0.318      .2220014   1.630239
_IdbpXma~111 |    .401376   .2205419   -1.66   0.097      .1367245   1.178302
------------------------------------------------------------------------------

. lrtest dbp_male .                                                          36

Likelihood-ratio test                                 LR chi2(6)  =      21.23
(Assumption: dbp_male nested in .)                    Prob > chi2 =     0.0017

. estimates store dbp_maleInteract

. lincom _Idbpgr_70 + male +  _IdbpXmal_70, hr                               37

 ( 1)  _Idbpgr_70 + male + _IdbpXmal_70 = 0

------------------------------------------------------------------------------
          _t | Haz. Ratio   Std. Err.      z    P>|z|     [95% Conf. Interval]
-------------+----------------------------------------------------------------
         (1) |   4.589761   1.595446    4.38   0.000      2.322223   9.071437
------------------------------------------------------------------------------

. lincom _Idbpgr_80 + male +_IdbpXmal_80, hr
```

Output omitted. See Table 7.3

```
. lincom _Idbpgr_90 + male + _IdbpXmal_90, hr
```

Output omitted. See Table 7.3

```
. lincom _Idbpgr_100 + male + _IdbpXmal_100, hr
                                            Output omitted. See Table 7.3
. lincom _Idbpgr_110 + male + _IdbpXmal_110, hr
                                            Output omitted. See Table 7.3
. lincom _Idbpgr_111 + male + _IdbpXmal_111, hr
                                            Output omitted. See Table 7.3
. *
. *  Adjust model for age, BMI and SCL.
. *
. xi: stcox  i.dbpgr*male age                                          38
                                                         Output omitted
. lrtest dbp_maleInteract .                                            39
Likelihood-ratio test                          LR chi2(1)  =    259.09
(Assumption: dbp_maleInte~t nested in .)       Prob > chi2 =    0.0000
. xi: stcox  i.dbpgr*male age if !missing(bmi) & !missing(scl)         40
                                                         Output omitted

No. of subjects =         4658                Number of obs   =      4658
No. of failures =         1465
Time at risk    =  102895.0938
                                              LR chi2(14)     =    628.25
Log likelihood  =   -11444.759                Prob > chi2     =    0.0000
                                                         Output omitted
. estimates store dbp_maleInteract_age
. xi: stcox  i.dbpgr*male age bmi scl                                  41
                                                         Output omitted
Log likelihood  =   -11382.132                 Prob > chi2     =    0.0000
```

| _t | Haz. Ratio | Std. Err. | z | P>\|z\| | [95% Conf. | Interval] |
|---|---|---|---|---|---|---|
| _Idbpgr_70 | 1.514961 | .5334695 | 1.18 | 0.238 | .7597392 | 3.020916 |
| _Idbpgr_80 | 1.654264 | .5669665 | 1.47 | 0.142 | .8450299 | 3.238451 |
| _Idbpgr_90 | 1.911763 | .6566924 | 1.89 | 0.059 | .9750921 | 3.748199 |
| _Idbpgr_100 | 1.936029 | .6796612 | 1.88 | 0.060 | .9729479 | 3.852425 |
| _Idbpgr_110 | 3.097614 | 1.123672 | 3.12 | 0.002 | 1.521425 | 6.306727 |
| _Idbpgr_111 | 5.269096 | 1.988701 | 4.40 | 0.000 | 2.514603 | 11.04086 |
| male | 1.984033 | .9355668 | 1.45 | 0.146 | .7873473 | 4.999554 |
| _IdbpXmal_70 | 1.173058 | .5802796 | 0.32 | 0.747 | .4448907 | 3.09304 |
| _IdbpXmal_80 | 1.18152 | .5693995 | 0.35 | 0.729 | .4594405 | 3.038457 |
| _IdbpXmal_90 | .8769476 | .4230106 | -0.27 | 0.785 | .3407078 | 2.257175 |

```
_IdbpXma~100 |  1.265976   .6179759    0.48   0.629    .4863156   3.295585
_IdbpXma~110 |  1.023429   .5215766    0.05   0.964    .3769245   2.778823
_IdbpXma~111 |  .6125694   .3371363   -0.89   0.373    .2082976   1.801467
         age |   1.04863    .003559   13.99   0.000    1.041677   1.055628
         bmi |  1.038651   .0070125    5.62   0.000    1.024998   1.052487
         scl |  1.005788   .0005883    9.87   0.000    1.004635   1.006941
-------------------------------------------------------------------------

. lrtest dbp_maleInteract_age .                                              42
Likelihood-ratio test                               LR chi2(2)  =     125.25
(Assumption: dbp_maleInte~e nested in .)            Prob > chi2 =     0.0000

. lincom  _Idbpgr_70 + male +  _IdbpXmal_70, hr
                                                 Output omitted. See Table 7.4
. lincom  _Idbpgr_80 + male + _IdbpXmal_80, hr
                                                 Output omitted. See Table 7.4
. lincom  _Idbpgr_90 + male + _IdbpXmal_90, hr
                                                 Output omitted. See Table 7.4
. lincom  _Idbpgr_100 + male +  _IdbpXmal_100, hr
                                                 Output omitted. See Table 7.4
. lincom  _Idbpgr_110 + male + _IdbpXmal_110, hr
                                                 Output omitted. See Table 7.4
. lincom  _Idbpgr_111 + male + _IdbpXmal_111, hr
                                                 Output omitted. See Table 7.4
. log close
```

### Comments

1 By default, Stata reserves at least one megabyte of memory for its calculations (Stata/IC reserves one megabyte, Stata/SE and Stata/MP reserve more). Calculating some statistics on large data sets may require more memory. The log-rank test given below is an example of such a calculation. The *set memory* command specifies the memory size. The argument may be either an integer or an integer followed by the letter "m", indicating kilobytes or megabytes, respectively. This command increases the memory to 2000 kilobytes or 2 megabytes. Equivalently we could have written 2m rather than 2000 to reserve this memory. The *set memory* command may not be used when a data set is open. There is no point-and-click version of this command.

2 This *histogram* command draws Figure 7.1. The *start(39)* and *width(2)* options causes the data to be grouped in bins of width 2 with the first bin starting at 39. The *frequency* option specifies that the *y*-axis will be the number of subjects in each bin. In the point-and-click version of this

command the bin width and starting value are specified by the *Width of bins* and *Lower limit of first bin* fields on the *Main* tab of the *histogram* dialogue box.

3 Define *dbpgr* to be a categorical variable based on *dbp*. The *recode* function sets

$$dbpgr = \begin{cases} 60: & \text{if } dbp \le 60 \\ 70: & \text{if } 60 < dbp \le 70 \\ \vdots & \\ 110: & \text{if } 100 < dbp \le 110 \\ 111: & \text{if } 110 < dbp. \end{cases}$$

4 This command tabulates *dbpgr* by *chdfate*. Note that the proportion of patients with subsequent CHD increases with increasing blood pressure. I recommend that you produce simple tabulations of your results frequently as a crosscheck on your more complicated statistics.

5 To make our graphs more intelligible we define *time* to be patient follow-up in years.

6 This command produces a Kaplan–Meier survival graph that is similar to Figure 7.2. It differs in that it places the figure legend in the lower left-hand corner of the graph, while in Figure 7.2 I labeled the survival curves by hand with a graphics editor.

7 The *color(gray)* suboption of the *plot2opts* option colors the second plot line gray. This is the survival curve for patients with a baseline DBP of 61–70 mm Hg. It is solid by default since no *lpattern* suboption is given. To implement the point-and-click version of this option fill in the *Main* tab of the *sts graph* dialog box as explained on page 303. Then fill in the *Plot* tab as follows: Plot Select plot: *Plot 2* [Edit] [Line properties] Color: *gray* [Accept] [Accept] [Submit].

8 The sixth line is gray and has a long dash pattern

9 The *lpattern("_-")* suboption creates a line pattern consisting of alternating long and medium length dashes.

10 This *sts test* command performs a log-rank test on the groups of patients defined by *dbpgr*. The highlighted *P*-value for this test is <0.000 05.

11 This log-rank test is restricted to patients with *dbpgr* equal to 60 or 70. In other words, this command tests whether the survival curves for patients with DBPs ≤60 and DBPs between 60 and 70 are equal. The *P*-value associated with this test equals 0.0052.

12 The next five commands test the equality of the other adjacent pairs of survival curves in Figure 7.2.

13 Under this simple model the relative risk of CHD associated with a unit rise in DBP is 1.032. This elevation in risk is of overwhelming statistical significance.

14 As is the case following other types of regression commands, the *xb* option of the *predict* command defines a new variable that equals the model's linear predictor. In this instance, *loghaz* is the linear predictor, which equals $\hat{\beta}(dbp_i - 60)$.

15 The *hr* option of this *predict* command defines *relhaz1* to be the exponentiated value of the linear predictor. In this example *relhaz1* is the relative risk given by Equation (7.5)

16 We have also used this command before following linear and logistic regression commands. The *stdp* option defines *se* to equal the standard error of the linear predictor.

17 The variables *cil* and *ciu* are the lower and upper bounds of the 95% confidence interval for *relhaz1* defined by Equation (7.6)

18 The subsequent *twoway* plot commands require that the data be sorted by *dbp*.

19 This command draws a graph that is similar to Figure 7.3. The 95% confidence band in this figure becomes very wide for high blood pressures. For this reason I used a graphics editor to truncate this figure above a relative risk of 16.

20 Proportional hazards regression models involving restricted cubic splines are fit in exactly the same way as for linear or logistic regression models. This command fits Model (7.8).

The *nohr* option causes the model's coefficients to be displayed. This option is implemented in the point-and-click version of this command by filling in the *stcox* dialog box as explained on page 311, selecting the *Reporting* tab, and checking the box labeled *Report coefficients, not hazard ratios.*

21 This likelihood ratio test evaluates the change in model deviance between the simple and RCS models. (Recall that the results of the simple model were stored under the name *simple* by the previous *estimate store* command.) Note that we are unable to reject the simple model using this test ($P = 0.18$).

22 Note that in the three-knot model, the parameter for the second spline covariate is an order of magnitude smaller than that for the first spline covariate and is not significantly different from zero ($P = 0.558$). There really is no statistical evidence to reject the simple model.

23 Testing the change in model deviance between the simple and three-knot models is equivalent to testing the null hypothesis that the parameter

associated with the second spline covariate is zero. Note that the likelihood ratio $P$-value highlighted here is very close to the Wald $P$-value highlighted in the preceding comment. In a large study such as this one we would expect these $P$-values to be very similar.

24 This is the model used to generate Figure 7.4.

25 This graph generates a figure that is similar to Figure 7.4. In this figure a graphics editor was used to truncate the 95% confidence interval for high blood pressures.

26 The syntax of the *xi:* prefix for the *stcox* command works in exactly the same way as in logistic regression. See Sections 5.10 and 5.23 for a detailed explanation. This command performs the proportional hazards regression analysis specified by Model (7.12). The variables *_Idbpgr_70*, *_Idbpgr_80*, ..., *_Idbpgr_111* are dichotomous classification variables that are created by this command. In Model (7.12) $dbp_{i2}$ = *_Idbpgr_70*, $dbp_{i3}$ = *_Idbpgr_80*, etcetera.

27 The column titled *Haz. Ratio* contains relative risks under the proportional hazards model. The relative risk estimates and 95% confidence intervals presented in Table 7.1 are highlighted. For example, $\exp[\beta_2] = 1.968\,764$, which is the relative risk of people in DBP Group 2 relative to DBP Group 1.

28 The *failure* option of the *sts graph* command produces a cumulative morbidity plot. The resulting graph is similar to Figure 7.5.

29 The log-rank test of the CHD morbidity curves for men and women is of overwhelming statistical significance.

30 In the database, *sex* is coded as 1 for men and 2 for women. As men have the higher risk of CHD we will treat male sex as a positive risk factor. (Alternatively, we could have treated female sex as a protective risk factor.) To do this in Stata, we need to give men a higher code than women. The logical value *sex* == 1 is true (equals 1) when the subject is a man (*sex* = 1), and is false (equals 0) when she is a woman (*sex* = 2). Hence the effect of this *generate* command is to define the variable *male* as equaling 0 or 1 for women or men, respectively.

A danger of using the command

```
generate male = sex==1
```

is that if *sex* were missing, *sex==1* would be false and hence *male* would equal zero. This would classify patients as female whose gender was, in fact, unknown. In this particular example, this does not matter since *sex* is never missing. However, it is a good habit to include the qualifier *if !missing(sex)* in *generate* commands such as this one. Had there been any patients whose value of *sex* was missing, then *!missing(sex)* would be false and hence *male* would also be assigned a missing value.

31 This command performs the simple proportional hazards regression specified by Model (7.14). It estimates that men have 1.90 times the risk of CHD as women. The 95% confidence interval for this risk is also given.

32 This command performs the proportional hazards regression specified by Model (7.15). In this command *male* specifies the covariate $male_i$ in Model (7.15). The highlighted relative risks and confidence intervals are also given in Table 7.2. Note that since *male* is already dichotomous, it is not necessary to create a new variable using the *i.male* syntax.

33 This command calculates the likelihood ratio $\chi^2$ statistic that equals the change in model deviance between Model (7.12) and Model (7.15). This statistic equals 133.07 with one degree of freedom and is of overwhelming statistical significance.

34 The covariates *_Idbpgr_70* and *male* equal $dbp_{i2}$ and $male_i$, respectively in Model (7.15). The coefficients associated with these covariates are $\beta_2$ and $\gamma$. The *hr* option of the *lincom* command has the same effect as the *or* option. That is, it exponentiates the desired expression and then calculates a confidence interval using Equation (5.32). The only difference between the *or* and *hr* options is that the column heading of the resulting output "*Odds Ratio*" is replaced by "*Haz. Ratio*". This *lincom* command calculates $\exp[\hat{\beta}_2 + \hat{\gamma}] = \exp[\hat{\beta}_2] \times \exp[\hat{\gamma}] = 1.911\,621 \times 1.833\,729 = 3.505\,395$, which is the relative risk for a man in DBP Group 2 relative to women in DBP Group 1. (See Comment 6 on page 231 for additional explanation.) This and the next five *lincom* commands provide the relative risks and confidence intervals needed to complete Table 7.2.

35 This command regresses CHD free survival against DBP and gender using Model (7.16). See Section 5.23 for a detailed explanation of this syntax. The names of the dichotomous classification variables created by this command are indicated in the first two lines of output. For example, in Model (7.16) $dbp_{i2}$ equals *_Idbpgr_70*, $male_i$ equals *male*, and $dbp_{i2} \times male_i$ equals *_IdbpXmal_70*. Note that the names of the interaction covariates are truncated to 12 characters in the table of hazard ratios. Hence, *_IdbpXma~100* denotes *_IdbpXmal_100*, etcetera. The highlighted relative risks and confidence intervals are also given in Table 7.3.

36 This likelihood ratio test allows us to reject the multiplicative Model (7.15) with $P = 0.0017$.

37 This *lincom* command calculates $\exp[\hat{\beta}_2 + \hat{\gamma} + \hat{\delta}_2] = 4.589\,761$, which is the relative risk of men in DBP Group 2 relative to women from

DBP Group 1 under Model (7.16). This and the following five *lincom* commands calculate the relative risks needed to complete Table 7.3.

38 This command regresses CHD free survival against DBP and gender adjusted for age using Model (7.17).

39 Adding *age* to the model greatly reduces the model deviance.

40 We next wish to add *bmi* and *scl* to our model and assess the impact of these variables on our model deviance. Some patients, however, have missing values of *bmi* and *scl*, which prevents Model (7.17) from being perfectly nested within Model (7.18) or Model (7.18) from being perfectly nested within Model (7.19). To make these nesting relationships true we refit Model (7.17) excluding patients with missing values of *bmi* or *scl*.

41 This command regresses CHD free survival against DBP and gender adjusted for age, BMI, and SCL using Model (7.19). The highlighted relative risks and confidence intervals are entered into Table 7.4. The subsequent *lincom* commands are used to complete this table.

42 The change in model deviance between Models (7.17) and (7.19), restricted to patients with known values of all covariates in Model (7.19) is also highly significant. Adding BMI and SCL to the model greatly improves the model fit. If we had added age, BMI, and SCL separately in successive models we would have seen that each of these variables significantly improves the model fit.

## 7.7. Stratified proportional hazards models

In Section 7.1, we defined the hazard for the $i^{\text{th}}$ patient at time $t$ by Equation (7.1). This hazard function obeys the proportional hazards assumption. In Section 7.9 we will discuss ways of evaluating the validity of this assumption for your data. There are two alternatives to consider when the proportional hazards model is inappropriate. One of these is to use a **stratified proportional hazards model**. In this approach, we subdivide the patients into $j = 1, 2, \ldots J$ strata defined by the patient's covariates. We then define the hazard for the $i^{\text{th}}$ patient from the $j^{\text{th}}$ stratum at time $t$ to be

$$\lambda_{ij}[t] = \lambda_{0j}[t]\exp[\beta_1 x_{ij1} + \beta_2 x_{ij2} + \cdots + \beta_q x_{ijq}], \tag{7.20}$$

where $x_{ij1}, x_{ij2}, \ldots, x_{ijq}$, are the covariate values for this patient, and $\lambda_{0j}[t]$ is the baseline hazard for patients from the $j^{\text{th}}$ stratum. Model (7.20) makes no assumptions about the shapes of the $J$ baseline hazard functions. Within each stratum the proportional hazards assumption applies. However, patients from different strata need not have proportional hazards.

For example, suppose that we were interested in the risk of CHD due to smoking in women and men. We might stratify the patients by gender, letting $j = 1$ or 2 designate men or women, respectively.

Let

$$x_{ij} = \begin{cases} 1: & \text{if } i^{\text{th}} \text{ patient from the } j^{\text{th}} \text{ stratum smokes} \\ 0: & \text{otherwise, and} \end{cases}$$

$\lambda_{ij}[t]$ be the CHD hazard for the $i^{\text{th}}$ patient from the $j^{\text{th}}$ stratum.

Then Model (7.20) reduces to

$$\lambda_{ij}[t] = \lambda_{0j}[t] \exp[\beta x_{ij}]. \tag{7.21}$$

In this model, $\lambda_{01}[t]$ and $\lambda_{02}[t]$ represent the CHD hazard for men and women who do not smoke, while $\lambda_{01}[t]\, e^{\beta}$ and $\lambda_{02}[t]\, e^{\beta}$ represents this hazard for men and women who do. By an argument similar to that given in Section 7.2, the within-strata relative risk of CHD in smokers relative to non-smokers is $e^{\beta}$. That is, smoking women have $e^{\beta}$ times the CHD risk of non-smoking women while smoking men have $e^{\beta}$ times the CHD risk of non-smoking men. Model (7.21) makes no assumptions about how CHD risk varies with time among non-smoking men or women. It does, however, imply that the relative CHD risk of smoking is the same among men as it is among women.

In Stata, a stratified proportional hazards model is indicated by the *strata(varnames)* option of the *stcox* command. Model (7.21) might be implemented by a command such as

```
stcox smoke, strata(sex)
```

where *smoke* equals 1 or 0 for patients who did or did not smoke, respectively.

The other alternative to the proportional hazards model is to use a model with time-dependent covariates (see Section 7.10).

## 7.8. Survival analysis with ragged study entry

Usually the time variable in a survival analysis measures follow-up time from some event. This event may be recruitment into a cohort, diagnosis of cancer, etcetera. In such studies everyone is at risk at time zero, when they enter the cohort. Sometimes, however, we may wish to use the patient's age as the time variable rather than follow-up time. Both Kaplan–Meier survival curves and hazard regression analyses can be easily adapted to this situation. The key difference is that when age is the time variable, patients are not observed to fail until after they reach the age when they enter the cohort. Hence, it is possible that no one will enter the study at age zero, and that subjects will enter the analysis at different "times" when they reach their age at recruitment. These analyses must be interpreted as the effect of age and other covariates on the risk of failure conditioned on the fact that each patient had not failed before her age of recruitment.

### 7.8.1. Kaplan–Meier survival curve and the log-rank test with ragged entry

In Section 6.3, we defined the Kaplan–Meier survival curve $\hat{S}(t)$ to be a product of probabilities $p_i$ on each death day before time $t$. Each probability $p_i = (n_i - d_i)/n_i$, where $n_i$ are the number of patients at risk at the beginning of the $i^{\text{th}}$ death day and $d_i$ are the number of deaths on this day. In a traditional survival curve, $n_i$ must decrease with increasing $i$ since the entire cohort is at risk at time 0 and death or censoring can only decrease this number with time. With ragged entry, $\hat{S}(t)$ is calculated in the same way only now the number of patients at risk can increase as well as decrease; $n_i$ equals the total number of people to be recruited before time $t$ minus the total number of people who die or are censored before this time. The cumulative mortality curve is $\hat{D}[t] = 1 - \hat{S}[t]$, as was the case in Section 6.3.

The log-rank test is performed in exactly the same way as in Section 6.8. The only difference is that now the number of patients at risk at the beginning of each death day equals the number of patients recruited before that day minus the number of patients who have previously died or been censored.

### 7.8.2. Age, sex, and CHD in the Framingham Heart Study

Figure 7.6 shows that the distribution of age at entry in the Framingham Heart Study was very wide. This means that at any specific follow-up time in Figure 7.5, we are comparing men and women with a wide variation in ages. Figure 7.7 shows the cumulative CHD mortality in men and women as a function of age rather than years since recruitment. This figure reveals an aspect of CHD epidemiology that is missed in Figure 7.5. The morbidity curves for men and women diverge most rapidly before age sixty. Thereafter, they remain relatively parallel. This indicates that the protective effects of female gender on CHD are greatest in the pre- and perimenopausal ages, and that this protective effect is largely lost a decade or more after the menopause. This interaction between age and sex on CHD is not apparent in the Kaplan–Meier curves in Figure 7.5 that were plotted as a function of time since recruitment.

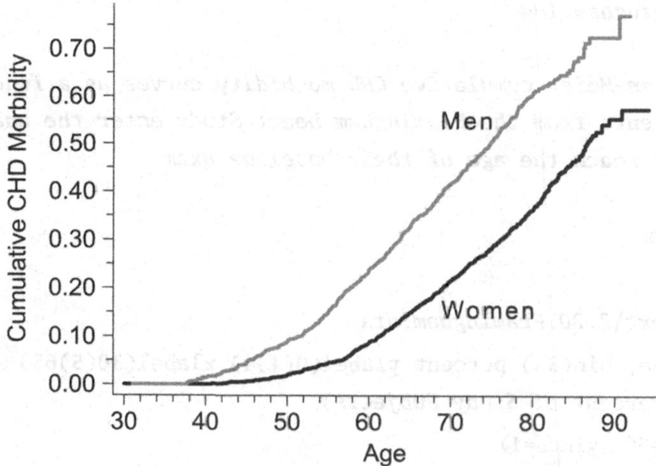


Figure 7.7 Cumulative coronary heart disease (CHD) morbidity with increasing age among men and women from the Framingham Heart Study (Levy et al., 1999).

### 7.8.3. Proportional hazards regression analysis with ragged entry

Proportional hazards regression analysis also focuses on the number of patients at risk and the number of deaths on each death day. For this reason, they are easily adapted for analyses of data with ragged study entry. A simple example of such a proportional hazards model is

$$\lambda_i[age] = \lambda_0[age] \exp[\beta \times male_i], \tag{7.22}$$

where *age* is a specific age for the $i^{\text{th}}$ subject, $\lambda_0[age]$ is the CHD hazard for women at this age, $male_i$ equals 1 if the $i^{\text{th}}$ subject is a man and equals 0 if she is a woman, and $\lambda_i[age]$ is the CHD hazard for the $i^{\text{th}}$ study subject at the indicated age. Model (7.22) differs from Model (7.14) only in that in Model (7.14) $t$ represents time since entry while in Model (7.22) *age* represents the subject's age. Under Model (7.22), a man's hazard is $\lambda_0[age]\exp[\beta]$. Hence, the age-adjusted relative risk of CHD in men compared with women is $\exp[\beta]$. Applying Model (7.22) to the Framingham Heart Study data gives this relative risk of CHD for men to be 2.01 with a 95% confidence interval of (1.8–2.2). Note, however, that Model (7.22) assumes that the relative risk of CHD between men and women remains constant with age. This assumption is rather unsatisfactory in view of the evidence from Figure 7.7 that this relative risk diminishes after age 60.

### 7.8.4. Survival analysis with ragged entry using Stata

The following log file and comments illustrate how to perform the analyses discussed above using Stata.

```
. * 7.8.4.Framingham.log
. *
. *  Plot Kaplan-Meier cumulative CHD morbidity curves as a function of
. *  age. Patients from the Framingham Heart Study enter the analysis
. *  when they reach the age of their baseline exam.
. *
. set memory 2m
(2048k)
. use C:\WDDtext\2.20.Framingham.dta
. histogram age, bin(38) percent ylabel(0(1)4) xlabel(30(5)65)
>     ytitle(Percent of Study Subjects)
(bin=38, start=30, width=1)
. generate time= followup/365.25
. generate male = sex == 1
. label define male 0 "Women" 1 "Men"
. label values male male
. label variable time "Follow-up in Years"
. generate exitage = age + time                                        1
. stset exitage, enter(time age) failure(chdfate)                      2

     failure event:  chdfate != 0 & chdfate < .
obs. time interval:  (0, exitage]
 enter on or after:  time age
 exit on or before:  failure

------------------------------------------------------------------------------
     4699  total obs.
        0  exclusions
------------------------------------------------------------------------------
     4699  obs. remaining, representing
     1473  failures in single record/single failure data
 103710.1  total analysis time at risk, at risk from t =         0
                             earliest observed entry t =        30
                                  last observed exit t =        94

. sts graph, by(male) failure plot2opts(color(gray))                   3
>     ytitle(Cumulative CHD Morbidity) xtitle(Age)
>     ylabel(0(.1).7) ymtick(0(.05).75) xlabel(30(10)90)
>     xmtick(30(2)90) legend(off) title(" ",size(zero)) noorigin       4

         failure _d:  chdfate
   analysis time _t:  exitage
  enter on or after:  time age
```

```
. *
. *  Calculate the logrank test corresponding to these morbidity functions
. *
. sts test male                                                              5

         failure _d:  chdfate
   analysis time _t:  exitage
  enter on or after:  time age

Log-rank test for equality of survivor functions

       |  Events        Events
male   |  observed      expected
-------+-------------------------
Women  |    650          901.92
Men    |    823          571.08
-------+-------------------------
Total  |   1473         1473.00

             chi2(1) =     182.91
             Pr>chi2 =     0.0000

. *
. *  Calculate the relative risk of CHD for men relative to women using
. *  age as the time variable.
. *
. stcox male                                                                 6

         failure _d:  chdfate
   analysis time _t:  exitage
  enter on or after:  time age

                                                               Output omitted

No. of subjects =          4699                    Number of obs    =      4699
No. of failures =          1473
Time at risk    =   103710.0914
                                                   LR chi2(1)       =    177.15
Log likelihood  =    -11218.785                    Prob > chi2      =    0.0000

------------------------------------------------------------------------------
          _t | Haz. Ratio   Std. Err.      z    P>|z|     [95% Conf. Interval]
-------------+----------------------------------------------------------------
        male |   2.011662   .1060464    13.26   0.000     1.814192    2.230626
------------------------------------------------------------------------------
```

**Comments**

1 We define *exitage* to be the patient's age at exit. This is the age when she either suffered CHD or was censored.

2 This command specifies the survival-time and fate variables for the subsequent survival commands. It defines *exitage* to be the time (age) when the subject's follow-up ends, *age* to be the time (age) when she is recruited into the cohort, and *chdfate* to be her fate at exit. Recall that *age* is the patient's age at her baseline exam and that she was free of CHD at that time (see Section 3.11).

To invoke the equivalent point-and-click command follow the instructions on page 302 and then enter ⌡ Options ⌊ ┌ Specify when subjects first enters study — Enter time expression: *age* ┘ [Submit].

3 This command plots cumulative CHD morbidity as a function of age for men and women. Strictly speaking, these plots are for people who are free of CHD at age 30, since this is the earliest age at recruitment. However, since CHD is rare before age 30, these plots closely approximate the cumulative morbidity curves from birth.

4 The *noorigin* option starts the $x$-axis at the first exit time. By default, these graphs start at time zero. This graph is similar to Figure 7.7. In this figure I have annotated the survival curves by hand with a graphics editor.

To specify the *noorigin* option with a point-and-click command select the *Options* tab of the *sts graph* dialogue box and enter ┌ Origin — ⦿ Begin survivor (failure) curve at first exit time ┘ .

5 The log-rank text is performed in exactly the same way as in Section 7.6. Changing the survival-time variable from years of follow-up to age increases the statistical significance of this test.

6 This command performs the proportional hazards regression defined by Model (7.22).

## 7.9. Predicted survival, log–log plots and the proportional hazards assumption

We need to assess whether the proportional hazards model is appropriate for our data (see Section 7.1). The proportional hazards assumption implies that the relative risk of the outcome of interest remains constant over time. In Figure 7.7 the separation between the cumulative morbidity curves for men and women increases until about age 60. Thereafter, these curves are roughly parallel. This suggests that the relative risk of CHD in men relative to women is greater before age 60 than after, which violates the proportional hazards assumption of Equation (7.22). The first step in evaluating this

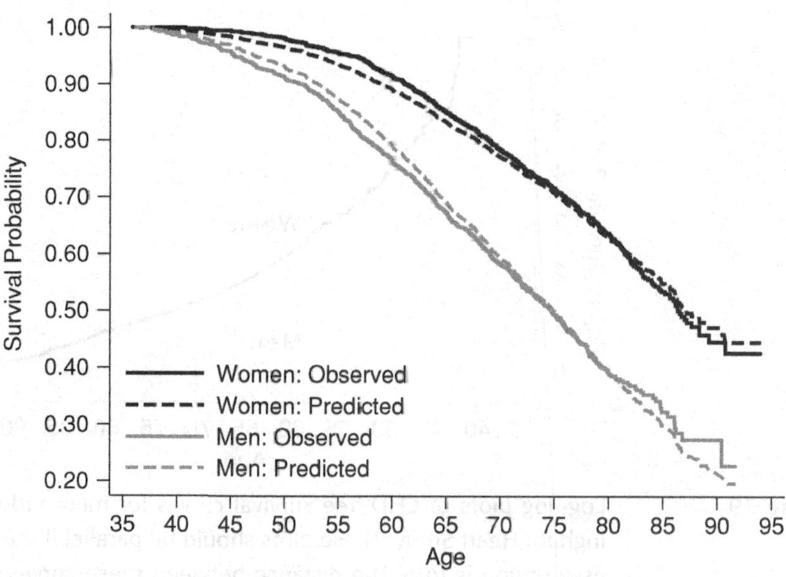


Figure 7.8 In this graph the solid lines are the unrestricted Kaplan–Meier CHD-free survival curves for men and women, while the dotted lines are the best fitting survival curves for these two groups under the proportional hazards assumption. These plots suggest that for younger subjects that male morbidity is higher and female morbidity is lower than we would expect if the proportional hazards assumption were true.

assumption is to compare the unrestricted Kaplan–Meier survival curves for men and women with the best-fitting curves for these two groups under the proportional hazards assumption. These plots are given in Figure 7.8. In this figure, the dashed lines give the best fit under the proportional hazards assumption while the solid lines give the unrestricted fit. At first glance the proportional hazards model appears to be quite good in that the dashed lines for men and women track the solid lines fairly closely. However, at younger ages the proportional hazards model gives a higher CHD-free survival probability for men and a lower probability for women. In their forties and fifties, the cumulative CHD morbidity for women expressed as a percentage of the cumulative morbidity for men of the same age is substantially less under the proportional hazards model than under an unrestricted model. It is not always easy to assess the reasonableness of the proportional hazards assumption by looking only at survival curves.

Suppose that the proportional hazards assumption given in Equation (7.1) is correct and let $\Lambda_0[t] = \int_0^t \lambda_0[u]\,du$ be the cumulative baseline hazard function for a patient whose linear predictor equals zero. That is, $\Lambda_0[t]$ is the area under the curve $\lambda_0[u]$ between 0 and $t$. Then it can be shown that

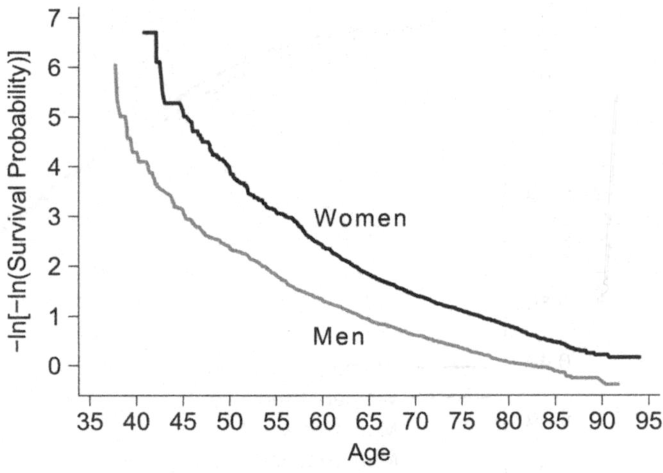


Figure 7.9 Log–log plots of CHD-free survival curves for men and women in the Framingham Heart Study. These plots should be parallel if the proportional hazards assumption is true. The distance between these curves drops from 2.0 units at age 45 to 0.28 units at age 85. This graph suggests that the hazard ratio for men relative to women decreases with increasing age.

the proportional hazards Model (7.1) implies that the survival function for the $i^{\text{th}}$ patient at time $t$ equals

$$S_i[t] = \exp\left[-\Lambda_0[t]\exp[\beta_1 x_{i1} + \beta_2 x_{i2} + \cdots + \beta_q x_{iq}]\right].$$

Taking logarithms of both sides of this equation twice gives that

$$\log[-\log[S_i[t]]] = \log[-\Lambda_0[t]] + \beta_1 x_{i1} + \beta_2 x_{i2} + \cdots + \beta_q x_{iq}. \qquad (7.23)$$

If we plot Equation (7.23) as a function of $t$ for two distinct values of the linear predictor $\beta_1 x_{i1} + \beta_2 x_{i2} + \cdots + \beta_q x_{iq}$ we obtain parallel curves. The distance between these curves will equal the difference between these linear predictors. For example, in Model (7.22) the difference between $\log[-\log[S_i[t]]]$ for men and women will equal $\beta$. A useful graphical method of evaluating the proportional hazards assumption is to plot estimates of $-\log[-\log[S_i[t]]]$ for different covariate values. Figure 7.9 shows plots of

$$-\log\left[-\log\left[\hat{S}_f[t]\right]\right] \text{ and } -\log\left[-\log\left[\hat{S}_m[t]\right]\right]$$

where $\hat{S}_f[t]$ and $\hat{S}_m[t]$ are the Kaplan–Meier survival curve estimates derived for women and men, respectively. Note that the separation between these curves is much greater for people in their forties than for people in their eighties. If the proportional hazards assumption were true, these curves would be parallel. The fact that they are not parallel suggests that we should test the proportional hazards assumption and consider models in which the CHD hazard in men relative to women is allowed to vary with age.

## 7.9.1. Evaluating the proportional hazards assumption with Stata

The *7.8.4.Framingham.log* file continues as follows. It illustrates how to contrast Kaplan–Meier curves with the optimal survival curves under the proportional hazards assumption, and how to draw log–log plots.

```
. *
. *  Compare Kaplan-Meier curve with best-fitting survival
. *  curves under the proportional hazards model.
. *
. stcoxkm, by(male) xtitle(Age) obs1opts(symbol(none))                1
>     pred1opts(symbol(none) lpattern(dash))
>     obs2opts( symbol(none) color(gray))
>     pred2opts(symbol(none) color(gray) lpattern(dash))              2
>     legend(ring(0) position(7) col(1) order(1 "Women: Observed"
>         3 "Women: Predicted" 2 "Men: Observed" 4 "Men: Predicted"))

         failure _d:  chdfate
   analysis time _t:  exitage
  enter on or after:  time age

. *
. *  Draw log-log plots to assess the proportional hazards assumption.
. *
. stphplot, by(male) nolntime plot1opts(symbol(none))                 3
>     plot2opts(symbol(none) color(gray)) xtitle(Age) legend(off)

         failure _d:  chdfate
   analysis time _t:  exitage
  enter on or after:  time age
```

**Comments**

1 This *stcoxkm* command draws Figure 7.8. Two survival plots are drawn for each distinct value of *male*. One of these is the unrestricted Kaplan–Meier survival plot and the other is the best-fitting survival plot under the proportional hazards assumption. The *obs1opts* option controls the

appearance of the first unrestricted survival curve. In this example, the plot symbol for this curve is suppressed. A *stset* command must be given before this command to define the time and fate variables (see Section 7.8.4).

2 The *pred2opts* option controls the appearance of the second survival curve drawn under the proportional hazards model. The *obs#opts* and *pred#opts* options take the same suboptions. The *symbol*, *color* and *lpattern* suboptions determine the plot symbol, line color, and line pattern for these plots. This example specifies a gray dashed line for the second restricted survival curve.

A point-and-click version of this command that uses the default legend and axes labels and titles is Graphics ▶ Survival analysis graphs ▶ Compare Kaplan–Meier and Cox survival curves ⌋Main⌊ Independent variable: *male* ⌋Observed plot⌊ [Edit] [Marker properties] ⌋Main⌊ ┌ Marker properties — Symbol: *None* ⌋ [Accept] [Accept] Select plot: *Plot 2* [Edit] [Line Properties] Color: *Gray* [Accept] [Marker properties] ⌋Main⌊ ┌ Marker properties — Symbol: *None* ⌋ [Accept] [Accept] ⌋Predicted plot⌊ [Edit] [Line properties] Pattern: *Dash* [Accept] [Marker properties] ⌋Main⌊ ┌ Marker properties — Symbol: *None* ⌋ [Accept] [Accept] Select plot: *Plot 2* [Edit] [Line properties] Color: *Gray* , Pattern: *Dash* [Accept] [Marker properties] ⌋Main⌊ ┌ Marker properties — Symbol: *None* ⌋ [Accept] [Accept] [Submit].

3 This *stphplot* command draws a log–log plot of the Kaplan–Meier survival plots for men and women (groups of subjects with distinct values of the variable *male*). The resulting figure is identical to Figure 7.9 except that in this figure I annotated the curves by hand. These curves may be adjusted for the average values of the other covariates by using the **adjust(*varlist*)** option. By default the *x*-axis is log analysis time. The *nolntime* option makes the time axis linear.

The point-and-click version of this command is Graphics ▶ Survival analysis graphs ▶ Assess proportional-hazards assumption ⌋Main⌊ Independent variable: *male* ⌋Options⌊ ⊙ Plot curves against analysis time ⌋Plot⌊ [Edit] [Marker properties] ⌋Main⌊ ┌ Marker properties — Symbol: *None* ⌋ [Accept] [Accept]

Select plot: *Plot 2* [Edit] [Line Properties] Color: *Gray* [Accept] [Marker properties] ⌋Main⌊ ⌈ Marker properties — Symbol: *None* ⌋ [Accept] [Accept] ⌋X axis⌊ Title: *Age* [Submit].

## 7.10. Hazard regression models with time-dependent covariates

Sometimes the relative risk between two groups varies appreciably with time. In this case, the proportional hazards assumption is invalid. We can weaken this assumption by using **time-dependent covariates**. That is, we assume that the $i^{\text{th}}$ patient has $q$ covariates $x_{i1}[t], x_{i2}[t], \ldots, x_{iq}[t]$ that are themselves functions of time $t$. The hazard function for this patient is

$$\lambda_i[t] = \lambda_0[t] \exp[x_{i1}[t]\beta_1 + x_{i2}[t]\beta_2 + \cdots + x_{iq}[t]\beta_q]. \tag{7.24}$$

The simplest time-dependent covariates are **step-functions.** For example, in Figure 7.9 we saw strong evidence that the protective effect for a woman against CHD diminishes with age. To estimate how the relative risk of being male varies with age we could define the following covariate step functions:

$$male_{i1}[age] = \begin{cases} 1: & i^{\text{th}} \text{ patient is a man age } \leq 50 \\ 0: & \text{otherwise,} \end{cases}$$

$$male_{i2}[age] = \begin{cases} 1: & i^{\text{th}} \text{ patient is a man and } 50 < \text{age} \leq 60 \\ 0: & \text{otherwise,} \end{cases}$$

$$male_{i3}[age] = \begin{cases} 1: & i^{\text{th}} \text{ patient is a man and } 60 < \text{age} \leq 70 \\ 0: & \text{otherwise,} \end{cases}$$

$$male_{i4}[age] = \begin{cases} 1: & i^{\text{th}} \text{ patient is a man and } 70 < \text{age} \leq 80 \\ 0: & \text{otherwise,} \end{cases}$$

$$male_{i5}[age] = \begin{cases} 1: & i^{\text{th}} \text{ patient is a man age } > 80 \\ 0: & \text{otherwise.} \end{cases}$$

They are called step-functions because they equal 1 on one age interval and then step down to 0 for ages outside this interval. For women, these step functions are uniformly equal to 0 for all ages. For men exactly one of these functions will equal 1 depending on the patient's age. We consider the hazard regression model

$$\lambda_i[age] = \lambda_0[age] \exp[male_{i1}[age]\beta_1 + male_{i2}[age]\beta_2 + \cdots + male_{i5}[age]\beta_5]. \tag{7.25}$$

The functions $male_{i1}[age]$ through $male_{i5}[age]$ are associated with five parameters $\beta_1, \beta_2, \ldots, \beta_5$ that assess the effect of male gender on CHD risk before age 50, during each decade of life between 50 and 80, and after age 80. Note that $\beta_1$ has no effect on CHD hazard after age 50 since, for $age > 50$, $x_{i1}[age] = 0$ regardless of the patient's sex. Similarly, $\beta_2$ has no effect on CHD hazard except for men between the ages of 50 and 60, and $\beta_3$, $\beta_4$, and $\beta_5$ only influence the hazard for men in their sixties, seventies, and after age 80, respectively. Hence, the hazard for men equals

$\lambda_0[age] \exp[\beta_1]$ before age 50,
$\lambda_0[age] \exp[\beta_2]$ between the ages of 50 and 60,
$\lambda_0[age] \exp[\beta_3]$ between the ages of 60 and 70,
$\lambda_0[age] \exp[\beta_4]$ between the ages of 70 and 80, and
$\lambda_0[age] \exp[\beta_5]$ after age 80.

The hazard for women at any age is $\lambda_0[age]$. Therefore, the age-adjusted relative risk of CHD in men compared with women equals $\exp[\beta_1]$ before age 50; equals $\exp[\beta_2]$, $\exp[\beta_3]$, and $\exp[\beta_4]$ in the sixth, seventh, and eighth decades of life, respectively; and equals $\exp[\beta_5]$ after age 80. If $\beta_1 = \beta_2 = \cdots = \beta_5 = \beta$ then the hazard for men at any age is $\lambda_0[age] \exp[\beta]$ and the proportional hazards assumption holds. Of course, the true hazard presumably is a continuous function of age. However, hazard functions with step-function covariates are often useful approximations that have the advantage of providing relevant relative risk estimates.

Applying Model (7.25) to the Framingham data set gives estimates of the $\beta$ parameters and their associated standard errors shown in Table 7.5. For example, in this table $\hat{\beta}_3 = 0.5668$. Hence, the age-adjusted relative risk of CHD in men age 60–70 compared with women is $\exp[\beta_3] = e^{0.5668} = 1.763$.

**Table 7.5.** Age-specific relative risks of coronary heart disease in men relative to women of the same age. The Framingham Heart Study data were analyzed using Model (7.25).

| Age | $j$ | $\hat{\beta}_j$ | $\hat{se}_j$ | Relative risk | 95% confidence interval |
|---|---|---|---|---|---|
| ≤50 | 1 | 1.4421 | 0.224 | 4.229 | (2.73–6.56) |
| 50–60 | 2 | 0.9083 | 0.107 | 2.480 | (2.01–3.06) |
| 60–70 | 3 | 0.5668 | 0.083 | 1.763 | (1.50–2.07) |
| 70–80 | 4 | 0.6318 | 0.113 | 1.881 | (1.51–2.35) |
| >80 | 5 | 0.0471 | 0.246 | 1.048 | (0.65–1.70) |

The 95% confidence interval for this relative risk is $\exp[0.5668 \pm 1.96 \times 0.083] = (1.50 - 2.07)$.

### 7.10.1. Testing the proportional hazards assumption

If the proportional hazards assumption is true, then $\beta_1 = \beta_2 = \cdots = \beta_5$ in Model (7.25), and this model reduces to the proportional hazards Model (7.22). Hence, we can test the proportional hazards assumption by testing the null hypothesis that $\beta_1 = \beta_2 = \cdots = \beta_5$. In the Framingham study, this test yields a $\chi^2$ statistic with four degrees of freedom that equals 24.74. This statistic is highly significant with $P = 0.0001$. Thus, the Framingham data set provides compelling evidence that the protection women enjoy against CHD diminishes with age. It is also of interest to determine whether the relative risks in consecutive age intervals in Table 7.5 are significantly different from each other. We do this by testing the separate null hypotheses

$\beta_1 = \beta_2$ to determine if men aged $\leq 50$ have a different relative risk from men in their sixth decade,

$\beta_2 = \beta_3$ to determine if men in their sixth decade have a different relative risk from men in their seventh decade,

$\beta_3 = \beta_4$ to determine if men in their seventh decade have a different relative risk from men in their eighth decade, and

$\beta_4 = \beta_5$ to determine if men in their eighth decade have a different relative risk from men aged over 80.

Tests of these four null hypotheses yield $z$ statistics whose $P$-values are 0.032, 0.012, 0.64, and 0.031, respectively. Hence, there is no evidence that the CHD risk of men compared to women varies between their seventh and eighth decade ($P = 0.64$) but in other consecutive age groups these risks differ significantly. In Table 7.5 the estimated relative risk for men in their eighth decade is slightly greater than their risk in their seventh decade, which goes against the trend of decreasing relative risk with increasing age. In view of this and the lack of significance between the risks in the seventh and eighth decade we could simplify our model by combining these two decades into a single epoch. This would give us a reasonable model that used four parameters to account for the varying effect of age on the relative CHD hazard between men and women (see Exercise 6).

Model (7.25) assumes that within each age interval the proportional hazards assumption holds. Figure 7.10 is identical to Figure 7.9 except that vertical lines have been drawn at the boundaries between the age epochs in

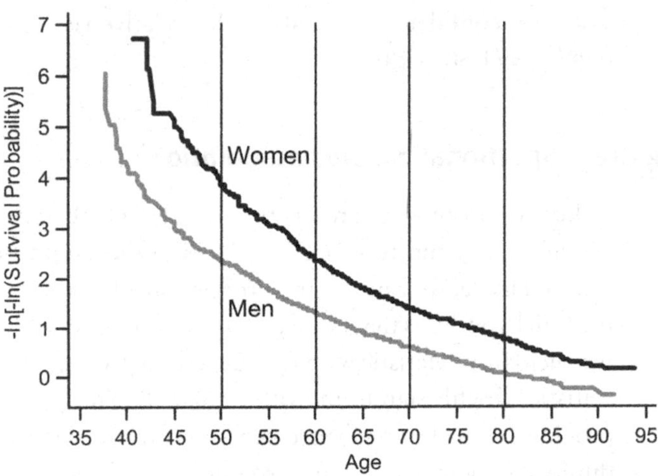


Figure 7.10 Log–log plots of CHD-free survival curves for men and women from the Framingham Heart Study. The vertical lines mark the boundaries between the age epochs in Model (7.25). Within each epoch the curves are fairly close to being parallel. This suggests that Model (7.25), which assumes proportional hazards within each age epoch, is reasonable for these data.

the model. If the model fit perfectly, the curves for men and women would be parallel within each epoch and would be discontinuous at the vertical lines. While this is not the case, the variation in the distance between these lines within each age epoch is much less than it is over the entire age range of the study. This indicates that Model (7.25) fits these data much better than the simple proportional hazards Model (7.22).

## 7.10.2. Modeling time-dependent covariates with Stata

Stata can analyze hazard regression models with time-dependent covariates that are step-functions. To do this, we must first define multiple data records per patient in such a way that the covariate functions for the patient are constant for the period covered by each record. This is best explained by an example. Suppose that we wished to analyze Model (7.25). In the Framingham data set, patient 924 is a man who entered the study at age 32 and exited with CHD at age 63. For this patient $id = 924$, $male = 1$, $age = 32$, $exitage = 63$, and $chdfate = 1$. We replace the record for this patient with three records. The first of these records describes his covariates from age 32 to age 50, the second describes his covariates from age 50 to 60, and the third describes his covariates from age 60 to 63. We define new

**Table 7.6.** Reformatting of the data for Framingham patient 924 that is required to analyze Model (7.25). For time-dependent hazard regression models the data must be split into multiple records per patient in such a way that the covariates remain constant over the time period covered by each record (see text)

| *id* | *male1* | *male2* | *male3* | *enter* | *exit* | *fate* |
|---|---|---|---|---|---|---|
| 924 | 1 | 0 | 0 | 32 | 50 | 0 |
| 924 | 0 | 1 | 0 | 50 | 60 | 0 |
| 924 | 0 | 0 | 1 | 60 | 63 | 1 |

variables *male1*, *male2*, *male3*, *enter*, *exit*, and *fate* whose values are shown in Table 7.6. The variables *male1*, *male2*, and *male3* describe the values of $male_{i1}[age]$, $male_{i2}[age]$, and $male_{i3}[age]$ for this patient in Model (7.25), respectively. In the first epoch from age 32 to 50, $male_{i1}[age] = male\ 1 = 1$ while $male_{i2}[age] = male\ 2 = male_{i3}[age] = male\ 3 = 0$. The variables *enter* and *exit* describe the subject's age at entry and exit from the first epoch, which are 32 and 50 years, respectively. The variable *fate* gives the patient's CHD status at the end of the epoch. Since we know that he has not had a CHD event by age 50, this variable equals 0. The second record in Table 7.6 describes the patient in his second epoch from age 50 to 60. Here $male_{i2}[age] = male\ 2 = 1$ while the other time-dependent covariates equal zero. The variables *enter* and *exit* give his age at entry and exit from the second epoch, which are 50 and 60, respectively; *fate* again equals zero since the subject had not had CHD by age 60. The final record describes the patient's status in the third epoch. Since the patient has an event at age 63, $exit = 63$ and $fate = 1$. We will also need to define covariates *male 4* and *male 5* to cover the last two epochs. For patient 924 these covariates will equal zero in each of his records since his follow-up ceased before the beginning of the fourth epoch. After reformatting, each patient will have one record for each epoch that includes some of his follow-up time. Patients whose follow-up lies entirely within one epoch will have only one record. Patients whose follow-up starts in the first epoch (before age 50) and ends in the fifth (after age 80) will have five records.

The only tricky part of a time-dependent hazard regression analysis is defining the data records as described above. Once this is done, the analysis is straightforward. We illustrate how to modify the data file and do this analysis below. The log file *7.8.4.Framingham.log* continues as follows.

```
. *
. * Perform hazard regression with time dependent covariates for sex
. *
. tabulate chdfate male                                                  1

 Coronary  |
     Heart |          male
   Disease |     Women        Men |     Total
-----------+----------------------+----------
  Censored |     2,000      1,226 |     3,226
       CHD |       650        823 |     1,473
-----------+----------------------+----------
     Total |     2,650      2,049 |     4,699

. *
. *  Split each patient's record into one or more records so that each
. *  record describes one epoch with constant covariates for the epoch.
. *
. generate exit = exitage                                                2
. stset exit, id(id) enter(time age) failure(chdfate)                    3
                                                          Output omitted
. list id male age exit chdfate if id == 924                             4

       +---------------------------------------+
       |  id   male   age       exit   chdfate |
       |---------------------------------------|
3182.  | 924    Men    32   63.23888       CHD |
       +---------------------------------------+

. stsplit enter, at(50 60 70 80)                                         5
(8717 observations (episodes) created)
. list id male enter exit chdfate if id == 924                           6

       +-----------------------------------------+
       |  id   male   enter       exit   chdfate |
       |-----------------------------------------|
7940.  | 924    Men       0         50         . |
7941.  | 924    Men      50         60         . |
7942.  | 924    Men      60   63.23888       CHD |
       +-----------------------------------------+

. replace enter = age if id != id[`n-1]                                  7
(4451 real changes made)
. generate male1 = male*(exit <= 50)                                     8
```

```
. generate male2 = male*(enter >= 50 & exit <= 60)
. generate male3 = male*(enter >= 60 & exit <= 70)
. generate male4 = male*(enter >= 70 & exit <= 80)
. generate male5 = male*(enter >= 80)
. list id male? enter exit chdfate if id == 924                              9

       +------------------------------------------------------------------------+
       | id   male1   male2   male3   male4   male5   enter       exit   chdfate |
       |------------------------------------------------------------------------|
7940.  | 924      1       0       0       0       0      32         50         . |
7941.  | 924      0       1       0       0       0      50         60         . |
7942.  | 924      0       0       1       0       0      60   63.23888       CHD |
       +------------------------------------------------------------------------+

. generate testmale = male1 + male2 + male3 + male4 + male5
. tabulate chdfate testmale, missing                                         10

  Coronary |
     Heart |       testmale
   Disease |         0          1 |     Total
-----------+----------------------+----------
  Censored |     2,000      1,226 |     3,226
       CHD |       650        823 |     1,473
         . |     5,217      3,500 |     8,717
-----------+----------------------+----------
     Total |     7,867      5,549 |    13,416

. stset exit, id(id) enter(time enter) failure(chdfate)                      11
                id:  id
     failure event:  chdfate != 0 & chdfate < .
obs. time interval:  (exit[_n-1], exit]
 enter on or after:  time enter
 exit on or before:  failure

-------------------------------------------------------------------------
    13416  total obs.
        0  exclusions
-------------------------------------------------------------------------
    13416  obs. remaining, representing
     4699  subjects
     1473  failures in single failure-per-subject data
 103710.1  total analysis time at risk, at risk from t =         0
                             earliest observed entry t =        30
                                  last observed exit t =        94
```

```
. stcox male?                                                            12

        failure _d:  chdfate
  analysis time _t:  exit
 enter on or after:  time enter
                id:  id
                                                               Output omitted
Cox regression -- Breslow method for ties

No. of subjects =         4699              Number of obs   =      13416
No. of failures =         1473
Time at risk    =  103710.0914
                                            LR chi2(5)      =     203.92
Log likelihood  =   -11205.396              Prob > chi2     =     0.0000

------------------------------------------------------------------------------
          _t | Haz. Ratio   Std. Err.      z    P>|z|     [95% Conf. Interval]
-------------+----------------------------------------------------------------
       male1 |    4.22961   .9479718     6.43   0.000      2.72598    6.562631
       male2 |   2.480204    .264424     8.52   0.000     2.012508    3.056591
       male3 |   1.762634   .1465087     6.82   0.000     1.497652    2.074499
       male4 |   1.880939   .2127479     5.59   0.000     1.506946     2.34775
       male5 |   1.048225   .2579044     0.19   0.848     .6471809    1.697788
------------------------------------------------------------------------------

. test male1 = male2 = male3 = male4 = male5                             13

 ( 1)  male1 - male2 = 0
 ( 2)  male1 - male3 = 0
 ( 3)  male1 - male4 = 0
 ( 4)  male1 - male5 = 0

          chi2(  4) =    24.74
        Prob > chi2 =    0.0001

. lincom male1 - male2                                                   14

 ( 1)  male1 - male2 = 0

------------------------------------------------------------------------------
          _t |      Coef.   Std. Err.      z    P>|z|     [95% Conf. Interval]
-------------+----------------------------------------------------------------
         (1) |   .5337688   .2481927     2.15   0.032     .0473199    1.020218
------------------------------------------------------------------------------

. lincom male2 - male3

 ( 1)  male2 - male3 = 0
```

```
-----------------------------------------------------------------------------
          _t |      Coef.   Std. Err.      z    P>|z|     [95% Conf. Interval]
-------------+---------------------------------------------------------------
         (1) |   .3415319   .1351862    2.53   0.012     .0765719    .6064919
-----------------------------------------------------------------------------

. lincom male3 - male4

 ( 1)  male3 - male4 = 0

-----------------------------------------------------------------------------
          _t |      Coef.   Std. Err.      z    P>|z|     [95% Conf. Interval]
-------------+---------------------------------------------------------------
         (1) |  -.0649622    .140364    -0.4   0.643    -.3400706    .2101463
-----------------------------------------------------------------------------

. lincom male4 - male5

 ( 1)  male4 - male5 = 0

-----------------------------------------------------------------------------
          _t |      Coef.   Std. Err.      z    P>|z|     [95% Conf. Interval]
-------------+---------------------------------------------------------------
         (1) |   .5846729   .2707924    2.16   0.031     .0539295    1.115416
-----------------------------------------------------------------------------

. log close
```

## Comments

1 The next few commands will create the multiple records per patient that we need for this time-dependent hazard regression analysis. It is prudent to be cautious doing this and to create before and after tables to confirm that we have done what we intended.

2 We will define *exit* to equal the patient's age at the end of each age epoch. Initially we set *exit* equal to the patient's age at the end of follow-up.

3 Hazard regression analyses with time-dependent step-function covariates require multiple records per patient. The *id* option of the *stset* command tells Stata the name of the variable (in this example *id*) that identifies multiple records as belonging to the same patient. In the point-and-click version of this command (see page 302) you must check the *Multiple-record ID variable* box on the *Main* tab of the *stset* dialogue box and enter the name of the ID variable.

4 Patient 924 is a man who enters the study at age 32 and exits at age 63.2 with coronary heart disease.

5 The *stsplit* command defines the time epochs for this analysis and creates a separate record for each epoch that contains some follow-up time for

each patient. These records are sorted in chronological order. In this example we are using the patient's age as the time variable. The age epochs are defined by the *at* option and are from age 0 to 50, 50 to 60, 60 to 70, 70 to 80, and 80 until the end of follow-up. The variable *enter* is set equal to the patient's age at the beginning of each epoch.

The equivalent point-and-click command is Statistics ▶ Survival Analysis ▶ Setup and utilities ▶ Split time-span records ⌡Main⌊ ┌ Variable to record time interval to which each new observation belongs — *enter* New variable name ┘ ┌ Analysis times at which the records are to be split — *50 60 70 80* Analysis time ┘ Submit.

6 This command shows the records for patient 924 after the preceding *stsplit* command has been executed. There are three records corresponding to the three epochs spanned by this patient's follow-up. In the first two records, *exit* equals the patient's age at the end of the first and second epoch, respectively. In the last record it equals the patient's age at the end of follow-up. The variable *enter* equals the patient's age at the beginning of each epoch; *chdfate* equals the patient's true fate on his last record and is set to missing on his earlier records. The *stcox* program will consider patients with missing values of the fate variable as being censored at this time.

7 In this example the patient's age is the time variable and patients enter the study at different ages. We need to set *enter* to equal the patient's entry age in the first epoch when they are followed. For patient 924 we need to change *enter* from 0 in his first record to 32.

Stata maintains a special variable *_n* which equals the record number of the current record. The value of *id*[*_n* − 1] is the value of *id* in the record that precedes the current record. Note that the data set is sorted by *id* and by *enter* within records of the same patient. Hence, *id*! = *id*[*_n* − 1] will be true if the current value of *id* is different from the preceding value. In other words, *id*! = *id*[*_n* − 1] is true for the first record of each patient, which describes her earliest epoch. This command changes the value of these records from the beginning of the epoch to the beginning of the patient's follow-up. Note that this command would not be needed if the time variable was time since recruitment, in which case all patients would enter the first epoch at time zero.

8 We set *male1* = 1 if and only if the subject is male and the record describes a patient in the first age epoch. Otherwise, *male1* = 0. The variables *male2* through *male5* are similarly defined for epochs two through five.

9 This table shows the values *male1* through *male5*, *enter*, *exit*, and *chdfate* for all records of patient 924 Compare this table with Table 7.6. The syntax *male?* specifies all variables that start with the letters *male* and end with a single additional character. Hence, *male?* specifies *male1* through *male5* but excludes *male*.

10 The *missing* option of this *tabulate* command specifies that the number of missing values of *chdfate* and *testmale* should be displayed. The variable *testmale* should equal zero or one for all records. This table should be compared with the earlier table of *chdfate* by *male* that we generated before the *stsplit* command. Note that the number of CHD events in men and women has not changed. Also, the number of men and women who were censored at exit is the same. We have added 1473 records for patients whose follow-up spanned multiple records. The consistency of these before and after tables increase our confidence that we have expanded the data set correctly.

The corresponding point-and-click command is Statistics ▶ Summaries, tables, and tests ▶ Tables ▶ Two-way tables with measures of association ⌋Main⌊ Row variable: *chdfate* , Column variable: *testmale* , [✓] Treat missing values like other values [Submit].

11 We need to give a final *stset* command that changes the entry time variable from *age* to *enter*. That is, the entry time variable is now the patient's age when he first enters the current epoch rather than his age when he is recruited into the study. The output from this command includes the number of subjects under study, which has not changed.

If we were analyzing a model with time-dependent covariates in which the time variable was time since recruitment then all patients would enter the study at time 0. In this case, the *stset* command would not require an *enter* option.

12 Finally, we perform a hazard regression analysis with the time-dependent covariates *male1* through *male5*. The age-adjusted relative risks of CHD and their confidence intervals are highlighted and agree with those given in Table 7.5.

13 This *test* command tests the null hypothesis that $\beta_1 = \beta_2 = \cdots = \beta_5$ in Model (7.25). The *P*-value for this test equals 0.0001, providing strong evidence that the proportional hazards assumption is false for these data. The point-and-click version of this command is Statistics ▶ Postestimation ▶ Tests ▶ Test linear hypotheses ⌋Main⌊ ┌ test type for specification 1 — ⊙ Linear expressions are equal

⌋ Specification1, linear expression: *male1* = *male2* = *male3* = *male4* = *male5* [Submit].

14 This *lincom* command tests the hypothesis that $\beta_1 = \beta_2$. This test gives $P = 0.032$ and provides evidence that the age-adjusted relative risk of CHD in men relative to women is greater in the first epoch than the second. That is, it is greater for men before age 50 than for men in their fifth decade. Subsequent *lincom* commands perform this same test for the other consecutive age epochs (see Section 7.10.1).

## 7.11. Additional reading

See Section 6.18 for some standard references on hazard regression analysis.

Fleming and Harrington (1991) and

Therneau and Grambsch (2000) are advanced texts on survival analysis with extensive discussions of methods of model selection and residual analysis.

## 7.12. Exercises

1 Using Model (7.16) estimate the risk of CHD of men in each DBP group relative to women in the same group. Calculate 95% confidence intervals for these relative risks.

2 Fit a multiplicative model similar to Model (7.19) but without the interaction terms for sex and blood pressure. Do the interaction terms in Model (7.19) significantly improve the model fit over the multiplicative model that you have just created? How does your answer affect which model you would use if you were publishing these results?

3 The relative risk obtained from Model (7.22) is age-adjusted while the relative risk derived from Model (7.14) is not. Explain why this is so.

4 Fit a simple proportional hazards regression model of the effects of baseline diastolic blood pressure on CHD risk by using *dbp* as the sole covariate in the model. Under this model, what is the relative risk of CHD for a subject whose baseline DBP is 85 compared with someone with a baseline DBP of 60? What is a 95% confidence interval for this relative risk? Contrast this model with Model (7.12). What are the strengths and weaknesses of these two models? Is your answer consistent with the relative risks in Table 7.1? (Hint: under your model, what is the hazard function for a patient with a DBP of 85? What is the hazard function for a patient with a DBP of 60? Divide the first hazard function by the second to obtain the desired relative risk. In your Stata program, after

you have run your hazard regression analysis, use the *lincom* command to obtain the desired relative risk and confidence interval. Remember that the *lincom* command can be used to calculate the exponentiated value of any weighted sum of model coefficients.)

5 Draw a graph of the relative risk of CHD as a function of baseline DBP using the model in Exercise 4. Make the denominator of the relative risks in this graph be patients with a DBP of 60 mm Hg. Display the 95% confidence band for these risks on this graph (hint: use the *predictnl* command). Compare your answer to Figure 7.3.

6 Re-analyze the time-dependent hazard regression model of CHD described in Section 7.10, only combining men between the ages of 60 and 80 into a single stratum. Test the proportional hazards assumption for this model. If you were publishing this data which model would you use?

The following questions concern the *6.ex.breast.dta* data set introduced in the exercises for Chapter 6. In Questions 7 through 10 use time since entry biopsy as the time variable. Use proportional hazards regression models for all questions except Question 13.

7 Calculate the relative risks of breast cancer among women with AH and PDWA compared with women without PD. Adjust for age by including age at entry biopsy as a covariate in your model. Calculate the 95% confidence intervals for these risks. Does this model give a better estimate of these risks than the model used in Question 4 in Chapter 6? If so, why?

8 Repeat Question 7 only this time adjust for age using a categorical variable that groups age at biopsy as follows: ≤30, 31–40, 41–50, 51–60, >60. Compare your answers to these questions. What are the strengths and weaknesses of these methods of age adjustment?

9 Repeat Question 7, but this time adjust for age by using a three-knot restricted cubic spline model. (Use the default knot locations.) Compare your answers with those to Questions 7 and 8. What are the strengths and weaknesses of these methods of age adjustment?

10 Build a proportional hazards model of the effects of entry biopsy diagnosis and family history on the risk of breast cancer. Adjust for age at biopsy by including *entage* as a covariate in your model. Treat *pd* and *fh* as categorical variables and include appropriate interaction terms. Fill in the following table. What is the risk of women with both AH and FH relative to women with FH but without PD? What is a 95% confidence interval for this risk?

| | First degree family history of breast cancer | | | |
|---|---|---|---|---|
| | No | | Yes | |
| Entry histology | Relative risk | 95% confidence interval | Relative risk | 95% confidence interval |
| No PD | 1.0* | | | |
| PDWA | | | | |
| AH | | | | |

*Denominator of relative risk

11 Calculate the relative risks of breast cancer among women with AH and PDWA compared with women without PD. Use the patient's age as the time variable. Calculate the 95% confidence intervals for these risks. Contrast your answer with that for Question 7. How do the model assumptions differ for these two questions?

12 Draw log–log plots of breast cancer-free survival in women without PD, with PDWA, and with AH in the model used in Question 7. Adjust these plots for the patient's average age at biopsy. Do these plots suggest that the proportional hazards assumption is reasonable for these data?

13 What are the relative risks of AH and PDWA compared with No PD in the first ten years after biopsy? What are these risks after ten years for women who remain free of breast cancer for the first ten years following biopsy? To answer this question, build the following hazard regression model with time-dependent covariates. Define two step functions: the first should equal 1 on the interval 0–10 and 0 elsewhere; the second should equal 0 on the interval 0–10 and 1 elsewhere. Adjust for age at biopsy by including *entage* as a covariate in the model. Include two parameters to model the risk of AH in the first ten years and thereafter. Include another two parameters to model these risks for PDWA. Note that in this question, all patients enter at time 0 when they have their entry biopsy. This is the default entry time used by the *stsplit* command for patients in their first epoch. Also, since all patients enter the study at time 0, you do not need to include the *enter* option in your *stset* command. (Reference: Dupont and Page, 1989.)

14 Use your model for Question 8 to test the proportional hazards assumption for the model used in Question 6. Is this assumption reasonable?

8

# Introduction to Poisson regression: inferences on morbidity and mortality rates

In previous chapters the basic unit of observation has been the individual patient. Sometimes, however, it makes more sense to analyze events per person–year of observation. This may be either because the data come to us in this form or because survival methods using suitable models are too complex and numerically intensive. For example, analyzing large cohorts with hazard regression models that have many time-dependent covariates can require substantial computation time. In this situation, converting the data to events per person–year of observation can greatly simplify the analysis. If the event rate per unit of time is low, then an excellent approach to consider is Poisson regression. We will introduce this technique in the next two chapters.

## 8.1. Elementary statistics involving rates

The **incidence** $I$ of an event is the expected number of events during 100 000 person–years of follow-up. Suppose that we observe $d$ independent events during $n$ person–years of observation, where $d$ is small compared with $n$. Then the **observed incidence** of the event is $\hat{I} = 100\,000 \times d/n$, which is the observed number of events per 100 000 patient–years of follow-up. For example, Table 8.1 is derived from the 4699 patients in the didactic data set from the Framingham Heart Study (Levy, 1999). This data set contains a total of 104 461 person–years of follow-up. Let $d_i$ be the number of CHD events observed in $n_i$ person–years of follow-up among men ($i = 1$) and women ($i = 0$), respectively. The observed incidence of coronary heart disease (CHD) in men is $\hat{I}_1 = 100\,000 \times d_1/n_1 = 100\,000 \times 823/42\,688 = 1927.9$, while the corresponding incidence in women is $\hat{I}_0 = 100\,000 \times d_0/n_0 = 100\,000 \times 650/61\,773 = 1052.2$. Incidence rates are always expressed as the observed or expected number of events in a specified number of patients during a specified interval of time. For

**Table 8.1.** Coronary heart disease and patient–years of follow-up in the Framingham Heart Study (Levy, 1999)

| | Men | Women | Total |
|---|---|---|---|
| Cases of coronary heart disease | $d_1 =$ 823 | $d_0 =$ 650 | 1473 |
| Person–years of follow-up | $n_1 =$ 42 688 | $n_0 =$ 61 773 | 104 461 |

example, an incidence rate might also be expressed as the expected number of events per thousand person–months of observation.

Suppose that the incidences of some event are $I_0$ and $I_1$ in patients from Groups 0 and 1, respectively. Then the **relative risk** of the event in Group 1 compared with Group 0 is

$$R = I_1/I_0, \tag{8.1}$$

which is the ratio of the incidence rates in the two groups. We estimate this relative risk by $\hat{R} = \hat{I}_1/\hat{I}_0$. For example, the estimated relative risk of CHD in men compared with women in Table 8.1 is $\hat{R} = \hat{I}_1/\hat{I}_0 = 1927.9/1052.2 = 1.832$.

The logarithm of $\hat{R}$ has an approximately normal distribution whose variance is estimated by

$$s^2_{\log(\hat{R})} = \frac{1}{d_0} + \frac{1}{d_1}. \tag{8.2}$$

Hence, a 95% confidence interval for $R$ is

$$\hat{R}\exp[\pm 1.96 s_{\log(\hat{R})}]. \tag{8.3}$$

For the patients from the Framingham Heart Study, $s^2_{\log(\hat{R})} = \frac{1}{823} + \frac{1}{650} = 0.002\,754$. Hence, a 95% confidence interval for the risk of CHD in men relative to women is

$$\hat{R} = (1.832\exp[-1.96 \times \sqrt{0.002\,754}], 1.832\exp[1.96 \times \sqrt{0.002\,754}])$$

$$= (1.65, 2.03).$$

## 8.2. Calculating relative risks from incidence data using Stata

The following log file and comments illustrate how to calculate relative risks from incidence data using Stata.

```
. * 8.2.Framingham.log
. *
. * Estimate the crude (unadjusted) relative risk of
. * coronary heart disease in men compared with women using
. * person-year data from the Framingham Heart Study.
. *
. iri 823 650 42688 61773                                        1

                 |   Exposed   Unexposed  |      Total
-----------------+------------------------+------------
           Cases |       823         650  |       1473
     Person-time |     42688       61773  |     104461
-----------------+------------------------+------------
                 |                        |
  Incidence Rate |  .0192794    .0105224  |    .014101
                 |                        |
                 |      Point estimate    |    [95% Conf. Interval]
                 |------------------------+------------------------
 Inc. rate diff. |           .008757      |   .0072113    .0103028
 Inc. rate ratio |          1.832227      |   1.651137    2.033836 (exact)
 Attr. frac. ex. |          .4542162      |   .3943566    .5083183 (exact)
 Attr. frac. pop |          .2537814      |
                 +-------------------------------------------------
                   (midp)   Pr(k>=823) =                  0.0000 (exact)
                   (midp) 2*Pr(k>=823) =                  0.0000 (exact)
. log close
```

**Comment**

1 The *ir* command is used for incidence rate data. Shown here is the immediate version of this command, called *iri*, which analyses the four data values given in the command line. These data are the number of exposed and unexposed cases together with the person–years of follow-up of exposed and unexposed subjects. In this example, "exposed" patients are male and "unexposed" patients are female. Cases are people who develop CHD. The arguments of the *iri* command are the number of men with CHD (exposed cases), the number of women with CHD (unexposed cases), and the number of person–years of follow-up in men and women, respectively. The relative risk of CHD in men compared with women is labeled "Inc. rate ratio". This relative risk, together with its 95% confidence interval, have been highlighted. They agree with Equations (8.1) and (8.3) to three significant figures. Stata uses an exact confidence interval that has a more complicated formula than Equation (8.3) and provides slightly wider intervals.

The point-and-click version of this command is Statistics ▶ Epidemiology and related ▶ Tables for epidemiologists ▶ Incidence-rate ratios calculator

| | Exposed | Unexposed |
|---|---|---|
| Cases | *823* | *650* |
| Person-time | *42688* | *61773* |

Submit.

## 8.3. The binomial and Poisson distributions

Suppose that $d$ unrelated deaths are observed among $n$ patients. Let $\pi$ be the probability that any individual patient dies. Then $d$ has a binomial distribution with parameters $n$ and $\pi$. The probability of observing $d$ deaths is

$$\Pr[d \text{ deaths}] = \frac{n!}{(n-d)!d!}\pi^d(1-\pi)^{(n-d)}. \tag{8.4}$$

In Equation (8.4) $d$ can take any integer value between 0 and $n$. The expected number of deaths is $E[d_i] = n\pi$, and the variance of $d$ is $\text{var}[d_i] = n\pi(1-\pi)$ (see Section 4.4). Poisson (1781–1849) showed that when $n$ is large and $\pi$ is small the distribution of $d$ is closely approximated by a **Poisson distribution**. If $n\pi$ approaches $\lambda$ as $n$ gets very large then the distribution of $d$ approaches

$$\Pr[d \text{ deaths}] = \frac{e^{-\lambda}(\lambda)^d}{d!}, \tag{8.5}$$

where $d$ can be any non-negative integer. Under a Poisson distribution the expected value and variance of $d$ both equal $\lambda$. Although it is not obvious from these formulas, the convergence of the binomial distribution to the Poisson is quite rapid. Figure 8.1 shows a Poisson distribution with expected value $\lambda = 5$. Binomial distributions are also shown with expected value $n\pi = 5$ for $n = 10$, 20, and 50. Note that the binomial distribution with $n = 50$ and $\pi = 0.1$ is very similar to the Poisson distribution with $\lambda = 5$.

## 8.4. Simple Poisson regression for 2×2 tables

Suppose that we have two groups of subjects who either are or are not exposed to some risk factor of interest. Let

$n_i$ be the number of patients or patient–years of observation of subjects who are ($i = 1$) or are not ($i = 0$) exposed,

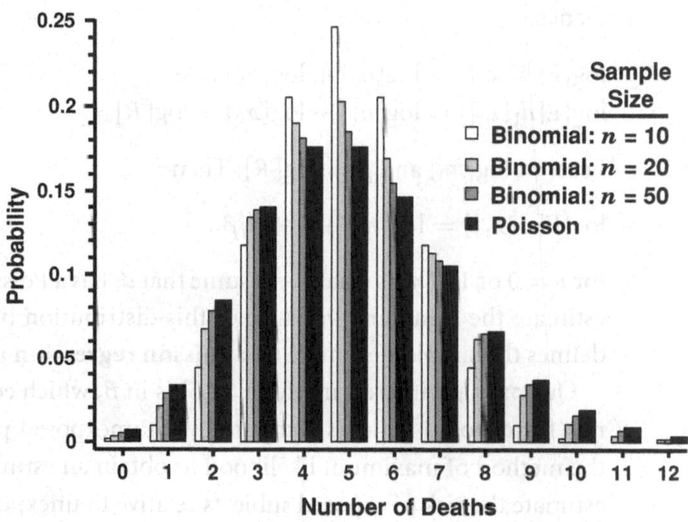


Figure 8.1 This graph illustrates the convergence of the binomial distribution to the Poisson distribution with increasing sample size ($n$) but constant expected value. The depicted distributions all have expected value five. By the time $n = 50$, the binomial distribution closely approximates the Poisson distribution with the same expected value.

$d_i$ be the number of deaths among exposed ($i = 1$) and unexposed ($i = 0$) subjects,

$\pi_i$ be the true death rate in exposed ($i = 1$) and unexposed ($i = 0$) people, and

$x_i = 1$ or 0 be a covariate that indicates patients who are ($i = 1$) or are not ($i = 0$) exposed.

Then

$R = \pi_1/\pi_0$ is the relative risk of death associated with exposure, and

$\hat{\pi}_i = d_i/n_i$ is the estimated death rate in exposed ($i = 1$) or unexposed ($i = 0$) people.

The expected number of deaths in Group $i$ is $\mathrm{E}[d_i \mid x_i] = n_i\pi_i$. Also $\mathrm{E}[\hat{\pi}_i \mid x_i] = \mathrm{E}[(d_i/n_i) \mid x_i] = \mathrm{E}[d_i \mid x_i]/n_i = \pi_i$, which implies that $\log[\pi_0] = \log[\mathrm{E}[d_0|x_0]] - \log[n_0]$ and $\log[\pi_1] = \log[\mathrm{E}[d_1|x_i]] - \log[n_1]$. Now since $R = \pi_1/\pi_0$, we also have that $\log[\pi_1] = \log[R] + \log[\pi_0]$.

Hence,

$$\log[\mathrm{E}[d_0|x_0]] = \log[n_0] + \log[\pi_0] \text{ and}$$
$$\log[\mathrm{E}[d_1|x_0]] = \log[n_1] + \log[\pi_0] + \log[R].$$

Let $\alpha = \log[\pi_0]$ and $\beta = \log[R]$. Then

$$\log[\mathrm{E}[d_i|x_i]] = \log[n_i] + \alpha + x_i\beta \qquad (8.6)$$

for $i = 0$ or 1. If $\pi_i$ is small we assume that $d_i$ has a Poisson distribution. We estimate the mean and variance of this distribution by $d_i$. Equation (8.6) defines the simplest example of a **Poisson regression model**.

Our primary interest in Model (8.6) is in $\beta$, which equals the log relative risk for exposed patients compared with unexposed patients. We will use the method of maximum likelihood to obtain an estimate $\hat{\beta}$ of $\beta$. We then estimate the risk of exposed subjects relative to unexposed subjects by

$$\hat{R} = e^{\hat{\beta}}. \qquad (8.7)$$

The maximum likelihood technique also provides us with an estimate of the standard error of $\hat{\beta}$ which we will denote se$[\hat{R}]$. A 95% confidence interval for $\hat{R}$ is therefore

$$(\hat{R} \times \exp[-1.96\ \mathrm{se}[\hat{\beta}]],\ \hat{R} \times \exp[1.96\ \mathrm{se}[\hat{\beta}]]). \qquad (8.8)$$

The $\alpha$ coefficient in Model (8.6) is called a **nuisance parameter**. This is one that is required by the model but is not used to calculate interesting statistics. An **offset** is a known quantity that must be included in a model. The term $\log[n_i]$ in Model (8.6) is an example of an offset.

Let us apply Model (8.6) to the Framingham Heart Study data in Table 8.1. Let $x_0 = 0$ and $x_1 = 1$ for person–years of follow-up in women and men, respectively. Regressing CHD against gender with this model gives estimates $\hat{\beta} = 0.6055$ and se$[\hat{\beta}] = 0.052\,47$. Applying Equations (8.7) and (8.8) to these values gives a relative risk estimate of CHD in men relative to women to be $\hat{R} = 1.832$. The 95% confidence interval for this risk is (1.65, 2.03). This relative risk and confidence interval are identical to the classical estimates obtained in Section 8.1.

## 8.5. Poisson regression and the generalized linear model

Poisson regression is another example of a generalized linear model. Recall that any generalized linear model is characterized by a random component, a linear predictor, and a link function (see Section 4.6). In Poisson regression the random component is the number of events $d_i$ in the $i^{\text{th}}$ group of

$n_i$ patients or patient–years of observation. The linear predictor is $\log[n_i] + \alpha + x_i\beta$. The expected number of deaths in Group $i$, $E[d_i|x_i]$, is related to the linear predictor through a logarithmic link function.

## 8.6. Contrast between Poisson, logistic, and linear regression

The models for simple linear, logistic, and Poisson regression are as follows:

$E[y_i \mid x_i] = \alpha + \beta x_i$ for $i = 1, 2, \ldots, n$ defines the linear model;
$\text{logit}[E[d_i \mid x_i]/n_i] = \alpha + \beta x_i$ for $i = 1, 2, \ldots, n$ defines the logistic model; and
$\log[E[d_i \mid x_i]] = \log[n_i] + \alpha + \beta x_i$ for $i = 0$ or $1$ defines the Poisson model.

In linear regression, the random component is $y_i$, which has a normal distribution. The standard deviation of $y_i$ given $x_i$ is $\sigma$. The linear predictor is $\alpha + \beta x_i$ and the link function is the identity function $I[x] = x$. The sample size $n$ must be fairly large since we must estimate $\sigma$ before we can estimate $\alpha$ or $\beta$. In logistic regression, the random component is $d_i$ events observed in $n_i$ trials. This random component has a binomial distribution. The linear predictor is $\alpha + \beta x_i$ and the model has a logit link function. In Poisson regression, the random component is also $d_i$ events observed in $n_i$ trials or person–years of observation. This random component has a Poisson distribution. The linear predictor is $\log(n_i) + \alpha + \beta x_i$ and the model has a logarithmic link function. In the simple Poisson regression $i$ takes only two values. This may also be the case for simple logistic regression. It is possible to estimate $\beta$ in these situations since we have reasonable estimates of the mean and variance of $d_i$ given $x_i$ for both of these models.

## 8.7. Simple Poisson regression with Stata

We apply a simple Poisson regression model to the data in Table 8.1 as follows.

```
. *  8.7.Framingham.log
. *
. *  Simple Poisson regression analysis of the effect of gender on
. *  coronary heart disease in the Framingham Heart Study.
. *
. use  C:\WDDtext\8.7.Framingham.dta, clear
. list                                                          1
```

|    | chd | per_yrs | male |
|---|---|---|---|
| 1. | 650 | 61773 | 0 |
| 2. | 823 | 42688 | 1 |

```
. glm chd male, family(poisson) link(log) lnoffset(per_yrs)
```
2

Output omitted

```
                                                   AIC              =  10.43307
Log likelihood   = -8.433070809                    BIC              =  6.53e-14
```

| chd | Coef. (OIM) | Std. Err. | z | P>\|z\| | [95% Conf. | Interval] |
|---|---|---|---|---|---|---|
| male | .6055324 | .0524741 | 11.54 | 0.000 | .5026851 | .7083797 |
| _cons | -4.554249 | .0392232 | -116.11 | 0.000 | -4.631125 | -4.477373 |
| per_yrs | (exposure) | | | | | |

```
. lincom male,irr
 ( 1)  [chd]male = 0
```
3

| chd | IRR | Std. Err. | z | P>\|z\| | [95% Conf. | Interval] |
|---|---|---|---|---|---|---|
| (1) | 1.832227 | .0961444 | 11.54 | 0.000 | 1.653154 | 2.030698 |

```
. log close
```

### Comments

1 The data in Table 8.1 are stored in two records of *8.7.Framingham.dta.* These records contain the number of patient–years of follow-up in women (*male* = 0) and men (*male* = 1), respectively. The variable *chd* records the number of cases of coronary heart disease observed during follow-up.

2 This *glm* command regresses *chd* against *male* using model (8.6). The *family(poisson)* and *link(log)* options specify that *chd* has a Poisson distribution and that a logarithmic link function is to be used. The *lnoffset(per_yrs)* option specifies that the logarithm of *per_yrs* is to be included as an offset in the model.

The equivalent point-and-click command is Statistics ▶ Generalized linear models (GLM) ▶ Generalized linear model (GLM) ⌋ Model ⌊ Dependent variable: *chd* , Independent variables: *male* , Family and link choices: {Log ⦿ Poisson} ⌋ Model 2 ⌊ ⌈ Options — ⦿ Exposure variable: *per_yrs* ⌋ Submit .

3 The *irr* option of this *lincom* command has the same effect as the *or* and *hr* options. That is, it exponentiates the coefficient associated with *male* to obtain the estimated relative risk of CHD in men relative to women (see page 231). It differs only in that it labels the second column of output IRR, which stands for incidence rate ratio. This rate ratio is our estimated relative risk. It and its associated confidence interval are in exact agreement with those obtained from Equations (8.7) and (8.8).

## 8.8. Poisson regression and survival analysis

For large data sets, Poisson regression is much faster than hazard regression analysis with time-dependent covariates. If we have reason to believe that the proportional hazards assumption is false, it makes sense to do our exploratory analyses using Poisson regression. Before we can do this we must first convert the data from survival format to person–year format.

### 8.8.1. Recoding survival data on patients as patient–year data

Table 8.2 shows a survival data set consisting of entry age, exit age, treatment, and fate on five patients. The conversion of this survival data set to a patient–year data set is illustrated in Figure 8.2. Individual patients contribute person–years of follow-up to a number of different ages. For

**Table 8.2.** This table shows survival data for five hypothetical patients. Each patient contributes person–years of follow-up to several strata defined by age and treatment. The conversion of this data set into a person–year data set for Poisson regression analysis is depicted in Figure 8.2.

| Patient ID | Entry age | Exit age | Treatment | Fate |
|---|---|---|---|---|
| A | 1 | 4 | 1 | Alive |
| B | 3 | 5 | 1 | Dead |
| C | 3 | 6 | 2 | Alive |
| D | 2 | 3 | 2 | Dead |
| E | 1 | 3 | 2 | Dead |

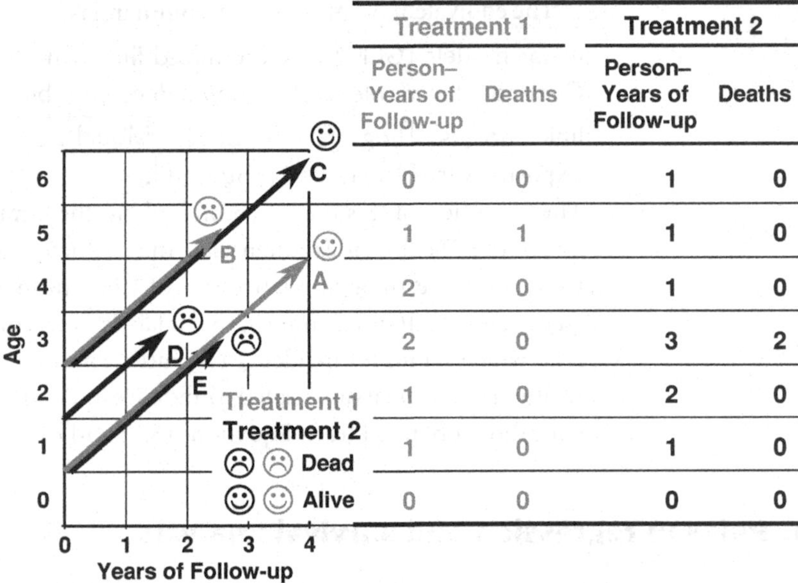


| Age | Treatment 1 Person–Years of Follow-up | Treatment 1 Deaths | Treatment 2 Person–Years of Follow-up | Treatment 2 Deaths |
|---|---|---|---|---|
| 6 | 0 | 0 | 1 | 0 |
| 5 | 1 | 1 | 1 | 0 |
| 4 | 2 | 0 | 1 | 0 |
| 3 | 2 | 0 | 3 | 2 |
| 2 | 1 | 0 | 2 | 0 |
| 1 | 1 | 0 | 1 | 0 |
| 0 | 0 | 0 | 0 | 0 |

Figure 8.2 The survival data from Table 8.2 are depicted in the graph on the left of this figure. As the study subjects age during follow-up, they contribute person–years of observation to strata defined by age and treatment. Before performing Poisson regression, the survival data must be converted into a table of person–year data such as that given on the right of this figure. For example, three patients (B, C, and A) contribute follow-up to four-year-old patients. Two of them (B and A) are in Treatment 1 and one (C) is in Treatment 2. No deaths were observed at this age. Patients D and E do not contribute to this age because they died at age three.

example, Patient B enters the study on her third birthday and dies at age 5. She contributes one year of follow-up at age 3, one at age 4, and a fraction of a year at age 5. (We will count a full year of follow-up for the year in which a patient dies.) To create the corresponding person–year data set we need to determine the number of patient–years of follow-up and number of deaths for each age in each treatment. This is done by summing across the columns of Figure 8.2. For example, consider age 3. There are three person–years of follow-up in Treatment 2 at this age that are contributed by patients C, D, and E. Deaths occur in two of these patient–years (Patients D and E). In Treatment 1 there are two person–years of follow-up for age 3 and no deaths (Patients B and A). The remainder of the table on the right side of Figure 8.2 is completed in a similar fashion. Note that the five patient survival records are converted into 14 records in the person–year file.

## 8.8.2. Converting survival records to person–years of follow-up using Stata

The following program may be used as a template to convert survival records on individual patients into records giving person–years of follow-up. It also demonstrates many of the ways in which data may be manipulated with Stata.

```
. *   8.8.2.Survival_to_PersonYears.log
. *
. *   Convert survival data to person-year data.
. *   The survival data set must have the following variables:
. *       id      = patient id,
. *       age_in  = age at start of follow-up,
. *       age_out = age at end of follow-up,
. *       fate    = fate at exit:  censored = 0, dead = 1,
. *       treat   = treatment variable.
. *
. *   The person-year data set created below will contain one
. *   record per unique combination of treatment and age.
. *
. *   Variables in the person-year data set that must not be in the
. *   original survival data set are
. *       age_now = a variable that takes values between age_in and age_out,
. *       pt_yrs  = number of patient-years of observations of people
. *                 who are age_now years old,
. *       deaths  = number of events (fate=1) occurring in pt_yrs of
. *                 follow-up for this group of patients.
. *
. use C:\WDDtext\8.8.2.Survival.dta
. list
```

|  | id | age_in | age_out | treat | fate |
|---|---|---|---|---|---|
| 1. | A | 1 | 4 | 1 | 0 |
| 2. | B | 3 | 5 | 1 | 1 |
| 3. | C | 3 | 6 | 2 | 0 |
| 4. | D | 2 | 3 | 2 | 1 |
| 5. | E | 1 | 3 | 2 | 1 |

```
. generate exit = age_out + 1                                              1
```

```
. stset exit, id(id) enter(time age_in) failure(fate)

                id:  id
     failure event:  fate != 0 & fate < .
obs. time interval:  (exit[_n-1], exit]
 enter on or after:  time age_in
 exit on or before:  failure

------------------------------------------------------------------------------
        5  total obs.
        0  exclusions
------------------------------------------------------------------------------
        5  obs. remaining, representing
        5  subjects
        3  failures in single failure-per-subject data
       16  total analysis time at risk, at risk from t =         0
                             earliest observed entry t =         1
                                  last observed exit t =         7

. stsplit age_now, at(0(1)6)                                                    2
(11 observations (episodes) created)

. list  id age_in age_out treat fate exit age_now                               3
```

| | id | age_in | age_out | treat | fate | exit | age_now |
|---|---|---|---|---|---|---|---|
| 1. | A | 1 | 4 | 1 | . | 2 | 1 |
| 2. | A | 1 | 4 | 1 | . | 3 | 2 |
| 3. | A | 1 | 4 | 1 | . | 4 | 3 |
| 4. | A | 1 | 4 | 1 | 0 | 5 | 4 |
| 5. | B | 3 | 5 | 1 | . | 4 | 3 |
| 6. | B | 3 | 5 | 1 | . | 5 | 4 |
| 7. | B | 3 | 5 | 1 | 1 | 6 | 5 |
| 8. | C | 3 | 6 | 2 | . | 4 | 3 |
| 9. | C | 3 | 6 | 2 | . | 5 | 4 |
| 10. | C | 3 | 6 | 2 | . | 6 | 5 |
| 11. | C | 3 | 6 | 2 | 0 | 7 | 6 |
| 12. | D | 2 | 3 | 2 | . | 3 | 2 |
| 13. | D | 2 | 3 | 2 | 1 | 4 | 3 |
| 14. | E | 1 | 3 | 2 | . | 2 | 1 |
| 15. | E | 1 | 3 | 2 | . | 3 | 2 |
| 16. | E | 1 | 3 | 2 | 1 | 4 | 3 |

```
. sort treat age_now
. collapse (count) pt_yrs = age_in (sum) deaths = fate                    4
>    , by(treat age_now)
. list treat age_now pt_yrs deaths                                        5

     treat   age_now   pt_yrs   deaths

  1.     1         1        1        0
  2.     1         2        1        0
  3.     1         3        2        0
  4.     1         4        2        0
  5.     1         5        1        1

  6.     2         1        1        0
  7.     2         2        2        0
  8.     2         3        3        2
  9.     2         4        1        0
 10.     2         5        1        0

 11.     2         6        1        0

. save 8.8.2.Person-Years.dta, replace                                    6
file 8.8.2.Person-Years.dta saved

. log close
```

**Comments**

1 A patient who is *age_out* years old at his end of follow-up will be in his *age_out* plus 1st year of life at that time. We define *exit* to be the patient's year of life at the end of follow-up.

2 This command, in combination with the preceding *stset* command, expands the data set so that there is one record for each patient–year of follow-up. The effects of this command are illustrated by the following *list* command. See also page 367.

3 There is now one record for each year of life that each patient had complete or partial follow-up. The variable *age_now* equals *age_in* in each patient's first record and is incremented sequentially in subsequent records. It equals *age_out* at the last record.

The variable *fate* is the patientís true fate in his last record and is missing for other records; *stsplit* divides the observed follow-up into one-year epochs with one record per epoch. Each epoch starts at *age_now* and ends at *exit*; *fate* gives the patient's fate at the end of the epoch.

4 This statement collapses all records with identical values of *treat* and *age_now* into a single record; *pt_yrs* is set equal to the number of records collapsed. (More precisely, it is the count of collapsed records with non-missing values of *age_in*.) The variable *deaths* is set equal to the number of deaths (the sum of non-missing values of *fate* over these records). All variables are deleted from memory except *treat*, *age_now*, *pt_yrs*, and *deaths*.

The equivalent point-and-click command is Data ▶ Create or change variables ▶ Other variable transformation commands ▶ Make dataset of means, medians, etc. ⌋ Main ⌊ ⌈ Statistics to collapse — Statistic 1: *Count nonmissing* , Variables *pt_years = age_in* , ☑ Statistic 2: *Sum* , Variables *deaths = fate* ⌋ ⌋ Options ⌊ Grouping variables: *treat age_now* Submit .

5 The data set now corresponds to the right-hand side of Figure 8.2. Note, however, that the program only creates records for which there is at least one person–year of follow-up. The reason why there are 11 rather than 14 records in the file is that there are no person–years of follow-up for 6 year-old patients on treatment 1 or for patients on either treatment in their first year of life.

6 The data set is saved for future Poisson regression analysis.

**N.B.** If you are working on a large data set with many covariates, you can reduce the computing time by keeping only those covariates that you will need in your model(s) before you start to convert to patient–year data. It is a good idea to check that you have not changed the number of deaths or number of years of follow-up in your program. See the *8.9.Framingham.log* file in the next section for an example of how this can be done.

## 8.9. Converting the Framingham survival data set to person–time data

The following Stata log file and comments illustrate how to convert a real survival data set for Poisson regression analysis.

```
. *  8.9.Framingham.log
. *
. *  Convert Framingham survival data setset to person-year data for
. *  Poisson regression analysis.
. *
. set memory 20m                                                          1
(20480k)

. use  C:\WDDtext\2.20.Framingham.dta
. *  Poisson regression analysis.
. *  Convert bmi, scl and dbp into categorical variables that
. *  subdivide the data set into quartiles for each of these
. *  variables.
. *
. centile bmi dbp scl, centile(25,50,75)                                  2

                                                      — Binom. Interp. —
    Variable |     Obs  Percentile      Centile      [95% Conf. Interval]
-------------+------------------------------------------------------------
         bmi |    4690         25          22.8           22.7         23
             |                 50          25.2           25.1   25.36161
             |                 75            28           27.9       28.1
         dbp |    4699         25            74             74         74
             |                 50            80             80         82
             |                 75            90             90         90
         scl |    4666         25           197            196        199
             |                 50           225            222        225
             |                 75           255            252        256

. generate bmi_gr = recode(bmi, 22.8, 25.2, 28, 29)
(9 missing values generated)

. generate dbp_gr = recode(dbp, 74,80,90,91)

. generate scl_gr = recode(scl, 197, 225, 255, 256)
(33 missing values generated)

. *
. *  Calculate years of follow-up for each patient.
. *  Round to nearest year for censored patients.
. *  Round up to next year when patients exit with CHD.
. *
. generate years = int(followup/365.25) + 1 if chdfate                    3
(3226 missing values generated)
```

```
. replace years = round(followup/365.25, 1) if !chdfate                    4
(3226 real changes made)
. table sex dbp_gr, contents(sum years) row col                            5
```

| Sex | dbp_gr 74 | 80 | 90 | 91 | Total |
|---|---|---|---|---|---|
| Men | 10663 | 10405 | 12795 | 8825 | 42688 |
| Women | 21176 | 14680 | 15348 | 10569 | 61773 |
| Total | 31839 | 25085 | 28143 | 19394 | 104461 |

6

```
. table sex dbp_gr, contents(sum chdfate) row col                          7
```

| Sex | dbp_gr 74 | 80 | 90 | 91 | Total |
|---|---|---|---|---|---|
| Men | 161 | 194 | 222 | 246 | 823 |
| Women | 128 | 136 | 182 | 204 | 650 |
| Total | 289 | 330 | 404 | 450 | 1473 |

```
. generate age_in = age
. generate exit = age + years
. summarize age_in exit
```

| Variable | Obs | Mean | Std. Dev. | Min | Max |
|---|---|---|---|---|---|
| age_in | 4699 | 46.04107 | 8.504363 | 30 | 68 |
| exit | 4699 | 68.27155 | 10.09031 | 36 | 94 |

```
. *
. * Transform data set so that there is one record per patient-year of
. * follow-up. Define age_now to be the patient's age in each record.
. *
. stset exit, id(id) enter(time age_in) failure(chdfate)

                id:  id
     failure event:  chdfate != 0 & chdfate < .
obs. time interval:  (exit[_n-1], exit]
 enter on or after:  time age_in
```

```
exit on or before:  failure
```

Output omitted

```
. stsplit age_now, at(30(1)94)
(99762 observations (episodes) created)
. list id age_in years exit age_now chdfate  in 278/282
```
8

|  | id | age_in | years | exit | age_now | chdfate |
|---|---|---|---|---|---|---|
| 278. | 4075 | 59 | 3 | 62 | 61 | CHD |
| 279. | 4182 | 41 | 3 | 42 | 41 | . |
| 280. | 4182 | 41 | 3 | 43 | 42 | . |
| 281. | 4182 | 41 | 3 | 44 | 43 | Censored |
| 282. | 1730 | 46 | 3 | 47 | 46 | . |

```
. generate age_gr = recode(age_now, 45,50,55,60,65,70,75,80,81)
. label define age 45 "<= 45" 50 "45-50" 55 "50-55" 60 "55-60" 65
>      "60-65" 70 "65-70" 75 "70-75" 80 "75-80" 81 "> 80"
. label values age_gr age
. sort sex bmi_gr scl_gr dbp_gr age_gr
. *
. *  Combine records with identical values of
. *  sex bmi_gr scl_gr dbp_gr and age_gr.
. *
. collapse (count) pt_yrs = age_in (sum) chd_cnt = chdfate
>      , by(sex bmi_gr scl_gr dbp_gr age_gr)
. list sex bmi_gr scl_gr dbp_gr age_gr pt_yrs chd_cnt in 310/315
```
9

10

|  | sex | bmi_gr | scl_gr | dbp_gr | age_gr | pt_yrs | chd_cnt |
|---|---|---|---|---|---|---|---|
| 310. | Men | 28 | 197 | 90 | 45-50 | 124 | 0 |
| 311. | Men | 28 | 197 | 90 | 50-55 | 150 | 1 |
| 312. | Men | 28 | 197 | 90 | 55-60 | 158 | 2 |
| 313. | Men | 28 | 197 | 90 | 60-65 | 161 | 4 |
| 314. | Men | 28 | 197 | 90 | 65-70 | 100 | 2 |
| 315. | Men | 28 | 197 | 90 | 70-75 | 55 | 1 |

11

```
. table sex dbp_gr, contents(sum pt_yrs) row col
```
12

| Sex | dbp_gr 74 | 80 | 90 | 91 | Total |
|---|---|---|---|---|---|
| Men | 10663 | 10405 | 12795 | 8825 | 42688 |
| Women | 21176 | 14680 | 15348 | 10569 | 61773 |
| Total | 31839 | 25085 | 28143 | 19394 | 104461 |

```
. table sex dbp_gr, contents(sum chd_cnt) row col
```
13

| Sex | dbp_gr 74 | 80 | 90 | 91 | Total |
|---|---|---|---|---|---|
| Men | 161 | 194 | 222 | 246 | 823 |
| Women | 128 | 136 | 182 | 204 | 650 |
| Total | 289 | 330 | 404 | 450 | 1473 |

```
. generate male = sex == 1 if !missing(sex)
```
14

```
. display _N
1267
```
15

```
. save 8.12.Framingham.dta, replace
file 8.12.Framingham.dta saved
```
16

```
. log close
```

**Comments**

1 This data conversion requires 20 megabytes of memory.

2 The *centile* command gives percentiles for the indicated variables. The *centile* option specifies the percentiles of these variables that are to be listed, which in this example are the 25th, 50th, and 75th. The equivalent point-and-click command is Statistics ▶ Summaries, tables, and tests ▶ Summary and descriptive statistics ▶ Centiles with CIs [Main] Variables: (leave empty for all) *bmi dbp scl*, Centiles: *25 50 75* [Submit].

These percentiles are used as arguments in the *recode* function to define the categorical variables *bmi_gr*, *dbp_gr*, and *scl_gr*. In the next chapter we will consider body mass index, serum cholesterol, and diastolic blood pressure as confounding variables in our analyses. We convert these data into categorical variables grouped by quartiles.

3 The last follow-up interval for most patients is a fraction of a year. If the patient's follow-up was terminated because of a CHD event, we include the patient's entire last year as part of her follow-up. The *int* function facilitates this by truncating follow-up in years to a whole integer. We then add 1 to this number to include the entire last year of follow-up.

4 If the patient is censored at the end to follow-up, we round this number to the nearest integer using the *round* function; *round(x,1)* rounds *x* to the nearest integer.

5 So far, we haven't added any records or modified any of the original variables. Before doing this it is a good idea to tabulate the number of person–years of follow-up and CHD events in the data set. At the end of the transformation we can recalculate these tables to ensure that we have not lost or added any spurious years of follow-up or CHD events. These tables show these data cross-tabulated by *sex* and *dbp_gr*. The *contents(sum years)* option causes *years* to be summed over every unique combination of values of *sex* and *dbp_gr* and displayed in the table. The equivalent point-and-click command is Statistics ▶ Summaries, tables, and tests ▶ Tables ▶ Table of summary statistics (table) ⌡Main⌊ Row variable: *sex* ⌐ ☑ Column variable — *dbp_gr* ⌋ Statistics 1 *Sum* , Variable *chdfate* ⌡Options⌊ ☑ Add row totals , ☑ Add column totals [Submit].

6 For example, the sum of the *years* variable for men with *dbp_gr* = 90 is 12 795. This means that there are 12 795 person–years of follow-up for men with baseline diastolic blood pressures between 80 and 90 mm Hg.

7 This table shows the number of CHD events by sex and DBP group.

8 The expansion of the data set by the *stset* and *stsplit* commands, and the definitions of *age_now* and *exit* are done in the same way as in Section 8.8.2. This *list* command shows the effects of these transformations. Note that patient 4182 enters the study at age 41 and exits at age 44 (after the end of her forty-third year) when she is censored. The expanded data set contains one record for each of these three years; *age_now* increases from 41 to 43 in these records. Initially, *chdfate* was coded as 0 or 1 for patients who were censored or developed CHD at the end of follow-up, respectively. These values, 0 and 1, were assigned the value labels *Censored* and *CHD*, respectively. After the *stsplit* command *chdfate* is missing in the first two records of patient 4182 and equals 0 in her final record.

9 Recode *age_now* into 5-year age groups.

10 Collapse records with identical values of *sex*, *bmi_gr*, *scl_gr*, *dbp_gr*, and *age_gr*. The syntax *(count) newvar = oldvar* creates *newvar* which contains the number on non-missing values of *oldvar* in records with identical values of the *by* variables. In this example, *pt_yrs* records the number of patient–years of follow-up associated with each record while *chd_cnt* records the corresponding number of CHD events.

11 For example, the subsequent listing shows that there were 161 patient–years of follow-up in men aged 61 to 65 with body mass indexes between 25.3 and 28, serum cholesterols less than or equal to 197, and diastolic blood pressures between 81 and 90 on their baseline exams. Four CHD events occurred in these patients during these years of follow-up.

12 This table shows total person–years of follow-up cross-tabulated by *sex* and *dbp_gr*. Note that this table is identical to the one produced before the data transformation.

13 This table shows CHD events of follow-up cross-tabulated by *sex* and *dbp_gr*. This table is also identical to its pre-transformation version and provides evidence that we have successfully transformed the data in the way we intended.

14 Define *male* to equal 1 for men and 0 for women. There are no missing values of *sex* in this data set. However, if there were, this *if* command qualifier would would ensure that the resulting values of *male* would also be missing rather than 0.

In later analyses male gender will be treated as a risk factor for coronary heart disease.

15 We have created a data set with 1267 records. There is one record for each unique combination of covariate values for the variables *sex*, *bmi_gr*, *scl_gr*, *dbp_gr*, and *age_gr*.

16 The person–year data set is stored away for future analysis. We will use this data set in Section 8.12 and in Chapter 9.

**N.B.** It is very important that you specify a new name for the transformed data set. If you use the original name, you will lose the original data set. It is also a very good idea to keep back-up copies of your original data sets in case you accidentally destroy the copy that you are working with.

## 8.10. Simple Poisson regression with multiple data records

In Section 8.9, we created a data set from the Framingham Heart Study with 1267 records. Each of these records describes a number of person–years of follow-up and number of CHD events associated with study subjects with a specific value for each of the covariates. Suppose that we wanted to repeat the analysis of the effect of gender on CHD from Section 8.4 using this data set. The model for this analysis is

$$\log[\mathrm{E}[d_i \mid x_i]] = \log[n_i] + \alpha + x_i\beta, \qquad (8.9)$$

where

$n_i$ is the number of person–years of follow-up in the $i^{\text{th}}$ record of this data set,

$d_i$ is the number of CHD events observed in these $n_i$ person–years of follow-up, and

$$x_i = \begin{cases} 1: & \text{if the } i^{\text{th}} \text{ record describes follow-up of men} \\ 0: & \text{if the } i^{\text{th}} \text{ record describes follow-up of women.} \end{cases}$$

Note that models (8.9) and (8.6) are almost identical. In Model (8.6) there are only two records and $n_0$ and $n_1$ equal the total number of person–years of follow-up in women and men, respectively. In model (8.9) there are 1267 records and $n_i$ equals the total number of person–years of follow-up in the $i^{\text{th}}$ record. The person–years of follow-up and CHD events in women and men from Model (8.6) have been distributed over a much larger number of records in Model (8.9). This difference in data organization has no effect on our estimate of the relative risk of CHD in men compared with women. Regressing CHD against gender using Model (8.9) gives a relative risk estimate of $\hat{R} = 1.832$, with a 95% confidence interval of (1.65, 2.03). This estimate and confidence interval are identical to those obtained from Model (8.6) in Section 8.4. Model (8.9) will work as long as the division of person–years of follow-up is done in such a way that each record describes follow-up in a subgroup of men or a subgroup of women (but not of both genders combined).

## 8.11. Poisson regression with a classification variable

Suppose that we wished to determine the crude relative risks of CHD among subjects whose body mass index (BMI) is in the second, third, and fourth quartiles relative to subjects in the first BMI quartile. We do this in much the same way as we did for logistic regression (see Section 5.8). Suppose that the data are organized so that each record describes person–years of follow-up and CHD events in subjects whose BMIs are in the same quartile. Consider the model

$$\log[\mathrm{E}[d_i \mid ij]] = \log[n_i] + \alpha + \beta_2 \times bmi_{i2} + \beta_3 \times bmi_{i3} + \beta_4 \times bmi_{i4}, \qquad (8.10)$$

where $n_i$ and $d_i$ describe the number of person–years of follow-up and CHD events in the $i^{th}$ record,

$j$ is the BMI quartile of patients from the $i^{th}$ record,

$$bmi_{ih} = \begin{cases} 1: & \text{if patients from the } i^{th} \text{ record are in the } h^{th} \text{ BMI quartile} \\ 0: & \text{otherwise.} \end{cases}$$

Let $\pi_j$ be the CHD event rate of patients in the $j^{th}$ BMI quartile, and let $R_j = \pi_j/\pi_1$ be the relative risk of people in the $j^{th}$ quartile compared with the first. Then for records describing patients in the first BMI quartile, Model (8.10) reduces to

$$\log[\mathrm{E}[d_i \mid i1]] = \log[n_i] + \alpha. \tag{8.11}$$

Subtracting $\log[n_i]$ from both sides of Equation (8.11) gives us

$$\log[\mathrm{E}[d_i \mid i1]] - \log[n_i] = \log[\mathrm{E}[d_i/n_i \mid i1]] = \log[\pi_1] = \alpha. \tag{8.12}$$

For records of patients from the fourth BMI quartile Model (8.10) reduces to

$$\log[\mathrm{E}[d_i \mid i4]] = \log[n_i] + \alpha + \beta_4. \tag{8.13}$$

Subtracting $\log[n_i]$ from both sides of Equation (8.13) gives us

$$\log[\mathrm{E}[d_i|i4]] - \log[n_i] = \log[\mathrm{E}[d_i/n_i|i4]] = \log[\pi_4] = \alpha + \beta_4. \tag{8.14}$$

Subtracting Equation (8.12) from Equation (8.14) gives us

$$\log[\pi_4] - \log[\pi_1] = \log[\pi_4/\pi_1] = \log[R_4] = \beta_4.$$

**Table 8.3.** Effect of baseline body mass index on coronary heart disease. The Framingham Heart Study data were analyzed using Model (8.10).

| Baseline body mass index | | Person–years of | Patients with coronary | Relative | 95% confidence |
|---|---|---|---|---|---|
| Quartile | Range | follow-up | heart disease | risk | interval |
| 1 | ≤22.8 kg/m$^2$ | 27 924 | 239 | 1* | |
| 2 | 22.8–25.2 kg/m$^2$ | 26 696 | 337 | 1.47 | (1.2–1.7) |
| 3 | 25.2–28 kg/m$^2$ | 26 729 | 443 | 1.94 | (1.7–2.3) |
| 4 | >28 kg/m$^2$ | 22 977 | 453 | 2.30 | (2.0–2.7) |
| Total | | 104 326 | 1472 | | |

* Denominator of relative risk

Hence, $\beta_4$ is the log relative risk of CHD for people in the fourth BMI quartile relative to people in the first BMI quartile. By a similar argument, $\beta_2$ and $\beta_3$ estimate the log relative risks of people in the second and third BMI quartiles, respectively. Applying Model (8.10) to the Framingham Heart Study data reformatted in Section 8.9 gives the relative risk estimates and confidence intervals presented in Table 8.3.

## 8.12. Applying simple Poisson regression to the Framingham data

The following log file and comments illustrate how to perform the analysis of models (8.9) and (8.10) using Stata.

```
. *   8.12.Framingham.log
. *
. *   Analysis of the effects of gender and body mass index
. *   on coronary heart disease using person-year data from the
. *   Framingham Heart Study.
. *
. use C:\WDDtext\8.12.Framingham.dta
. *
. *   Regress CHD against gender using model 8.9.
. *
. poisson chd_cnt male, exposure(pt_yrs) irr                              1

                                                            Output omitted

Poisson regression                              Number of obs   =      1267
                                                LR chi2(1)      =    134.30
                                                Prob > chi2     =    0.0000
Log likelihood = -1841.3756                     Pseudo R2       =    0.0352

------------------------------------------------------------------------------
     chd_cnt |       IRR   Std. Err.      z    P>|z|     [95% Conf. Interval]
-------------+----------------------------------------------------------------
        male |  1.832227   .0961444   11.54   0.000     1.653154    2.030698
      pt_yrs |  (exposure)
------------------------------------------------------------------------------

. table bmi_gr, contents(sum pt_yrs sum chd_cnt) row                      2
```

| bmi_gr | sum(pt_yrs) | sum(chd_cnt) |
|---|---|---|
| 22.8 | 27924 | 239 |
| 25.2 | 26696 | 337 |
| 28 | 26729 | 443 |
| 29 | 22977 | 453 |
| Total | 104326 | 1472 |

```
. *
. *  Regress CHD against BMI using model 8.10.
. *
. xi: poisson chd_cnt i.bmi_gr, exposure(pt_yrs) irr
i.bmi_gr          _Ibmi_gr_1-4        (_Ibmi_gr_1 for bmi~r==22.79999923706055
> omitted)
```

3

Output omitted

```
Poisson regression                            Number of obs   =       1234
                                              LR chi2(3)      =     131.76
                                              Prob > chi2     =     0.0000
Log likelihood = -1837.5816                   Pseudo R2       =     0.0346
```

| chd_cnt | IRR | Std. Err. | z | P>\|z\| | [95% Conf. | Interval] |
|---|---|---|---|---|---|---|
| _Ibmi_gr_2 | 1.474902 | .124727 | 4.60 | 0.000 | 1.249627 | 1.740789 |
| _Ibmi_gr_3 | 1.936424 | .1554146 | 8.23 | 0.000 | 1.654567 | 2.266297 |
| _Ibmi_gr_4 | 2.30348 | .1841575 | 10.44 | 0.000 | 1.969396 | 2.694237 |
| pt_yrs | (exposure) | | | | | |

4

```
. log close
```

**Comments**

1 The *poisson* command provides an alternative method of doing Poisson regression. It fits the same model as the *glm* command when the latter uses the *family(poisson)*, *link(log)*, and *lnoffset(pt_yrs)* options. The option *exposure(pt_yrs)* adds the logarithm of the variable *pt_yrs* as an offset to the model. The number of CHD events in each record, *chd_cnt*, is regressed against *male* using Model (8.9). The variable *pt_yrs* gives the number of patient–years of follow-up per record. The *irr* option specifies that the estimate of the model coefficient for the covariate *male* is to be

exponentiated. This gives an estimate of the relative risk of CHD in men without having to use a *lincom* command. The heading IRR stands for incidence rate ratio, which is a synonym for relative risk. The highlighted relative risk and confidence interval are identical to those obtained in Section 8.7 from Model (8.6). The equivalent point-and-click command is Statistics ▶ Count outcomes ▶ Poisson regression ⌋ Model ⌊ Dependent variable: *chd_cnt* , Independent variables: *male* ⌈ Options — ⦿ Exposure variable: *pt_yrs* ⌋ ⌋ Reporting ⌊ ⦿ Report incidence-rate ratios Submit.

2 Create a table of the number of patient–years of follow-up and CHD events among patients in each quartile of BMI. A separate row of the table is generated for each distinct value of *bmi_gr*. The *contents(sum pt_yrs sum chd_cnt)* option sums and lists the value of *pt_yrs* and *chd_cnt* over all records with the same value of *bmi_gr*. The *row* option provides the total number of patient–years of follow-up and CHD events among patients whose BMI is known. These totals are less than that given in Table 8.1 because some patients have missing BMIs. This output is entered in Table 8.3.

3 The *xi* prefix works exactly the same way for the *glm* and *poisson* commands as for the *logistic* command. The term *i.bmi_gr* creates separate indicator variables for all but the first value of the classification variable *bmi_gr*. In Section 8.9, we defined *dbp_gr* to take the values 22.8, 25.2, 28, and 29 for patients whose BMI was in the first, second, third, and fourth quartile, respectively. The indicator variables that are generated are called *_Ibmi_gr_2*, *_Ibmi_gr_3*, and *_Ibmi_gr_4*. *_Ibmi_gr_2* equals 1 for patients whose BMI is in the second quartile and equals 0 otherwise. *_Ibmi_gr_3* and *_Ibmi_gr_4* are similarly defined for patients whose BMIs are in the third and fourth quartiles, respectively. These covariates are entered into the model. In other words, *i.bmi_gr* enters the terms $\beta_2 \times bmi_{i2} + \beta_3 \times bmi_{i3} + \beta_4 \times bmi_{i4}$ from Model (8.10). Thus, the entire command regresses CHD against BMI using Model (8.10).

4 The highlighted relative risks and confidence intervals were used to create Table 8.3.

## 8.13. Additional reading

Rothman and Greenland (1998) discuss classical methods of estimating relative risks from incidence data.

Breslow and Day (1987) provides an excellent discussion of Poisson regression. I recommend this text to readers who are interested in the mathematical underpinnings of this technique.

McCullagh and Nelder (1989) is a standard reference that discusses Poisson regression within the framework of the generalized linear model.

## 8.14. Exercises

Scholer et al. (1997) studied a large cohort of children from Tennessee with known risk factors for injuries (see also the exercises from Chapter 5). Children were followed until their fifth birthday. Data from a subset of this study are posted on my web site in a file called *8.ex.InjuryDeath.dta.* There is one record in this data file for each distinct combination of the following covariates from the original file. These covariates are defined as follows:

| | |
|---|---|
| *age* | Child's age in years |
| *age_mom* | Mother's age in years when her child was born, categorized as |
| | 19: $\text{age} < 20$ |
| | 24: $20 \le \text{age} \le 24$ |
| | 29: $25 \le \text{age} \le 29$ |
| | 30: $\text{age} > 29$ |
| *lbw* | Birth weight, categorized as |
| | 0: $\ge$2500 g |
| | 1: $<$2500 g |
| *educ_mom* | Mother's years of education, categorized as |
| | 11: $<$12 years |
| | 12: 12 years |
| | 15: 13–15 years |
| | 16: $>$15 years |
| *income* | Maternal neighborhood's average income, categorized by quintiles |
| *illegit* | Maternal marital status at time of birth, categorized as |
| | 0: Married |
| | 1: Single |
| *oth_chld* | Number of other children, categorized as |
| | 0: No siblings |
| | 1: 1 sibling |
| | 2: 2 siblings |

| | | |
|---|---|---|
| | 3: | 3 siblings |
| | 4: | 4 or more siblings |
| *race_mom* | Race of mother, categorized as | |
| | 0: | White |
| | 1: | Black |
| *pnclate* | Late or absent prenatal care, categorized as | |
| | 0: | Care in first 4 months of pregnancy |
| | 1: | No care in first 4 months of pregnancy. |

Also included in each record is

*childyrs* The number of child–years of observation among children with the specified covariate values

*inj_dth* The number of injury deaths observed in these child–years of observation

1 Using the *8.ex.InjuryDeath.dta* data set, fill in the following table of person–years of follow-up in the Tennessee Children's Cohort, subdivided by the mother's marital status and injury deaths in the first five years of life.

| | Marital status of mother | | |
|---|---|---|---|
| | Not married | Married | Total |
| Injury deaths | | | |
| Child-years of follow-up | | | |

2 Using classical methods, estimate the risk of injury deaths in children born to unmarried mothers relative to children born to married mothers. Calculate a 95% confidence interval for this relative risk. How does your answer differ from the relative risk for illegitimacy that you calculated in Question 4 of Chapter 5? Explain any differences you observe.

3 Use Poisson regression to complete the following table. How does your estimate of the relative risk of injury death associated with illegitimacy compare to your answer to Question 2?

| Numerator of relative risk | Denominator of relative risk | Crude relative risk* | 95% confidence interval |
|---|---|---|---|
| Maternal age 25–29 | Maternal age > 29 | | |
| Maternal age 20–24 | Maternal age > 29 | | |
| Maternal age < 20 | Maternal age > 29 | | |
| Birth weight < 2500 g | Birth weight ≥ 2500 g | | |
| Mother's education 13–15 yrs | Mother's ed. > 15 yrs | | |
| Mother's education = 12 yrs | Mother's ed. > 15 yrs | | |
| Mother's education < 12 yrs | Mother's ed. > 15 yrs | | |
| Income in lowest quintile | Income in highest quintile | | |
| Income in 2nd quintile | Income in highest quintile | | |
| Income in 3rd quintile | Income in highest quintile | | |
| Income in 4th quintile | Income in highest quintile | | |
| Unmarried mother | Married mother | | |
| One sibling | No siblings | | |
| Two siblings | No siblings | | |
| Three siblings | No siblings | | |
| >3 siblings | No siblings | | |
| Black mother | White mother | | |
| Late/no prenatal care | Adequate prenatal care | | |
| 1st year of life | 3-year-old | | |
| 1-year-old | 3-year-old | | |
| 2-year-old | 3-year-old | | |
| 4-year-old | 3-year-old | | |

* Unadjusted for other covariates

9

# Multiple Poisson regression

Simple Poisson regression generalizes to multiple Poisson regression in the same way that simple logistic regression generalizes to multiple logistic regression. The response variable is a number of events observed in a given number of person–years of observation. We regress this response variable against several covariates, using the logarithm of the number of person–years of observation as an offset in the model. This allows us to estimate event rates that are adjusted for confounding variables or to determine how specific variables interact to affect these rates. We can add interaction terms to our model in exactly the same way as in the other regression techniques discussed in this text.

The methods used in this chapter are very similar to those used in Chapter 5 for multiple logistic regression. You will find this chapter easier to read if you have read Chapter 5 first.

## 9.1. Multiple Poisson regression model

Suppose that data on patient–years of follow-up can be logically grouped into $J$ strata based on age or other factors, and that there are $K$ exposure categories that affect morbidity or mortality in the population. For $j = 1, \ldots, J$ and $k = 1, \ldots, K$ let

$n_{jk}$ be the number of person–years of follow-up observed among patients in the $j^{\text{th}}$ stratum who are in the $k^{\text{th}}$ exposure category,

$d_{jk}$ be the number of morbid or mortal events observed in these $n_{jk}$ person–years of follow-up,

$x_{jk1}, x_{jk2}, \ldots, x_{jkq}$ be explanatory variables that describe the $k^{\text{th}}$ exposure group of patients in stratum $j$, and

$\mathbf{x}_{jk} = (x_{jk1}, x_{jk2}, \ldots, x_{jkq})$ denote the values of all of the covariates for patients in the $j^{\text{th}}$ stratum and $k^{\text{th}}$ exposure category.

**Table 9.1.** This table shows the relationships between the age strata, the exposure categories and the covariates of Model (9.2)

| | | Exposure category | | | |
|---|---|---|---|---|---|
| | | $k = 1$ | $k = 2$ | $k = 3$ | $k = 4$ |
| | $K = 4$<br>$J = 5$<br>$p = 2$ | Light drinker<br>light smoker<br>$x_{j11} = 0, x_{j12} = 0$ | Light drinker<br>heavy smoker<br>$x_{j21} = 0, x_{j22} = 1$ | Heavy drinker<br>light smoker<br>$x_{j31} = 1, x_{j32} = 0$ | Heavy drinker<br>heavy smoker<br>$x_{j41} = 1, x_{j42} = 1$ |
| Age Stratum | $j = 1$ | $x_{111} = 0, x_{112} = 0$ | $x_{121} = 0, x_{122} = 1$ | $x_{131} = 1, x_{132} = 0$ | $x_{141} = 1, x_{142} = 1$ |
| | $j = 2$ | $x_{211} = 0, x_{212} = 0$ | $x_{221} = 0, x_{222} = 1$ | $x_{231} = 1, x_{232} = 0$ | $x_{241} = 1, x_{242} = 1$ |
| | $j = 3$ | $x_{311} = 0, x_{312} = 0$ | $x_{321} = 0, x_{322} = 1$ | $x_{331} = 1, x_{332} = 0$ | $x_{341} = 1, x_{342} = 1$ |
| | $j = 4$ | $x_{411} = 0, x_{412} = 0$ | $x_{421} = 0, x_{422} = 1$ | $x_{431} = 1, x_{432} = 0$ | $x_{441} = 1, x_{442} = 1$ |
| | $j = 5$ | $x_{511} = 0, x_{512} = 0$ | $x_{521} = 0, x_{522} = 1$ | $x_{531} = 1, x_{532} = 0$ | $x_{541} = 1, x_{542} = 1$ |

Then the **multiple Poisson regression** model assumes that

$$\log[\mathrm{E}[d_{jk} \mid \mathbf{x}_{jk}]] = \log[n_{jk}] + \alpha_j + \beta_1 x_{jk1} + \beta_2 x_{jk2} + \cdots + \beta_q x_{jkq}, \quad (9.1)$$

where

$\alpha_1, \ldots, \alpha_J$ are unknown nuisance parameters, and
$\beta_1, \beta_2, \ldots, \beta_q$ are unknown parameters of interest.

For example, suppose that there are $J = 5$ age strata, and that patients are classified as light or heavy drinkers and light or heavy smokers in each stratum. Then there are $K = 4$ exposure categories (two drinking categories by two smoking categories). We might choose $q = 2$ and let

$$x_{jk1} = \begin{cases} 1\text{: for patients who are heavy drinkers} \\ 0\text{: for patients who are light drinkers,} \end{cases}$$

$$x_{jk2} = \begin{cases} 1\text{: for patients who are heavy smokers} \\ 0\text{: for patients who are light smokers.} \end{cases}$$

Then Model (9.1) reduces to

$$\log[\mathrm{E}[d_{jk} \mid \mathbf{x}_{jk}]] = \log[n_{jk}] + \alpha_j + \beta_1 x_{jk1} + \beta_2 x_{jk2}. \quad (9.2)$$

The relationship between the age strata, exposure categories, and covariates of this model is clarified in Table 9.1.

Let $\lambda_{jk} = \mathrm{E}[d_{jk}/n_{jk} \mid \mathbf{x}_{jk}]$ be the expected morbidity incidence rate for people from stratum $j$ who are in exposure category $k$. If we subtract

$\log(n_{jk})$ from both sides of Model (9.1) we get

$$\log[\mathrm{E}[d_{jk} \mid \mathbf{x}_{jk}]/n_{jk}] = \log[\mathrm{E}[d_{jk}/n_{jk} \mid \mathbf{x}_{jk}]] = \log[\lambda_{jk}]$$
$$= \alpha_j + \beta_1 x_{jk1} + \beta_2 x_{jk2} + \cdots + \beta_q x_{jkq}. \qquad (9.3)$$

In other words, Model (9.1) imposes a log–linear relationship between the expected morbidity rates and the model covariates. Note that this model permits people in the same exposure category to have different morbidity rates in different strata. This is one of the more powerful features of Poisson regression in that it makes it easy to model incidence rates that vary with time.

Suppose that two groups of patients from the $j^{\text{th}}$ stratum have been subject to exposure categories $f$ and $g$. Then the relative risk of an event for patients in category $f$ compared with category $g$ is $\lambda_{jf}/\lambda_{jg}$. Equation (9.3) gives us that

$$\log[\lambda_{jf}] = \alpha_j + x_{jf1}\beta_1 + x_{jf2}\beta_2 + \cdots + x_{jfq}\beta_q, \text{ and} \qquad (9.4)$$

$$\log[\lambda_{jg}] = \alpha_j + x_{jg1}\beta_1 + x_{jg2}\beta_2 + \cdots + x_{jgq}\beta_q. \qquad (9.5)$$

Subtracting Equation (9.5) from Equation (9.4) gives that the within-stratum log relative risk of group $f$ subjects relative to group $g$ subjects is

$$\log[\lambda_{jf}/\lambda_{jg}] = (x_{jf1} - x_{jg1})\beta_1 + (x_{jf2} - x_{jg2})\beta_2 + \cdots + (x_{jfq} - x_{jgq})\beta_q. \qquad (9.6)$$

Thus, we can estimate log relative risks in Poisson regression models in precisely the same way that we estimated log odds ratios in logistic regression. Indeed, the only difference is that in logistic regression weighted sums of model coefficients are interpreted as log odds ratios while in Poisson regression they are interpreted as log relative risks. An important feature of Equation (9.6) is that the relative risk $\lambda_{jf}/\lambda_{jg}$ may vary between the different strata.

The nuisance parameters $\alpha_1, \alpha_2, \ldots, \alpha_J$ are handled in the same way that we handle any parameters associated with a categorical variable. That is, for any two values of $j$ and $h$ between 1 and $J$ we let

$$strata_{jh} = \begin{cases} 1: & \text{if } j = h \\ 0: & \text{otherwise.} \end{cases}$$

Then Model (9.1) can be rewritten as

$$\log[\mathrm{E}[d_{jk} \mid \mathbf{x}_{jk}]] = \log[n_{jk}] + \sum_{h=1}^{J} \alpha_h \times strata_{jh} + \beta_1 x_{jk1} + \beta_2 x_{jk2} + \cdots + \beta_q x_{jkq}. \tag{9.7}$$

Models (9.1) and (9.7) are algebraically identical. We usually write the simpler form (9.1) when the strata are defined by confounding variables that are not of primary interest. However, in Stata these models are always specified in a way that is analogous to Equation (9.7).

We derive maximum likelihood estimates $\hat{\alpha}_j$ for $\alpha_j$ and $\hat{\beta}_1, \ldots, \hat{\beta}_q$ for $\beta_1, \ldots, \beta_q$. Inferences about these parameter estimates are made in the same way as in Section 5.13 through 5.15. Again the only difference is that in Section 5.14 weighted sums of parameter estimates were interpreted as estimates of log odds ratios, while here they are interpreted as log relative risks. Suppose that $f$ is a weighted sum of parameters that corresponds to a log relative risk of interest, $\hat{f}$ is the corresponding weighted sum of parameter estimates from a large study, and $s_f$ is the estimated standard error of $\hat{f}$. Then under the null hypothesis that the relative risk $\exp[f] = 1$, the test statistic

$$z = \hat{f}/s_f \tag{9.8}$$

will have an approximately standard normal distribution if the sample size is large. A 95% confidence interval for this relative risk is given by

$$(\exp[\hat{f} - 1.96 s_f], \exp[\hat{f} + 1.96 s_f]). \tag{9.9}$$

## 9.2. An example: the Framingham Heart Study

In Section 8.9 we created a person–year data set from the Framingham Heart Study for Poisson regression analysis. Patients were divided into strata based on age, body mass index, serum cholesterol, and baseline diastolic blood pressure. Age was classified into nine strata. The first and last consisted of people ≤45 years of age, and people older than 80 years, respectively. The inner strata consisted of people 46–50, 51–55, . . . , and 76–80 years of age. The values of the other variables were divided into strata defined by quartiles. Each record in this data set consists of a number of person–years of follow-up of people of the same gender who are in the same strata for age, body mass index, serum cholesterol, and diastolic blood pressure. Let $n_k$ be the number of person–years of follow-up in the $k^{\text{th}}$ record of this file and let $d_k$ be the number of cases of coronary heart disease observed during these $n_k$ person–years of follow-up. Let

$$male_k = \begin{cases} 1: & \text{if record } k \text{ describes men} \\ 0: & \text{if it describes women,} \end{cases}$$

$$age_{jk} = \begin{cases} 1: & \text{if record } k \text{ describes people from the } j^{\text{th}} \text{ age stratum} \\ 0: & \text{otherwise,} \end{cases}$$

$$bmi_{jk} = \begin{cases} 1: & \text{if record } k \text{ describes people from the } j^{\text{th}} \text{ BMI quartile} \\ 0: & \text{otherwise,} \end{cases}$$

$$scl_{jk} = \begin{cases} 1: & \text{if record } k \text{ describes people from the } j^{\text{th}} \text{ SCL quartile} \\ 0: & \text{otherwise, and} \end{cases}$$

$$dbp_{jk} = \begin{cases} 1: & \text{if record } k \text{ describes people from the } j^{\text{th}} \text{ DBP quartile} \\ 0: & \text{otherwise.} \end{cases}$$

For any model that we will consider let

$\mathbf{x}_k = (x_{jk1}, x_{jk2}, \ldots, x_{jkq})$ denote the values of all of the covariates of people in the $k^{\text{th}}$ record that are included in the model,

$\lambda_k = \mathrm{E}[d_k/n_k \mid \mathbf{x}_k]$ be the expected CHD incidence rate for people in the $k^{\text{th}}$ record given their covariates $\mathbf{x}_k$. We will now build several models with these data.

### 9.2.1. A multiplicative model of gender, age and coronary heart disease

Consider the model

$$\log[\mathrm{E}[d_k \mid \mathbf{x}_k]] = \log[n_k] + \alpha + \sum_{j=2}^{9} \beta_j \times age_{jk} + \gamma \times male_k, \tag{9.10}$$

where $\alpha$, $\beta_2$, $\beta_3, \ldots, \beta_9$ and $\gamma$ are parameters in the model. Subtracting $\log[n_k]$ from both sides of Equation (9.10) gives that

$$\log[\lambda_k] = \alpha + \sum_{j=2}^{9} \beta_j \times age_{jk} + \gamma \times male_k. \tag{9.11}$$

If record $f$ describes women from the first age stratum then Equation (9.11) reduces to

$$\log[\lambda_f] = \alpha. \tag{9.12}$$

If record $g$ describes men from the first age stratum then Equation (9.11) reduces to

$$\log[\lambda_g] = \alpha + \gamma. \tag{9.13}$$

Subtracting Equation (9.12) from Equation (9.13) gives that

$$\log[\lambda_g] - \log[\lambda_f] = \log[\lambda_g/\lambda_f] = (\alpha + \gamma) - \alpha = \gamma.$$

In other words, $\gamma$ is the log relative risk of CHD for men compared with women within the first age stratum. Similarly, if records $f$ and $g$ now describe women and men, respectively, from the $j^{\text{th}}$ age stratum with $j > 1$ then

$$\log[\lambda_f] = \alpha + \beta_j \text{ and} \tag{9.14}$$

$$\log[\lambda_g] = \alpha + \beta_j + \gamma. \tag{9.15}$$

Subtracting Equation (9.14) from (9.15) again yields that

$$\log[\lambda_g/\lambda_f] = \gamma.$$

Hence, $\gamma$ is the within-stratum (i.e., age-adjusted) log relative risk of CHD for men compared with women for all age strata. We have gone through virtually identical arguments many times in previous chapters. By subtracting appropriate pairs of log incidence rates you should also be able to show that $\beta_j$ is the sex-adjusted log relative risk of CHD for people from the $j^{\text{th}}$ age stratum compared with the first age stratum, and that $\beta_j + \gamma$ is the log relative risk of CHD for men from the $j^{\text{th}}$ age stratum compared with women from the first. Hence, the age-adjusted risk for men relative to women is $\exp[\gamma]$, the sex-adjusted risk of people from the $j^{\text{th}}$ age stratum relative to the first is $\exp[\beta_j]$, and the risk for men from the $j^{\text{th}}$ age stratum relative to women from the first is $\exp[\gamma] \times \exp[\beta_j]$. Model (9.10) is called a multiplicative model because this latter relative risk equals the risk for men relative to women times the risk for people from the $j^{\text{th}}$ stratum relative to people from the first.

The maximum likelihood estimate of $\gamma$ in (9.10) is $\hat{\gamma} = 0.6912$. Hence, the age-adjusted estimate of the relative risk of CHD in men compared with women from this model is $\exp[0.6912] = 2.00$. The standard error of $\hat{\gamma}$ is 0.0527. Therefore, from Equation (9.9), the 95% confidence interval for this relative risk is $(\exp[0.6912 - 1.96 \times 0.0527], \exp[0.6912 + 1.96 \times 0.0527]) = (1.8, 2.2)$. This risk estimate is virtually identical to the estimate we obtained from Model (7.22), which was a proportional hazards model with ragged entry.

Model (9.10) is not of great practical interest because we know from Chapter 7 that the risk of CHD in men relative to women is greater for premenopausal ages than for postmenopausal ages. The incidence of CHD

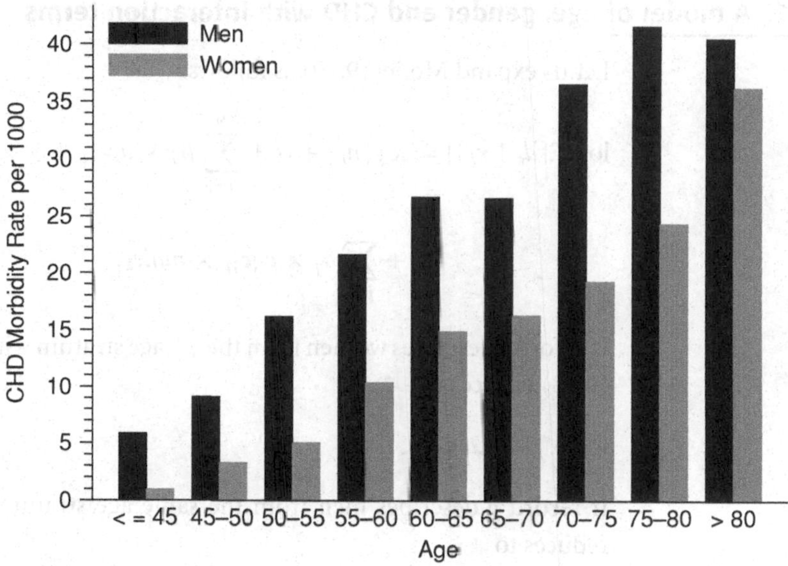


Figure 9.1 Age–sex specific incidence of coronary heart disease (CHD) in people from the Framingham Heart Study (Levy, 1999).

in women in the $j^{\text{th}}$ stratum is the sum of all CHD events in women from this stratum divided by the total number of women–years of follow-up in this stratum. That is, this incidence is

$$\hat{I}_{0j} = \sum_{\{k:\ male_k = 0,\ age_{jk} = 1\}} d_k \Big/ \sum_{\{k:\ male_k = 0,\ age_{jk} = 1\}} n_k. \tag{9.16}$$

Similarly, the incidence of CHD in men from the $j^{\text{th}}$ age stratum can be estimated by

$$\hat{I}_{1j} = \sum_{\{k:\ male_k = 1,\ age_{jk} = 1\}} d_k \Big/ \sum_{\{k:\ male_k = 1,\ age_{jk} = 1\}} n_k. \tag{9.17}$$

Equations (9.16) and (9.17) are used in Figure 9.1 to plot the age-specific incidence of CHD in men and women from the Framingham Heart Study. This figure shows dramatic differences in CHD rates between men and women; the ratio of these rates at each age diminishes as people grow older. To model these rates effectively we need to add interaction terms into our model.

### 9.2.2. A model of age, gender and CHD with interaction terms

Let us expand Model (9.10) as follows:

$$\log[\mathrm{E}[d_k \mid \mathbf{x}_k]] = \log[n_k] + \alpha + \sum_{j=2}^{9} \beta_j \times age_{jk} + \gamma \times male_k$$

$$+ \sum_{j=2}^{9} \delta_j \times age_{jk} \times male_k. \tag{9.18}$$

If record $f$ describes women from the $j^{\text{th}}$ age stratum with $j > 1$ then Model (9.18) reduces to

$$\log[\lambda_f] = \alpha + \beta_j. \tag{9.19}$$

If record $g$ describes men from the same age stratum then Model (9.18) reduces to

$$\log[\lambda_g] = \alpha + \beta_j + \gamma + \delta_j. \tag{9.20}$$

Subtracting Equation (9.19) from Equation (9.20) gives the log relative risk of CHD for men versus women in the $j^{\text{th}}$ age stratum to be

$$\log[\lambda_g/\lambda_f] = \gamma + \delta_j. \tag{9.21}$$

Hence, we estimate this relative risk by

$$\exp[\hat{\gamma} + \hat{\delta}_j]. \tag{9.22}$$

A similar argument gives that the estimated relative risk of men compared with women in the first age stratum is

$$\exp[\hat{\gamma}]. \tag{9.23}$$

Equations (9.22) and (9.23) are used in Table 9.2 to estimate the age-specific relative risks of CHD in men versus women. Ninety-five percent confidence intervals are calculated for these estimates using Equation (9.9).

When Models (9.10) and (9.18) are fitted to the Framingham Heart Study data they produce model deviances of 1391.3 and 1361.6, respectively. Note that Model (9.10) is nested within Model (9.18) (see Section 5.24). Hence, under the null hypothesis that the multiplicative Model (9.10) is correct, the change in deviance will have a chi-squared distribution with as many degrees of freedom as there are extra parameters in Model (9.18). As there are eight more parameters in Model (9.18) than Model (9.10) this

**Table 9.2.** Age-specific relative risks of coronary heart disease (CHD) in men compared with women from the Framingham Heart Study (Levy, 1999). These relative risk estimates were obtained from Model (9.18). Five-year age intervals are used. Similar relative risks from contiguous age strata have been highlighted

| | Patient–years of follow-up | | CHD events | | | |
|---|---|---|---|---|---|---|
| Age | Men | Women | Men | Women | Relative risk | 95% confidence interval |
| ≤45 | 7370 | 9205 | 43 | 9 | 5.97 | 2.9–12 |
| 46–50 | 5835 | 7595 | 53 | 25 | 2.76 | 1.7–4.4 |
| 51–55 | 6814 | 9113 | 110 | 46 | 3.20 | 2.3–4.5 |
| 56–60 | 7184 | 10139 | 155 | 105 | 2.08 | 1.6–2.7 |
| 61–65 | 6678 | 9946 | 178 | 148 | 1.79 | 1.4–2.2 |
| 66–70 | 4557 | 7385 | 121 | 120 | 1.63 | 1.3–2.1 |
| 71–75 | 2575 | 4579 | 94 | 88 | 1.90 | 1.4–2.5 |
| 76–80 | 1205 | 2428 | 50 | 59 | 1.71 | 1.2–2.5 |
| ≥81 | 470 | 1383 | 19 | 50 | 1.12 | 0.66–1.9 |

chi-squared statistic will have eight degrees of freedom. The probability that this statistic will exceed $1391.3 - 1361.6 = 29.7$ is $P = 0.0002$. Hence, these data allow us to reject the multiplicative model with a high level of statistical significance.

Table 9.2 shows a marked drop in the risk of CHD in men relative to women with increasing age. Note, however, that the relative risks for ages 46–50 and ages 51–55 are similar, as are the relative risks for ages 61–65 through 76–80. Hence, we can reduce the number of age strata from nine to five with little loss in explanatory power by lumping ages 46–55 into one stratum and ages 61–80 into another. This reduces the number of parameters in Model (9.18) by eight (four age parameters plus four interaction parameters). Refitting Model (9.18) with only these five condensed age strata rather than the original nine gives the results presented in Table 9.3. Note that the age-specific relative risk of men versus women in this table diminishes with age but remains significantly different from one for all ages less than 80. Gender does not have a significant influence on the risk of CHD in people older than 80. These data are consistent with the hypothesis that endogenous sex hormones play a cardioprotective role in premenopausal women.

**Table 9.3.** Age-specific relative risks of coronary heart disease (CHD) in men compared with women from the Framingham Heart Study (Levy, 1999). Age intervals from Table 9.2 that had similar relative risks have been combined in this figure giving age intervals with variable widths

| | Patient–years of follow-up | | CHD events | | | |
|---|---|---|---|---|---|---|
| Age | Men | Women | Men | Women | Relative risk | 95% confidence interval |
| ≤45 | 7370 | 9205 | 43 | 9 | 5.97 | 2.9–12 |
| 46–55 | 12649 | 16708 | 163 | 71 | 3.03 | 2.3–4.0 |
| 56–60 | 7184 | 10139 | 155 | 105 | 2.08 | 1.6–2.7 |
| 61–80 | 15015 | 24338 | 443 | 415 | 1.73 | 1.5–2.0 |
| ≥81 | 470 | 1383 | 19 | 50 | 1.12 | 0.66–1.9 |

## 9.2.3. Adding confounding variables to the model

Let us now consider the effect of possibly confounding variables on our estimates in Table 9.3. The variables that we will consider are body mass index, serum cholesterol, and diastolic blood pressure. We will add these variables one at a time in order to gauge their influence on the model deviance. As we will see in Section 9.3, all of these variables have an overwhelmingly significant effect on the change in model deviance. The final model that we will consider is

$$\log[\mathrm{E}[d_k \mid \mathbf{x}_k]] = \log[n_k] + \alpha + \sum_{j=2}^{5} \beta_j \times age_{jk} + \gamma \times male_k + \sum_{j=2}^{5} \delta_j \times age_{jk} \times male_k + \sum_{f=2}^{4} \theta_f \times bmi_{fk} + \sum_{g=2}^{4} \phi_g \times scl_{gk} + \sum_{h=2}^{4} \psi_h \times dbp_{hk}, \tag{9.24}$$

where the age strata are those given in Table 9.3 rather than those given at the beginning of Section 9.2. Recall that $bmi_{fk}$, $scl_{gk}$, and $dbp_{hk}$ are indicator covariates corresponding to the four quartiles of body mass index, serum cholesterol, and diastolic blood pressure, respectively. By the usual argument, the age-specific CHD risk for men relative to women adjusted for body mass index, serum cholesterol, and diastolic blood pressure is either

$$\exp[\gamma] \tag{9.25}$$

**Table 9.4.** Age-specific relative risks of coronary heart disease (CHD) in men compared with women adjusted for body mass index, serum cholesterol, and baseline diastolic blood pressure (Levy, 1999). These risks were derived using Model (9.24). They should be compared with those from Table 9.3

| Age | Adjusted relative risk | 95% confidence interval |
|---|---|---|
| ≤45 | 4.64 | 2.3–9.5 |
| 46–55 | 2.60 | 2.0–3.4 |
| 56–60 | 1.96 | 1.5–2.5 |
| 61–80 | 1.79 | 1.6–2.0 |
| ≥81 | 1.25 | 0.73–2.1 |

for the first age stratum or

$$\exp[\gamma + \delta_j] \tag{9.26}$$

for the other age strata. Substituting the maximum likelihood estimates of $\gamma$ and $\delta_j$ into Equations (9.25) and (9.26) gives the adjusted relative risk estimates presented in Table 9.4. Comparing these results with those of Table 9.3 indicates that adjusting for body mass index, serum cholesterol, and diastolic blood pressure does reduce the age-specific relative risk of CHD in men versus women who are less than 56 years of age.

## 9.3. Using Stata to perform Poisson regression

The following log file and comments illustrate how to perform the Poisson regressions of the Framingham Heart Study data that were described in Section 9.2. You should be familiar with how to use the *glm* and *logistic* commands to perform logistic regression before reading this section (see Chapters 4 and 5).

```
. *  9.3.Framingham.log
. *
. *  Estimate the effect of age and gender on coronary heart disease
. * (CHD) using several Poisson regression models
. *
. use  C:\WDDtext\8.12.Framingham.dta, clear
. *
. *  Fit a multiplicative model of the effect of gender and age on CHD
. *
```

```
. xi: poisson chd_cnt  i.age_gr male, exposure(pt_yrs) irr                    1
                                                                  Output omitted
i.age_gr          _Iage_gr_45-81      (naturally coded; _Iage_gr_45 omitted)
Poisson regression                              Number of obs   =       1267
                                                LR chi2(9)      =     698.64
                                                Prob > chi2     =     0.0000
Log likelihood = -1559.2065                     Pseudo R2       =     0.1830

------------------------------------------------------------------------------
     chd_cnt |        IRR   Std. Err.      z    P>|z|     [95% Conf. Interval]
-------------+----------------------------------------------------------------
 _Iage_gr_50 |   1.864355   .3337745     3.48   0.001     1.312618    2.648005
 _Iage_gr_55 |   3.158729   .5058088     7.18   0.000     2.307858    4.323303
 _Iage_gr_60 |   4.885053   .7421312    10.44   0.000     3.627069    6.579347
 _Iage_gr_65 |    6.44168   .9620181    12.47   0.000     4.807047    8.632168
 _Iage_gr_70 |   6.725369   1.028591    12.46   0.000     4.983469    9.076127
 _Iage_gr_75 |   8.612712   1.354852    13.69   0.000     6.327596    11.72306
 _Iage_gr_80 |   10.37219   1.749287    13.87   0.000     7.452702    14.43534
 _Iage_gr_81 |   13.67189   2.515296    14.22   0.000     9.532967    19.60781
        male |   1.996012   .1051841    13.12   0.000     1.800144    2.213192   2
      pt_yrs | (exposure)
------------------------------------------------------------------------------

. estimates store age_male
. *
. * Tabulate patient-years of follow-up and number of
. * CHD events by sex and age group.
. *
. table sex, contents(sum pt_yrs sum chd_cnt) by(age_gr)                      3

----------------------------------------
age_gr      |
and Sex     | sum(pt_yrs)   sum(chd_cnt)
------------+---------------------------
<= 45       |
        Men |        7370             43
      Women |        9205              9
------------+---------------------------
45-50       |
        Men |        5835             53
      Women |        7595             25
----------------------------------------
```

Output omitted

```
75-80
      Men          1205          50
    Women          2428          59

> 80
      Men           470          19
    Women          1383          50

. *
. * Calculate age-sex specific incidence of CHD
. *
. collapse (sum) patients = pt_yrs chd = chd_cnt, by(age_gr male)
. generate rate = 1000*chd/patients                                   4
. generate men = rate if male == 1                                    5
(9 missing values generated)
. generate women = rate if male == 0
(9 missing values generated)
. graph bar men women, over(age_gr)                                   6
>     ytitle(CHD Morbidity Rate per 1000) ylabel(0(5)40)
>     ymtick(0 (1) 41) subtitle(Age, position(6))                     7
>     bar(1, color(black)) bar(2, color(gray))                        8
>     legend(order(1 "Men" 2 "Women")
>         ring(0) position(11) col(1))

. use 8.12.Framingham.dta, clear                                      9
. *
. * Add interaction terms to the model
. *
. xi: poisson chd_cnt i.age_gr*male, exposure(pt_yrs)                 10
i.age_gr          _Iage_gr_45-81     (naturally coded; _Iage_gr_45 omitted)
i.age_gr*male     _IageXmale_#       (coded as above)
```

Output omitted

```
Poisson regression                          Number of obs   =      1267
                                            LR chi2(17)     =    728.41
                                            Prob > chi2     =    0.0000
Log likelihood = -1544.3226                 Pseudo R2       =    0.1908
```

| chd_cnt | Coef. | Std. Err. | z | P>\|z\| | [95% Conf. | Interval] |
|---|---|---|---|---|---|---|
| _Iage_gr_50 | 1.213908 | .3887301 | 3.12 | 0.002 | .4520111 | 1.975805 |
| _Iage_gr_55 | 1.641461 | .3644862 | 4.50 | 0.000 | .9270816 | 2.355841 |
| _Iage_gr_60 | 2.360093 | .3473254 | 6.80 | 0.000 | 1.679348 | 3.040838 |
| _Iage_gr_65 | 2.722564 | .3433189 | 7.93 | 0.000 | 2.049671 | 3.395457 |
| _Iage_gr_70 | 2.810563 | .3456073 | 8.13 | 0.000 | 2.133185 | 3.487941 |
| _Iage_gr_75 | 2.978378 | .3499639 | 8.51 | 0.000 | 2.292462 | 3.664295 |
| _Iage_gr_80 | 3.212992 | .3578551 | 8.98 | 0.000 | 2.511609 | 3.914375 |
| _Iage_gr_81 | 3.61029 | .3620927 | 9.97 | 0.000 | 2.900601 | 4.319979 |
| male | 1.786304 | .3665609 | 4.87 | 0.000 | 1.067858 | 2.504751 |
| _IageXmal~50 | -.7712728 | .4395848 | -1.75 | 0.079 | -1.632843 | .0902976 |
| _IageXmal~55 | -.6237429 | .4064443 | -1.53 | 0.125 | -1.420359 | .1728733 |
| _IageXmal~60 | -1.052307 | .38774 | -2.71 | 0.007 | -1.812263 | -.2923502 |
| _IageXmal~65 | -1.203381 | .3830687 | -3.14 | 0.002 | -1.954182 | -.4525804 |
| _IageXmal~70 | -1.295219 | .3885418 | -3.33 | 0.001 | -2.056747 | -.5336914 |
| _IageXmal~75 | -1.144715 | .395435 | -2.89 | 0.004 | -1.919754 | -.369677 |
| _IageXmal~80 | -1.251231 | .4139034 | -3.02 | 0.003 | -2.062466 | -.4399948 |
| _IageXmal~81 | -1.674611 | .4549709 | -3.68 | 0.000 | -2.566337 | -.7828844 |
| _cons | -6.930277 | .3333333 | -20.79 | 0.000 | -7.583599 | -6.276956 |
| pt_yrs | (exposure) | | | | | |

**. lincom *male*, irr**

( 1) [chd_cnt]male = 0

| chd_cnt | IRR | Std. Err. | z | P>\|z\| | [95% Conf. | Interval] |
|---|---|---|---|---|---|---|
| (1) | 5.967359 | 2.187401 | 4.87 | 0.000 | 2.909142 | 12.24051 |

**. lincom *male* + *_IageXmale_50*, irr** 11

( 1) [chd_cnt]male + [chd_cnt]_IageXmale_50 = 0

| chd_cnt | IRR | Std. Err. | z | P>\|z\| | [95% Conf. | Interval] |
|---|---|---|---|---|---|---|
| (1) | 2.759451 | .6695175 | 4.18 | 0.000 | 1.715134 | 4.439634 |

```
. lincom male + _IageXmale_55, irr
```

Output omitted. See Table 9.2.

```
. lincom male + _IageXmale_60, irr
```

Output omitted. See Table 9.2.

```
. lincom male + _IageXmale_65, irr
```

Output omitted. See Table 9.2.

```
. lincom male + _IageXmale_70, irr
```

Output omitted. See Table 9.2.

```
. lincom male + _IageXmale_75, irr
```

Output omitted. See Table 9.2.

```
. lincom male + _IageXmale_80, irr
```

Output omitted. See Table 9.2.

```
. lincom male + _IageXmale_81, irr
 ( 1)  [chd_cnt]male + [chd_cnt]_IageXmale_81 = 0

------------------------------------------------------------------------------
     chd_cnt |        IRR   Std. Err.      z    P>|z|     [95% Conf. Interval]
-------------+----------------------------------------------------------------
         (1) |    1.11817   .3013496     0.41   0.679     .6593363    1.896308
------------------------------------------------------------------------------

. lrtest age_male .                                                          12

Likelihood-ratio test                                 LR chi2(8)  =      29.77
(Assumption: age_male nested in .)                    Prob > chi2 =     0.0002

. *
. *  Refit model with interaction terms using fewer parameters.
. *
. generate age_gr2 = recode(age_gr, 45,55,60,80,81)

. xi: poisson chd_cnt i.age_gr2*male, exposure(pt_yrs) irr                   13

i.age_gr2         _Iage_gr2_45-81     (naturally coded; _Iage_gr2_45 omitted)
i.age_gr2*male    _IageXmale_#        (coded as above)
```

Output omitted

```
Poisson regression                                Number of obs   =       1267
                                                  LR chi2(9)      =     689.40
                                                  Prob > chi2     =     0.0000
Log likelihood = -1563.8267                       Pseudo R2       =     0.1806
```

| chd_cnt | IRR | Std. Err. | z | P>\|z\| | [95% Conf. | Interval] |
|---|---|---|---|---|---|---|
| _Iage_gr2_55 | 4.346254 | 1.537835 | 4.15 | 0.000 | 2.172374 | 8.695522 |
| _Iage_gr2_60 | 10.59194 | 3.678848 | 6.80 | 0.000 | 5.362058 | 20.92277 |
| _Iage_gr2_80 | 17.43992 | 5.876003 | 8.48 | 0.000 | 9.010533 | 33.75502 |
| _Iage_gr2_81 | 36.97678 | 13.38902 | 9.97 | 0.000 | 18.18508 | 75.18702 |
| male | 5.967359 | 2.187401 | 4.87 | 0.000 | 2.909142 | 12.24051 |
| _IageXmal~55 | .5081774 | .1998025 | -1.72 | 0.085 | .2351497 | 1.098212 |
| _IageXmal~60 | .3491315 | .1353723 | -2.71 | 0.007 | .1632842 | .7465071 |
| _IageXmal~80 | .2899566 | .1081168 | -3.32 | 0.001 | .1396186 | .6021749 |
| _IageXmal~81 | .1873811 | .0852529 | -3.68 | 0.000 | .0768164 | .4570857 |
| pt_yrs | (exposure) | | | | | |

```
. lincom male + _IageXmale_55, irr                                    14
 ( 1)  [chd_cnt]male + [chd_cnt]_IageXmale_55 = 0
```

| chd_cnt | IRR | Std. Err. | z | P>\|z\| | [95% Conf. | Interval] |
|---|---|---|---|---|---|---|
| (1) | 3.032477 | .4312037 | 7.80 | 0.000 | 2.294884 | 4.007138 |

```
. lincom male + _IageXmale_60, irr
```

Output omitted. See Table 9.3.

```
. lincom male + _IageXmale_80, irr
```

Output omitted. See Table 9.3.

```
. lincom male + _IageXmale_81, irr
```

Output omitted. See Table 9.3.

```
. *
. *  Repeat previous analysis restricted to records with
. *  non-missing bmi values.
. *
. quietly xi: poisson chd_cnt i.age_gr2*male if !missing(bmi_gr)      15
>      , exposure(pt_yrs)

. estimates store age_male_interact                                   16

. *
. *  Adjust analysis for body mass index (BMI)
. *
```

```
. xi: poisson chd_cnt i.age_gr2*male i.bmi_gr, exposure(pt_yrs)                17
i.age_gr2         _Iage_gr2_45-81    (naturally coded; _Iage_gr2_45 omitted)
i.age_gr2*male    _IageXmale_#       (coded as above)
i.bmi_gr          _Ibmi_gr_1-4       (_Ibmi_gr_1 for bmi~r==22.79999923706055
> omitted)
                                                                   Output omitted

Poisson regression                              Number of obs   =       1234
                                                LR chi2(12)     =     754.20
                                                Prob > chi2     =     0.0000
Log likelihood = -1526.3585                     Pseudo R2       =     0.1981

------------------------------------------------------------------------------
     chd_cnt |      Coef.   Std. Err.      z    P>|z|     [95% Conf. Interval]
-------------+----------------------------------------------------------------
 _Iage_gr2_55 |   1.426595   .3538794     4.03   0.000     .7330039    2.120186
 _Iage_gr2_60 |   2.293218   .3474423     6.60   0.000     1.612244    2.974193
 _Iage_gr2_80 |   2.768015   .3371378     8.21   0.000     2.107237    3.428793
 _Iage_gr2_81 |   3.473889   .3625129     9.58   0.000     2.763377    4.184401
        male |   1.665895   .3669203     4.54   0.000     .9467446    2.385046
_IageXmal~55 |  -.6387423   .3932103    -1.62   0.104     -1.40942    .1319357
_IageXmal~60 |  -.9880223   .3878331    -2.55   0.011    -1.748161   -.2278834
_IageXmal~80 |  -1.147882   .3730498    -3.08   0.002    -1.879046   -.4167178
_IageXmal~81 |  -1.585361   .4584837    -3.46   0.001    -2.483972   -.6867493
  _Ibmi_gr_2 |    .231835     .08482     2.73   0.006     .0655909    .3980791
  _Ibmi_gr_3 |   .4071791   .0810946     5.02   0.000     .2482366    .5661216
  _Ibmi_gr_4 |   .6120817   .0803788     7.61   0.000     .4545421    .7696213
       _cons |  -7.165097   .3365738   -21.29   0.000    -7.824769   -6.505424
      pt_yrs | (exposure)
------------------------------------------------------------------------------

. lrtest age_male_interact .                                                   18
Likelihood-ratio test                               LR chi2(3)  =      66.90
(Assumption: age_male_int~t nested in .)            Prob > chi2 =     0.0000

. quietly xi: poisson chd_cnt i.age_gr2*male i.bmi_gr
>     if !missing(scl_gr) , exposure(pt_yrs)

. estimates store age_male_interact_bmi

. *
. * Adjust estimates for BMI and serum cholesterol
. *
. xi: poisson chd_cnt i.age_gr2*male i.bmi_gr  i.scl_gr                        19
```

```
>       , exposure(pt_yrs)
i.age_gr2           _Iage_gr2_45-81     (naturally coded; _Iage_gr2_45 omitted)
i.age_gr2*male      _IageXmale_#        (coded as above)
i.bmi_gr            _Ibmi_gr_1-4        (_Ibmi_gr_1 for bmi~r==22.79999923706055
> omitted)
i.scl_gr            _Iscl_gr_197-256    (naturally coded; _Iscl_gr_197 omitted)
```

Output omitted

```
Poisson regression                            Number of obs   =       1134
                                              LR chi2(15)     =     827.10
                                              Prob > chi2     =     0.0000
Log likelihood = -1460.2162                   Pseudo R2       =     0.2207
```

| chd_cnt | Coef. | Std. Err. | z | P>\|z\| | [95% Conf. | Interval] |
|---|---|---|---|---|---|---|
| _Iage_gr2_55 | 1.355069 | .3539889 | 3.83 | 0.000 | .6612635 | 2.048875 |
| _Iage_gr2_60 | 2.177978 | .3477139 | 6.26 | 0.000 | 1.496471 | 2.859485 |
| _Iage_gr2_80 | 2.606269 | .3376422 | 7.72 | 0.000 | 1.944502 | 3.268035 |
| _Iage_gr2_81 | 3.254861 | .3634038 | 8.96 | 0.000 | 2.542603 | 3.96712 |
| male | 1.569233 | .3671214 | 4.27 | 0.000 | .8496882 | 2.288778 |
| _IageXmal~55 | -.5924098 | .3933743 | -1.51 | 0.132 | -1.363409 | .1785897 |
| _IageXmal~60 | -.8886688 | .3881041 | -2.29 | 0.022 | -1.649339 | -.1279989 |
| _IageXmal~80 | -.994868 | .3734877 | -2.66 | 0.008 | -1.72689 | -.2628454 |
| _IageXmal~81 | -1.40099 | .4590461 | -3.05 | 0.002 | -2.300704 | -.501276 |
| _Ibmi_gr_2 | .1929941 | .0849164 | 2.27 | 0.023 | .0265609 | .3594273 |
| _Ibmi_gr_3 | .334175 | .0814824 | 4.10 | 0.000 | .1744724 | .4938776 |
| _Ibmi_gr_4 | .5230984 | .0809496 | 6.46 | 0.000 | .3644401 | .6817566 |
| _Iscl_gr_225 | .192923 | .0843228 | 2.29 | 0.022 | .0276532 | .3581927 |
| _Iscl_gr_255 | .5262667 | .0810581 | 6.49 | 0.000 | .3673957 | .6851377 |
| _Iscl_gr_256 | .6128653 | .0814661 | 7.52 | 0.000 | .4531947 | .7725359 |
| _cons | -7.340656 | .3392161 | -21.64 | 0.000 | -8.005507 | -6.675804 |
| pt_yrs | (exposure) | | | | | |

```
. lrtest age_male_interact_bmi .
Likelihood-ratio test                                 LR chi2(3)  =      80.05
(Assumption: age_male_int~i nested in .)              Prob > chi2 =     0.0000
. estimates store age_male_interact_bmi_scl

. *
. *  Adjust estimates for BMI, serum cholesterol and
```

```
. *   diastolic blood pressure
. *
. xi: poisson chd_cnt i.age_gr2*male i.bmi_gr  i.scl_gr  i.dbp_gr          20
>     , exposure(pt_yrs) irr

i.age_gr2         _Iage_gr2_45-81      (naturally coded; _Iage_gr2_45 omitted)
i.age_gr2*male    _IageXmale_#         (coded as above)
i.bmi_gr          _Ibmi_gr_1-4         (_Ibmi_gr_1 for bmi~r==22.79999923706055
> omitted)
i.scl_gr          _Iscl_gr_197-256     (naturally coded; _Iscl_gr_197 omitted)
i.dbp_gr          _Idbp_gr_74-91       (naturally coded; _Idbp_gr_74 omitted)
                                                                  Output omitted

Poisson regression                                Number of obs   =      1134
                                                  LR chi2(18)     =    873.98
                                                  Prob > chi2     =    0.0000
Log likelihood = -1436.7742                       Pseudo R2       =    0.2332

------------------------------------------------------------------------------
     chd_cnt |        IRR   Std. Err.      z    P>|z|     [95% Conf. Interval]
-------------+----------------------------------------------------------------
 _Iage_gr2_55 |   3.757542   1.330346     3.74   0.000     1.877322    7.520886
 _Iage_gr2_60 |   8.411822   2.926015     6.12   0.000     4.254057    16.63324
 _Iage_gr2_80 |   12.78982   4.320504     7.54   0.000     6.596625    24.79746
 _Iage_gr2_81 |   23.92786   8.701239     8.73   0.000     11.73192    48.80213
        male |    4.63766   1.703033     4.18   0.000     2.257991    9.525233
 _IageXmal~55 |   .5610104   .2207002    -1.47   0.142     .2594838    1.212918
 _IageXmal~60 |   .4230948   .1642325    -2.22   0.027     .1977093    .9054161
 _IageXmal~80 |   .3851574   .1438922    -2.55   0.011     .1851975    .8010164
 _IageXmal~81 |   .2688894   .1234925    -2.86   0.004     .1093058    .6614605
   _Ibmi_gr_2 |   1.159495   .0991218     1.73   0.083     .9806235    1.370994
   _Ibmi_gr_3 |   1.298532   .1077862     3.15   0.002     1.103564    1.527944
   _Ibmi_gr_4 |   1.479603   .1251218     4.63   0.000     1.253614    1.746332
 _Iscl_gr_225 |   1.189835   .1004557     2.06   0.040     1.008374    1.403952
 _Iscl_gr_255 |   1.649807   .1339827     6.16   0.000     1.407039    1.934462
 _Iscl_gr_256 |   1.793581   .1466507     7.15   0.000     1.527999    2.105323
  _Idbp_gr_80 |    1.18517   .0962869     2.09   0.037     1.010709    1.389744
  _Idbp_gr_90 |   1.122983   .0892217     1.46   0.144     .9610473    1.312205
  _Idbp_gr_91 |   1.638383   .1302205     6.21   0.000     1.402041    1.914564
      pt_yrs |  (exposure)
------------------------------------------------------------------------------
```

```
. lincom male + _IageXmale_55, irr                                        21
 ( 1)  [chd_cnt]male + [chd_cnt]_IageXmale_55 = 0

------------------------------------------------------------------------------
     chd_cnt |        IRR   Std. Err.      z    P>|z|     [95% Conf. Interval]
-------------+----------------------------------------------------------------
         (1) |   2.601775   .3722797     6.68   0.000     1.965505    3.444019
------------------------------------------------------------------------------

. lincom male + _IageXmale_60, irr
                                         Output omitted.  See Table 9.4
. lincom male + _IageXmale_80, irr
                                         Output omitted.  See Table 9.4
. lincom male + _IageXmale_81, irr
                                         Output omitted.  See Table 9.4
. lrtest age_male_interact_bmi_scl                                         22
Likelihood-ratio test                                 LR chi2(3)  =     46.88
(Assumption: age_male_int~l nested in .)              Prob > chi2 =    0.0000
```

### Comments

1 This *poisson* command analyzes Model (9.10). The variables *chd_cnt*, *male*, and *pt_yrs* give the values of $d_k$, $male_k$, and $n_k$, respectively. The syntax of *i.age_gr* is explained in Section 5.10 and generates the indicator variables $age_{jk}$ in Model (9.10). These variables are called *_Iage_gr_50*, *_Iage_gr_55*, . . . , and *_Iage_gr_81* by Stata.

2 The highlighted value in this column equals $\exp[\hat{\gamma}]$, which is the estimated age-adjusted CHD risk for men relative to women. The other values in this column are sex-adjusted risks of CHD in people of the indicated age strata relative to people from the first age stratum. The 95% confidence interval for the age-adjusted relative risk for men is also highlighted.

3 This *table* command sums the number of patient–years of follow-up and CHD events in groups of people defined by sex and age strata. The values tabulated in this table are the denominators and numerators of Equations (9.16) and (9.17). They are also given in Table 9.2. The output for ages 51–55, 56–60, 61–65, 66–70 and 71–75 have been deleted from this log file.

4 This *generate* command calculates the age–gender-specific CHD incidence rates using Equations (9.16) and (9.17). They are expressed as rates per thousand person–years of follow-up.

5 The variable *men* is missing for records that describe women.

6 This *graph bar* command produces the grouped bar chart of *men* and *women* shown in Figure 9.1. The *over(age_gr)* option specifies that separate bars will be drawn for each value of *age_gr*. The lengths of the bars are proportional to the mean of the variables *men* and *women* in records with the same value of *age_gr*. However, the preceding *collapse* and *generate* commands have ensured that there is only one non-missing value of *men* and *women* for each age stratum. Hence, the bar lengths are proportional to the age and gender specific CHD morbidity rates.

The point-and-click command that generates this graph is Graphics ▶ Bar chart ┘Main└ ┌ Statistics to plot — Variables ☑ 1: *men* ☑ 2: *women* ┘ ┘Categories└ ┌ ☑ Group 1 — Grouping variable: *age_gr* ┘ ┘Bars└ ┌ Bar properties — Bars: *Bar for variable 2* Edit Fill color: *Gray* , Outline color: *Gray* Accept ┘ ┘Y axis└ Title: *CHD Morbidity Rate per 1000* Minor tick/label properties ┘Rule└ ┌ Axis rule — ⦿ Suggest # between major ticks ┘ Accept ┘Titles└ Subtitle: *Age* Properties ┌ Placement — Position: *6 o'clock* ┘ Accept ┘Legend└ ┌ ☑ Override default keys — Specific order of keys and optionally change labels: *1 " Men " 2 " Women "* ┘ Organization/Appearance ┘Organization└ ┌ Organization — Rows/Columns: *Columns* ┘ Accept Placement Position: *11 o'clock* , ☑ Place legend inside plot region Accept Submit.

7 This *subtitle* option places the subtitle *Age* at the six o'clock position. That is, *Age* is centered below the graph.

8 These bar options color the bars for *men* and *women* black and white, respectively; *bar(1, color(black))* specifies that the bars for the first variable in the variable list (i.e. *men*) will be colored black.

9 The previous collapse command altered the data set. We reload the *8.12.Framingham.dta* data set before proceeding with additional analyses.

10 This *poisson* command specifies Model (9.18). The syntax of *i.age_gr*male* is analogous to that used for the logistic command in Section 5.23. This term specifies the covariates and parameters to the right of the offset term in Equation (9.18). Note that since *male* is already a zero–one indicator variable, it is not necessary to write *i.age_gr*i.male* to specify this part of the model. This latter syntax would, however, have generated the same model.

In this command I did not specify the *irr* option in order to output the parameter estimates. Note that the interaction terms become increasingly more negative with increasing age. This has the effect of reducing the age-specific relative risk of CHD in men versus women as their age increases.

11 This *lincom* statement calculates the CHD risk for men relative to women from the second age stratum (ages 46–50) using Equation (9.21). The following *lincom* commands calculate this relative risk for the other age strata. The output from these commands has been omitted here but has been entered into Table 9.2.

12 This command calculates the likelihood ratio test associated with the change in model deviance between Models (9.10) and (9.18).

13 This command analyzes the model used to produce Table 9.3. It differs from Model (9.18) only in that it uses five age strata rather than nine. These five age strata are specified by *age_gr2*. The highlighted relative risk estimate and confidence interval is also given for the first stratum in Table 9.3.

14 This and subsequent *lincom* commands provide the remaining relative risk estimates in Table 9.3.

15 There are a few missing values of *bmi_gr*. To assess the impact of BMI on our model fit, we eliminate records with these missing values to obtain properly nested models. The *quietly* prefix runs the indicated model but suppresses all output.

16 This command stores (among other things) the model deviance from the preceding regression command. It will be used by the next *lrtest* command.

17 The term *i.bmi_gr* adds

$$\sum_{f=2}^{4} \theta_f \times bmi_{fk}$$

to our model. It adjusts our risk estimates for the effect of body mass index as a confounding variable.

18 The change in model deviance due to adding BMI to our model is highly significant.

19 The term *i.scl_gr* adds

$$\sum_{g=2}^{4} \phi_g \times scl_{gk}$$

to our model. It adjusts our risk estimates for the effect of serum cholesterol as a confounding variable.

20 This *poisson* command implements Model (9.24). The term *i.dbp_gr* adds

$$\sum_{h=2}^{4} \psi_h \times dbp_{hk}$$

to the preceding model. The highlighted relative risk in the output is that for men versus women from the first stratum adjusted for body mass index, serum cholesterol, and diastolic blood pressure. This risk and its confidence interval are also given in Table 9.4.

21 This *lincom* command calculates the CHD risk for men relative to women from the second age stratum adjusted for body mass index, serum cholesterol, and diastolic blood pressure. The highlighted output is also given in Table 9.4. The output from the subsequent *lincom* commands completes this table.

22 This and the preceding likelihood ratio tests show that the model fit is greatly improved by adding MBI, serum cholesterol, and DBP to the model as confounding variables. Note that there are no records with missing values of *dbp_gr*. Hence, the model with BMI and SCL as confounding variables is properly nested within Model 9.24 and our likelihood ratio test is valid (see Comment 15 above).

## 9.4. Residual analyses for Poisson regression models

A good way to check the adequacy of a Poisson regression model is to graph a scatter plot of standardized residuals against estimated expected incidence rates. As with logistic regression, such plots can identify covariate patterns that fit the model poorly. In order to best identify outlying covariate patterns, you should always condense your data set so that there is only one record per covariate pattern. That is, you should sum the values of $d_k$ and $n_k$ over all records for which the covariate patterns from your model are identical. We will let $d_i$ and $n_i$ denote the number of observed events and person–years of follow-up associated with the $i^{\text{th}}$ distinct covariate pattern in the model.

### 9.4.1. Deviance residuals

An excellent residual for use with either Poisson or logistic regression is the deviance residual. The model deviance can be written in the form $D = \sum_i c_i$, where $c_i$ is a non-negative value that represents the contribution to the deviance of the $i^{\text{th}}$ group of patients with identical covariate values (see

Section 5.24). Let

$$r_i = \text{sign}[d_i/n_i - \hat{\lambda}_i]\sqrt{c_i} = \begin{cases} \sqrt{c_i} : \text{if } d_i/n_i \geq \hat{\lambda}_i \\ -\sqrt{c_i} : \text{if } d_i/n_i < \hat{\lambda}_i, \end{cases} \tag{9.27}$$

where $\hat{\lambda}_i$ is the estimated incidence rate for people with the $i^{\text{th}}$ covariate pattern under the model. Then $r_i$ is the **deviance residual** for this covariate pattern and

$$D = \sum_i r_i^2.$$

If the model is correct then the overwhelming majority of these residuals should fall between $\pm 2$. The magnitude of $r_i$ increases as $d_i/n_i$ diverges from $\hat{\lambda}_i$, and a large value of $r_i$ indicates a poor fit of the associated group of patients to the model.

As with Pearson residuals, deviance residuals are affected by varying degrees of leverage associated with the different covariate patterns (see Section 5.28). This leverage tends to shorten the residual by pulling the estimate of $\lambda_i$ in the direction of $d_i/n_i$. We can adjust for this shrinkage by calculating the **standardized deviance residual** for the $i^{\text{th}}$ covariate pattern, which is

$$r_{sj} = r_i/\sqrt{1 - h_i}. \tag{9.28}$$

In Equation (9.28), $h_i$ is the leverage of the $i^{\text{th}}$ covariate pattern. If the model is correct, roughly 95% of these residuals should lie between $\pm 2$. A residual plot provides evidence of poor model fit if substantially more than 5% of the residuals have an absolute value greater than two or if the average residual value varies with the estimated incidence of the disease.

Figure 9.2 shows a plot of standardized deviance residuals against expected CHD incidence from Model (9.24). A lowess regression curve of this residual versus CHD incidence is also plotted in this figure. If the model is correct, this curve should be flat and near zero for the great majority of residuals. In Figure 9.2 the lowess regression curve is very close to zero for incidence rates that range from about 10 to 35, and is never too far from zero outside this range. This figure indicates a good fit for this model to the Framingham Heart Study data.

## 9.5. Residual analysis of Poisson regression models using Stata

A residual analysis of Model (9.24) is illustrated below. The Stata log file *9.3.Framingham.log* continues as follows.

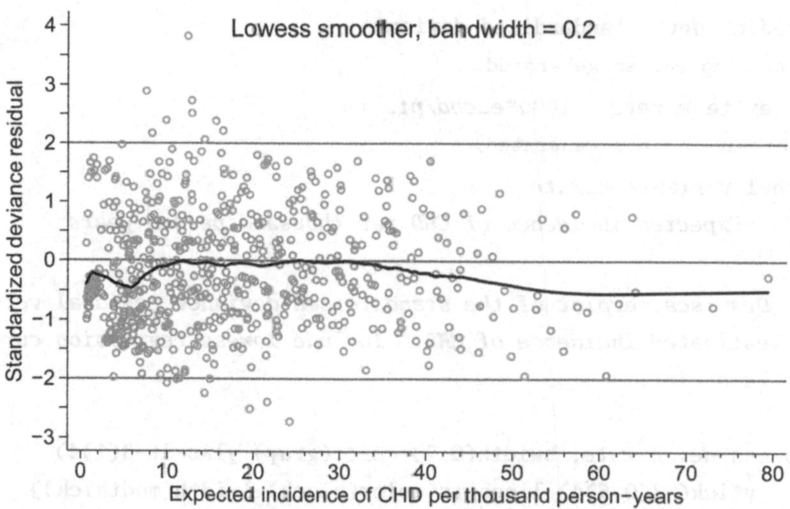


Figure 9.2 Plot of standardized deviance residuals against expected incidence of coronary heart disease (CHD) from Model (9.24). A plot of the lowess regression line of these residuals versus the expected incidence of CHD is also given. This graph indicates a good fit for these data. If Model (9.24) is correct, we would expect that roughly 95% of the standardized deviance residuals would lie between ±2; the lowess regression line should be flat and lie near zero.

```
. *
. *  Compress data set for residual plot
. *
. sort male bmi_gr scl_gr dbp_gr age_gr2
. collapse (sum) pt_yrs = pt_yrs chd_cnt = chd_cnt                    1
>      , by(male bmi_gr scl_gr dbp_gr age_gr2)
. *
. *  Re-analyze model (9.24)
. *
. xi: glm chd_cnt i.age_gr2*male i.bmi_gr  i.scl_gr  i.dbp_gr          2
>      , family(poisson) link(log) lnoffset(pt_yrs)
                         Output omitted.  See previous analysis of this model
. *
. *  Estimate the expected number of CHD events and the
. *  standardized deviance residual for each record in the data set.
. *
. predict e_chd, mu                                                     3
(82 missing values generated)
```

```
. predict dev, standardized deviance                                    4
(82 missing values generated)
. generate e_rate = 1000*e_chd/pt_yrs                                   5
(82 missing values generated)
. label variable e_rate
>      "Expected incidence of CHD per thousand person-years"
. *
. * Draw scatterplot of the standardized deviance residual versus the
. * estimated incidence of CHD. Include lowess regression curve on
. * this plot.
. *
. lowess dev e_rate, bwidth(0.2) color(gray) ylabel(-3(1)4)            6
>      ytick(-3(0.5)4) lineopts(color(black) lwidth(medthick))
>      yline(-2 0 2) xlabel(0(10)80) xmtick(0(2)80)
. log close
```

**Comments**

1 This *collapse* command produces one record for each unique combination of the values of the covariates from Model (9.24).

2 We need to repeat the analysis of this model to calculate the standardized deviance residuals from the compressed data set. The parameter estimates from this model are identical to those of the previous *poisson* command. We use the *glm* command here to be able to use the post-estimation commands described below.

3 This *predict* command calculates *e_chd* to equal $\hat{E}[d_i \mid \mathbf{x}_i]$, which is the estimated expected number of CHD events in people with the $i^{th}$ combination of covariate values. The equivalent point-and-click command is Statistics ▶ Postestimation ▶ Predictions, residuals, etc. ⌡Main⌊ New variable name: *e_chd* [Submit].

4 This command sets *dev* equal to the standardized deviance residual for each combination of covariate values. The equivalent point-and-click command is Statistics ▶ Postestimation ▶ Predictions, residuals, etc. ⌡Main⌊ New variable name: *dev* ┌ Produce: — ⦿ Deviance residuals ┘ ⌡Options⌊ [✓] Multiply residual by 1/sqrt(1-hat) [Submit].

5 This command calculates *e_rate* to be the estimated incidence of CHD per thousand person–years among patients with the $i^{th}$ combination of covariate values.

6 This *lowess* command produces a scatter plot of the standardized deviance residual versus the expected incidence of CHD, together with a lowess regression curve for these two variables. The *bwidth* option sets the band width for this regression. This graph is similar to Figure 9.2. An equivalent way of generating this graph using the *twoway lowess* command is discussed on page 65.

## 9.6. Additional reading

Breslow and Day (1987) is an excellent reference on Poisson regression that I highly recommend to readers with at least an intermediate level background in biostatistics. These authors provide an extensive theoretical and practical discussion of this topic.

McCullagh and Nelder (1989) is a more theoretical reference that discusses Poisson regression in the context of the generalized linear model. This text also discusses deviance residuals.

Hosmer and Lemeshow (2000) also provide an excellent discussion of deviance residuals in the context of logistic regression.

Levy (1999) provides a thorough description of the Framingham Heart Study.

## 9.7. Exercises

The following exercises are concerned with the child injury death data set *8.ex.InjuryDeath.dta* from Chapter 8.

1 Fit a multiplicative Poisson regression model that includes the covariates maternal age, birth weight, mother's education, income, mother's marital status at time of birth, number of siblings, mother's race, late or absent prenatal care, and age of child. Complete the following table; each relative risk should be adjusted for all of the other risk factors in your model.

| Numerator of relative risk | Denominator of relative risk | Adjusted relative risk | 95% confidence interval |
|---|---|---|---|
| Maternal age 25–29 | Maternal age > 29 | | |
| Maternal age 20–24 | Maternal age > 29 | | |
| Maternal age < 20 | Maternal age > 29 | | |
| Birth weight < 2500 g | Birth weight ≥ 2500 g | | |
| Mother's ed. 13–15 yrs | Mother's education > 15 yrs | | |
| Mother's ed. = 12 yrs | Mother's education > 15 yrs | | |
| Mother's ed. < 12 yrs | Mother's education > 15 yrs | | |
| Income in lowest quintile | Income in highest quintile | | |
| Income in 2nd quintile | Income in highest quintile | | |
| Income in 3rd quintile | Income in highest quintile | | |
| Income in 4th quintile | Income in highest quintile | | |
| Unmarried mother | Married mother | | |
| One sibling | No siblings | | |
| Two siblings | No siblings | | |
| Three siblings | No siblings | | |
| >3 siblings | No siblings | | |
| Black mother | White mother | | |
| Late/no prenatal care | Adequate prenatal care | | |
| 1st year of life | 3 year old | | |
| 1-year-old | 3 year old | | |
| 2-year-old | 3 year old | | |
| 4-year-old | 3 year old | | |

2 Contrast your answers to those of Question 3 in Chapter 8. In particular, what can you say about the relationship between race, prenatal care, and the risk of injury death?

3 Graph a scatter plot of the standardized deviance residuals against the corresponding expected incidence of injury deaths from your model. Plot the lowess regression curve of the deviance residuals against the expected incidence of mortal injuries on this graph. What proportion of the residuals have an absolute value greater than two? List the standardized deviance residual, expected incidence of injury deaths, observed number of injury deaths, and number of child–years of follow-up for all records with a deviance residual greater than two and at least two child injury deaths. Comment on the adequacy of the model. What might you do to improve the fit?

# 10

# Fixed effects analysis of variance

The term **analysis of variance** refers to a very large body of statistical methods for regressing a dependent variable against indicator covariates associated with one or more categorical variables. Much of the literature on this topic is concerned with sophisticated study designs that could be evaluated using the mechanical or electric calculators of the last century. These designs are now of reduced utility in medical statistics. This is, in part, because the enormous computational power of modern computers makes the computational simplicity of these methods irrelevant, but also because we are often unable to exert the level of experimental control over human subjects that is needed by these methods. As a consequence, regression methods using categorical variables have replaced classical analyses of variance in many medical experiments today.

In this chapter we introduce traditional analysis of variance from a regression perspective. In these methods, each patient is observed only once. As a result, it is reasonable to assume that the model errors for different patients are mutually independent. These techniques are called **fixed-effects** methods because each observation is assumed to equal the sum of a fixed expected value and an independent error term. Each of these expected values is a function of fixed population parameters and the patient's covariates. In Chapter 11, we will discuss more complex designs in which multiple observations are made on each patient, and it is no longer reasonable to assume that different error terms for the same patient are independent.

## 10.1. One-way analysis of variance

A **one-way analysis of variance** is a generalization of the independent $t$ test. Suppose that patients are divided into $k$ groups on the basis of some categorical variable. Let $n_i$ be the number of subjects in the $i^{\text{th}}$ group, $n = \sum n_i$ be the total number of study subjects, and $y_{ij}$ be a continuous response variable on the $j^{\text{th}}$ patient from the $i^{\text{th}}$ group. We assume for

$i = 1, 2, \ldots, k; j = 1, 2, \ldots, n_i$ that

$$y_{ij} = \beta_i + \varepsilon_{ij}, \tag{10.1}$$

where

$\beta_1, \beta_2, \ldots, \beta_k$ are unknown parameters, and
$\varepsilon_{ij}$ are mutually independent, normally distributed error terms with mean 0 and standard deviation $\sigma$.

Under this model, the expected value of $y_{ij}$ is $E[y_{ij}|i] = \beta_i$. Models like (10.1) are called **fixed-effects** models because the parameters $\beta_1, \beta_2, \ldots, \beta_k$ are fixed constants that are attributes of the underlying population. The response $y_{ij}$ differs from $\beta_i$ only because of the error term $\varepsilon_{ij}$. Let

$b_1, b_2, \ldots, b_k$ be the least squares estimates of $\beta_1, \beta_2, \ldots, \beta_k$, respectively,

$\bar{y}_i = \sum_{j=1}^{n_i} y_{ij}/n_i$ be the sample mean for the $i^{\text{th}}$ group,

$n = \sum n_i$, and

$$s^2 = \sum_{i=1}^{k} \sum_{j=1}^{n_i} (y_{ij} - \bar{y}_i)^2/(n - k) \tag{10.2}$$

be the mean squared error (MSE) estimate of $\sigma^2$. Equation (10.2) is analogous to Equation (3.5). We estimate $\sigma$ by $s$, which is called the root MSE. It can be shown that $E[y_{ij}|i] = b_i = \bar{y}_i$, and $E[s^2] = \sigma^2$. A 95% confidence interval for $\beta_i$ is given by

$$\bar{y}_i \pm t_{n-k,0.025}(s/\sqrt{n_i}). \tag{10.3}$$

Note that Model (10.1) assumes that the standard deviation of $\varepsilon_{ij}$ is the same for all groups. If it appears that there is appreciable variation in this standard deviation among groups then the 95% confidence interval for $\beta_i$ should be estimated by

$$\bar{y}_i \pm t_{n_i-1,0.025}(s_i/\sqrt{n_i}), \tag{10.4}$$

where $s_i$ is the sample standard deviation of $y_{ij}$ within the $i^{\text{th}}$ group.

We wish to test the null hypothesis that the expected response is the same in all groups. That is, we wish to test whether

$$\beta_1 = \beta_2 = \cdots = \beta_k. \tag{10.5}$$

We can calculate a statistic that has an ***F* distribution** with $k - 1$ and $n - k$ degrees of freedom when this null hypothesis is true. The $F$ distribution is another family of standard distributions like the chi-squared family. However, while a chi-squared distribution is determined by a single parameter that gives its degrees of freedom, an $F$ distribution is uniquely characterized by two separate degrees of freedom. These are called the numerator and denominator degrees of freedom, respectively. We reject the null hypothesis in favor of a multisided alternative hypothesis when the $F$ statistic is sufficiently large. The $P$-value associated with this test is the probability that this statistic exceeds the observed value when this null hypothesis is true.

When there are just two groups, the $F$ statistic will have 1 and $n - 2$ degrees of freedom. In this case, the one-way analysis of variance is equivalent to an independent $t$ test. The square root of this $F$ statistic equals the absolute value of the $t$ statistic given by Equation (1.11). The square of a $t$ statistic with $n$ degrees of freedom equals an $F$ statistic with numerator and denominator degrees of freedom of 1 and $n$, respectively.

Bartlett (1937) proposed a test of the assumption that the standard deviations of $\varepsilon_{ij}$ are equal within each group. This test, which is calculated by Stata's *oneway* command, is sensitive to departures from normality of the model's error terms. Levene (1960) proposed a more robust test of this hypothesis. If Levene's test is significant, or if there is considerable variation in the values of $s_i$, then you should use Equation (10.4) rather than Equation (10.3) to calculate confidence intervals for the group means.

## 10.2. Multiple comparisons

In a one-way analysis of variance we are interested in knowing not only if the group means are all equal, but also which means are different. For example, we may wish to separately test whether $\beta_1 = \beta_2, \beta_2 = \beta_3, \ldots$, or $\beta_{k-1} = \beta_k$. For any individual test, a $P$-value of 0.05 means that we have a 5% probability of false rejection of the null hypothesis. However, if we have multiple tests, the probability of false rejection of at least one test will be greater than 0.05. A mindless data-dredging exercise that calculates many $P$-values is likely to produce some spurious tests of significance. Various methods are available that adjust the $P$-values of an experiment in such a way that the probability of false rejection of one or more of the associated null hypotheses is not greater than 0.05. Such $P$-values are said to be adjusted for **multiple comparisons**. Discussion of these methods can be found in Armitage et al. (2002) and Steel and Torrie (1980). An alternative approach, which we will use, is known as **Fisher's protected LSD procedure**. (Here, LSD stands for "least significant difference" rather than Fisher's favorite psychotropic medicine – see Steel and Torrie, 1980.) This approach proceeds as follows. We perform a one-way analysis of variance to test if all of the means are equal. If this test is not significant, we say that there is not sufficient statistical evidence to claim that there are any differences in the group means. If, however, the analysis of variance $F$ statistic is significant, then we have evidence from a single test that at least some of these means must differ from some others. We can use this evidence as justification for looking at pair-wise differences between the group means without adjusting for multiple comparisons. Comparisons between any two groups are performed by calculating a $t$ statistic. If the standard deviations within the $k$ groups appear similar we can increase the power of the test that $\beta_i = \beta_j$ by using the formula

$$t_{n-k} = (\bar{y}_i - \bar{y}_j) \Big/ \left( s\sqrt{\frac{1}{n_i} + \frac{1}{n_j}} \right), \qquad (10.6)$$

where $s$ is the root MSE estimate of $\sigma$ obtained from the analysis of variance. Under the null hypothesis that $\beta_i = \beta_j$, Equation (10.6) will have a $t$ distribution with $n - k$ degrees of freedom. This test is usually more powerful than the independent $t$ test because it uses all of the data to estimate $\sigma$ (see Section 1.4.12). On the other hand, the independent $t$ test is more robust than Equation (10.6) since it makes no assumptions about the homogeneity of the standard deviations of groups other than $i$ and $j$.

A 95% confidence interval for the difference in population means between groups $i$ and $j$ is

$$\bar{y}_i - \bar{y}_j \pm t_{n-k,0.025} \left( s\sqrt{\frac{1}{n_i} + \frac{1}{n_j}} \right). \qquad (10.7)$$

Alternatively, a confidence interval based on the independent $t$ test may be used if it appears unreasonable to assume a uniform standard deviation in all groups (see Equations (1.12) and (1.15)).

There is considerable controversy about the best way to deal with multiple comparisons. Fisher's protected LSD approach works best when the hypothesized differences between the groups are predicted before the experiment is performed, when the number of groups is fairly small, or when there is some natural ordering of the groups. It should be noted, however, that if we are comparing groups receiving $k$ unrelated treatments, then there are $k(k-1)$ possible contrasts between pairs of treatments. If $k$ is large then the chance of false rejection of at least some of these null hypotheses may be much greater than 0.05 even when the overall $F$ statistic is significant. In this situation, it is prudent to make a multiple comparisons adjustment to these $P$-values.

A problem with multiple comparisons adjustment relates to how $P$-values are used. Although a $P$-value is, by definition, a probability, we use it as a measure of strength of evidence. That is, suppose we have two completely unrelated experiments comparing, say, survival among breast cancer patients and blood pressure reduction among hypertensive patients. If the log-rank and $t$ test $P$-values from these two studies are equal, then we would like to conclude that the evidence against their respective null hypotheses is similar. In a large clinical study, we typically have a small number of primary hypotheses that are stipulated in advance. Such studies are very expensive and it makes sense to perform careful exploratory analyses to learn as much as possible about the treatments under study. This typically involves many sub-analyses. If we performed multiple comparisons adjustments on all of these analyses we would greatly reduce or eliminate the statistical significance of our tests of the primary hypotheses of interest. Moreover, these adjusted $P$-values would not be comparable with $P$-values of similar magnitude from experiments with fewer comparisons. In my opinion, it is usually best to report unadjusted $P$-values and confidence intervals, but to make it very clear which hypotheses were specified in advance and which are the result of exploratory analyses. The latter results will need to be confirmed by other studies but may be of great value in suggesting the direction of future research. Also, investigators need to use good judgment and common sense in deciding which sub-analyses to report. Investigators are in no way obligated to report an implausible finding merely because its unadjusted $P$-value is less than 0.05.

Classical methods of statistical inference almost always lead to sensible conclusions when applied with some common sense. There are, however, some fundamental problems with the philosophical foundations of classical statistical inference. An excellent review of these problems is given by Royall (1997), who discusses multiple comparisons in the context of the deeper problems of classical statistical inference. Dupont (1983, 1986) gives two examples of how classical inference can lead to unsatisfactory conclusions.

## 10.3. Reformulating analysis of variance as a linear regression model

A one-way analysis of variance is, in fact, a special case of the multiple regression model we considered in Chapter 3. Let $y_h$ denote the response from the $h^{\text{th}}$ study subject, $h = 1, 2, \ldots, n$, and let

$$x_{hi} = \begin{cases} 1\text{: if the } h^{\text{th}} \text{ patient is in the } i^{\text{th}} \text{ group} \\ 0\text{: otherwise.} \end{cases}$$

Then Model (10.1) can be rewritten

$$y_h = \alpha + \beta_2 x_{h2} + \beta_3 x_{h3} + \cdots + \beta_k x_{hk} + \varepsilon_h, \qquad (10.8)$$

where $\varepsilon_h$ are mutually independent, normally distributed error terms with mean 0 and standard deviation $\sigma$. Note that Model (10.8) is a special case of Model (3.1). Thus, this analysis of variance is also a regression analysis in which all of the covariates are zero–one indicator variables. Also,

$$\mathrm{E}\left[y_h | x_{hi}\right] = \begin{cases} \alpha & \text{if the } h^{\text{th}} \text{ patient is from group 1} \\ \alpha + \beta_i & \text{if the } h^{\text{th}} \text{ patient is from group } i > 1. \end{cases}$$

Thus, $\alpha$ is the expected response of patients in the first group and $\beta_i$ is the expected difference in the response of patients in the $i^{\text{th}}$ and first groups. The least squares estimates of $\alpha$ and $\beta_i$ are $\bar{y}_1$ and $\bar{y}_i - \bar{y}_1$, respectively. We can use any multiple linear regression program to perform a one-way analysis of variance, although most software packages have a separate procedure for this task.

## 10.4. Non-parametric methods

The methods that we have considered in this text so far assume a specific form for the distribution of the response variable that is determined by one or more parameters. These techniques are called **parametric methods.** For example, in Model (10.1) we assume that $y_{ij}$ is normally distributed with mean $\beta_i$ and standard deviation $\sigma$. Our inferences are not greatly affected by minor violations of these distributional assumptions. However, if the true model differs radically from the one that we have chosen our conclusions may be misleading. In Section 2.17 we discussed transforming the dependent and independent variables to achieve a better model fit. Another approach is to use a method that makes fewer assumptions about the distribution of the response variable. These are called **non-parametric methods.** When the data are normally distributed, these methods are less powerful than their parametric counterparts. Also, they are often not useful for estimating attributes of the population of interest. They do, however, lead to robust tests of statistical significance when the distributional assumptions of the analogous parametric methods are wrong. They are particularly useful when there are extreme outliers in some of the groups or when the within-group distribution of the response variable is highly skewed. Lehmann (2006) provides an excellent introduction to non-parametric statistics.

## 10.5. Kruskal–Wallis test

The **Kruskal–Wallis** test is the non-parametric analog of the one-way analysis of variance (Kruskal and Wallis, 1952). Model (10.1) assumes that the $\varepsilon_{ij}$ terms are normally distributed and have the same standard deviation. If either of these assumptions is badly violated then the Kruskal–Wallis test should be used. Suppose that patients are divided into $k$ groups as in Model (10.1) and that $y_{ij}$ is a continuous response variable on the $j^{\text{th}}$ patient from the $i^{\text{th}}$ group. The null hypothesis of this test is that the distributions of the response variables are the same in each group. Let $n_i$ be the number of subjects in the $i^{\text{th}}$ group, and $n = \sum n_i$ be the total number of study subjects. We rank the values of $y_{ij}$ from lowest to highest and let $R_i$ be the sum of the ranks for the patients from the $i^{\text{th}}$ group. If all of the values of $y_{ij}$ are distinct (no ties) then the Kruskal–Wallis test statistic is

$$H = \frac{12}{n(n+1)}\left(\sum \frac{R_i^2}{n_i}\right) - 3(n+1). \tag{10.9}$$

When there are ties a slightly more complicated formula is used (see Steel and Torrie, 1980). Under the null hypothesis, $H$ will have a chi-squared distribution with $k-1$ degrees of freedom as long as the number of patients in each group is reasonably large. Note that the value of $H$ will be the same for any two data sets in which the data values have the same ranks. Increasing the largest observation or decreasing the smallest observation will have no effect on $H$. Hence, extreme outliers will not unduly affect this test.

The non-parametric analog of the independent $t$-test is the **Wilcoxon–Mann–Whitney rank-sum test.** This rank-sum test and the Kruskal–Wallis test are equivalent when there are only two groups of patients. (The non-parametric analog of the paired $t$-test is the **Wilcoxon signed-rank test,** which is described in most introductory biostatistics texts, including Pagano and Gauvreau 2000.)

## 10.6. Example: a polymorphism in the estrogen receptor gene

The human estrogen receptor gene contains a two-allele restriction fragment length polymorphism that can be detected by Southern blots of DNA digested with the PuvII restriction endonuclease. Bands at 1.6 kb and/or

**Table 10.1.** Effect of estrogen receptor genotype on age at diagnosis among 59 breast cancer patients (Parl et al., 1989)

| | Genotype* | | | |
|---|---|---|---|---|
| | 1.6/1.6 | 1.6/0.7 | 0.7/0.7 | Total |
| *Number of patients* | 14 | 29 | 16 | 59 |
| *Age at breast cancer diagnosis* | | | | |
| Mean | 64.643 | 64.379 | 50.375 | 60.644 |
| Standard deviation | 11.18 | 13.26 | 10.64 | 13.49 |
| 95% confidence interval | | | | |
| Equation (10.3) | (58.1–71.1) | (59.9–68.9) | (44.3–56.5) | |
| Equation (10.4) | (58.2–71.1) | (59.3–69.4) | (44.7–56.0) | (57.1–64.2) |

*The numbers 0.7 and 1.6 identify the alleles of the estrogen receptor genes that were studied (see text). Patients were homozygous for the 1.6 kb pattern allele (had two copies of the same allele), heterozygous (had one copy of each allele), or homozygous for the 0.7 kb pattern allele.

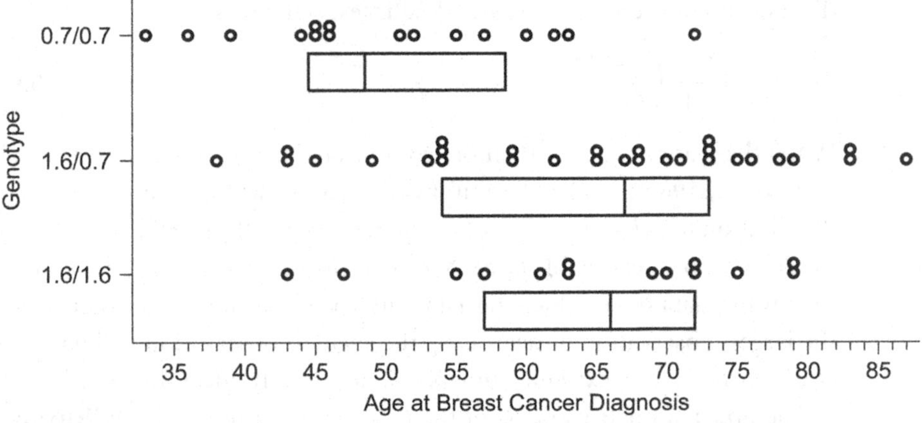


Figure 10.1 Dot and (whiskerless) box plots of the age at breast cancer diagnosis subdivided by estrogen receptor genotype in the study by Parl et al. (1989). Women who were homozygous for the 0.7 pattern allele had a significantly younger age of breast cancer diagnosis than did women in the other two groups.

0.7 kb identify the genotype for these alleles. Parl et al. (1989) studied the relationship between this genotype and age of diagnosis among 59 breast cancer patients. Table 10.1 shows the average age of breast cancer diagnosis among these patients subdivided by genotype. Figure 10.1 shows dot plots and box plots (minus whiskers) for these ages. The average age of diagnosis for patients who are homozygous for the 0.7 kb pattern allele was about

14 years younger than that of patients who were homozygous for the 1.6 kb pattern allele or who were heterozygous. To test the null hypothesis that the age at diagnosis does not vary with genotype, we perform a one-way analysis of variance on the ages of patients in these three groups using Model (10.1). In this analysis, $n = 59$, $k = 3$, and $\beta_1$, $\beta_2$, and $\beta_3$ represent the expected age of breast cancer diagnosis among patients with the 1.6/1.6, 1.6/0.7, and 0.7/0.7 genotypes, respectively. The estimates of these parameters are the average ages given in Table 10.1. The $F$ statistic from this analysis equals 7.86. This statistic has $k - 1 = 2$ and $n - k = 56$ degrees of freedom. The $P$-value associated with this test equals 0.001. Hence, we can reject the null hypothesis that these three population means are equal.

The root MSE estimate of $\sigma$ from this analysis of variance is $s = \sqrt{147.25} = 12.135$. The critical value $t_{56,0.025}$ equals 2.003. Substituting these values into Equation (10.3) gives a 95% confidence interval for the age of diagnosis of women with the 1.6/0.7 genotype of $64.38 \pm 2.003 \times 12.135/\sqrt{29} = (59.9, 68.9)$. The within-group standard deviations shown in this table are quite similar, and Levene's test of the equality of these standard deviations is not significant ($P = 0.44$). Hence, it is reasonable to use Equation (10.3) rather than Equation (10.4) to calculate the confidence intervals for the mean age at diagnosis for each genotype. In Table 10.1, these intervals are calculated for each genotype using both of these equations. Note that, in this example, these equations produce similar estimates. If the equal standard deviations assumption is true, then Equation (10.3) will provide more accurate confidence intervals than Equation (10.4) since it uses all of the data to calculate the common standard deviation estimate $s$. However, Equation (10.4) is more robust than Equation (10.3) since it does not make any assumptions about the standard deviation within each patient group.

The $F$ test from the analysis of variance permits us to reject the null hypothesis that the mean age of diagnosis is the same for each group. Hence, it is reasonable to investigate if there are pair-wise differences in these ages (see Section 10.2). This can be done using either independent $t$-tests or Equation (10.6). For example, the difference in average age of diagnosis between women with the 0.7/0.7 genotype and those with the 1.6/1.6 genotype is −14.268. From Equation (10.6), the $t$ statistic to test whether this difference is significantly different from zero is $t = -14.268/(12.135\sqrt{1/14 + 1/16}) = -3.21$. The $P$-value for this statistic, which has 56 degrees of freedom, is 0.002. The 95% confidence interval for this difference using Equation (10.7) is $-14.268 \pm 2.003 \times 12.135 \times \sqrt{1/14 + 1/16} = (-23.2, -5.37)$. Table 10.2 gives estimates of the difference between the mean ages of these

**Table 10.2.** Comparison of mean age of breast cancer diagnosis among patients with the three estrogen receptor genotypes studied by Parl et al. (1989). The one-way analysis of variance of these data shows that there is a significant difference between the mean age of diagnosis among women with these three genotypes ($P = 0.001$)

| Comparison | Difference in mean age of diagnosis | 95% confidence interval | *P* value | |
|---|---|---|---|---|
| | | | Eq. (10.6) | Rank-sum* |
| 1.6/0.7 vs. 1.6/1.6 | −0.264 | (−8.17 to 7.65) | 0.95 | 0.96 |
| 0.7/0.7 vs. 1.6/1.6 | −14.268 | (−23.2 to −5.37) | 0.002 | 0.003 |
| 0.7/0.7 vs. 1.6/0.7 | −14.004 | (−21.6 to −6.43) | <0.0005 | 0.002 |

*Wilcoxon–Mann–Whitney rank-sum test

three groups. In this table, confidence intervals are derived using Equation (10.7) and $P$-values are calculated using Equation (10.6). It is clear that the age of diagnosis among women who are homozygous for the 0.7 kb pattern allele is less than that of women with the other two genotypes.

Although the age distributions in Figure 10.1 are mildly asymmetric, it is unlikely that the normality assumptions of the analysis of variance are sufficiently violated to invalidate this method of analysis. Of course, the Kruskal–Wallis analysis of variance is also valid and avoids these normality assumptions. The Kruskal–Wallis test statistic for these data is $H = 12.1$. Under the null hypothesis that the age distributions of the three patient groups are the same, $H$ will have a chi-squared distribution with $k - 1 = 2$ degrees of freedom. The $P$-value for this test is 0.0024, which allows us to reject this hypothesis. Note that this $P$-value is larger (less statistically significant) than that obtained from the analogous conventional analysis of variance. This illustrates the slight loss of statistical power of the Kruskal–Wallis test, which is the cost of avoiding the normality assumptions of the conventional analysis of variance. Table 10.2 also gives the $P$-values from pair-wise comparisons of the three groups using the Wilcoxon–Mann–Whitney rank-sum test. These tests lead to the same conclusions that we obtained from the conventional analysis of variance.

## 10.7. User contributed software in Stata

There is an active community of Stata users who contribute Stata programs. Access to these programs can greatly increase our options for both analyses and graphic displays. For example, although the Stata canon contains programs for drawing box plots and dot plots, there is no official program that makes it easy to draw graphs like Figure 10.1. However, Nicholas J. Cox from Durham University has provided precisely such a program. A real strength of Stata is the ease with which such programs can be found and integrated into our personal versions of Stata.

The first step in obtaining such programs is to use the *findit* command in the Command Window to search the Internet for suitable software. For example, the command

```
findit dot plot
```

generates a list of commands and command descriptions associated with the key words *dot plots.* Part of this output is as follows:

```
stripplot from http://fmwww.bc.edu/RePEc/bocode/s
'STRIPPLOT': module for strip plots (one-way dot plots)/stripplot plots data
as a series of marks against a single magnitude axis, horizontal or vertical.
```

The first line of this output gives the name of a command and the web URL where it is stored. Clicking on this line gives a more detailed description of the *stripplot* command. Included in this output is a link that says *(click here to install).* Clicking on this link installs the *stripplot* command and its associated documentation on your computer. I will use this command in the following Stata example.

## 10.8. One-way analyses of variance using Stata

The following Stata log file and comments illustrate how to perform the one-way analysis of variance discussed in the preceding section.

```
. *  10.8.ERpolymorphism.log
. *
. *  Do a one-way analysis of variance to determine whether age
. *  at breast cancer diagnosis varies with estrogen receptor (ER)
. *  genotype using the data of Parl et al. 1989.
. *
. use C:\WDDtext\10.8.ERpolymorphism.dta                                   1
. ci age                                                                   2

    Variable |        Obs        Mean    Std. Err.       [95% Conf. Interval]
-------------+---------------------------------------------------------------
         age |         59    60.64407    1.756804        57.12744    64.16069
```

```
. by genotype: ci age                                                    3

-> genotype = 1.6/1.6

    Variable |        Obs        Mean    Std. Err.       [95% Conf. Interval]
-------------+---------------------------------------------------------------
         age |         14    64.64286    2.988269        58.1871    71.09862

-> genotype = 1.6/0.7

    Variable |        Obs        Mean    Std. Err.       [95% Conf. Interval]
-------------+---------------------------------------------------------------
         age |         29    64.37931    2.462234       59.33565    69.42297

-> genotype = 0.7/0.7

    Variable |        Obs        Mean    Std. Err.       [95% Conf. Interval]
-------------+---------------------------------------------------------------
         age |         16      50.375    2.659691         44.706      56.044
. *
. *  The following stripplot command must be downloaded from the web
. *  prior to use.  See Section 10.7
. *
. stripplot age, over(genotype)  boffset(-0.2) stack height(0.1)         4
>     box(lwidth(medthick)   barwidth(0.2))                               5
>     xtitle(Age at Breast Cancer Diagnosis)
>     xlabel(35(5)85) xmtick(33(1)87) xsize(5)
. oneway age genotype                                                    6

                        Analysis of Variance
    Source              SS         df      MS            F     Prob > F
------------------------------------------------------------------------
Between groups     2315.73355       2   1157.86678      7.86     0.0010   7
 Within groups     8245.79187      56   147.246283                        8
------------------------------------------------------------------------
    Total          10561.5254      58   182.095266
Bartlett's test for equal variances:  chi2(2) =   1.0798  Prob>chi2 = 0.583   9
. *
. *  Test whether the standard deviations of age are equal in
. *  patients with different genotypes.
. *
. robvar age, by(genotype)                                              10
```

```
            |     Summary of Age at Diagnosis
   Genotype |        Mean   Std. Dev.       Freq.
------------+------------------------------------
    1.6/1.6 |   64.642857   11.181077          14
    1.6/0.7 |    64.37931   13.259535          29
    0.7/0.7 |      50.375   10.638766          16
------------+------------------------------------
      Total |   60.644068   13.494268          59
W0  =  0.83032671   df(2, 56)     Pr > F = 0.44120161

W50 =  0.60460508   df(2, 56)     Pr > F = 0.54981692

W10 =  0.79381598   df(2, 56)     Pr > F = 0.45713722
. *
. * Repeat analysis using linear regression
. *
. xi: regress age i.genotype                                                11
i.genotype        _Igenotype_1-3      (naturally coded; _Igenotype_1 omitted)
      Source |       SS       df       MS              Number of obs =      59
-------------+------------------------------           F(  2,    56) =    7.86
       Model |  2315.73355     2  1157.86678           Prob > F      =  0.0010
    Residual |  8245.79187    56  147.246283           R-squared     =  0.2193
-------------+------------------------------           Adj R-squared =  0.1914
       Total |  10561.5254    58  182.095266           Root MSE      =  12.135

------------------------------------------------------------------------------
         age |      Coef.   Std. Err.      t    P>|t|     [95% Conf. Interval]
-------------+----------------------------------------------------------------
 _Igenotype_2|  -.2635468   3.949057    -0.07   0.947    -8.174458    7.647365   12
 _Igenotype_3|  -14.26786   4.440775    -3.21   0.002    -23.1638    -5.371915
       _cons |   64.64286   3.243084    19.93   0.000     58.14618    71.13953   13
------------------------------------------------------------------------------

. lincom _cons + _Igenotype_2                                                14

 ( 1)  _Igenotype_2 + _cons = 0

------------------------------------------------------------------------------
         age |      Coef.   Std. Err.      t    P>|t|     [95% Conf. Interval]
-------------+----------------------------------------------------------------
         (1) |   64.37931   2.253322    28.57   0.000     59.86536    68.89326   15
------------------------------------------------------------------------------
```

```
. lincom _cons + _Igenotype_3
 ( 1)  _Igenotype_3 + _cons = 0
```

| age | Coef. | Std. Err. | t | P>\|t\| | [95% Conf. | Interval] |
|---|---|---|---|---|---|---|
| (1) | 50.375 | 3.033627 | 16.61 | 0.000 | 44.29791 | 56.45209 |

```
. lincom _Igenotype_3 - _Igenotype_2
 ( 1) - _Igenotype_2 + _Igenotype_3 = 0
```
16

| age | Coef. | Std. Err. | t | P>\|t\| | [95% Conf. | Interval] |
|---|---|---|---|---|---|---|
| (1) | -14.00431 | 3.778935 | -3.71 | 0.000 | -21.57443 | -6.434194 |

```
. *
. *  Perform a Kruskal-Wallis analysis of variance
. *
. kwallis age, by(genotype)
Test: Equality of populations (Kruskal-Wallis test)
```
17

| genotype | Obs | Rank Sum |
|---|---|---|
| 1.6/1.6 | 14 | 494.00 |
| 1.6/0.7 | 29 | 999.50 |
| 0.7/0.7 | 16 | 276.50 |

```
chi-squared =     12.060 with 2 d.f.
probability =      0.0024

chi-squared with ties =     12.073 with 2 d.f.
probability =      0.0024
. ranksum age if genotype !=3, by(genotype)
Two-sample Wilcoxon rank-sum (Mann-Whitney) test
```
18

| genotype | obs | rank sum | expected |
|---|---|---|---|
| 1.6/1.6 | 14 | 310 | 308 |
| 1.6/0.7 | 29 | 636 | 638 |
| combined | 43 | 946 | 946 |

```
unadjusted variance       1488.67
adjustment for ties         -2.70
                          ----------
adjusted variance         1485.97

Ho: age(genotype==1.6/1.6) = age(genotype==1.6/0.7)
             z =   0.052
    Prob > |z| =   0.9586

. ranksum age if genotype !=2, by(genotype)

Two-sample Wilcoxon rank-sum (Mann-Whitney) test

    genotype |      obs    rank sum    expected
-------------+---------------------------------
     1.6/1.6 |       14         289         217
     0.7/0.7 |       16         176         248
-------------+---------------------------------
    combined |       30         465         465

unadjusted variance        578.67
adjustment for ties         -1.67
                          ----------
adjusted variance          576.99

Ho: age(genotype==1.6/1.6) = age(genotype==0.7/0.7)
             z =   2.997
    Prob > |z| =   0.0027

. ranksum age if genotype !=1, by(genotype)

Two-sample Wilcoxon rank-sum (Mann-Whitney) test

    genotype |      obs    rank sum    expected
-------------+---------------------------------
     1.6/0.7 |       29       798.5         667
     0.7/0.7 |       16       236.5         368
-------------+---------------------------------
    combined |       45        1035        1035

unadjusted variance       1778.67
adjustment for ties         -2.23
                          ----------
adjusted variance         1776.44

Ho: age(genotype==1.6/0.7) = age(genotype==0.7/0.7)
             z =   3.120
    Prob > |z| =   0.0018

. kwallis age if genotype !=1, by(genotype)                              19
```

```
Test: Equality of populations (Kruskal-Wallis test)
```

| genotype | Obs | Rank Sum |
|---|---|---|
| 1.6/0.7 | 29 | 798.50 |
| 0.7/0.7 | 16 | 236.50 |

```
chi-squared =       9.722 with 1 d.f.
probability =       0.0018

chi-squared with ties =      9.734 with 1 d.f.
probability =       0.0018

. log close
```

**Comments**

1 This data set contains the age of diagnosis and estrogen receptor genotype of the 59 breast cancer patients studied by Parl et al. (1989). The genotypes 1.6/1.6, 1.6/0.7 and 0.7/0.7 are coded 1, 2 and 3 in the variable *genotype*, respectively.

2 This *ci* command calculates the mean age of diagnosis (*age*) together with the associated 95% confidence interval. This confidence interval is calculated by combining all patients into a single group and using Equation (10.4). The estimated standard error of the mean and the number of patients with non-missing ages is also given.

3 The command prefix *by genotype:* specifies that means and 95% confidence intervals are to be calculated for each of the three genotypes. The highlighted output from this and the preceding command are given in Table 10.1. The sample standard deviations are obtained by multiplying each standard error estimate by the square root of its sample size. (Alternatively, we could have used the *summarize* command.)

4 This command produces a graph that is similar to Figure 10.1. Separate dot plots and box plots of *age* are generated for each value of *genotype*. The *boffset* option controls the distance between each pair of box and dot plots. The *stack* option shows observations with identical values as separate circles stacked on top of each other; *height* controls the vertical spacing between stacked observations. This program must be downloaded from the Internet before use (see Section 10.7).

5 The *box* option controls the appearance of the box plots; *lwidth(medthick)* draws boxes with medium thick lines while *barwidth(0.2)* controls the thickness of the boxes.

6 This *oneway* command performs a one-way analysis of variance of *age* with respect to the three distinct values of *genotype.* The equivalent point-and-click command is Statistics ▶ Linear models and related ▶ ANOVA/MANOVA ▶ One-way ANOVA Main Response variable: *age* , Factor variable: *genotype* Submit .

7 The $F$ statistic from this analysis equals 7.86. If the mean age of diagnosis in the target population is the same for all three genotypes, this statistic will have an $F$ distribution with $k - 1 = 3 - 1 = 2$ and $n - k = 59 - 3 = 56$ degrees of freedom. The probability that this statistic exceeds 7.86 is 0.001.

8 The MSE estimate of $\sigma^2$ is $s^2 = 147.246$.

9 Bartlett's test for equal variances (i.e. equal standard deviations) gives a $P$-value of 0.58.

10 The *robvar* command also tests the null hypothesis that the variances of *age* within groups defined by *genotype* are equal. W0 is Levene's test statistic for this hypothesis while W50 and W10 are refinements of Levene's test proposed by Brown and Forsythe (1974). In this example, these three tests are mutually consistent and agree with Bartlett's test. The data provide little or no evidence that the standard deviation of age varies among genotypes.

The equivalent point-and-click command is Statistics ▶ Summaries, tables, and tests ▶ Classical tests of hypotheses ▶ Robust equal variance test Main Variable: *age* , Variable defining two comparison groups: *genotype* Submit .

11 This *regress* command performs exactly the same one-way analysis of variance as the *oneway* command given above. Note that the $F$ statistic, the $P$-value for this statistic and the MSE estimate of $\sigma^2$ are identical to that given by the *oneway* command. The syntax of the *xi:* prefix is explained in Section 5.10. The model used by this command is Equation (10.8) with $k = 3$.

12 The estimates of $\beta_2$ and $\beta_3$ in this example are $\bar{y}_2 - \bar{y}_1 = 64.379 - -64.643 = -0.264$ and $\bar{y}_3 - \bar{y}_1 = 50.375 - 64.643 = -14.268$, respectively. They are highlighted in the column labeled *Coef.* The 95% confidence intervals for $\beta_2$ and $\beta_3$ are calculated using Equation (10.7). The $t$ statistics for testing the null hypotheses that $\beta_2 = 0$ and $\beta_3 = 0$ are $-0.07$ and $-3.21$, respectively. They are calculated using Equation (10.6). The highlighted values in this output are also given in Table 10.2.

13 The estimate of $\alpha$ is $\bar{y}_1 = 64.643$. The 95% confidence interval for $\alpha$ is calculated using Equation (10.3). These statistics are also given in Table 10.1.

14 This *lincom* command estimates $\alpha + \beta_2$ by $\hat{\alpha} + \hat{\beta}_2 = \bar{y}_2$. A 95% confidence interval for this estimate is also given. Note that $\alpha + \beta_2$ equals the population mean age of diagnosis among women with the 1.6/0.7 genotype. Output from this and the next *lincom* command is also given in Table 10.1.

15 This confidence interval is calculated using Equation (10.3).

16 This command estimates $\beta_3 - \beta_2$ by $\hat{\beta}_3 - \hat{\beta}_2 = \bar{y}_3 - \bar{y}_2 = 50.375 - 64.379 = -14.004$. The null hypothesis that $\beta_3 = \beta_2$ is the same as the hypothesis that the mean age of diagnosis in Groups 2 and 3 are equal. The confidence interval for $\beta_3 - \beta_2$ is calculated using Equation (10.7). The highlighted values are also given in Table 10.2.

17 This *kwallis* command performs a Kruskal–Wallis test of *age* by *genotype*. The test statistic, adjusted for ties, equals 12.073. The associated $P$-value equal 0.0024. The equivalent point-and-click command is Statistics ▶ Nonparametric analysis ▶ Tests of hypotheses ▶ Kruskal-Wallis rank test ⌡Main⌊ Outcome variable: *age*, Variable defining groups: *genotype* [Submit].

18 This command performs a Wilcoxon–Mann–Whitney rank-sum test on the age of diagnosis of women with the 1.6/1.6 genotype versus the 1.6/0.7 genotype. The $P$-value for this test is 0.96. The next two commands perform the other two pair-wise comparisons of age by genotype using this rank-sum test. The highlighted $P$-values are included in Table 10.2. The equivalent point-and-click command is Statistics ▶ Nonparametric analysis ▶ Tests of hypotheses ▶ Wilcoxon rank sum test ⌡Main⌊ Variable: *age*, Grouping variable: *genotype* ⌡by/if/in⌊ ┌ Restrict observations — If: (expression) *genotype !=3* ┘ [Submit].

19 This command repeats the preceding command using the Kruskal–Wallis test. This test is equivalent to the rank-sum test when only two groups are being compared. Note that the $P$-values from these tests both equal 0.0018.

## 10.9. Two-way analysis of variance, analysis of covariance, and other models

Fixed-effects analyses of variance generalize to a wide variety of complex models. For example, suppose that hypertensive patients were treated with a placebo, or a diuretic alone, or a beta-blocker alone, or both a diuretic and a beta-blocker. Then a model of the effect of treatment on diastolic blood pressure (DBP) might be

$$y_i = \alpha + \beta_1 x_{i1} + \beta_2 x_{i2} + \varepsilon_i, \tag{10.10}$$

where

$\alpha$, $\beta_1$, and $\beta_2$ are unknown parameters,

$$x_{i1} = \begin{cases} 1: & i^{\text{th}} \text{ patient is on a diuretic} \\ 0: & \text{otherwise,} \end{cases}$$

$$x_{i2} = \begin{cases} 1: & i^{\text{th}} \text{ patient is on a beta-blocker} \\ 0: & \text{otherwise,} \end{cases}$$

$y_i$ is the DBP of the $i^{\text{th}}$ patient after some standard interval of therapy, and $\varepsilon_i$ are error terms that are independently and normally distributed with mean zero and standard deviation $\sigma$.

Model (10.10) is an example of a fixed-effects, **two-way analysis of variance**. It is called two-way because each patient is simultaneously influenced by two covariates – in this case whether she did or did not receive a diuretic or a beta-blocker. A critical feature of this model is that each patient's blood pressure is only observed once. It is this feature that makes the independence assumption for the error term reasonable and makes this a fixed-effects model. In this model, $\alpha$ is the mean DBP of patients on placebo, $\alpha + \beta_1$ is the mean DBP of patients on the diuretic alone, and $\alpha + \beta_2$ is the mean DBP of patients on the beta-blocker alone. The model is additive since it assumes that the mean DBP of patients on both drugs is $\alpha + \beta_1 + \beta_2$. If this assumption is unreasonable we can add an interaction term as in Section 3.13.

Another possibility is to mix continuous and indicator variables in the same model. Inference from these models is called **analysis of covariance**. For example, we could add the patient's age to Model (10.10). This gives

$$y_i = \alpha + \beta_1 x_{i1} + \beta_2 x_{i2} + \beta_3 \times age_i + \varepsilon_i, \tag{10.11}$$

where $age_i$ is the $i^{\text{th}}$ patient's age, $\beta_3$ is the parameter associated with age, and the other terms are as defined in Model (10.10). The analysis of Model (10.11) would be an example of analysis of covariance. There is a vast statistical literature on the analysis of variance and covariance. The interested reader will find references to some good texts on this topic in Section 10.10. Note, however, that Models (10.10) and (10.11) are both special cases of Model (3.1). Thus, we can usually reformulate any fixed-effects analysis of variance or covariance problem as a multiple linear regression problem by choosing suitably defined indicator and continuous covariates.

## 10.10. Additional reading

Armitage et al. (2002) and

Steel and Torrie (1980) provide additional discussion of fixed-effects analysis of variance and covariance.

Cochran and Cox (1957) is a classic text that documents the extraordinary ingenuity and effort that was devoted in the last century to devising methods of experimental design and analysis of variance that could be implemented with mechanical or electric calculators.

Lehmann (2006) is a graduate level text on non-parametric statistical methods.

Searle (1987) is a more mathematically advanced text on linear models, including analysis of variance.

Parl et al. (1989) studied the relationship between age of breast cancer diagnosis and a polymorphism in the estrogen receptor gene. We use their data to illustrate fixed-effects one-way analysis of variance.

Royall (1997) provides an excellent introduction to the foundations of statistical inference. This introduction is written from a likelihood perspective, of which Royall is a leading advocate.

Cox and Hinkley (1974) provide a concise summary of the different fundamental approaches to statistical inference.

Dupont (1983, 1986) provides two examples of how classical inference can lead to unsatisfactory conclusions.

Bartlett (1937) is the original reference for Bartlett's test of equal standard deviations.

Levene (1960) is the original reference for Levene's test of equal standard deviations.

Brown and Forsythe (1974) proposed variants of Levene's test and conducted simulation studies to assess the properties of these tests under various assumptions.

Kruskal and Wallis (1952) is the original reference for the Kruskal–Wallis test.

Wilcoxon (1945) and

Mann and Whitney (1947) are the original references on the Wilcoxon–Mann–Whitney rank-sum test.

## 10.11. Exercises

1 Perform a one-way analysis of variance on the age of entry biopsy in the three different diagnostic groups of women from the Nashville Breast

Cohort (see Section 6.19). In Question 5 of Chapter 6 you were also asked to compare these ages. If you answered this previous question by performing $t$ tests, what additional information does the analysis of variance provide you that the individual $t$ tests did not?

2 Draw box plots of the age of entry biopsy in the Nashville Breast Cohort subdivided by diagnosis. In view of these plots, is a one-way analysis of variance a reasonable approach to analyzing these data? Perform Levene's test of the equality of variances among these diagnostic groups.

3 Perform a Kruskal–Wallis analysis of variance for the age of entry biopsy in these three groups. Contrast your answer with that for question 1.

4 Perform Wilcoxon–Mann–Whitney rank-sum tests of the age of biopsy for each pair of diagnostic groups in the Nashville Breast Cohort. Contrast your answer with that for Question 5 of Chapter 6.

# 11

# Repeated-measures analysis of variance

**Repeated-measures** analysis of variance is concerned with study designs in which the same patient is observed repeatedly over time. Such data are also referred to as **longitudinal** data, or **panel** data. In analyzing these data, we must take into consideration the fact that the error components of repeated observations on the same patient are usually correlated. This is a critical difference between repeated-measures and fixed-effects designs. In a repeated-measures experiment, the fundamental unit of observation is the patient. We seek to make inferences about members of a target population who are treated in the same way as our study subjects. Using a fixed-effects method of analysis on repeated-measures data can lead to wildly exaggerated levels of statistical significance since we have many more observations than patients. For this reason, it is essential that studies with repeated-measures designs be always analyzed with methods that account for the repeated measurements on study subjects.

## 11.1. Example: effect of race and dose of isoproterenol on blood flow

Lang et al. (1995) studied the effect of isoproterenol, a $\beta$-adrenergic agonist, on forearm blood flow in a group of 22 normotensive men. Nine of the study subjects were black and 13 were white. Each subject's blood flow was measured at baseline and then at escalating doses of isoproterenol. Figure 11.1 shows the mean blood flow at each dose subdivided by race. The standard deviations of these flows are also shown.

At first glance, the data in Figure 11.1 look very much like that from a fixed-effects two-way analysis of variance in that each blood flow measurement is simultaneously affected by the patient's race and isoproterenol dose. The fixed-effects model, however, provides a poor fit because each patient is observed at each dose. Observations on the same patient are likely to be correlated, and the closer the dose, the higher the correlation is likely to be. In a fixed-effects model, all of the error terms are assumed to be independent. This implies that the probability that a patient's response is greater than the

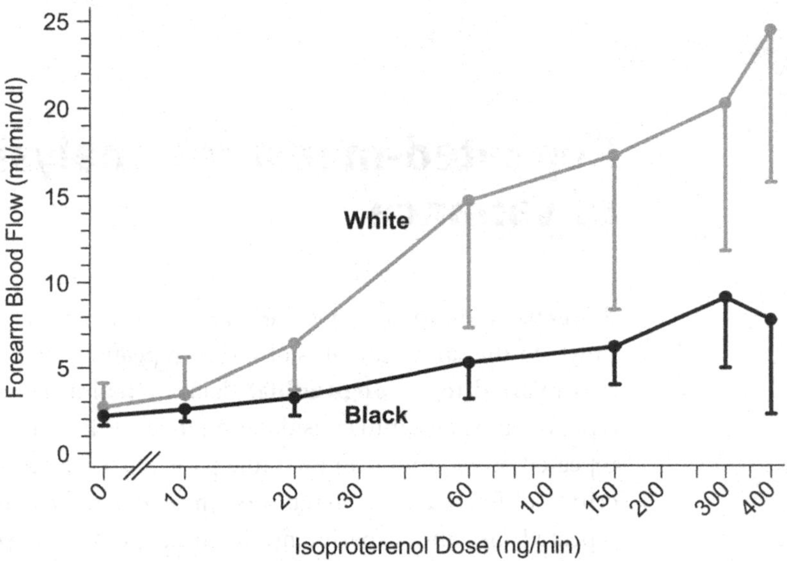


Figure 11.1 Mean rates of forearm blood flow in normotensive white and black men in response to different doses of isoproterenol. The vertical bars indicate the estimated standard deviations within each racial group at each dose (Lang et al., 1995).

mean value for his race at the specified dose is in no way affected by his response at an earlier dose. In fact, if a patient's response at one dose is well above average, his response at the next is more likely to be above average than below. This invalidates the independence assumption of the fixed-effects model. It is important to obtain an intuitive feel for the correlation structure of data from individual patients. One way to do this is shown in Figure 11.2. In this figure, straight lines connect observations from the same patient. Note, that these lines usually do not cross, indicating a high degree of correlation between observations from the same patient. Both Figures 11.1 and 11.2 suggest that the response of men to escalating doses of isoproterenol tends to be greater in whites than in blacks.

Graphs like Figure 11.2 can become unintelligible when the number of subjects is large. In this situation, it is best to connect the observations from a representative sub-sample of patients. For example, we might calculate the mean response for each patient. We could then identify those patients with the lowest and highest mean response as well as those patients whose mean response corresponds to the $5^{th}$, $10^{th}$, $20^{th}$, $30^{th}$, $40^{th}$, $50^{th}$, $60^{th}$, $70^{th}$, $80^{th}$, $90^{th}$, and $95^{th}$ percentile of the entire sample. Connecting the observations for these 13 patients gives a feel for the degree of correlation of observations

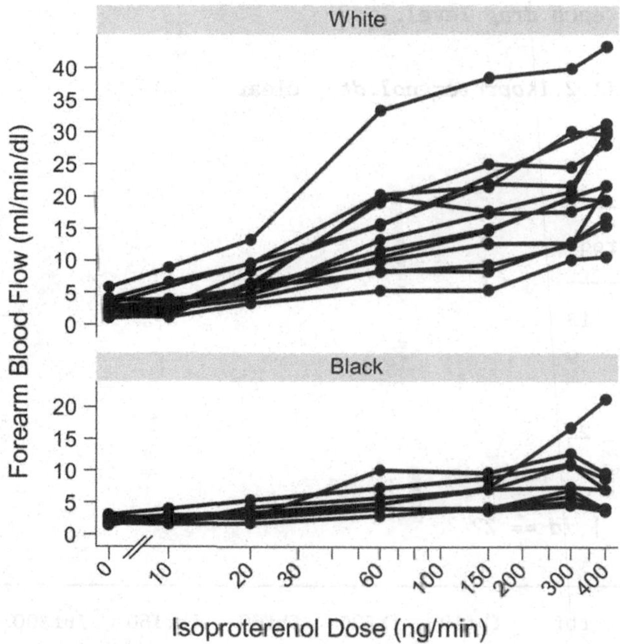


Figure 11.2 Plots of forearm blood flow against isoproterenol dose for white and black men. Straight lines connect observations from the same study subjects. Note that patients who have high, medium, or low flows at one dose tend to have high, medium, or low flows at other doses, respectively. This indicates that blood flows from the same patient are strongly correlated (Lang et al., 1995).

from the same subject without overwhelming the graph with interconnecting lines. Diggle et al. (2002) provide an excellent discussion of exploratory methods of graphing repeated measures data.

## 11.2. Exploratory analysis of repeated measures data using Stata

The following log file and comments illustrates how to produce graphs similar to Figures 11.1 and 11.2. It also reformats the data from one record per patient to one record per observation. This latter format will facilitate the analysis of these data.

```
. * 11.2.Isoproterenol.log
. *
. * Plot mean forearm blood flow by race and log dose of isoproternol
. * using the data of Lang et al. (1995).  Show standard deviation for
```

```
. *  each race at each drug level.
. *
. use C:\WDDtext\11.2.Isoproterenol.dta, clear

. table race, row                                                    1

  Race       Freq.

 White          13
 Black           9

 Total          22

. list if id == 1 | id == 22                                         2

        id   race   fbf0   fbf10   fbf20   fbf60   fbf150   fbf300   fbf400

  1.     1   White     1     1.4     6.4    19.1       25     24.6       28
 22.    22   Black   2.1     1.9       3     4.8      7.4     16.7     21.2

. generate baseline = fbf0                                           3

. *
. * Convert data from one record per patient to one record per
. * observation.
. *
. reshape long fbf, i(id) j(dose)                                    4
(note: j = 0 10 20 60 150 300 400)

Data                                  wide   ->   long
------------------------------------------------------------------------
Number of obs.                          22   ->    154
Number of variables                     10   ->      5
j variable (7 values)                        ->   dose
xij variables:
                     fbf0 fbf10 ... fbf400   ->   fbf
------------------------------------------------------------------------

. list if id == 1 | id == 22                                         5
```

```
     +--------------------------------------+
     | id   dose   race    fbf   baseline   |
     |--------------------------------------|
  1. |  1      0   White     1          1   |
  2. |  1     10   White   1.4          1   |
  3. |  1     20   White   6.4          1   |
  4. |  1     60   White  19.1          1   |
  5. |  1    150   White    25          1   |
     |--------------------------------------|
  6. |  1    300   White  24.6          1   |
  7. |  1    400   White    28          1   |
148. | 22      0   Black   2.1        2.1   |
149. | 22     10   Black   1.9        2.1   |
150. | 22     20   Black     3        2.1   |
     |--------------------------------------|
151. | 22     60   Black   4.8        2.1   |
152. | 22    150   Black   7.4        2.1   |
153. | 22    300   Black  16.7        2.1   |
154. | 22    400   Black  21.2        2.1   |
     +--------------------------------------+
. generate delta_fbf = fbf - baseline
(4 missing values generated)
. label variable delta_fbf "Change in Forearm Blood Flow"
. label variable dose "Isoproterenol Dose (ng/min)"
. generate plotdose = dose
. replace plotdose = 6    if dose == 0                                    6
(22 real changes made)
. label variable plotdose "Isoproterenol Dose (ng/min)"
. generate logdose = log(dose)
(22 missing values generated)
. label variable logdose "Log Isoproterenol Dose"
. *
. *  Save long format of data for subsequent analyses
. *
. save 11.2.Long.Isoproterenol.dta, replace
file 11.2.Long.Isoproterenol.dta saved
. *
. *  Generate Figure 11.1
```

```
. *
. collapse (mean) fbfbar = fbf (sd) sd = fbf, by(race plotdose)          7
. generate whitefbf = fbfbar if race == 1                               8
(7 missing values generated)
. generate blackfbf = fbfbar if race == 2
(7 missing values generated)
. generate blacksd = sd if race == 2
(7 missing values generated)
. generate whitesd = sd if race == 1
(7 missing values generated)
. label variable whitefbf "Forearm Blood Flow (ml/min/dl)"
. label variable blackfbf "Forearm Blood Flow (ml/min/dl)"
. generate wsdbar = whitefbf - whitesd                                  9
(7 missing values generated)
. generate bsdbar = blackfbf - blacksd
(7 missing values generated)
. replace wsdbar = whitefbf + whitesd if plotdose < 20                  10
(2 real changes made)
. twoway connected whitefbf plotdose, color(gray) symbol(circle)        11
>       || rcap whitefbf wsdbar plotdose, color(gray)
>       || connected blackfbf plotdose, color(black) symbol(circle)
>       || rcap blackfbf bsdbar plotdose, color(black)
>       ||, ytitle(Forearm Blood Flow (ml/min/dl))
>           xtitle(Isoproterenol Dose (ng/min)) xscale(log)             12
>           xlabel(10 20 30 60 100 150 200 300 400, angle(45))          13
>           xtick(40(10)90 250 350) legend(off)                         14

. *
. *         Plot individual responses for white and black patients
. *
. use 11.2.Long.Isoproterenol.dta, clear                                15
. sort id plotdose
. twoway connected fbf plotdose, connect(L) symbol(circle)              16
>     xlabel(10 20 30 60 100 150 200 300 400, angle(45))
>     xtick(40(10)90 250 350) ylabel(0(5)40) xscale(log) ysize(5.5)
>     ytitle(Forearm Blood Flow (ml/min/dl)) by(race, cols(1))          17
. log close
```

**Comments**

1 *11.2.Isoproterenol.dta* contains one record (row of variable values) per patient. Lang et al. (1995) studied 13 white subjects and 9 black subjects.

2 We list the variables in the first and last record of this file. In addition to race and patient identification number there are seven variables recording the patient's forearm blood flow at different doses: *fbf0* records the baseline blood-flow, *fbf10* the blood flow at 10 ng/min, *fbf20* the blood flow at 20 ng/min, etcetera.

3 We set baseline equal to *fbf0* for use in subsequent calculations.

4 The *reshape long* command converts data from one record per patient to one record per observation. In this command, *i*(*id*) specifies that the *id* variable identifies observations from the same subject. The variable *fbf* is the first three letters of variables *fbf0*, *fbf10*, . . . , *fbf400*; *j*(*dose*) defines *dose* to be a new variable whose values are the trailing digits in the names of the variables *fbf0*, *fbf10*, . . . , *fbf400*. That is, *dose* will take the values 0, 10, 20, . . . , 300, 400. One record will be created for each value of *fbf0*, *fbf10*, . . . , *fbf400*. Other variables in the file that are not included in this command (like *race* or *baseline*) are assumed not to vary with *dose* and are replicated in each record for each specific patient.

The equivalent point-and-click command is Data ▶ Create or change variables ▶ Other variable transformation commands ▶ Convert data between wide and long | Main | ID variable(s) - the i() option: *id* , Subobservation identifier variable - the j() option: *dose*, Base (stub) names of X_ij variables: *fbf* | Submit |.

5 This *list* command shows the effect of the preceding *reshape long* command. There are now seven records that record the data for the patient with $id = 1$; *fbf* records the forearm blood pressure for this patient at the different doses of isoproterenol. Note that the values of *race* and *baseline* remain constant in all records with the same value of *id*.

6 We want to create Figures 11.1 and 11.2 that plot dose on a logarithmic scale. We also want to include the baseline dose of zero on these figures. Since the logarithm of zero is undefined, we create a new variable called *plotdose* that equals *dose* for all values greater than zero and equals 6 when $dose = 0$. We will use a graphics editor to relabel this value zero with a break in the *x*-axis when we create these figures.

7 This *collapse* command compresses the data to a single record for each unique combination of *race* and *dose*. Two new variables called *fbfbar* and *sd* are created. The variable *fbfbar* equals the mean of all values of *fbf* that

have identical values of *race* and *plotdose*; *sd* is the standard deviation of these values. Hence, *fbfbar* and *sd* record the mean and standard deviation of the forearm blood flow at each dose within each race. The point-and-click version of this command is similar to that described on page 386 except that on the *Main* tab we enter ┌ Statistics to collapse — Variables 1: *fbfbar* = *fbf* , Statistic [✓] 2: *Standard deviation* , Variables *sd* = *fbf* ┘ .

8 The variable *whitefbf* equals the mean forearm blood flow for white subjects and is missing for black subjects; *blackfbf* is similarly defined for black subjects. The variables *blacksd* and *whitesd* give the standard deviations for black and white subjects, respectively.

9 The distance between *whitefbf* and *wsdbar* equals the standard deviation of the forearm blood flow for white subjects at each dose; *bsdbar* is similarly defined for black patients.

10 In Figure 11.1 we will draw bars indicating standard deviations, which will hang from the associated mean forearm blood flows. This works well except for the baseline and 10 ng doses, where the mean values for blacks and whites are very close. To avoid collisions between the standard deviation bars for the two races, we will draw the white standard deviations extending above the means for these two doses. This *replace* command accomplishes this task.

11 This *twoway connected* graph draws a plot symbol at each observed value of *whitefbf* and *plotdose* and also connects these observations with straight lines. The same effect could be obtained by superimposing a *scatter* plot with a *line* plot of these variables.

12 The *xscale(log)* option of this command causes the *x*-axis to be drawn on a logarithmic scale.

13 The *angle(45)* suboption of the *xlabel* option writes the *x*-axis labels at a 45 degree angle for increased legibility.

Suppose we wanted to plot *whitefbf* against *plotdose* with connected circles at the observations, a logarithmic scale on the *x*-axis, and *x*-axis labels written at a 45 degree angle. Using the pull-down menus we would proceed as follows: Graphics ▶ Twoway graph (Scatter, line, etc.) ┘Plots└ [Create] ┘Plot└ ┌ Choose a plot category and type — Basic plots: (Select type) *Connected* ┘ ┌ Plot type: (connected line plot) — Y variable: *whitefbf*, X variable: *plotdose* [Marker properties] ┘Main└ ┌ Marker properties — Symbol: *Circle* ┘ [Accept] ┘ [Accept] ┘X axis└ [Major tick/label properties] ┘Labels└ ┌ Labels — Angle: *45 degrees* ⌟ Accept Axis scale properties ✓ Use logarithmic scale Accept Submit.

14 This command creates a graph that is similar to Figure 11.1. In this figure I used a graphics editor to relabel the baseline dose 0, break the *x*-axis between 0 and 10, and label the two curves *White* and *Black*.

15 We restore the long form of the data set. Note that this data set was destroyed in memory by the preceding *collapse* command.

16 This *connect(L)* option specifies that straight lines are to connect consecutive observations in the scatter plot as long as the values of the *x*-variable, *plotdose*, are increasing. Otherwise the points are not connected. Note that in the preceding command we sorted the data set by *id* and *plotdose*. This has the effect of grouping all observations on the same patient together and of ordering the values on each patient by increasing values of *plotdose*. Hence, *connect(L)* will connect the values for each patient but will not connect the last value of one patient with the first value of the next. The result is shown in Figure 11.2.

17 This *cols(1)* suboption of the *by* option causes the separate plots for white and black subjects to be plotted in a single column instead of side by side. The resulting graph is similar to Figure 11.2.

Suppose we wanted to draw of scatter plot of *fbf* by *plotdose* with lines connecting observations on the same patient. We could generate this graph with the pull-down menus as follows: Graphics ▶ Twoway graph (Scatter, line, etc.) ⌟ Plots ⌞ Create ⌟ Plot ⌞ ⌜ Choose a plot category and type — Basic plots: (Select type) *Connected* ⌟ ⌜ Plot type: (connected line plot) — Y variable: *fbf*, X variable: *plotdose* Line properties Connecting method: *Ascending* Accept ⌟ Accept Submit.

## 11.3. Response feature analysis

The simplest approach to analyzing repeated measures data is a **response feature analysis** (Crowder and Hand 1990). This approach is also called a **two-stage analysis** (Diggle et al. 2002). The basic idea is to reduce the multiple responses on each patient to a single biologically meaningful response that captures the patient attribute of greatest interest. This response measure is then analyzed in a fixed-effects one-way analysis of variance. Examples of response features that may be useful are an area under the curve or a regression slope derived from the observations on an individual patient, or the number of events that occur to an individual patient. The great advantage of this approach is that since we analyze a single value per patient we do not need to worry about the correlation structure on the multiple observations on each patient. We do need to assume that the observations on separate patients are independent, but this is usually reasonable. Another advantage is its simplicity. It is easy for non-statisticians to understand a response feature analysis. More complex analyses may appear to your colleagues as a black box from which *P*-values and confidence intervals magically arise. Also, more complex methods can be misleading if they are based on models that fit the data poorly. Another advantage of this method is that it can handle situations where some patients have missing values on some observations. The disadvantage of the response feature analysis is that we may lose some power by ignoring information that is available in the correlation structure of observations from individual patients.

## 11.4. Example: the isoproterenol data set

Figure 11.2 suggests that there is a linear relationship between forearm blood flow and the log dose of isoproterenol in both black and white patients. The hypothesis of greatest interest in this data set is whether white patients are, in general, more responsive to increasing doses of isoproterenol than black patients. There is a small degree of variation in the baseline blood flow levels and the average baseline blood flow is slightly larger in white patients than black patients (see Figure 11.1). In order to keep these facts from complicating the interpretation of our analysis, we will use as our dependent variable the change in blood flow from baseline for each patient. Figure 11.3 shows a scatter plot of the responses for the first patient ($id = 1$) together with the linear regression line for change in blood flow against log dose of isoproterenol. As can be seen from this figure, this model provides an excellent fit for this patient. The quality of the model fit for the other patients is similar. The estimate of the regression slope parameter for this patient is 7.18. We calculate the corresponding slope estimates for all the other patients in this experiment. These slopes are shown as dot plots for black and white subjects in Figure 11.4. Box plots (without whiskers) for black and white patients are also shown. The difference in response of black and white patients is quite marked. There are only two black subjects whose slopes are higher than the lowest slope for a white patient. There are outliers in both the black and white subject groups. For this reason we will analyze these slopes using the Wilcoxon–Mann–Whitney rank-sum test. (Had there been three or more racial groups we would have used a one-way analysis of variance or a Kruskal–Wallis test.) The Wilcoxon–Mann–Whitney test gives

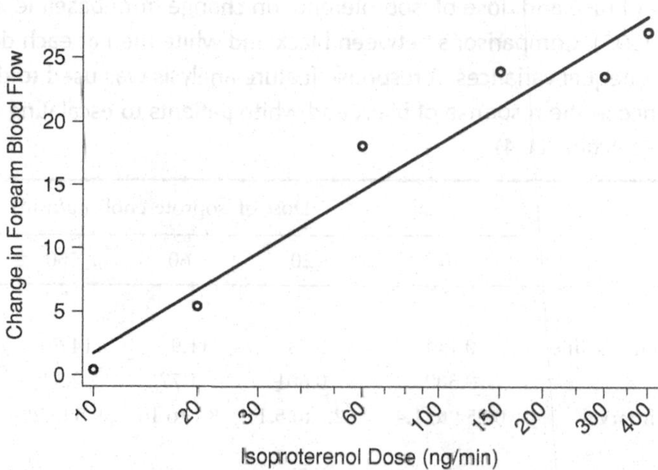


Figure 11.3 Scatter plot of change from baseline forearm blood flow in response to escalating isoproterenol dose for a single patient (*id* = 1). Note that dose is plotted on a logarithmic scale. The linear regression line of change in blood flow against log dose is also plotted and fits these data well. The slope of this regression line for this patient is 7.18. We calculate a similar slope for every patient in the study. These slopes are plotted in Figure 11.4.

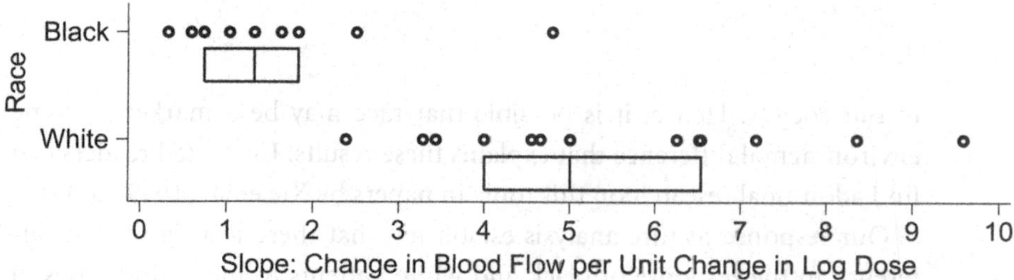


Figure 11.4 Dot and (whiskerless) box plots of the individual regression slopes in white and black patients treated with escalating doses of isoproterenol by Lang et al. (1995). Each circle represents the regression slope of change in forearm blood flow against log dose of isoproterenol for an individual subject. These slopes were analyzed using the Wilcoxon–Mann–Whitney rank-sum test, which showed that slopes for white study subjects were significantly higher than those for black study subjects ($P = 0.0006$).

a *P*-value of 0.0006. Hence, it is clear that the markedly stronger response of white patients to increasing doses of isoproterenol can not be explained by chance. Of course, one needs to be very cautious about inferring that this difference in response between black and white patients is of genetic origin. This is because genetic and environmental factors are highly confounded

**Table 11.1.** Effect of race and dose of isoproterenol on change from baseline in forearm blood flow (Lang et al., 1995). Comparisons between black and white men at each dose were made using $t$ tests with unequal variances. A response feature analysis was used to demonstrate a significant difference in the response of black and white patients to escalating doses of isoproterenol (see Section 11.4)

| | Dose of isoproterenol (ng/min) | | | | | |
|---|---|---|---|---|---|---|
| | 10 | 20 | 60 | 150 | 300 | 400 |
| *White subjects* | | | | | | |
| Mean change from baseline | 0.734 | 3.78 | 11.9 | 14.6 | 17.5 | 21.7 |
| Standard error | 0.309 | 0.601 | 1.77 | 2.32 | 2.13 | 2.16 |
| 95% confidence interval | 0.054 to 1.4 | 2.5 to 5.1 | 8.1 to 16 | 9.5 to 20 | 13 to 22 | 17 to 26 |
| *Black subjects* | | | | | | |
| Mean change from baseline | 0.397 | 1.03 | 3.12 | 4.05 | 6.88 | 5.59 |
| Standard error | 0.207 | 0.313 | 0.607 | 0.651 | 1.30 | 1.80 |
| 95% confidence interval | −0.081 to 0.87 | 0.31 to 1.8 | 1.7 to 4.5 | 2.6 to 5.6 | 3.9 to 9.9 | 1.4 to 9.7 |
| *Mean difference* | | | | | | |
| White – black | 0.338 | 2.75 | 8.82 | 10.5 | 10.6 | 16.1 |
| 95% confidence interval | −0.44 to 1.1 | 1.3 to 4.2 | 4.8 to 13 | 5.3 to 16 | 5.4 to 16 | 10 to 22 |
| *P*-value | 0.38 | 0.0009 | 0.0003 | 0.0008 | 0.0005 | <0.0001 |

in our society. Hence, it is possible that race may be a marker of some environmental difference that explains these results. Interested readers can find additional research on this topic in papers by Xie et al. (1999, 2000).

Our response feature analysis establishes that there is a significant difference in the response of black and white patients to increasing doses of isoproterenol. This justifies determining which doses induce a significant effect using the same logic as in Fisher's protected LSD procedure (see Section 10.2). Table 11.1 shows the results of these sub-analyses. The differences in change from baseline between black and white patients at each dose in this table are assessed using independent $t$ tests. The standard errors for black patients tend to be lower than for whites and Levene's test for equal variances is significant at doses 20, 60, and 150. For this reason, we use Satterthwaite's $t$ test, which assumes unequal variances (see Section 1.4.13). Equations (1.13) and (1.15) are used to derive the $P$-values and confidence intervals, respectively, for the differences in change from baseline given in Table 11.1. This table provides convincing evidence that the response to treatment is greater for white patients than for black patients at all doses greater than or equal to 20 ng/min.

## 11.5. Response feature analysis using Stata

The following log file and comments illustrate how to perform the response feature analysis described in the preceding section. The *11.2.Long.Isoproterenol.dta* data set was created in Section 11.2.

```
. * 11.5.Isoproterenol.log
. *
. * Perform a response feature analysis of the effect of race and dose
. * of isoproterenol on blood flow using the data of Lang et al.
. * (1995). For each patient, we will perform separate linear
. * regressions of change in blood flow against log dose of
. * isoproterenol. The response feature that we will use is the
. * slope of each individual regression curve.
. *
. use C:\wddtext\11.2.Long.Isoproterenol.dta
. *
. * Calculate the regression slope for the first patient
. *
. regress delta_fbf logdose if id == 1                                  1

      Source |       SS       df       MS              Number of obs =       6
-------------+------------------------------           F(  1,     4) =   71.86
       Model |  570.114431     1  570.114431           Prob > F      =  0.0011
    Residual |  31.7339077     4  7.93347694           R-squared     =  0.9473
-------------+------------------------------           Adj R-squared =  0.9341
       Total |  601.848339     5  120.369668           Root MSE      =  2.8166

------------------------------------------------------------------------------
   delta_fbf |      Coef.   Std. Err.      t    P>|t|     [95% Conf. Interval]
-------------+----------------------------------------------------------------
     logdose |   7.181315   .8471392     8.48   0.001      4.82928    9.533351
       _cons |  -14.82031   3.860099    -3.84   0.018    -25.53767    -4.10296
------------------------------------------------------------------------------

. predict yhat
(option xb assumed; fitted values)
(22 missing values generated)
. scatter delta_fbf dose if dose !=0 & id == 1                          2
>     || line yhat dose  if dose !=0 & id == 1
>     , ylabel(0 5 10 15 20 25)
>       ytitle(Change in Forearm Blood Flow) xscale(log)
```

```
>       xlabel(10 20 30 60 100 150 200 300 400, angle(45))
>       xmtick(10(10)90 250 350) legend(off)
.  *
.  * Calculate regression slopes for each patient.
.  * Reduce data set to one record per patient.
.  * The variable slope contains the regression slopes; race
.  * is included in the by option of the statsby command to
.  * keep this variable in the data file.
.  *
. statsby slope = _b[logdose], by(id race) clear :
>     regress delta_fbf logdose
```
3

```
(running regress on estimation sample)

      command:  regress delta_fbf logdose
        slope:  _b[logdose]
           by:  id race

Statsby groups
```
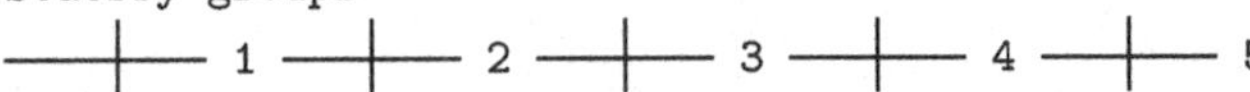

```
......................
```

```
. list id slope race
```
4

|  | id | slope | race |
|---|---|---|---|
| 1. | 1 | 7.181315 | White |
| 2. | 2 | 6.539237 | White |
| 3. | 3 | 3.999704 | White |
| 4. | 4 | 4.665485 | White |
| 5. | 5 | 4.557809 | White |
| 6. | 6 | 6.252436 | White |
| 7. | 7 | 2.385183 | White |
| 8. | 8 | 8.354769 | White |
| 9. | 9 | 9.590916 | White |
| 10. | 10 | 6.515281 | White |
| 11. | 11 | 3.280572 | White |
| 12. | 12 | 3.434072 | White |
| 13. | 13 | 5.004545 | White |
| 14. | 14 | .5887727 | Black |
| 15. | 15 | 1.828892 | Black |

```
     +---------------------------+
16.  | 16   .3241574    Black    |
17.  | 17    1.31807    Black    |
18.  | 18   1.630882    Black    |
19.  | 19   .7392463    Black    |
20.  | 20   2.513615    Black    |
     |---------------------------|
21.  | 21   1.031773    Black    |
22.  | 22   4.805952    Black    |
     +---------------------------+

. stripplot slope, over(race) boffset(-0.1)                                    5
>     box(lwidth(medthick)  barwidth(0.1)) xsize(5)
>     xtitle(Slope: Change in Blood Flow per Unit Change in Log Dose)
. *
. * Do ranksum test on slopes.
. *
. ranksum slope, by(race)                                                      6

Two-sample Wilcoxon rank-sum (Mann-Whitney) test

        race |      obs    rank sum    expected
-------------+---------------------------------
       White |       13         201       149.5
       Black |        9          52       103.5
-------------+---------------------------------
    combined |       22         253         253

unadjusted variance      224.25
adjustment for ties       -0.00
                         ----------
adjusted variance        224.25

Ho: slope(race==White) = slope(race==Black)
             z =   3.439
    Prob > |z| =   0.0006
. *
. * Do t tests comparing change in blood flow in blacks and whites at
. * different doses
. *
. use C:\wddtext\11.2.Long.Isoproterenol.dta, clear                            7
. sort dose
. drop if dose == 0
(22 observations deleted)
```

```
. by dose: ttest delta_fbf , by(race) unequal
```
8

```
-> dose = 10

Two-sample t test with unequal variances

   Group |     Obs        Mean    Std. Err.   Std. Dev.   [95% Conf. Interval]
---------+--------------------------------------------------------------------
   White |      12    .7341667    .3088259    1.069804    .0544455    1.413888
   Black |       9    .3966667    .2071634    .6214902    -.081053    .8743863
---------+--------------------------------------------------------------------
combined |      21    .5895238    .1967903    .9018064    .1790265    1.000021
---------+--------------------------------------------------------------------
    diff |               .3375    .3718737               -.4434982    1.118498
------------------------------------------------------------------------------
    diff = mean(White) - mean(Black)                              t =   0.9076
Ho: diff = 0                     Satterthwaite's degrees of freedom =  18.0903

    Ha: diff < 0                 Ha: diff != 0                 Ha: diff > 0
 Pr(T < t) = 0.8120         Pr(|T| > |t|) = 0.3760          Pr(T > t) = 0.1880
------------------------------------------------------------------------------
-> dose = 20

Two-sample t test with unequal variances

   Group |     Obs        Mean    Std. Err.   Std. Dev.   [95% Conf. Interval]
---------+--------------------------------------------------------------------
   White |      12    3.775833    .6011875    2.082575    2.452628    5.099038
   Black |       9        1.03    .3130229    .9390686     .308168    1.751832
---------+--------------------------------------------------------------------
combined |      21    2.599048    .4719216    2.162616    1.614636    3.583459
---------+--------------------------------------------------------------------
    diff |            2.745833    .6777977                1.309989    4.181677
------------------------------------------------------------------------------
    diff = mean(White) - mean(Black)                              t =   4.0511
Ho: diff = 0                     Satterthwaite's degrees of freedom =  16.1415

    Ha: diff < 0                 Ha: diff != 0                 Ha: diff > 0
 Pr(T < t) = 0.9995         Pr(|T| > |t|) = 0.0009          Pr(T > t) = 0.0005
------------------------------------------------------------------------------
```

Output omitted. See Table 11.1

```
-> dose = 400

Two-sample t test with unequal variances

------------------------------------------------------------------------------
   Group |     Obs        Mean    Std. Err.   Std. Dev.   [95% Conf. Interval]
---------+--------------------------------------------------------------------
   White |      13    21.69308    2.163637    7.801104    16.97892    26.40724
   Black |       9    5.586667     1.80355    5.410649    1.427673     9.74566
---------+--------------------------------------------------------------------
combined |      22    15.10409    2.252517    10.56524    10.41972    19.78846
---------+--------------------------------------------------------------------
    diff |            16.10641    2.816756                 10.2306    21.98222
------------------------------------------------------------------------------
    diff = mean(White) - mean(Black)                              t =   5.7181
Ho: diff = 0                     Satterthwaite's degrees of freedom =  19.9917

    Ha: diff < 0                 Ha: diff != 0                 Ha: diff > 0
 Pr(T < t) = 1.0000         Pr(|T| > |t|) = 0.0000          Pr(T > t) = 0.0000

. log close
```

**Comments**

1 We regress change in blood flow against log dose of isoproterenol for the observations from the first patient. Note that *logdose* is missing when *dose* = 0. Hence, only the six positive doses are included in this analysis. The regression slope for this patient is 7.18. We could obtain the slopes for all 22 patients with the command

**by id: regress *delta_fbf logdose***

However, this would require extracting the slope estimates by hand and re-entering them into Stata. This is somewhat tedious to do and is prone to transcription error. Alternatively, we can use the *statsby* command described below.

2 This graph shows the regression line and individual data points for the first patient. It is similar to Figure 11.3.

3 This *statsby* command regresses *delta_fbf* against *logdose* for each combination of distinct values of *id* and *race* (i.e. for each individual patient). The original dataset in memory is deleted! In its place is a dataset with one record per distinct combination of values of the *by* variables. In addition, a new variable, *slope*, is created which equals the estimated slope coefficient from the regression for each separate patient. Note that including *race* in the *by* option in addition to *id* does not affect the regressions performed here since a patient's race does not change during the study. We include

*race* in this *by* option in order to keep this variable in the subsequent dataset.

The equivalent point-and-click command is Statistics ▶ Other ▶ Collect statistics for a command across a by list ⌋ Main ⌊ Stata command to run: *regress delta_fbf logdose* ⌈ List of statistics — Other statistical expressions: *slope = _b[logdose]* ⌋ Group variables: (required) *id race* Submit.

4 We list the individual slope estimates for each patient. Note that the highlighted slope estimate for the first patient is identical to the estimate obtained earlier with the *regress* command.
5 This graph, which is similar to Figure 11.4, highlights the difference in the distribution of slope estimates between black and white patients.
6 This *ranksum* command performs a Wilcoxon–Mann–Whitney rank sum test of the null hypothesis that the distribution of slopes is the same for both races. The test is highly significant, giving a *P*-value of 0.0006.
7 The preceding *statsby* command deleted most of the data. We must read in the data set before performing *t* tests at the different doses.
8 This *ttest* command performs independent *t* tests of *delta_fbf* in black and white patients at each dose of isoproterenol. Unequal variances between racial groups are assumed. The output for doses 60, 150, and 300 have been omitted. The highlighted output from this command is also given in Table 11.1.

## 11.6. The area-under-the-curve response feature

A response feature that is often useful in response feature analysis is the **area under the curve**. Suppose that $y_i(t)$ is the response from the $i^{\text{th}}$ patient at time $t$. Suppose further that we measure this response at times $t_1, t_2, \ldots, t_n$, and that $y_{ij} = y_i(t_j)$, for $j = 1, 2, \ldots, n$. We can estimate the area under the curve $y_i(t)$ between $t_1$ and $t_n$ as follows. Draw a scatter plot of $y_{ij}$ against $t_j$ for $j = 1, 2, \ldots, n$. Then, draw straight lines connecting the points $(t_1, y_{i1})$, $(t_2, y_{i2}), \ldots, (t_n, y_{in})$. We estimate the area under the curve to be the area under these lines. Specifically, the area under the line from $(t_j, y_{ij})$ to $(t_{j+1}, y_{i,j+1})$ is

$$\left(\frac{y_{ij} + y_{i,j+1}}{2}\right)(t_{j+1} - t_j). \tag{11.1}$$

Hence, the area under the entire curve is estimated by

$$\sum_{j=1}^{n-1}\left(\frac{y_{ij} + y_{i,j+1}}{2}\right)(t_{j+1} - t_j). \tag{11.2}$$

For example, if $n = 3$, $t_1 = 0$, $t_2 = 1$, $t_3 = 3$, $y_{i1} = 4$, $y_{i2} = 8$ and $y_{i3} = 6$ then Equation (11.2) reduces to

$$\left(\frac{4+8}{2}\right)(1-0) + \left(\frac{8+6}{2}\right)(3-1) = 20.$$

In a response feature analysis based on area under the curve, we use Equation (11.2) to calculate this area for each patient and then perform a one-way analysis of variance on these areas.

Equation (11.2) can be implemented in Stata as follows. Suppose that a Stata data set with repeated-measures data has one record per observation. Let the variables *id*, *time*, and *response* indicate the patient's identification number, time of observation, and response, respectively. Then the area under the response curve for study subjects can be calculated by using the following Stata code:

```
. sort id time
. *
. * Delete records with missing values for time or response
. *
. drop if missing(time) | missing(response)
(2 observations deleted)
. generate area = (response + response[_n+1])*(time[_n+1] - time)/2      1
>      if id == id[_n+1]
(2 missing values generated)
. collapse (sum) area, by(id)                                             2
```

**Comments**

1 The variable *area* is the area under the curve for the current patient between the current and next observation time (see Equation (11.1)). Note that for each patient there are one fewer areas between adjacent observation times than there are observation times; no area is defined for the last observation on each patient.

2 This *collapse* command sums all of the values of *area* for each patient. The resulting area under the curve is also called *area* (see Equation (11.2)). We could also have calculated this area using the syntax explained on page 257, in which case the command would have been

```
collapse (sum) area = area, by(id)
```

After the execution of this command the data file contains one record per patient.

## 11.7. Generalized estimating equations

There are a number of excellent methods for analyzing repeated measures data. One of these is **generalized estimating equations (GEE)** analysis. This approach extends the generalized linear model so that it can handle repeated measures data (Zeger and Liang, 1986). Suppose that we observe an unbiased sample of $n$ patients from some target population and that the $i^{th}$ patient is observed on $n_i$ separate occasions. Let $y_{ij}$ be the response of the $i^{th}$ patient at her $j^{th}$ observation and let $x_{ij1}, x_{ij2}, \ldots, x_{ijq}$ be $q$ covariates that are measured on her at this time. Let $\mathbf{x}_{ij} = (x_{ij1}, x_{ij2}, \ldots, x_{ijq})$ denote the values of all of the covariates for the $i^{th}$ patient at her $j^{th}$ observation. Then the model used by GEE analysis assumes that:

(i) The distribution of $y_{ij}$ belongs to the exponential family of distributions. This is a large family that includes the normal, binomial, and Poisson distributions; $y_{ij}$ is called the random component of the model.

(ii) The expected value of $y_{ij}$ given the patient's covariates $x_{ij1}, x_{ij2}, \ldots, x_{ijq}$ is related to the model parameters through an equation of the form

$$g[E[y_{ij} \mid \mathbf{x}_{ij}]] = \alpha + \beta_1 x_{ij1} + \beta_2 x_{ij2} + \cdots + \beta_q x_{ijq}. \tag{11.3}$$

In Equation (11.3), $\alpha$, $\beta_1$, $\beta_2, \ldots,$ and $\beta_q$ are unknown parameters and $g$ is a smooth function that is either always increasing or always decreasing over the range of $y_{ij}$. The function $g$ is the link function for the model; $\alpha + \beta_1 x_{ij1} + \beta_2 x_{ij2} + \cdots + \beta_q x_{ijq}$ is the linear predictor.

(iii) Responses from different patients are mutually independent.

When there is only one observation per patient ($n_i = 1$ for all $i$), Model (11.3) is, in fact, the generalized linear model. In this case, when $g$ is the identity function ($g[y] = y$), and $y_{ij}$ is normally distributed, (11.3) reduces to multiple linear regression; when $g$ is the logit function and $y_{ij}$ has a binomial distribution, (11.3) describes logistic regression; when $g$ is the logarithmic function and $y_{ij}$ has a Poisson distribution, this model becomes Poisson regression. Model (11.3) differs from the generalized linear model in that it does not make any assumptions about how observations on the same patient are correlated.

## 11.8. Common correlation structures

Let $\rho_{jk}$ denote the population correlation coefficient between the $j^{th}$ and $k^{th}$ observations on the same patient. If all patients have $n$ observations, we express the correlation structure for each patient's observations as the following square array of correlation coefficients:

$$\mathbf{R} = \begin{bmatrix} 1 & \rho_{12} & \rho_{13} & \cdots & \rho_{1n} \\ \rho_{21} & 1 & \rho_{23} & \cdots & \rho_{2n} \\ \rho_{31} & \rho_{32} & 1 & \cdots & \rho_{3n} \\ \vdots & \vdots & \vdots & \ddots & \vdots \\ \rho_{n1} & \rho_{n2} & \rho_{n3} & \cdots & 1 \end{bmatrix}. \tag{11.4}$$

**R** is called the **correlation matrix** for repeated observations on study subjects. In this matrix, the coefficient in the $j^{\text{th}}$ row and $k^{\text{th}}$ column is the correlation coefficient between the $j^{\text{th}}$ and $k^{\text{th}}$ observations. The diagonal elements are always 1 since any observation will be perfectly correlated with itself. Any correlation matrix will be symmetric about the diagonal that runs from upper left to lower right. This is because the correlation between the $j^{\text{th}}$ and $k^{\text{th}}$ observation equals the correlation between the $k^{\text{th}}$ and $j^{\text{th}}$ observation.

There are a number of special correlation structures that come up in various models. However, we will only need to mention two of these here. The first is the **unstructured correlation** matrix given by Equation (11.4). Although this matrix makes no assumptions about the correlation structure it requires $n(n-1)/2$ correlation parameters. Estimating this large number of parameters may be difficult if the number of observations per patient is large. The second is the **exchangeable correlation** structure, which assumes that

$$\mathbf{R} = \begin{bmatrix} 1 & \rho & \rho & \cdots & \rho \\ \rho & 1 & \rho & \cdots & \rho \\ \rho & \rho & 1 & \cdots & \rho \\ \vdots & \vdots & \vdots & \ddots & \vdots \\ \rho & \rho & \rho & \cdots & 1 \end{bmatrix}. \tag{11.5}$$

In other words, the exchangeable structure assumes that any two distinct observations from the same patient have the same correlation coefficient $\rho$. Many data sets have much more complicated correlation structures. In particular, observations on a patient taken closer in time are often more correlated than observations taken far apart. Also, the correlation structure is not necessarily the same for all patients. Nevertheless, the exchangeable correlation structure will meet our needs for GEE analysis. This is because a GEE analysis requires only a rough estimate of this structure to get started. Its final parameter estimates are not usually dependent on the accuracy of our initial assumptions about the correlation matrix.

## 11.9. GEE analysis and the Huber–White sandwich estimator

GEE analysis is computationally and methodologically complex (Diggle et al., 2002). However, the basic idea of the analysis can be summarized as follows.

1 We select a working correlation matrix $\mathbf{R}_i$ for each patient. $\mathbf{R}_i$, the matrix for the $i^{\text{th}}$ patient, can be quite complicated, but need not be. An exchangeable correlation structure usually works just fine. From this, we estimate the working variance–covariance matrix for the $i^{\text{th}}$ patient. This is a function of both the working correlation matrix and the link function $g$. For example, if we use an exchangeable correlation structure, the identity link function, and a normal random component then the working variance–covariance matrix specifies that $y_{ij}$ will have variance $\sigma^2$ and that the covariance between any two distinct observations on the $i^{\text{th}}$ patient will equal $\rho\sigma^2$.

2 Using the working variance–covariance structure we obtain estimates of the model parameters. This is done using a technique called **quasi-likelihood**, which is related to maximum likelihood estimation but does not require the likelihood function to be fully specified.

3 We estimate the variance–covariance matrix of our model parameters using a technique called the **Huber–White sandwich estimator**.

4 We use our parameter estimates and the Huber–White variance–covariance matrix to test hypotheses or construct confidence intervals from relevant weighted sums of the parameter estimates (see Sections 5.14 through 5.16).

What is truly amazing about this technique is that, under mild regularity conditions, the Huber–White variance–covariance estimate converges to the true variance–covariance matrix of the parameter estimates as $n$ gets large. This is so even when the working correlation matrix is incorrectly specified. Thus, we can specify a very simple working matrix such as the exchangeable correlation matrix for models in which none of the observations obey this structure and the correlation structure may vary for different study subjects. This result holds, however, "... only when there is a diminishing fraction of missing data or when the data are missing completely at random" (Zeger and Liang, 1986; page 125). For this reason, if there are only a small number of missing values that are concentrated in a few patients, and if the true variance–covariance structure is complicated, it can sometimes be prudent to drop patients with missing response values from the analysis. When there is a large proportion of patients who have at least one missing response value, dropping patients with missing values is not an option since it can lead to serious non-response bias as well as loss of power. If you include patients with missing values in your analysis, then the validity of your choice of working correlation matrix can become important; if the true correlation structure cannot be reasonably modeled by any of the working correlation matrices provided by your statistical software, then GEE may not be the best approach to analyzing your data. (See Exercises 6–8.)

## 11.10. Example: analyzing the isoproterenol data with GEE

Suppose that in Model (11.3), $y_{ij}$ is a normally distributed random component and $g[y] = y$ is the identity link function. Then Model (11.3) reduces to

$$E[y_{ij}|\mathbf{x}_{ij}] = \alpha + \beta_1 x_{ij1} + \beta_2 x_{ij2} + \cdots + \beta_q x_{ijq}. \tag{11.6}$$

Model (11.6) is a special case of the GEE model (11.3). We now analyze the blood flow, race and isoproterenol data set of Lang et al. (1995) using this model. Let

$y_{ij}$ be the change from baseline in forearm blood flow for the $i^{\text{th}}$ patient at the $j^{\text{th}}$ dose of isoproterenol,

$$white_i = \begin{cases} 1: & \text{if the } i^{\text{th}} \text{ patient is white} \\ 0: & \text{if he is black, and} \end{cases}$$

$$dose_{jk} = \begin{cases} 1: & \text{if } j = k \\ 0: & \text{otherwise.} \end{cases}$$

We will assume that $y_{ij}$ is normally distributed and

$$E[y_{ij} \mid white_i,\ j] = \alpha + \beta \times white_i + \sum_{k=2}^{6} (\gamma_k dose_{jk} + \delta_k \times white_i \times dose_{jk}), \tag{11.7}$$

where $\alpha, \beta, \{\gamma_k, \delta_k : k = 2, \ldots, 6\}$ are the model parameters. Model (11.7) is a special case of Model (11.6). Note that this model implies that the expected change in blood flow is

$\alpha$ for a black man on the first dose, (11.8)

$\alpha + \beta$ for a white man on the first dose, (11.9)

$\alpha + \gamma_j$ for a black man on the $j^{\text{th}}$ dose with $j > 1$, and (11.10)

$\alpha + \beta + \gamma_j + \delta_j$ for a white man on the $j^{\text{th}}$ dose with $j > 1$. (11.11)

It must be noted that patient 8 in this study has four missing blood flow measurements. This concentration of missing values in one patient causes the choice of the working correlation matrix to have an appreciable effect on our model estimates. Regardless of the working correlation matrix, the working variance for $y_{ij}$ in Model (11.6) is constant. Figure 11.2 suggests that this variance is greater for white than black patients and increases with increasing dose. Hence, it is troubling to have our parameter estimates affected by a working correlation matrix that we know is wrong. Also, the Huber–White variance–covariance estimate is only valid when the missing values are few and randomly distributed. For these reasons, we delete patient 8 from our analysis. This results in parameter estimates and a Huber–White variance–covariance estimate that are unaffected by our choice of the working correlation matrix.

Let $\hat{\alpha}, \hat{\beta}, \{\hat{\gamma}_k, \hat{\delta}_k : k = 2, \ldots, 6\}$ denote the GEE parameter estimates from the model. Then our estimates of the mean change in blood flow in black and white patients at the different doses are given by Equations (11.8) through (11.11) with the parameter estimates substituting for the true parameter values. Subtracting the estimate of Equation (11.8) from that for Equation (11.9) gives the estimated mean difference in change in flow between white and black patients at dose 1, which is

$$(\hat{\alpha} + \hat{\beta}) - \hat{\alpha} = \hat{\beta}. \tag{11.12}$$

Subtracting the estimate of Equation (11.10) from that for Equation (11.11) gives the estimated mean difference in change in flow between white and black patients at dose $j > 1$, which is

$$(\hat{\alpha} + \hat{\beta} + \hat{\gamma}_j + \hat{\delta}_j) - (\hat{\alpha} + \hat{\gamma}_j) = (\hat{\beta} + \hat{\delta}_j). \tag{11.13}$$

Tests of significance and 95% confidence intervals can be calculated for these estimates using the Huber–White variance–covariance matrix. This is done in the same way as was illustrated in Sections 5.14 through 5.16. These estimates, standard errors, confidence intervals, and *P*-values are given in Table 11.2.

Testing the null hypothesis that there is no interaction between race and dose on blood flow is equivalent to testing the null hypothesis that the effects of race and dose on blood flow are additive. In other words, we test the null hypothesis that $\delta_2 = \delta_3 = \delta_4 = \delta_5 = \delta_6 = 0$. Under this null hypothesis a chi-squared statistic can be calculated that has as many degrees of freedom as there are interaction parameters (in this case five). This statistic equals 40.41, which is highly significant ($P < 0.000\,05$). Hence, we can conclude that the observed interaction is certainly not due to chance.

**Table 11.2.** Effect of race and dose of isoproterenol on change from baseline in forearm blood flow (Lang et al., 1995). This table was produced using a generalized estimating equation (GEE) analysis. Note that the confidence intervals in this table are slightly narrower than the corresponding intervals in Table 11.1. This GEE analysis is slightly more powerful than the response feature analysis that produced Table 11.1

| | Dose of isoproterenol (ng/min) | | | | | |
|---|---|---|---|---|---|---|
| | 10 | 20 | 60 | 150 | 300 | 400 |
| *White subjects* | | | | | | |
| Mean change from baseline | 0.734 | 3.78 | 11.9 | 14.6 | 17.5 | 21.2 |
| Standard error | 0.303 | 0.590 | 1.88 | 2.27 | 2.09 | 2.23 |
| 95% confidence interval | 0.14 to 1.3 | 2.6 to 4.9 | 8.2 to 16 | 10 to 19 | 13 to 22 | 17 to 26 |
| *Black subjects* | | | | | | |
| Mean change from baseline | 0.397 | 1.03 | 3.12 | 4.05 | 6.88 | 5.59 |
| Standard error | 0.200 | 0.302 | 0.586 | 0.629 | 1.26 | 1.74 |
| 95% confidence interval | 0.0044 to 0.79 | 0.44 to 1.6 | 2.0 to 4.3 | 2.8 to 5.3 | 4.4 to 9.3 | 2.2 to 9.0 |
| *Mean difference* | | | | | | |
| White – black | 0.338 | 2.75 | 8.79 | 10.5 | 10.6 | 15.6 |
| 95% confidence interval | −0.37 to 1.0 | 1.4 to 4.0 | 4.9 to 13 | 5.9 to 15 | 5.9 to 15 | 10 to 21 |
| *P*-value | 0.35 | <0.0005 | <0.0005 | <0.0005 | <0.0005 | <0.0001 |

The GEE and response feature analysis (RFA) in Tables 11.2 and 11.1 should be compared. Note that the mean changes in blood flow in the two races and six dose levels are very similar. They would be identical except that patient 8 is excluded from the GEE analysis but is included in the RFA. This is a challenging data set to analyze in view of the fact that the standard deviation of the response variable increases with dose and differs between the races. The GEE analysis does an excellent job at modeling this variation. Note how the standard errors in Table 11.2 increase from black subjects to white subjects at any dose or from low dose to high dose within either race. Figure 11.5 compares the mean difference between black and white subjects at the six different doses. The white and gray bars are from the RFA and GEE analyses, respectively. Note that these two analyses provide very similar results for these data. The GEE analysis is slightly more powerful than the RFA as is indicated by the slightly narrower confidence intervals for its estimates. This increase in power is achieved at a cost of considerable methodological complexity in the GEE model. The GEE approach constitutes an impressive intellectual achievement and is a valuable tool for advanced statistical analysis. Nevertheless, RFA is a simple and easily understood approach to repeated

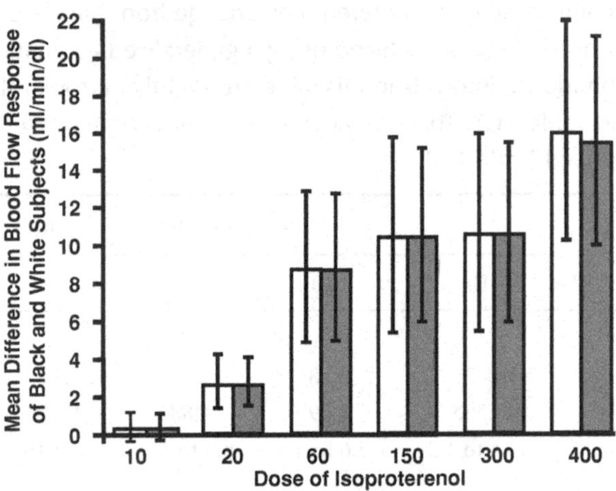


Figure 11.5 This graph shows the mean differences between black and white study subjects given at the bottom of Tables 11.1 and 11.2. The white and gray bars are from the response feature analysis (RFA) and generalized estimating equation (GEE) analysis, respectively. The vertical lines give the 95% confidence intervals for these differences. These analyses give very similar results. The GEE analysis is slightly more powerful than the RFA as is indicated by the slightly narrower confidence intervals of the GEE results.

measures analysis that can, as in this example, approach the power of a GEE analysis. At the very least, it is worth considering as a crosscheck against more sophisticated multiple regression models for repeated measures data.

## 11.11. Using Stata to analyze the isoproterenol data set using GEE

The following log file and comments illustrate how to perform the GEE analysis from Section 11.10 using Stata.

```
. *  11.11.Isoproterenol.log
. *
. *  Perform a GEE analysis of the effect of race and dose of
. *  isoproterenol on blood flow using the data of
. *  Lang et al. (1995).
. *
. use C:\WDDtext\11.2.Long.Isoproterenol.dta
```

```
. drop if dose == 0 | id == 8                                                  1
(28 observations deleted)

. generate white = race == 1

. *
. * Analyze data using classification variables with interaction
. *
. xi: xtgee delta_fbf i.dose*white, i(id) robust                               2
i.dose            _Idose_10-400       (naturally coded; _Idose_10 omitted)
i.dose*white      _IdosXwhi_#         (coded as above)

Iteration 1: tolerance = 2.066e-13

GEE population-averaged model                   Number of obs      =       126
Group variable:                         id      Number of groups   =        21
Link:                             identity      Obs per group: min =         6
Family:                           Gaussian                     avg =       6.0
Correlation:                  exchangeable                     max =         6
                                                Wald chi2(11)      =    506.86
Scale parameter:                  23.50629      Prob > chi2        =    0.0000

                                  (Std. Err. adjusted for clustering on id)

------------------------------------------------------------------------------
             |             Semi-robust
   delta_fbf |      Coef.   Std. Err.      z    P>|z|     [95% Conf. Interval]
-------------+----------------------------------------------------------------
    _Idose_20 |   .6333333   .2706638    2.34   0.019     .1028421    1.163825
    _Idose_60 |   2.724445   .6585882    4.14   0.000     1.433635    4.015254
   _Idose_150 |   3.656667   .7054437    5.18   0.000     2.274022    5.039311
   _Idose_300 |   6.478889   1.360126    4.76   0.000     3.813091    9.144687
   _Idose_400 |       5.19   1.830717    2.83   0.005     1.601861     8.77814
        white |      .3375    .363115    0.93   0.353    -.3741922    1.049192   3
  _IdosXwhi_20 |   2.408333   .5090358    4.73   0.000     1.410642    3.406025
  _IdosXwhi_60 |   8.450556   1.823352    4.63   0.000     4.876852    12.02426
  _IdosXwh~150 |   10.17667    2.20775    4.61   0.000     5.849557    14.50378
  _IdosXwh~300 |   10.30444   2.305474    4.47   0.000     5.785798    14.82309
  _IdosXwh~400 |   15.22667   2.748106    5.54   0.000     9.840479    20.61285
        _cons |   .3966667   .2001388    1.98   0.047     .0044017    .7889316   4
------------------------------------------------------------------------------
```

```
. lincom _cons + white                                                        5
( 1)  white + _cons = 0
```

| delta_fbf | Coef. | Std. Err. | z | P>\|z\| | [95% Conf. | Interval] |
|---|---|---|---|---|---|---|
| (1) | .7341667 | .30298 | 2.42 | 0.015 | .1403367 | 1.327997 |

```
. lincom _cons + _Idose_20                                                    6
( 1)  _Idose_20 + _cons = 0
```

| delta_fbf | Coef. | Std. Err. | z | P>\|z\| | [95% Conf. | Interval] |
|---|---|---|---|---|---|---|
| (1) | 1.03 | .3024088 | 3.41 | 0.001 | .4372896 | 1.62271 |

```
. lincom _cons + _Idose_20 + white +_IdosXwhi_20                              7
( 1)  _Idose_20 + white + _IdosXwhi_20 + _cons = 0
```

| delta_fbf | Coef. | Std. Err. | z | P>\|z\| | [95% Conf. | Interval] |
|---|---|---|---|---|---|---|
| (1) | 3.775833 | .5898076 | 6.40 | 0.000 | 2.619832 | 4.931835 |

```
. lincom                    white +_IdosXwhi_20                               8
( 1)  white + _IdosXwhi_20 = 0
```

| delta_fbf | Coef. | Std. Err. | z | P>\|z\| | [95% Conf. | Interval] |
|---|---|---|---|---|---|---|
| (1) | 2.745833 | .6628153 | 4.14 | 0.000 | 1.446739 | 4.044927 |

```
. lincom _cons + _Idose_60
```

Output omitted. See Table 11.2

```
. lincom _cons + _Idose_60 + white +_IdosXwhi_60
```

Output omitted. See Table 11.2

```
. lincom                    white +_IdosXwhi_60
```

Output omitted. See Table 11.2

```
. lincom _cons + _Idose_150
```

Output omitted. See Table 11.2

```
. lincom _cons + _Idose_150 + white +_IdosXwhi_150
```

Output omitted. See Table 11.2

```
. lincom                          white +_IdosXwhi_150
```

Output omitted. See Table 11.2

```
. lincom _cons + _Idose_300
```

Output omitted. See Table 11.2

```
. lincom _cons + _Idose_300 + white +_IdosXwhi_300
```

Output omitted. See Table 11.2

```
. lincom                          white +_IdosXwhi_300
```

Output omitted. See Table 11.2

```
. lincom _cons + _Idose_400
 ( 1)  _Idose_400 + _cons = 0
```

| delta_fbf | Coef. | Std. Err. | z | P>\|z\| | [95% Conf. | Interval] |
|---|---|---|---|---|---|---|
| (1) | 5.586667 | 1.742395 | 3.21 | 0.001 | 2.171636 | 9.001698 |

```
. lincom _cons + _Idose_400 + white +_IdosXwhi_400
 ( 1)  _Idose_400 + white + _IdosXwhi_400 + _cons = 0
```

| delta_fbf | Coef. | Std. Err. | z | P>\|z\| | [95% Conf. | Interval] |
|---|---|---|---|---|---|---|
| (1) | 21.15083 | 2.233954 | 9.47 | 0.000 | 16.77236 | 25.5293 |

```
. lincom                          white +_IdosXwhi_400
 ( 1)  white + _IdosXwhi_400 = 0
```

| delta_fbf | Coef. | Std. Err. | z | P>\|z\| | [95% Conf. | Interval] |
|---|---|---|---|---|---|---|
| (1) | 15.56417 | 2.833106 | 5.49 | 0.000 | 10.01138 | 21.11695 |

```
. test _IdosXwhi_20 _IdosXwhi_60 _IdosXwhi_150
>       _IdosXwhi_300 _IdosXwhi_400
 ( 1)  _IdosXwhi_20 = 0
 ( 2)  _IdosXwhi_60 = 0
 ( 3)  _IdosXwhi_150 = 0
 ( 4)  _IdosXwhi_300 = 0
 ( 5)  _IdosXwhi_400 = 0

           chi2(  5) =   40.41
         Prob > chi2 =    0.0000
. log close
```

9

**Comments**

1 We drop all records with *dose* = 0 or *id* = 8. When *dose* = 0, the change from baseline, *delta_fbf*, is, by definition, zero. We eliminate these records as they provide no useful information to our analyses. Patient 8 has four missing values. These missing values have an adverse effect on our analysis. For this reason we eliminate all observations on this patient (see Sections 11.9 and 11.10 and Question 8 in Section 11.14).

2 This *xtgee* command analyzes Model (11.7). The syntax of *i.dose***white* is analogous to that used for the *logistic* command in Section 5.23 (see also Comment 10 of Section 9.3). The default link function is the identity function. For the identity link function the default random component is the normal distribution. Hence, we do not need to specify either of these aspects of our model explicitly in this command. The *i(id)* option specifies *id* to be the variable that identifies all observations made on the same patient. The exchangeable correlation structure is the default working correlation structure, which we use here. The *robust* option specifies that the Huber–White sandwich estimator is to be used. The table of coefficients generated by this command is similar to that produced by other Stata regression commands.

   Note that if we had not used the *robust* option the model would have assumed that the exchangeable correlation structure was true. This would have led to inaccurate confidence intervals for our estimates. I strongly recommend that this option always be used in any GEE analysis.

   The equivalent point-and-click command is Statistics ▶ Generalized linear models ▶ Generalized estimating equations (GEE) Model Dependent variable: *delta_fbf* , Independent variables: *i.dose***i.white* Panel settings Main Panel ID variable: *id* OK Submit.

3 The highlighted terms are the estimated mean, *P*-value, and 95% confidence interval for the difference in response between white and black men on the first dose of isoproterenol (10 ng/min). The parameter estimate associated with the *white* covariate is $\hat{\beta} = 0.3375$ in Model (11.7). The highlighted values in this and in subsequent lines of output are entered into Table 11.2.

4 The highlighted terms are the estimated mean, standard error and 95% confidence interval for black men on the first dose of isoproterenol. The parameter estimate associated with *_cons* is $\hat{\alpha} = 0.3967$.

5 This command calculates $\hat{\alpha} + \hat{\beta}$, the mean response for white men at the first dose of isoproterenol, together with related statistics.

6 This command calculates $\hat{\alpha} + \hat{\gamma}_2$, the mean response for black men at the second dose of isoproterenol, together with related statistics.
7 This command calculates $\hat{\alpha} + \hat{\beta} + \hat{\gamma}_2 + \hat{\delta}_2$, the mean response for white men at the second dose of isoproterenol, together with related statistics.
8 This command calculates $\hat{\beta} + \hat{\delta}_2$, the mean difference in response between white and black men at the second dose of isoproterenol, together with related statistics. Analogous *lincom* commands are also given for doses 3, 4, 5, and 6.
9 This command tests the null hypothesis that the interaction parameters $\delta_2, \delta_3, \delta_4, \delta_5$, and $\delta_6$ are simultaneously equal to zero. That is, it tests the null hypothesis that the effects of race and dose on change in blood flow are additive. This test, which has five degrees of freedom, gives $P < 0.000\,05$, which allows us to reject the null hypothesis with overwhelming statistical significance.

## 11.12. GEE analyses with logistic or Poisson models

GEE analyses can be applied to any generalized linear model with repeated measures data. For logistic regression we use the logit link function and a binomial random component. For Poisson regression we use the logarithmic link function and a Poisson random component. In Stata, the syntax for specifying these terms is the same as in the *glm* command. For logistic regression, we use the *link(logit)* and *family(binomial)* options to specify the link function and random component, respectively. For Poisson regression, these options are *link(log)* and *family(poisson)*. Additional discussion on these techniques is given by Diggle et al. (2002).

## 11.13. Additional reading

Matthews et al. (1990) provide a nice discussion of response feature analysis. Like Diggle et al. they refer to it as two stage analysis.

Crowder and Hand (1990),

Diggle et al. (2002), and

Rabe-Hesketh and Skrondal (2005) are excellent texts on repeated measures data analysis. Diggle et al. (2002) is the definitive text on GEE analysis at this time. Rabe-Hesketh and Skrondal (2005) discuss many complex techniques for analyzing longitudinal data using Stata.

Lang et al. (1995) studied the effects of race and dose of isoproterenol on forearm blood flow. We used data from their study to illustrate repeated measures analyses of variance.

Xie et al. (1999) and
Xie et al. (2000) have done additional research on the relationship between blood flow and isoproterenol dose in different races.
Wishart (1938) is the earliest reference on response feature analysis that I have been able to find.
Liang and Zeger (1986) and
Zeger and Liang (1986) are the original references on generalized estimating equation analysis.
Huber (1967),
White (1980) and
White (1982) are the original references for the Huber–White sandwich estimator.

## 11.14. Exercises

1 Create a repeated measures data set in Stata with one record per patient. Calculate the area under the curve for these patients using code similar to that given in Section 11.6. Confirm by hand calculations that your program calculates this area properly. Explain why this code correctly calculates Equation (11.2).

2 In the Ibuprofen in Sepsis Study each patient's temperature was measured at baseline, after two and four hours, and then every four hours until 44 hours after entry into the study. Ibuprofen treatment in the intervention group was stopped at 44 hours. Three additional temperatures were recorded at 72, 96, and 120 hours after baseline (see the *11.ex.Sepsis.dta* data set). Draw exploratory graphs to investigate the relationship between treatment and body temperature in this study.

3 Perform a response feature analysis of body temperature and treatment in the Ibuprofen in Sepsis Study. What response feature do you think is most appropriate to use in this analysis?

4 For the response feature chosen in Question 3, draw box plots of this statistic for patients in the intervention and control groups. Calculate a 95% confidence interval for the difference in this response feature between patients in the ibuprofen and control groups. Can we conclude that ibuprofen changes the body temperature profile in septic patients?

5 At what times can we conclude that body temperature was reduced in the ibuprofen group compared with controls?

6 Repeat Question 3 using a GEE analysis. Do you get similar answers? Note that a sizable fraction of patients had at least one missing temperature reading. How have you dealt with these missing values in

your analysis? What are the strengths and weaknesses of these two approaches?

7 Experiment with different working correlation structures in your answer to Question 6 by specifying the *corr* option to the *xtgee* command. Does your choice of working correlation structure affect your answers?

8 Repeat the analysis in Section 11.11 but without dropping patient 8. Experiment with different working correlation structures. Contrast your answers to the results given in Section 11.11. How important is the choice of the working correlation matrix to your answers?

9 Repeat the analysis in Section 11.11 but omit the *robust* option from the *xtgee* command. This will cause the program to use your actual working correlation structure in your model. Contrast your answer to that obtained in Sections 11.11 and 11.5. Do you feel that using the Huber–White sandwich estimator is important in this example? Why?

10 Lang et al. (1995) reported impressive physiologic differences in the response of a group of white and black men to escalating doses of isoproterenol. Suppose that you wanted to determine whether these differences were due to genetic or environmental factors. What additional experiments might you wish to perform to try to settle this question? What sort of evidence would you consider to be conclusive that this difference has a genetic etiology?

A

# Summary of statistical models discussed in this text

The following tables summarize the types of data that are discussed in this text and the statistical models that may be used for their analyses. The pages where these methods are discussed are also given

**Table A.1.** Models for continuous response variables with one response per patient

| Model attributes | Method of analysis | Pages |
|---|---|---|
| Normally distributed response variable | | |
| Single continuous independent variable | | |
| Linear relationship between response and independent variable | Simple linear regression | 45–95 |
| Non-linear relationship between response and independent variable | Multiple linear regression using restricted cubic splines | 133–154 |
| | Transform response or independent variables and use simple linear regression | 70–79 |
| | Convert continuous independent variable to dichotomous variables and use multiple linear regression | 216–224, 97–157 |
| Single dichotomous independent variable | Independent *t*-test | 34–38 |
| Single categorical variable | Convert categorical variable to dichotomous variables and use multiple linear regression | 216–224, 97–157 |
| | One-way analysis of variance | 429–446 |
| Multiple independent variables | | |
| Independent variables have additive effects on response variable | Multiple linear regression model without interaction terms | 97–119 |
| Independent variables have non-additive effects on response variable | Include interaction terms in multiple linear regression model | 107–110 |
| Independent variables are categorical or have non-linear effects on the response variable | Multiple linear regression: see above for single independent variable | 97–157 |

**Table A.1.** Models for continuous response variables (*cont.*)

| Model attributes | Method of analysis | Pages |
|---|---|---|
| Two independent categorical variables | Two-way analysis of variance | 446–447 |
| Multiple categorical and continuous independent variables | Analysis of covariance. This is another name for multiple linear regression | 97–157 |
| Skewed response variable | | |
| Single dichotomous independent variable | Wilcoxon–Mann–Whitney rank-sum test | 435 |
| Single categorical independent variable | Kruskal–Wallis test | 435–435 |
| Any combination of independent variables | Apply normalizing transformation to response variable. Then see methods for linear regression noted above | 70–79 |

**Table A.2.** Models for dichotomous or categorical response variables with one response per patient

| Model attributes | Method of analysis | Pages |
|---|---|---|
| Dichotomous response variable | | |
| Single continuous independent variable | | |
| Linear relationship between log-odds of response and independent variable | Simple logistic regression | 159–199 |
| Non-linear relationship between log-odds of response and independent variable | Multiple logistic regression using restricted cubic splines | 265–278 |
| | Transform independent variable. Then use simple logistic regression | 70–79, 159–199 |
| | Convert continuous variable to dichotomous variables and use multiple logistic regression | 216–223 |
| Single dichotomous independent variable | $2 \times 2$ contingency table analysis. Calculate crude odds ratio | 187–190 |
| | Simple logistic regression | 191–196 |
| Single categorical variable | Convert categorical variable to dichotomous variables and use multiple logistic regression | 216–224 |
| Multiple independent variables | | |
| Two dichotomous independent variables with multiplicative effects on the odds ratios | Mantel–Haenszel odds-ratio and test for multiple $2 \times 2$ tables | 201–209 |
| | Multiple logistic regression | 212–217 |
| Independent variables have multiplicative effects on the odds-ratios | Multiple logistic regression model without interaction terms | 210–231 |

**Table A.2.** Models for dichotomous or categorical response variables (*cont.*)

| Model attributes | Method of analysis | Pages |
|---|---|---|
| Independent variables have non-multiplicative effects on the odds-ratios | Include interaction terms in multiple logistic regression model | 231–238 |
| Independent variables are categorical or have non- linear effects on the log odds | Multiple logistic regression. See above for single independent variable | 216–224, 265–278, 70–79 |
| Matched cases and controls | Conditional logistic regression | 258–258 |
| Categorical response variable | | |
| Response categories are ordered and proportional odds assumption is valid | Proportional odds logistic regression | 278–279 |
| Response categories not ordered or proportional odds assumption invalid | Polytomous logistic regression | 279–281 |
| Independent variables have non-multiplicative effects on the odds-ratios, are categorical or have non-linear effects on the log odds | See above for logistic regression | 231–238, 216–224, 265–278, 70–79 |

**Table A.3.** Models for survival data (follow-up time plus fate at exit observed on each patient)

| Model attributes | Method of analysis | Pages |
|---|---|---|
| Categorical independent variable | Kaplan–Meier survival curve | 290–296 |
| | Log-rank test | 296–305 |
| Proportional hazards assumption valid | | |
| Single continuous independent variable | | |
| Linear relationship between log-hazard and independent variable | Simple proportional hazards regression model | 306–312 |
| Non-linear relationship between log-hazard and independent variable | Multiple proportional hazards model using restricted cubic splines | 320–323, 331–348 |
| | Transform independent variable. Then use simple proportional hazards model | 70–79, 306–312 |
| | Convert continuous variable to dichotomous variables. Then use multiple proportional hazards regression model | 323–323, 331–348 |
| Time denotes age rather than time since recruitment | Proportional hazards regression analysis with ragged entry | 349–354 |

**Table A.3.** Models for survival data (*cont.*)

| Model attributes | Method of analysis | Pages |
|---|---|---|
| Single categorical independent variable | Convert categorical variable to dichotomous variables and use multiple proportional hazards regression model | 216–217, 323–323, 331–348 |
| Multiple independent variables | | 315–359 |
| Independent variables have non-multiplicative effects on the hazard ratios | Include interaction terms in multiple proportional hazards regression | 326–327, 331–348 |
| Independent variables are categorical or have non-linear effects on the log-hazard | Multiple proportional hazards regression. See above for single independent variable | 315–359 |
| Proportional hazards assumption invalid | Stratified proportional-hazards regression analysis | 348–349 |
| | Hazard regression analysis with time-dependent covariates | 359–370 |
| Events are rare and sample size is large | Poisson regression | 383–427 |
| Independent variables have non-multiplicative effects on the hazard ratios | Include interaction terms in time-dependent hazard regression model | 326–327, 359–370 |
| Independent variables have non-linear effects on the log-hazard | See above for a single continuous independent variable. Use a time-dependent hazard regression model | 320–323, 70–79, 359–370 |
| Independent variables are categorical | Convert categorical variables to dichotomous variables in time-dependent model | 323–323, 359–370 |
| Time denotes age rather than time since recruitment | Hazards regression analysis with time-dependent covariates and ragged entry | 349–354, 359–370 |

**Table A.4.** Models for response variables that are event rates or the number of events during a specified number of patient–years of follow-up. The event must be rare

| Model attributes | Method of analysis | Pages |
|---|---|---|
| Single dichotomous independent variable | Incident rate ratios | 373–376 |
| | Simple Poisson regression | 376–381 |
| Single categorical independent variable | Convert categorical variable to dichotomous variables and use multiple Poisson regression | 216–217, 404–423 |
| Multiple independent variables | | |
| Independent variables have multiplicative effects on the event rates | Multiple Poisson regression models without interaction terms | 401–407 |
| Independent variables have non-multiplicative effects on the event rates | Multiple Poisson regression models with interaction terms | 408–423 |
| Independent variables are categorical | Multiple Poisson regression. See above for single independent variable | 216–217, 404–423 |

**Table A.5.** Models with multiple observations per patient or matched or clustered patients

| Model attributes | Method of analysis | Pages |
|---|---|---|
| Continuous response measures | | |
| Dichotomous independent variable | Paired *t*-test | 30–34 |
| Multiple independent variables | | |
| | Response feature analysis: consider slopes of individual patient regressions or areas under individual patient curves | 459–469 |
| | GEE analysis with identity link function and normal random component | 470–481 |
| Dichotomous response measure | | |
| Multiple independent variables | Response feature analysis: consider within-patient event rate | 459 |
| | GEE analysis with logit link function and binomial random component | 481 |

B

# Summary of Stata commands used in this text

The following tables list the Stata commands and command components that are used in this text. A terse indication of the function of each command is also given. See the Stata reference manuals for a complete explanation of these commands. Page numbers show where the command is explained or first illustrated in this text.

**Table B.1.** Data manipulation and description

| Command | Function | Page |
|---|---|---|
| * *comment* | Any command that starts with an asterisk is ignored. | 10 |
| browse | View data in memory. | 10 |
| by *varlist*: egen *newvar* = *function*(*expression*) | Define *newvar* to equal some function of *expression* within groups defined by *varlist*. Acceptable functions include count, mean, sd, and sum. | 275 |
| codebook *varlist* | Describe variables in memory. | 33 |
| collapse (count) *newvar* = *varname*, by(*varlist*) | Make dataset with one record for each distinct combination of values in *varlist*; *newvar* equals the count of all non-missing values of *varname* in records with identical values of the variables in *varlist*. | 386, 392 |
| collapse (mean) *newvar* = *varname*, by(*varlist*) | Make dataset with one record for each distinct combination of values in *varlist*; *newvar* equals the mean of all values of *varname* in records with identical values of the variables in *varlist*. | 457 |
| collapse (sd) *newvar* = *varname*, by(*varlist*) | This command is similar to the preceding one except that now *newvar* equals the standard deviation of *varname* in records with identical values of the variables in *varlist*. | 457 |
| collapse (sum) *newvar* = *varname*, by(*varlist*) | This command is similar to the preceding one except that now *newvar* equals the sum of values of *varname*. | 386, 392 |

**Table B.1.** Data manipulation and description (*cont.*)

| Command | Function | Page |
|---|---|---|
| db *commandname* | Display the dialogue box for the *commandname* command. | 18 |
| describe *varlist* | Describe variables in memory (see also codebook). | 10 |
| drop if *expression* | Drop observations from memory where *expression* is true. | 120 |
| drop *varlist* | Drop variables in *varlist* from memory. | 133 |
| edit | Modify or add data in memory. | 118 |
| egen *newvar* = mean(*expression*) | Define *newvar* to equal the mean value of *expression*. | 275 |
| findit *keywords* | Search Internet for Stata programs related to *keywords*. | 438 |
| generate *newvar* = *expression* | Define a new variable equal to *expression*. | 37 |
| help *commandname* | Search for help on *commandname*. | 13 |
| keep if *expression* | Keep only observations where *expression* is true. | 33 |
| keep *varlist* | Keep *varlist* variables in memory. Drop all others. | 33 |
| label define *lblname* # "*label*" # "*label*" . . . # "*label*" | Define the value label *lblname*. | 194 |
| label values *varname lblname* | Assign a value label *lblname* to a variable *varname*. | 194 |
| label variable *varname* "*label*" | Assign a label to the variable *varname*. | 106 |
| log close | Close log file. | 22 |
| log using \ *foldername*\ *filename* | Open a log file called *filename* in the *foldername* folder (MS-Windows computers). | 21 |
| mkspline *stubname* = *var*, cubic displayknots | Generate cubic spline covariates for *var* to be used in a 5 knot RCS model with default knot locations. Print the knot values | 150 |
| mkspline *stubname* = *var*, cubic nknots(#) | Generate spline covariates for *var* to be used in a RCS model with # knots at their default locations. | 151 |
| mkspline *stubname* = *var*, cubic knots(#1 #2 . . . #*k*) | Generate spline covariates for *var* to be used in a RCS model with #*k* knots located at #1, #2, . . . , #*k*. | 153 |
| recode *varname* 1 3 = 10 5/7 = 11 * = 12 | Recode *varname* values 1 and 3 as 10, 5 through 7 as 11 and all other values as 12. | 230 |
| rename *oldvar newvar* | Change the name of the variable *oldvar* to *newvar*. | 194 |
| replace *oldvar* = *expression1* if *expression2* | Redefine values of *oldvar* if *expression2* is true. | 118 |
| reshape long *stubname*, i(*idvar*) j(*subvar*) | Convert data from wide to long data-structure; *idvar* identifies observations on the same patient; *subvar* identifies specific values on each patient. | 457 |
| save "*filename*", replace | Store memory data set in a file called *filename*. Overwrite any existing file with the same name. | 194 |

**Table B.1.** Data manipulation and description (*cont.*)

| Command | Function | Page |
|---|---|---|
| scalar *name* = *expression* | Define *name* to be a scalar that equals *expression*. | 86 |
| search *keywords* | Search for help on *keywords* in the Stata database (see also *findit*). | 13 |
| set memory # | Set memory size to # kilobytes. | 343 |
| set memory #m | Set memory size to # megabytes. | 343 |
| sort *varlist* | Sort data records in ascending order by values in *varlist*. | 78 |
| stset *exittime*, enter(time *entrytime*) failure(*failvar*) | Declare *entrytime*, *exittime*, and *failvar* to be the entry time, exit time, and failure variables, respectively. | 354 |
| stset *exittime*, id(*idvar*) enter(time *entrytime*) failure(*failvar*) | Declare *entrytime*, *exittime*, and *failvar* to be the entry time, exit time, and failure variables, respectively; id(*idvar*) is a patient identification variable needed for time-dependent hazard regression analysis. | 367 |
| stset *timevar*, failure(*failvar*) | Declare *timevar* and *failvar* to be time and failure variables, respectively; *failvar* $\neq 0$ denotes failure. | 302 |
| stsplit *varname*, at(#1 #2 . . . #k) | Create multiple records for time-dependent hazard regression or Poisson regression analyses; *at* defines the time epochs. A record is created for each epoch spanned by the patient's follow-up. | 367, 385 |
| use "*stata_data_file*", clear | Load new data file, purge old data from memory. | 10 |

**Table B.2.** Analysis commands

| Command | Function | Page |
|---|---|---|
| cc *var_case var_control*, woolf | Calculate odds-ratio for case–control study using Woolf's method to derive a confidence interval. | 196 |
| cc *var_case var_control*, by(*varcon*) | Calculate Mantel–Haenszel odds-ratio adjusted for *varcon*. | 209 |
| centile *varlist*, centile(*numlist*) | Produce a table of percentiles specified by *numlist* for the variables in *varlist*. | 390 |
| ci *varlist* | Calculate standard errors and confidence intervals for variables in *varlist*. | 444 |
| clogit *depvar varlist*, group(*groupvar*) | Conditional logistic regression: regress *depvar* against *varlist* with matching variable *groupvar*. | 258 |

**Table B.2.** Analysis commands (*cont.*)

| Command | Function | Page |
|---|---|---|
| display *expression* | Calculate *expression* and show result. | 70 |
| display *"text-1" expression-1* ... *"text-n" expression-n* | Display multiple expressions interspersed with text. | 86 |
| forvalues *index* = #1/#2 { Commands referring to '*index*' } | Loop through commands with *index* varying from #1 to #2 | 238 |
| glm *depvar varlist*, family(binomial) link(logit) | Logistic regression: Bernoulli dependent variable. | 172 |
| glm *depvar varlist*, family(poisson) link(log) lnoffset(*ptyears*) | Poisson regression with *depvar* events in *ptyears* patient–years of observation. | 380 |
| glm *nvar varlist*, family(binomial *dvar*) link(logit) | Logistic regression with *nvar* events in *dvar* trials. | 184 |
| iri *#a #b #Na #Nb* | Calculate relative risk from incidence data; *#a* and *#b* are the number of exposed and unexposed cases observed during *#Na* and *#Nb* person–years of follow-up. | 375 |
| kwallis *var*, by(*groupvar*) | Perform a Kruskal–Wallis test of *var* by *groupvar.* | 446 |
| list *varlist* | List values of variables in *varlist.* | 10 |
| logistic *depvar varlist* | Logistic regression: regress *depvar* against variables in *varlist.* | 176, 215 |
| oneway *depvar factorvar* | One-way analysis of variance of *depvar* in groups defined by *factorvar.* | 445 |
| poisson *depvar varlist*, exposure(*ptyears*) irr | Poisson regression with *depvar* events in *ptyears* patient–years of observation. Display the incidence rate ratios. | 396. |
| ranksum *var*, by(*groupvar*) | Perform a Wilcoxon–Mann–Whitney rank-sum test of *var* by *groupvar.* | 446 |
| regress *depvar xvar* | Simple linear regression: regress *depvar* against *xvar.* | 60 |
| regress *depvar varlist* | Multiple linear regression: regress *depvar* against variables in *varlist.* | 117 |
| robvar *varname*, by(*groupvar*) | Test equality of standard deviations of *varname* in groups of patients defined by *groupvar.* | 445 |
| statsby *svar* = _b[*xvar*], by(*varlist*) clear: regress *depvar xvar* | For each combination of values of *varlist*, regress *depvar* against *xvar* and store the slope coefficient as *svar.* Delete all variables except *svar* and the variables in *varlist.* | 445 |
| stcox *varlist* | Proportional hazard regression analysis with independent variables given by *varlist.* A *stset* statement defines failure. Exponentiated model coefficients are displayed. | 311 |

**Table B.2.** Analysis commands (*cont.*)

| Command | Function | Page |
|---|---|---|
| stcox *varlist*, nohr | Proportional hazard regression analysis with independent variables given by *varlist*. The model coefficients are displayed. | 345 |
| stcox *varlist1*, strata(*varlist2*) | Stratified proportional hazard regression analysis with strata defined by the values of variables in *varlist2*. | 349 |
| sts list, at(# . . . #) | List estimated survival function at specific times specified by #, . . . , # | 304 |
| sts list, by(*varlist*) | List estimated survival function by patient groups defined by unique combinations of values of *varlist*. | 303 |
| sts test *varlist* | Perform log-rank test on groups defined by the values of *varlist*. | 305, 354 |
| summarize *varlist*, detail | Summarize variables in *varlist*. | 21 |
| table *rowvar colvar*, contents(sum *varname*) | Create a table of sums of *varname* cross-tabulated by *rowvar* and *colvar*. | 391 |
| table *rowvar colvar*, row col | Two-way frequency tables with row and column totals. | 230 |
| table *rowvar colvar* | Two-way frequency tables of values of *rowvar* by *colvar*. | 208 |
| table *rowvar colvar*, by(*varlist*) | Two-way frequency tables of values of *rowvar* by *colvar* for each unique combination of values of *varlist*. | 209 |
| tabulate *varname1 varname2*, column row | Two-way frequency tables with row and column percentages. | 220 |
| tabulate *varname* | Frequency table of *varname* with percentages and cumulative percentages. | 132 |
| tabulate *varname*, missing | Frequency table of *varname* treating missing values like other values. | 369 |
| ttest *var1* = *var2* | Paired *t*-test of *var1* vs. *var2*. | 33 |
| ttest *var*, by(*groupvar*) | Independent *t*-test of *var* in groups defined by *groupvar*. | 38 |
| ttest *var*, by(*groupvar*) unequal | Independent *t*-test of *var* in groups defined by *groupvar*. Variances assumed unequal. | 38 |
| xi: glm *depvar* i.*var1*∗i.*var2*, family(*poisson*) link(*log*) lnoffset(*ptyears*) | Poisson regression using *glm* command with dichotomous indicator variables replacing categorical variables *var1*, *var2*. All two-way interaction terms are also generated. | 426 |

**Table B.2.** Analysis commands (*cont.*)

| Command | Function | Page |
|---|---|---|
| xi: logistic *depvar varlist* i.*var1*∗i.*var2* | Logistic regression with dichotomous indicator variables replacing categorical variables *var1* and *var2*. All two-way interaction terms are also generated. | 237 |
| xi: logistic *depvar varlist* i.*catvar* | Logistic regression with dichotomous indicator variables replacing a categorical variable *catvar*. | 217 |
| xi: poisson *depvar varlist* i.*catvar*, exposure(*ptyears*) | Poisson regression with dichotomous indicator variables replacing a categorical variable *catvar*. | 420 |
| xi: poisson *depvar varlist* i.*var1*∗i.*var2*, exposure(*ptyears*) | Poisson regression with dichotomous indicator variables replacing categorical variables *var1*, *var2*. All two-way interaction terms are also generated. | 421 |
| xi: regress *depvar* i.*catvar* | Linear regression with dichotomous indicator variables replacing a categorical variable *catvar*. See also *oneway*. | 445 |
| xi: stcox *varlist* i.*var1*∗i.*var2* | Proportional hazards regression with dichotomous indicator variables replacing categorical variables *var1* and *var2*. All two-way interaction terms are also generated. | 347 |
| xi: stcox *varlist* i.*varname* | Proportional hazards regression with dichotomous indicator variables replacing categorical variable *varname*. | 346 |
| xi: xtgee *depvar* i.*var1*∗i.*var2*, family(family) link(link) corr(correlation) i(*idname*) robust | Perform a generalized estimating equation analysis regressing *depvar* against categorical variables *var1* and *var2* with interaction terms. | 480 |
| xtgee *depvar varlist*, family(family) link(link) corr(correlation) i(*idname*) robust | Perform a generalized estimating equation analysis regressing *depvar* against the variables in *varlist*. | 480 |

**Table B.3.** Graph commands

| Command | Function | Page |
|---|---|---|
| dot plot *varname*, over(*groupvar*) center | Draw centered dot plots of *varname* by *groupvar*. | 22 |
| graph hbox *varname*, over(*groupvar*) | Draw horizontal box plots of *var* for each distinct value of *groupvar*. | 22 |
| graph bar *var1 var2*, over(*varstrat*) | Grouped bar graph of mean values of *var1* and *var2* stratified by *varstrat*. | 421 |
| graph bar *varname*, over(*varstrat*) bar(1, color(black)) | Bar graph of mean values of *varname* stratified by *varstrat*. Color bars for *varname* black. | 421 |
| graph matrix *varlist* | Plot matrix scatter plot of variables in *varlist*. | 107 |
| histogram | See also twoway histogram | |
| histogram *varname*, bin(#) | Draw histogram of *var* with # bars on each histogram. | 10 |
| histogram *varname*, by(*groupvar*)) | Draw histograms of *var* by *groupvar*. | 10 |
| histogram *varname*, discrete | Draw histogram of *varname*. Show a separate bar for each discrete value of *varname*. | 187 |
| histogram *varname*, frequency | Draw histogram of *varname*. Show number of observations on the *y*-axis. | 187 |
| histogram *varname*, percent | Draw histogram of *var*; *y*-axis is percent of subjects. | 10 |
| histogram *varname*, width(#1) start(#2) | Draw histogram of *varname*. Group data in bins of width #1 starting at #2. | 343 |
| lfitci | See twoway lfitci. | |
| lfit | See twoway lfit. | |
| line *yvar xvar* | Draw line plot of *yvar* against *xvar*. | 61 |
| line *yvar xvar, sort* | Draw line plot of *yvar* against *xvar*. Sort data by *xvar* prior to drawing the graph. | 79 |
| line *yvarlist xvar* | Draw line plots of the variables in *yvarlist* against *xvar*. | 153 |
| lowess *yvar xvar, bwidth(#)* | Draw a scatter plot of *yvar* vs. *xvar*. Overlay the lowess regression line of *yvar* vs. *xvar* using a bandwidth of #. | 132 |
| lowess | See also twoway lowess. | |
| rarea | See twoway rarea. | |
| rcap | See twoway rcap. | |
| scatter *yvar xvar* | Scatter plot of *yvar* vs. *xvar* | 59 |
| scatter *yvar1 xvar* \|\| line *yvar2 xvar* | Line plot of *yvar2* vs. *xvar* overlayed on a scatter plot of *yvar1* vs. *xvar* | 61 |
| scatter *yvar xvar*, connect(L) | Connect observations in scatter plot as long as consecutive values of *xvar* increase. | 459 |
| stcoxkm, by(*varname*) | Plot Kaplan–Meier survival curves together with best fitting survival curves under the proportional hazards model. Draw separate curves for each distinct value of *varname*. | 357 |

**Table B.3.** Graph commands (*cont.*)

| Command | Function | Page |
|---|---|---|
| stcoxkm, by(*varname*) obs#opts(symbol(none)) | Plot unrestricted and restricted survival curves. Do not use a plot symbol on the $\#^{th}$ unrestricted curve. | 357 |
| stcoxkm, by(*varname*) pred#opts(color(gray) lpattern(dash)) | Plot unrestricted and restricted survival curves. Use a dashed gray line for the $\#^{th}$ restricted curve. | 358 |
| stphplot, by(*varname*) | Plot log–log plots of the Kaplan–Meier survival curves against log analysis time. Draw separate curves for each distinct value of *varname*. | 358 |
| stphplot, by(*varname*) nolntime | Plot log–log plots of the Kaplan–Meier survival curves against analysis time. | 358 |
| stphplot, by(*varname*) adjust(varlist) | Plot log–log plots of the Kaplan–Meier survival curves against log analysis time. Adjust curves for the average value of the variables in *varlist*. | 358 |
| stripplot *varname*, over(*groupvar*) boffset(−0.2) stack box(barwidth(0.2)) | Plot separate dot and box plots of *varname* for each value of *groupvar*. Stack observations with identical values. | 444 |
| sts graph | Graph a Kaplan–Meier survival plot. Must be preceded by a *stset* statement. | 303 |
| sts graph, by(*varlist*) | Kaplan–Meier survival plots. Plot a separate curve for each combination of distinct values of the variables in *varlist*. | 303 |
| sts graph, by(*varlist*) byopts(title (" ", size(0)) | Kaplan–Meier survival plots with *by* option suppressing the graph title. | 304 |
| sts graph, by(*varlist*) byopts(legend(off)) | Kaplan–Meier survival plots with *by* option suppressing the figure legend. | 304 |
| sts graph, by(*varlist*) plot#opts(lpattern(dash)) | Kaplan–Meier survival plots. Use a dashed pattern for the $\#^{th}$ line | 344 |
| sts graph, by(*varlist*) plot#opts(lpattern(longdash)) | Kaplan–Meier survival plots. Use a pattern for the $\#^{th}$ line with long dashes. | 303 |
| sts graph, by(*varlist*) plot#opts(lpattern("_-")) | Kaplan–Meier survival plots. Use a pattern for the $\#^{th}$ line with alternating long and short dashes | 344 |
| sts graph, by(*varlist*) plot#opts(color(gray)) | Kaplan–Meier survival plots. Color the $\#^{th}$ line gray. | 344 |
| sts graph, by(*varlist*) separate | Kaplan–Meier survival plots. Plot a separate survival graph for each combination of distinct values of the variables in *varlist*. | 304 |
| sts graph, failure | Kaplan–Meier cumulative mortality plot. | 305 |
| sts graph, by(*varlist*) risktable | Kaplan–Meier survival plots with risk table. | 305 |

**Table B.3.** Graph commands (*cont.*)

| Command | Function | Page |
|---|---|---|
| sts graph, by(*varlist*) risktable(,order(#1 "*string1*" . . . #n "*string#n*")) | Kaplan–Meier survival plots with risk table specifying order and labels of the table rows. | 305 |
| sts graph, censored(single) | Kaplan–Meier survival plot showing hatch marks at each censoring time. | 304 |
| sts graph, ci | Kaplan–Meier survival plot with shaded 95% confidence interval. | 304 |
| sts graph, ci ciopts(lcolor(none)) | Kaplan–Meier survival plot with 95% confidence interval. The outline of this interval is suppressed. | 304 |
| sts graph, lost | Kaplan–Meier survival plot showing number of patients censored between consecutive death days. | 304 |
| sts graph, noorigin | Kaplan–Meier survival plot with *x*-axis starting at first exit time. | 354 |
| sts graph, title(" ", height(0)) | Kaplan–Meier survival plot. Suppress the default graph title. | 303 |
| sunflower *yvar xvar*, binwidth(#) | Draw a density-distribution sunflower plot of *yvar* vs. *xvar* using a bin width of # | 90 |
| sunflower *yvar xvar*, light(#1) dark(#2) | Draw a density-distribution sunflower plot of *yvar* vs. *xvar*. Set minimum number of observations in a light and dark sunflower to be #1 and #2, respectively. | 91 |
| sunflower *yvar xvar*, petalweight(#) | Draw a density-distribution sunflower plot of *yvar* vs. *xvar*. Set the number of observations represented by a dark petal to be #. | 91 |
| twoway connected *yvar xvar* | Overlay a *scatter* plot with a *line* plot of *yvar* vs. *xvar*. | 458 |
| twoway histogram *var*, discrete | Plot histogram of *var*. Draw a separate bar for each distinct value of *var*. | 276 |
| twoway histogram *var*, frequency | Plot histogram of *var*. Let the *y*-axis denote number of observations. | 276 |
| twoway histogram *var*, color(gray) | Plot histogram of *var*. Color the bars gray. | 276 |
| twoway histogram *var*, gap(#) | Plot histogram of *var*. Create a gap between the bars by reducing their width by #%. | 276 |
| twoway histogram *var* | Plot histogram of *var*. | 276 |
| twoway lfit *yvar xvar* | Plot the linear regression line of *yvar* vs. *xvar*. | 62 |
| twoway lfitci *yvar xvar* | Plot the linear regression line of *yvar* vs. *xvar* overlayed on a 95% confidence interval band for this line. | 62 |
| twoway lfitci *yvar xvar*, ciplot(rline) | Plot linear regression line and 95% confidence interval for *yvar* vs. *xvar*. Denote the confidence interval with lines instead of a shaded region. | 63 |

**Table B.3.** Graph commands (*cont.*)

| Command | Function | Page |
|---|---|---|
| twoway lfitci *yvar xvar*, stdf | Plot the linear regression line of *yvar* vs. *xvar* overlayed on a 95% prediction interval for a new patient. | 63 |
| twoway lowess *yvar xvar*, bwidth(#) | Plot the lowess regression line of *yvar* vs. *xvar* using a band width of #. The default bandwidth is 0.8. | 65 |
| twoway rarea *yvar1 yvar2 xvar* | Shade the region between the curves *yvar1* vs. *xvar* and *yvar2* vs. *xvar*. | 78 |
| twoway rcap *y1 y2 x* | Draw error bars connecting *y1* to *y2* as a function of *x*. | 185 |

**Table B.4.** Common options for graph commands (insert after comma)

| Command | Function | Page |
|---|---|---|
| by(*varlist*) | Make separate graphs for each distinct combination of values of *varlist*. | 85 |
| by(*varlist*, cols(1)) | Make separate graphs by *varlist* arranged vertically in one column. | 459 |
| by(*varlist*, legend(off)) | Make separate graphs for each distinct combination of values of *varlist*. Suppress graph legend. | 85 |
| color(gray) | Color plotted line, symbol, or shaded region gray. | 63 |
| color(gs#) | Color plotted line, symbol, or shaded region gray scale value #. | 78 |
| legend(off) | Suppress legend. | 62 |
| legend(ring(0) position(#)) | Insert legend within the *x*- and *y*-axes at clock position #. | 90 |
| legend(ring(1) position(#)) | Insert legend just outside of the *x*- and *y*-axes at clock position #. | 151 |
| legend(subtitle(*text*)) | Use *text* as the legend subtitle. | 152 |
| legend(cols(1)) | Insert legend keys in a single column. | 90 |
| legend(rows(1)) | Insert legend keys in a single row. | 154 |
| legend(order(#1 ... #n)) | Insert indicated legend keys in the specified order. | 90 |
| legend(order(#1 "*string1*" ... #n "*string#n*")) | Insert indicated legend keys in the specified order with the specified labels. | 152 |
| lpattern(dash) | Draw the line(s) specified by the graph command with dashes. | 85 |
| lpattern(longdash) | Draw the line(s) specified by the graph command with long dashes. | 151 |
| lpattern(shortdash) | Draw the line(s) specified by the graph command with short dashes. | 151 |

**Table B.4.** Common options for graph commands (*cont.*)

| Command | Function | Page |
|---|---|---|
| lpattern(solid) | Draw the line(s) specified by the graph command with a continuous line. | 63 |
| lpattern(_-) | Make the line(s) specified by the graph command with alternating long and medium dashes | 344 |
| lwidth(medthick) | Make the line(s) specified by the graph command of medium thickness. | 63 |
| lwidth(vvthin) | Make the line(s) specified by the graph command very thin. | 153 |
| mlwidth(thick) | Use a thick line for the outline of the plot symbol. | 256 |
| scale(#) | Magnify markers, labels and line-widths by 100 × (# − 1)%. | 77 |
| subtitle(*text*) | Add a subtitle to a graph. The position of this subtitle is specified in the same way as for the legend. | 153 |
| symbol(circle) | Use a solid circle as the plot symbol. | 185 |
| symbol(Oh) | Use a large open circle as the plot symbol. | 59 |
| symbol(oh) | Use a small open circle as the plot symbol. | 62 |
| title(*text*) | Add a title to a graph. See subtitle. | |
| xlabel( #1 (#2) #3) | Label *x*-axis from #1 to #3 in units of #2. | 59 |
| xlabel( #1 "L1" #2 "L2" ... #n "Ln") | Label *x*-axis at the values #1, #2, ... , #n with the labels "L1", "L2", ... , "Ln". | 78 |
| xlabel(# ... #) | Add specific numeric labels #, ... , # to the *x*-axis. | 79 |
| xlabel(# ... #, angle(45)) | Write labels at a 45 degree angle to the *x*-axis. | 458 |
| xline(# ... #) | Add vertical grid lines at values #, ... , #. | 59 |
| xmtick( #1 (#2) #3) | Add minor tick marks to the *y*-axis from #1 to #3 in units of #2. | 78 |
| xmtick(# ... #) | Add minor tick marks to the *x*-axis at #, ... , #. | 79 |
| xscale(log) | Plot the *x*-axis on a logarithmic scale. | 78 |
| xsize(#) | Make graph # inches wide. | 77 |
| xtick(#1 (#2) #3) | Add tick marks to the *x*-axis from #1 to #3 in units of #2. | 77 |
| xtick(# ... #) | Add tick marks to the *x*-axis at #, ... , #. | 79 |
| xtitle(*text-string*) | Give the *x*-axis the title *text-string*. | 79 |
| yaxis(2) | Define a second *y*-axis on the right of the graph | 173 |
| ylabel(#1 (#2) #3) | Label *y*-axis from #1 to #3 in units of #2. | 59 |
| ylabel(#1 (#2) #3, angle(0)) | Label *y*-axis from #1 to #3 in units of #2. Orient labels parallel to the *x*-axis. | 59 |
| ylabel(#1 "L1" #2 "L2" ... #n "Ln") | Label *y*-axis at the values #1, #2, ... , #n with the labels "L1", "L2", ... , "Ln". | 78 |
| ylabel(# ... #) | Add specific numeric labels #, ... , # to the *y*-axis. | 79 |
| ylabel(# ... #, valuelabel) | Add specific labels at #, ... , # to the *y*-axis. Use the value labels for the *y*-variable instead of the numeric values. | 173 |

**Table B.4.** Common options for graph commands (*cont.*)

| Command | Function | Page |
|---|---|---|
| yline(# . . . #) | Add horizontal grid lines at values #, . . . , #. | 59 |
| yline(# . . . #, lcolor(gray)) | Add horizontal grid lines at values #, . . . , #. Color these lines gray. | 70 |
| yline(# . . . #, lpattern(dash)) | Add horizontal dashed grid lines at values #, . . . , #. | 70 |
| ymtick(#1 (#2) #3) | Add minor tick marks to the $y$-axis from #1 to #3 in units of #2. | 77 |
| ymtick(# . . . #) | Add minor tick marks to the $y$-axis at #, . . . , #. | 79 |
| yscale(range(#1 #2)) | Extend the range of the $y$-axis from #1 to #2. | 70 |
| yscale(log) | Plot $y$-axis on a logarithmic scale. | 149 |
| yscale(titlegap(#)) | Move the title of the $y$-axis to the left or right from its default location. | 173 |
| ysize(#) | Make graph # inches tall. | 77 |
| ytick(#1 (#2) #3) | Add tick marks to the $x$-axis from #1 to #3 in units of #2. | 78 |
| ytick(# . . . #) | Add tick marks to the $y$-axis at #, . . . , #. | 79 |
| ytitle(*text-string*) | Give the $y$-axis the title *text-string*. | 62 |
| ytitle(, axis(2) color(gray)) | Color the default $y$-axis title gray. | 186 |

**Table B.5.** Post-estimation commands (affected by preceding regression-type command)

| Command | Function | Page |
|---|---|---|
| estat vce | Display variance–covariance matrix of last model. | 185 |
| estat gof | Calculate the Pearson chi-squared goodness-of-fit test after logistic regression. | 255 |
| estat gof, group(#) table | Calculate Hosmer–Lemeshow goodness-of-fit test with # groups. Display goodness-of-fit table. | 255 |
| estimates store *ename* | Store parameter estimates using the name *ename* | 276 |
| lincom *expression* | Calculate *expression* and a 95% CI associated with *expression*. | 231, 446 |
| lincom *expression*, or | Calculate exp[*expression*] with associated 95% CI. Label the second column “Odds Ratio”. | 231 |
| lincom *expression*, hr | Calculate exp[*expression*] with associated 95% CI. Label the second column “Haz. Ratio”. | 347 |
| lincom *expression*, irr | Calculate exp[*expression*] with associated 95% CI. Label the second column “IRR”. | 381 |

**Table B.5.** Post-estimation commands (*cont.*)

| Command | Function | Page |
|---|---|---|
| lrtest *ename* . | Perform a likelihood ratio test of model *ename* compared with the most recent model. | 276 |
| predict *newvar*, cooksd | Set *newvar* = Cook's *D*. | 133 |
| predict *newvar*, dbeta | Set *newvar* = delta beta influence statistic. | 256 |
| predict *newvar*, dfbeta(*varname*) | Set *newvar* = delta beta statistic for the *varname* covariate in the linear regression model. | 133 |
| predict *newvar*, dx2 | Set *newvar* = the square of the standardized Pearson-residual. | 255 |
| predict *newvar*, hr | Set *newvar* = relative risk of event after hazard regression. | 345 |
| predict *newvar*, mu | Set *newvar* = expected value of the random component after a *glm* command. Set *newvar* = number of events after Poisson regression. | 173, 426 |
| predict *newvar*, p | Set *newvar* = probability of event after logistic regression. | 255 |
| predict *newvar*, rstandard | Set *newvar* = standardized-residual, or standardized-Pearson-residual after linear or logistic regression, respectively. | 133, 255 |
| predict *newvar*, rstudent | Set *newvar* = studentized residual. | 70, 132 |
| predict *newvar*, standardized deviance | Set *newvar* = standardized deviance residual after *glm* command. | 426 |
| predict *newvar*, stdp | Set *newvar* = standard error of the linear predictor. | 78, 119, 153, 185, 345 |
| predict *newvar*, stdf | Set *newvar* = standard error of a forecasted value. | 119 |
| predict *newvar*, xb | Set *newvar* = linear predictor. | 61, 118, 150, 172, 345 |
| predictnl *newvar* = *var1* ∗ *est1* + *var2* ∗ *est2* + · · · + *var_k* ∗ *est_k*, se(*se_var*) | Define *newvar* to be a weighted sum of parameter estimates. Define *se_var* to be the standard error of *newvar*. | 277 |
| test *varlist* | Test the null hypothesis that the parameters associated with the variables in *varlist* are all simultaneously zero. | 154 |
| test *var1* = *var2* = · · · = *var_k* | Test the null hypothesis that the parameters associated with *var1* through *var_k* are all equal. | 369 |

**Table B.6.** Command prefixes

| Command | Function | Page |
|---|---|---|
| by *varlist*: | Repeat following command for each distinct value of *varlist*. The data must be sorted by *varlist*. | 21 |
| by *varlist*, sort: | Repeat following command for each distinct value of *varlist*. | 21 |
| quietly | Suppress output from the following command. | 422 |
| stepwise, pe(#): | Fit a model using the forward selection algorithm; pe(#) sets the entry threshold. | 121 |
| stepwise, pe(#) pr(#): | Fit a model using the backward stepwise selection algorithm; pe(#) and pr(#) set the entry and removal thresholds, respectively. | 123 |
| stepwise, pe(#) pr(#) forward: | Fit a model using the forward stepwise selection algorithm; pe(#) and pr(#) set the entry and removal thresholds, respectively. | 123 |
| stepwise, pr(#): | Fit a model using the backward selection algorithm; pr(#) sets the removal threshold. | 121 |
| xi: | Execute the following estimation command with categorical variables like i.*catvar* and i.*catvar1*∗ i.*catvar2*. | 217, 237 |

**Table B.7.** Command qualifiers (insert before comma)

| Qualifier | Function | Page |
|---|---|---|
| if *expression* | Apply command to observations where *expression* is true. | 33 |
| in *range* | Apply command to observations in *range*. | 10 |
| in 5/25 | Apply command to observations 5 through 25. | 10 |
| in −5/ − 1 | Apply command to fifth from last through last observation. | 133 |
| [freq = *varname*] | Weight each observation by the value of *varname* by replacing each record with *varname* identical records and doing an unweighted analysis. | 187, 196 |
| [weight =*varname*] | When used in a scatter plot, this qualifier makes the size of the plot symbol proportional to *varname*. | 256 |

**Table B.8.** Logical and relational operators and system variables (see Stata User's Guide)

| Operator or variable | Meaning | Page |
|---|---|---|
| 1 | true | 346 |
| 0 | false | 346 |
| > | greater than | 33 |
| < | less than | 33 |
| >= | greater than or equal to | 33 |
| <= | less than or equal to | 33 |
| == | equal to | 33 |
| != | not equal to | 33 |
| & | and | 33 |
| \| | or | 33 |
| ! | not | 33 |
| _n | Record number of current observation. When used with the *by id:* prefix, *_n* is reset to 1 whenever the value of *id* changes and equals *k* at the $k^{th}$ record with the same value of *id*. | 368 |
| _N | Total number of observations in the data set. When used with the *by id:* prefix, *_N* is the number of records with the current value of *id*. | 70 |
| *varname*[*expression*] | The value of variable *varname* in observation *expression*. | 368 |
| *var** | This is a terse way of referring to all variables in memory that start with the letters *var*. | 150 |
| *var?* | This is a terse way of referring to all variables in memory consisting of the letters *var* followed by exactly one other character. | 369 |

**Table B.9.** Functions (see Stata Data Management Manual)

| Function | Meaning | Page |
|---|---|---|
| abs($x$) | Absolute value of $x$ | 132 |
| exp($x$) | $e$ raised to the power $x$, where $e$ is the base of the natural logarithm. | 79 |
| int(*var*) | Truncate *var* to an integer. | 391 |
| invbinomial($m$, $d$, *gamma*) | Calculates $p$ such that the probability of $\leq d$ deaths in $m$ patients at mortal risk $p$ equals *gamma*. | 184 |
| invlogit($x$) | inverse logit of $x = e^x/(1 + e^x)$ | 185 |
| invttail(*df*, $\alpha$) | Critical value of size $\alpha$ for a $t$ distribution with *df* degrees of freedom. | 70 |
| log($x$) | Natural logarithm of $x$. | 1 |
| missing(*expression*) | *True* (i.e. 1) if expression evaluates to missing, *false* (i.e. 0) otherwise. | 265 |
| recode(*var*, $x_1, x_2, \ldots, x_n$) | Missing if *var* is missing; $x_1$ if $var \leq x_1$; $x_i$ if $x_{i-1} < var \leq x_i$ for $2 \leq i < n$; $x_n$ otherwise. | 344 |
| round($x$, #) | Round $x$ to nearest multiple of #. | 275 |
| sqrt($x$) | Square root of $x$. | 86 |
| ttail(*df*, #) | Probability that a $t$ statistic with *df* degrees of freedom exceeds #. | 87 |

# References


Agresti, A. *Categorical Data Analysis. 2nd Edn.* Hoboken, NJ: Wiley-Interscience, 2002.

Armitage, P., Berry, G., and Matthews, N.J.S. *Statistical Methods in Medical Research, 4th Edn.* Oxford: Blackwell Science, Inc., 2002.

Bartlett, M.S. Properties of sufficiency and statistical tests. *P. R. Soc. Lond. A Mat.* 1937; **160:** 268–82.

Bernard, G.R., Wheeler, A.P., Russell, J.A., Schein, R., Summer, W.R., Steinberg, K.P., et al. The effects of ibuprofen on the physiology and survival of patients with sepsis. The Ibuprofen in Sepsis Study Group. *N. Engl. J. Med.* 1997; **336:** 912–8.

Brent, J., McMartin, K., Phillips, S., Burkhart, K.K., Donovan, J.W., Wells, M., et al. Fomepizole for the treatment of ethylene glycol poisoning. Methylpyrazole for Toxic Alcohols Study Group. *N. Engl. J. Med.* 1999; **340:** 832–8.

Breslow, N.E. and Day, N.E. *Statistical Methods in Cancer Research: Vol. 1 – The Analysis of Case-Control Studies.* Lyon, France: IARC Scientific Publications, 1980.

Breslow, N.E. and Day, N.E. *Statistical Methods in Cancer Research: Vol. II – The Design and Analysis of Cohort Studies.* Lyon, France: IARC Scientific Publications, 1987.

Brown, M.B. and Forsythe, A.B. Robust tests for the equality of variances. *J. Am. Stat. Assoc.* 1974; **69:** 364–7.

Carr, D.B., Littlefield, R.J., Nicholson, W.L., and Littlefield, J.S. Scatterplot matrix techniques for large N. *J. Am. Stat. Assoc.* 1987; **82:** 424–36.

Clayton, D. and Hills, M. *Statistical Models in Epidemiology.* Oxford: Oxford University Press, 1993.

Cleveland, W.S. Robust locally weighted regression and smoothing scatterplots. *J. Am. Stat. Assoc.* 1979; **74:** 829–36.

Cleveland, W.S. *Visualizing Data.* Summit, NJ: Hobart Press, 1993.

Cleveland, W.S. and McGill, R. The many faces of a scatterplot. *J. Am. Stat. Assoc.* 1984; **79:** 807–22.

Cochran, W.G. and Cox, G.M. *Experimental Designs, 2nd Edn.* New York: Wiley, 1957.

Cook, R.D. Detection of influential observations in linear regression. *Technometrics* 1977; **19:** 15–8.

Cook, R.D. and Weisberg, S. *Applied Regression Including Computing and Graphics.* New York: Wiley, 1999.

Cox, D.R. Regression models and life-tables (with discussion). *J. R. Stat. Soc. Ser. B* 1972; **34:** 187–220.

Cox, D.R. and Hinkley, D.V. *Theoretical Statistics.* London: Chapman and Hall, 1974.

Cox, D.R. and Oakes, D. *Analysis of Survival Data.* London: Chapman and Hall, 1984.

Crowder, M.J. and Hand, D.J. *Analysis of Repeated Measures.* London: Chapman and Hall, 1990.

Devlin, T.F. and Weeks, B.J. Spline functions for logistic regression modeling. *Proceedings of the Eleventh Annual SAS Users Group International Conference.* Cary, NC: SAS Institute, 1986.

Diggle, P.J., Heagerty, P., Liang, K.-Y., and Zeger, S.L. *Analysis of Longitudinal Data, 2nd Edn.* Oxford: Oxford University Press, 2002.

Dobson, A.J. *Introduction to Generalized Linear Models, 2nd Edn.* Boca Raton, FL: Chapman & Hall/CRC, 2001.

Draper, N. and Smith, H. *Applied Regression Analysis, 3rd Edn.* New York: Wiley-Interscience, 1998.

Dupont, W.D. Sequential stopping rules and sequentially adjusted P values: does one require the other? *Control. Clin. Trials* 1983; **4:** 3–10.

Dupont, W.D. Sensitivity of Fisher's exact test to minor perturbations in $2 \times 2$ contingency tables. *Stat. Med.* 1986; **5:** 629–35.

Dupont, W.D. and Page, D.L. Risk factors for breast cancer in women with proliferative breast disease. *N. Engl. J. Med.* 1985; **312:** 146–51.

Dupont, W.D. and Page, D.L. Relative risk of breast cancer varies with time since diagnosis of atypical hyperplasia. *Hum. Pathol.* 1989; **20:** 723–5.

Dupont, W.D. and Plummer, W.D. Power and sample size calculations: a review and computer program. *Control. Clin. Trials* 1990; **11:** 116–28.

Dupont, W.D. and Plummer, W.D. Power and sample size calculations for studies involving linear regression. *Control. Clin. Trials* 1998; **19:** 589–601.

Dupont, W.D. and Plummer, W.D. Exact confidence intervals for odds ratio from case-control studies. *Stata Technical Bulletin* 1999; **52:** 12–6.

Dupont, W.D. and Plummer, W.D. Using density distribution sunflower plots to explore bivariate relationships in dense data. *Stata Journal* 2005; **5:** 371–84.

Durrleman, S. and Simon, R. Flexible regression models with cubic splines. *Stat. Med.* 1989; **8:** 551–61.

Eisenhofer, G., Lenders, J.W., Linehan, W.M., Walther, M.M., Goldstein, D.S., and Keiser, H.R. Plasma normetanephrine and metanephrine for detecting pheochromocytoma in von Hippel–Lindau disease and multiple endocrine neoplasia type 2. *N. Engl. J. Med.* 1999; **340:** 1872–9.

Fleiss, J.L., Levin, B., and Paik, M.C. *Statistical Methods for Rates and Proportions, 3rd Edn.* New York: John Wiley & Sons, 2003.

Fleming, T.R. and Harrington, D.P. *Counting Processes and Survival Analysis.* New York: Wiley-Interscience, 1991.

Framingham Heart Study. *The Framingham Study – 40 Year Public Use Data Set.* Bethesda, MD: National Heart, Lung, and Blood Institute, NIH, 1997.

Gordis, L. *Epidemiology, 3rd Edn.* Philadelphia: Saunders, 2004.

Greenwood, M. *The Natural Duration of Cancer: Reports on Public Health and Medical Subjects, No. 33.* London: His Majesty's Stationery Office, 1926.

Grizzle, J.E. Continuity correction in the $\chi^2$ test for 2 × 2 tables. *The American Statistician* 1967; **21:**(4) 28–32.

Gross, C.P., Anderson, G.F., and Rowe, N.R. The relation between funding by the National Institutes of Health and the burden of disease. *N. Engl. J. Med.* 1999; **340:** 1881–7.

Hamilton, L.C. *Regression with Graphics: A Second Course in Applied Statistics.* Pacific Grove, CA: Brooks/Cole Pub. Co., 1992.

Harrell, F.E. *Regression Modeling Strategies: With Applications to Linear Models, Logistic Regression, and Survival Analysis.* New York: Springer-Verlag, 2001.

Harrell, F.E., Jr., Lee, K.L., and Pollock, B. G. Regression models in clinical studies: determining relationships between predictors and response. *J Natl Cancer Inst.* 1988; **80:** 1198–202.

Hennekens, C.H. and Buring, J.E. *Epidemiology in Medicine.* Boston, MA: Little, Brown and Company, 1987.

Hosmer, D.W. and Lemeshow, S. A goodness-of-fit test for the multiple logistic regression model. *Commun. Stat.* 1980; **A10:** 1043–69.

Hosmer, D.W. and Lemeshow, S. *Applied Logistic Regression, 2nd Edn.* New York: John Wiley & Sons, 2000.

Huber, P.J. The behavior of maximum likelihood estimates under non-standard conditions. *Proceedings of the Fifth Berkeley Symposium on Mathematical Statistics and Probability.* Berkeley, CA: University of California Press, 1967; **5:** 221–3.

Kalbfleisch, J.D. and Prentice, R.L. *The Statistical Analysis of Failure Time Data, 2nd Edn.* New York: Wiley-Interscience, 2002.

Kaplan, E.L. and Meier, P. Nonparametric estimation from incomplete observations. *J. Am. Stat. Assoc.* 1958; **53:** 457–81.

Katz, M. *Study Design and Statistical Analysis: A Practical Guide for Clinicians.* Cambridge: Cambridge University Press, 2006.

Knaus, W.A., Harrell, F.E., Jr., Lynn, J., Goldman, L., Phillips, R.S., Connors, A.F., Jr. et al. The SUPPORT prognostic model. Objective estimates of survival for seriously ill hospitalized adults. Study to understand prognoses and preferences for outcomes and risks of treatments. *Ann Intern Med.* 1995; **122:** 191–203.

Kruskal, W.H. and Wallis, W.A. Use of ranks in one-criterion variance analysis. *J. Am. Stat. Assoc.* 1952; **47:** 583–621. Correction, *J. Am. Stat. Assoc.* 1953; **48:** 907–11.

Lang, C.C., Stein, C.M., Brown, R.M., Deegan, R., Nelson, R., He, H.B., et al. Attenuation of isoproterenol-mediated vasodilatation in blacks. *N. Engl. J. Med.* 1995; **333:** 155–60.

Lawless, J.F. *Statistical Models and Methods for Lifetime Data, 2nd Edn.* New York: John Wiley & Sons, 2002.

Lehmann, E.L. *Nonparametrics: Statistical Methods Based on Ranks, Revised Edn.* New York: Springer-Verlag, 2006.

Levene, H. Robust tests for equality of variances. In *Contributions to Probability and Statistics: Essays in Honor of Harold Hotelling.* Olkin, I. et al., eds., Menlo Park, CA: Stanford University Press, 1960; 278–92.

Levy, D. *50 Years of Discovery: Medical Milestones from the National Heart, Lung, and Blood Institute's Framingham Heart Study.* Hackensack, NJ: Center for Bio-Medical Communication Inc., 1999.

Liang, K.-Y. and Zeger, S. Longitudinal data analysis using generalized linear models. *Biometrika* 1986; **73:** 13–22.

Little, R.J.A. and Rubin, D.B. *Statistical Analysis with Missing Data, 2nd Edn.* Hoboken, NJ: Wiley, 2002.

Mann, H.B. and Whitney, D.R. On a test of whether one of two random variables is stochastically larger than the other. *Ann. Math. Stat.* 1947; **18:** 50–60.

Mantel, N. Evaluation of survival data and two new rank order statistics arising in its consideration. *Cancer Chemother. Rep.* 1966; **50:** 163–70.

Mantel, N. and Greenhouse, S.W. What is the continuity correction? *The American Statistician* 1968; **22:**(5) 27–30.

Mantel, N. and Haenszel, W. Statistical aspects of the analysis of data from retrospective studies of disease. *J. Natl Cancer Inst.* 1959; **22:** 719–48.

Marini, J.J. and Wheeler, A.P. *Critical Care Medicine: The Essentials, 2nd Edn.* Baltimore: Williams & Wilkins, 1997.

Matthews, J.N., Altman, D.G., Campbell, M.J., and Royston, P. Analysis of serial measurements in medical research. *Br. Med. J.* 1990; **300:** 230–5.

McCullagh, P. Regression models for ordinal data. *J. R. Stat. Soc. Ser. B.* 1980; **42:** 109–42.

McCullagh, P. and Nelder, J.A. *Generalized Linear Models, 2nd Edn.* London: Chapman and Hall, 1989.

O'Donnell, H.C., Rosand, J., Knudsen, K.A., Furie, K.L., Segal, A.Z., Chiu, R.I., et al. Apolipoprotein E genotype and the risk of recurrent lobar intracerebral hemorrhage. *N. Engl. J. Med.* 2000; **342:** 240–5.

Pagano, M. and Gauvreau, K. *Principles of Biostatistics, 2nd Edn.* Belmont, CA: Duxbury Thomson Learning, 2000.

Parl, F.F., Cavener, D.R., and Dupont, W.D. Genomic DNA analysis of the estrogen receptor gene in breast cancer. *Breast Cancer Res. Tr.* 1989; **14:** 57–64.

Peto, R. and Peto, J. Asymptotically efficient rank invariant test procedures. *J. R. Stat. Soc. Ser. A* 1972; **135:** 185–207.

Pregibon, D. Logistic regression diagnostics. *Ann. Stat.* 1981; **9:** 705–24.

Rabe-Hesketh, S. and Skrondal, A. *Multilevel and Longitudinal Modeling using Stata.* College Station, TX: Stata Press, 2005.

Robins, J., Breslow, N., and Greenland, S. Estimators of the Mantel–Haenszel variance consistent in both sparse data and large-strata limiting models. *Biometrics* 1986; **42:** 311–23.

Rothman, K.J. and Greenland, S. *Modern Epidemiology.* Philadelphia: Lippincott-Raven, 1998.

Royall, R.M. *Statistical Evidence: A Likelihood Paradigm.* London: Chapman & Hall, 1997.

Royston, P. Multiple imputation of missing values. *Stata J.* 2004; **4:** 227–41.

Royston, P. Multiple imputation of missing values: update. *Stata J.* 2005; **5:** 188–201.

Satterthwaite, F.E. An approximate distribution of estimates of variance components. *Biometrics Bulletin* 1946; **2:** 110–4.

Scholer, S.J., Hickson, G.B., Mitchel, E.F., and Ray, W.A. Persistently increased injury mortality rates in high-risk young children. *Arch. Pediatr. Adolesc. Med.* 1997; **151:** 1216–9.

Searle, S.R. *Linear Models for Unbalanced Data.* New York: Wiley, 1987.

StataCorp. *Stata Statistical Software: Release 10.0.* College Station, TX: StataCorp LP, 2007.

Steel, R.G.D. and Torrie, J.H. *Principles and Procedures of Statistics: A Biometrical Approach, 2nd Edn.* New York: McGraw-Hill Book Co., 1980.

Stone, C.J. and Koo, C.Y. Additive splines in statistics. *Proceedings of the Statistical Computing Section, American Statistical Association.* Washington DC: 1985; 45–8.

Student. The probable error of a mean. *Biometrika* 1908; **6:** 1–25.

Tarone, R.E. On heterogeneity tests based on efficient scores. *Biometrika* 1985; **72:** 91–5.

Therneau, T.M. and Grambsch, P.M. *Modeling Survival Data.* New York: Springer-Verlag, 2000.

Tuyns, A.J., Pequignot, G., and Jensen, O.M. Le cancer de l'oesophage en Ille-et-Vilaine en fonction des niveau de consommation d'alcool et de tabac. Des risques qui se multiplient. *Bull. Cancer* 1977; **64:** 45–60.

Van Buuren, S., Boshuizen, H.C., and Knook, D.L. Multiple imputation of missing blood pressure covariates in survival analysis. *Stat. Med.* 1999; **18:** 681–94.

Varmus, H. Evaluating the burden of disease and spending the research dollars of the National Institutes of Health. *N. Engl. J. Med.* 1999; **340:** 1914–5.

Wald, A. Tests of statistical hypotheses concerning several parameters when the number of observations is large. *T. Am. Math. Soc.* 1943; **54:** 426–82.

White, H. A heteroskedasticity-consistent covariance matrix estimator and a direct test for heteroskedasticity. *Econometrica* 1980; **48:** 817–30.

White, H. Maximum likelihood estimation of misspecified models. *Econometrica* 1982; **50:** 1–25.

Wilcoxon, F. Individual comparisons by ranking methods. *Biometrics Bulletin* 1945; **1:** 80–3.

Wishart, J. Growth-rate determinations in nutrition studies with the bacon pig, and their analysis. *Biometrika,* 1938; **30:** 16–28.

Woolf, B. On estimating the relationship between blood group and disease. *Ann. Hum. Genet.* 1955; **19:** 251–3.

Xie, H.G., Stein, C.M., Kim, R.B., Xiao, Z.S., He, N., Zhou, H.H., et al. Frequency of functionally important beta-2 adrenoceptor polymorphisms varies markedly among African-American, Caucasian and Chinese individuals. *Pharmacogenetics* 1999; **9:** 511–16.

Xie, H.G., Stein, C.M., Kim, R.B., Gainer, J.V., Sofowora, G., Dishy, V., et al. Human beta2-adrenergic receptor polymorphisms: no association with essential hypertension in black or white Americans. *Clin. Pharmacol. Ther.* 2000; **67:** 670–5.

Yates, F. Contingency tables involving small numbers and the chi-square test. *J. R. Stat. Soc. Suppl.* 1934; **1:** 217–35.

Zeger, S.L. and Liang, K.Y. Longitudinal data analysis for discrete and continuous outcomes. *Biometrics* 1986; **42:** 121–30.

# Index

Printed in the United States
By Bookmasters